COGNITIVE NEUROSCIENCE OF ATTENTION

COGNITIVE NEUROSCIENCE of ATTENTION

Edited by
MICHAEL I. POSNER

THE GUILFORD PRESS
New York   London

Library of Congress Cataloging-in-Publication Data
Cognitive neuroscience of attention / edited by Michael I. Posner.
     p. cm.
  Includes bibliographical references and index.
  ISBN 1-59385-048-4 (hardcover)
  1. Attention—Physiological aspects.   2. Cognitive neuroscience.   I. Posner, Michael I.
QP405.C7125 2004
153.7′33—dc22

                                                                                        2004006240

About the Editor

Michael I. Posner, PhD, is Professor of Psychology at the Institute of Neuroscience at the University of Oregon. He has written numerous articles involving studies of attention for over 40 years. Dr. Posner's studies involve cognitive, neuroimaging, electrical recording, developmental, and genetic methods. His model of attention, involving networks controlling alertness, orientation to sensory events, and executive control, has been influential in the field. Dr. Posner and his colleagues have developed methods for measuring each aspect of attention that have been widely used by many researchers. His work has been recognized by his election to the National Academy of Sciences and by several awards, including the first Grawemeyer Award (with Marc Raichle and Steven Petersen) and the Fyssen Foundation International Prize for 2003.

Contributors

Kimmo Alho, PhD, Department of Psychology, University of Helsinki, Helsinki, Finland

Lourdes Anllo-Vento, PhD, Neurosciences Program, University of California, San Diego, La Jolla, California

Serguei V. Astafiev, PhD, Visual Attention and Brain Recovery Laboratory, Department of Radiology, Washington University School of Medicine, St. Louis, Missouri

Gary Aston-Jones, PhD, Department of Psychology, University of Pennsylvania, Philadelphia, Pennsylvania

Melinda Beane, MS, Institute of Neuroscience, University of Oregon, Eugene, Oregon

Nadia Bolognini, PhD, Department of Psychology, University of Bologna, Bologna, Italy

Matthew Botvinick, MD, PhD, Department of Psychology, University of Pennsylvania, Philadelphia, Pennsylvania

Todd S. Braver, PhD, Department of Psychology, Washington University, St. Louis, Missouri

Borís Burle, PhD, Department of Psychology, University of Amsterdam, Amsterdam, The Netherlands, and National Center of Scientific Research, University of Provence, Marseille, France

George Bush, MD, Department of Psychiatry, Harvard Medical School, Boston, Massachusetts, and Psychiatric Neuroimaging Research, Massachusetts General Hospital, Charlestown, Massachusetts

Thomas H. Carr, PhD, Department of Psychology, Michigan State University, East Lansing, Michigan

Cameron S. Carter, MD, Department of Psychiatry, University of Pittsburgh, Pittsburgh, Pennsylvania

B. J. Casey, PhD, Sackler Institute for Developmental Psychology, Weill Medical College of Cornell University, New York, New York

F. Xavier Castellanos, MD, Department of Psychiatry, New York University School of Medicine, New York, New York

Patrick Cavanagh, PhD, Department of Psychology, Harvard University, Cambridge, Massachusetts

Jonathan D. Cohen, PhD, Department of Psychology, Princeton University, Princeton, New Jersey

Michael G. H. Coles, PhD, FC Donders Centre for Cognitive Neuroimaging, Nijmegen, The Netherlands, and University of Illinois at Urbana–Champaign, Urbana, Illinois

John Colombo, PhD, Department of Psychology, University of Kansas, Lawrence, Kansas

Maurizio Corbetta, MD, Department of Neurology, Radiology, and Anatomy and Neurobiology, Washington University School of Medicine, St. Louis, Missouri

Jeffrey W. Dalley, PhD, Department of Experimental Psychology, University of Cambridge, Cambridge, United Kingdom

Richard C. Deth, PhD, Department of Pharmaceutical Sciences, Northeastern University, Boston, Massachusetts

John Duncan, DPhil, MRC Cognition and Brain Sciences Unit, University of Cambridge, Cambridge, United Kingdom

Francesca Frassinetti, MD, PhD, Department of Psychology, University of Bologna, Bologna, Italy

Luis J. Fuentes, PhD, Department of Psychology, University of Almeria, Almeria, Spain

Mark S. Gilzenrat, MS, Department of Psychology, Princeton University, Princeton, New Jersey

David K. Grandy, MS, PhD, Departments of Cell and Developmental Biology and Physiology and Pharmacology, Oregon Health and Science University, Portland, Oregon

Pamela Greenwood, PhD, Cognitive Science Laboratory and Department of Psychology, Catholic University of America, Washington, DC

C. J. Han, PhD, Feinberg School of Medicine, Northwestern University, Chicago, Illinois

Steven A. Hillyard, PhD, Neurosciences Program, University of California, San Diego, La Jolla, California

Clay B. Holroyd, PhD, Department of Psychology, Princeton University, Princeton, New Jersey

Sabine Kastner, MD, PhD, Department of Psychology, Princeton University, Princeton, New Jersey

Raymond M. Klein, PhD, Department of Psychology, Dalhousie University, Halifax, Nova Scotia, Canada

Christof Koch, PhD, Koch Laboratory, Division of Biology, California Institute of Technology, Pasadena, California

Paul J. Kruzich, PhD, Department of Physiology and Pharmacology, Oregon Health and Science University, Portland, Oregon

Anna Kuznetsova, MS, Department of Pharmaceutical Sciences, Northeastern University, Boston, Massachusetts

Elisabetta Làdavas, PhD, Department of Psychology, University of Bologna, Bologna, Italy

Phan Luu, PhD, Electrical Geodesics, Inc., and Department of Psychology, University of Oregon, Eugene, Oregon

Richard Marrocco, PhD, Department of Psychology, Institute of Cognitive and Decision Sciences, University of Oregon, Eugene, Oregon

Rogier B. Mars, MS, Nijmegen Institute for Cognition and Information and FC Donders Centre for Cognitive Neuroimaging, Nijmegen, The Netherlands

Jean A. Milstein, BA, Department of Experimental Psychology, University of Cambridge, Cambridge, United Kingdom

Risto Näätänen, PhD, Cognitive Brain Research Unit, Department of Psychology, University of Helsinki, Helsinki, Finland

Sander Nieuwenhuis, PhD, Department of Cognitive Psychology, Vrije University, Amsterdam, The Netherlands

Joel Nigg, PhD, Department of Psychology, Michigan State University, East Lansing, Michigan

Anna Christina Nobre, PhD, Department of Experimental Psychology, University of Oxford, Oxford, United Kingdom

Colm M. O'Tuathaigh, BA, Department of Clinical Pharmacology, Royal College of Surgeons in Ireland, Dublin, Ireland

Raja Parasuraman, PhD, Department of Psychology, George Mason University, Fairfax, Virginia

Stacey M. Pederson, MA, Department of Psychology, University of Oregon, Eugene, Oregon

Seth D. Pollak, PhD, Department of Psychology, University of Wisconsin–Madison, Madison, Wisconsin

Michael I. Posner, PhD, Department of Psychology, Institute of Cognitive and Decision Sciences, University of Oregon, Eugene, Oregon

Amir Raz, PhD, Department of Psychiatry, Columbia University, New York, New York

John H. Reynolds, PhD, The Salk Institute for Biological Studies, La Jolla, California

John E. Richards, PhD, Department of Psychology, University of South Carolina, Columbia, South Carolina

K. Richard Ridderinkhof, PhD, Department of Psychology, University of Amsterdam, Amsterdam, The Netherlands, and Leiden University, Leiden, The Netherlands

Trevor W. Robbins, PhD, Department of Experimental Psychology, University of Cambridge, Cambridge, United Kingdom

Ian H. Robertson, PhD, Department of Psychology, Trinity College Dublin, Dublin, Ireland

Mircea A. Schoenfeld, MD, Department of Neurology, Otto Von Guericke University, Magdeburg, Germany

Gordon L. Shulman, PhD, Department of Neurology, Radiology, and Anatomy and Neurobiology, Washington University School of Medicine, St. Louis, Missouri

James M. Swanson, PhD, Department of Pediatrics, University of California, Irvine, California

Diane Swick, PhD, Department of Neurology, University of California, Davis, California, and Veterans Affairs Northern California Health Care System, Martinez, California

Eric Taylor, PhD, Department of Child and Adolescent Psychiatry, Institute of Psychiatry, King's College London, London, United Kingdom

Stephanie Tolley-Schell, MA, Department of Psychology, University of Wisconsin–Madison, Madison, Wisconsin

And U. Turken, PhD, Department of Psychology, Stanford University, Stanford, California

Markus Ullsperger, MD, Max Planck Institute of Cognitive Science, Leipzig, Germany

Wery P. M. van den Wildenberg, PhD, Department of Psychology, University of Amsterdam, Amsterdam, The Netherlands, and National Center of Scientific Research, University of Provence, Marseille, France

Nora D. Volkow, MD, National Institute on Drug Abuse, National Institutes of Health, Bethesda, Maryland

Mostafa Waly, PhD, Department of Biomedical Sciences, Northeastern University, Boston, Massachusetts

Jasper Wijnen, MA, Department of Psychology, University of Amsterdam, Amsterdam, The Netherlands

Nick Yeung, PhD, Department of Psychology, Princeton University, Princeton, New Jersey

Contents

I

INTRODUCTION

1

Progress in Attention Research

Michael I. Posner

Attention is being studied at the cognitive, neurosystem, cellular, synaptic, and genetic levels. No one of these levels provide an analysis of attention that both illuminates its role in tasks of daily life and prepares the way for a remediation of conditions. Only successful links between these levels can allow attention to be viewed as an organ system with its own anatomy, circuitry, functions, and deficits. This book is a snapshot of the rather amazing progress along all of these research lines in recent years.

It is often said that we do not have a better definition of attention than William James had a century ago, and in some sense that is probably true.

> Everyone knows what attention is. It is the taking possession of the mind in clear and vivid
> form of what seem several simultaneous objects or trains of thought. (1890, p. 403)

James's definition is largely subjective and gives us little hint of the mechanisms that underlie the vivid experience. Just as DNA research changed how we thought about life but did not really clarify the meaning of life, so the study of the anatomy, cellular structure and genetics of attention but has allowed us to view attention like any other organ system but not change its definition.

I believe that viewing attention as an organ system aids in answering many perplexing issues raised in cognitive psychology, psychiatry, and neurology. Like other organ systems, attention has its own anatomy, transmitters, and development. Each of these topics is represented in this volume.

The book has been divided into five sections based primarily on method. The divisions are somewhat arbitrary because so many of the authors draw on ideas and methods from other sections. None of the cognitive studies are purely cognitive. Sometimes they rest heavily on imaging (e.g., Cohen, Aston-Jones, & Gilzenrat, Chapter 6; Fuentes, Chapter 4) to complement the purely functional analysis. Others use concepts from cellular studies (Klein, Chapter 3) or an analysis of synaptic transmitters and modulators (Cohen et al.). It would be just as appropriate to group Cohen and colleagues and Botvinick and colleagues (Chapter 7) with the imaging studies of the anterior cingulate (Bush, Chapter 15; Luu & Pederson, Chapter 17; Holroyd, Nieuwenhuis, Mars, & Coles, Chapter 16) rather than in the section of cognitive studies as we have done.

COGNITIVE STUDIES

The cognitive category contains two studies that refer mainly to attention in dealing with sensory (mainly visual) input, what Petersen and I once named the posterior attention network (Posner & Petersen, 1990) but which I now prefer calling the function of orienting to sensory stimuli. Cavanagh deals with the functions that this network carries out within the visual system, extending these functions in ways that are just beginning to be dealt with in physiological terms (e.g., Ito & Gilbert, 1999). Klein addresses instead the brain areas that carry out attention orienting, what I have called the sources of the attentional effects. His chapter is fully informed of the anatomical overlap between the systems that carry out eye movements and covert attention, yet he argues from cognitive data that the functions are separable and shows why this might be so in terms of the requirements of vision. These efforts show why the cognitive approach is not dying in the era of imaging and genetics. Rather, cognitive studies carve out new domains of study and discover interesting differences between the brain areas involved and the logic of how computations carried out in these areas fit together.

Fuentes (Chapter 4) and Carr (Chapter 5) both provide interesting similarities between the sensory orienting discussed in Chapters 2 and 3 and more anterior functions such as control of semantics, by showing commonalities and difference in the functions carried out in these two systems. Both chapters refer to inhibition in the sense of a reduction in the speed of processing some event over a baseline condition. The problem of working out links between facilitation and inhibition in reaction time, increases and decreases in activation as revealed in imaging studies, and inhibitory and excitatory potentials in cellular studies remains a major difficulty in making the links between areas. Inhibition within the cognitive system may be carried out by activation of networks of brain areas as revealed by imaging studies. Activation in imaging can be based on either excitatory or inhibitory cellular activity. It is important to keep these ideas separate to understand chapters in this volume.

Chapters 6 (Cohen et al.) and 7 (Botvinick et al.) discuss cognitive control in more detail. Issues of cognitive control appear to be separable from orienting to sensory stimuli in the sense they are carried out by different anatomical areas, although, as pointed out in Chapters 4 (Fuentes) and 5 (Carr) they can have analogous functions. Anatomically, Chapters 6 and 7 both identify critical control functions performed by the anterior cingulate.

IMAGING

The imaging sections bring together hemodynamic, electrical and cellular methods to explore the anatomy of orienting to sensory events and the control of cognitive processes. Hemodynamic methods (now largely functional magnetic resonance imaging [fMRI]) have shown that a wide variety of cognitive tasks can be seen as activating a distributed set of neural areas each of which can be identified with specific mental operations (Posner & Raichle, 1994, 1998).

The areas of activation have been more consistent for the study of attention, particularly for orienting to sensory stimuli, than for any other cognitive system. The hemodynamic chapters in this section (Chapters 9, 11, and 12) lay out a common network of brain areas active when people or monkeys orient to sensory events. Although the sources of the orienting network are discussed primarily for vision, there is evidence that a similar network is involved for other sensory modalities (e.g., Làdavas, Bolognini, & Frassinetti, Chapter 28; see also Driver & Spence, 1998). Several areas of the parietal lobe (e.g., superior parietal lobe and temporal parietal junction) play a very crucial role in this process; however, it would be inaccurate to label the network as solely posterior as we did in 1990 (Posner & Petersen, 1990), because it clearly involves frontal areas as well.

While the sources of orienting effects activate a common brain network, the sites where attention influences sensory processing differ between vision (Reynolds, Chapter 10; Anllo-Vento, Schoenfeld, & Hillyard, Chapter 13) and audition (Näätänen & Alho, Chapter 14). Differences would arise in studies using different modalities because of the sites at which attention operates, even if, as appears to be the case, the sources were similar.

There is impressive convergence on the brain areas found active in a wide variety of tasks involving sensory orienting. These brain areas provide a common top-down effect on different sensory systems. However, the relative importance of bottom-up and top-down processes in attention remains controversial. Duncan (Chapter 8) develops a view of selective attention that arises out of conflict within each sensory area and top-down control, while recognized, is not emphasized. In contrast, Chapters 15 (Bush), 16 (Holroyd et al.), and 17 (Luu & Pederson) strongly emphasize the role of top-down mechanisms in controlling conflict between neural systems.

The chapters using electrophysiology either in the form of scalp potentials linked to neural generators by imaging studies (Anllo-Vento et al., Chapter 13; Holroyd et al., Chapter 16; Luu & Pederson, Chapter 17) or by cellular recording (Reynolds, Chapter 10) provide more detailed information on the time course of computations and on their microcircuitry. Anllo-Vento and colleagues show that primary visual cortex activity is amplified by attention only after attentional influences are shown in prestriate areas. The mechanism by which attention amplifies visual information is shown both at the cellular (Reynolds) and the systems level (Anllo-Vento et al.) to involve very similar mechanisms. The extent of convergence between methods in the area of visual orienting allows for more mechanistic cognitive models to develop.

The study of cognitive control is not yet as advanced as sensory orienting, but at least one part of the network involved is explored in some detail in Chapters 15–17. Bush (Chapter 15) describes convergence between the frequency of cells of different types found in the anterior cingulate and the results of imaging of the region. Both hemodynamic and electrical methods can probe the time course and rhythmic activity involving this area. There is little question that conflict tasks are excellent for activation of this region (Carr, Chapter 5; Cohen et al., Chapter 6), but the role of the cingulate in reward, error detection, and regulation of thought and behavior (Chapters 5 and 15) provides important links between the studies of imaging and those of genetic control (Grandy & Kruzich, Chapter 19; Han, O'Tuathaigh, & Koch, Chapter 22; Deth, Kuznetsova, & Waly, Chapter 20) described in the next section of the book.

GENES AND SYNAPSES

In some cases it has been possible to connect attention to underlying molecular events. This approach holds the promise of linking networks of attention to the genes and environmental events of early development. It also makes possible connecting the differences found between people in the efficiency of attention with variations in the underlying genome (Fan, Fossella, Summer, & Posner, 2003). Recently this approach has found that differences in the efficiency of attention relate to variation in the genes underlying the cholinergic (Parasuraman & Greenwood, Chapter 18) and dopaminergic systems (Deth et al., Chapter 20; Fossella et al., 2002). Pharmacological studies described by Beane and Marrocco (Chapter 23) link the cholinergic system to orienting and studies described in Chapters 20 (Deth et al.) and 21 (Robbins, Milstein, & Dalley) link dopminergic activity to the anterior cingulate gyrus.

These pharmacological results have made it possible to search economically for candidate genes relating specifically to the functioning of specific attentional networks. Alleles of the CHRNA4 gene, related to cholinergic function, are shown by Parasuraman and Greenwood (Chapter 18) to modulate efficiency of visual orienting and related working memory tasks. This approach was used to show that alleles of two genes (MAOA and DRD4), both of which influence the dopaminergic system (although not uniquely) relate to individual differences in the ability to control conflict (Fossella et al., 2002) and to the strength of activation of the anterior cingulate when performing the attention network test (Fan et al., 2003). These individual differences in normals may also be related to the link between one of these molecules (DRD4) and attention-deficit/hyperactivity disorder (ADHD) (Deth et al., Chapter 20; Swanson et al., Chapter 32).

Grandy and Kruzich (Chapter 19) have shown that knockout mice, who are missing the DRD4 gene, produce predictable changes in their behavior that relates to hyperactivity. The potential specificity of the behavioral assays on knockout mice is shown by Han and colleagues (Chapter 22), who found that trace but not delayed conditioning activates the anterior cingulate gyrus. Examining the comparative effects of genetic variation on different mammalian species may soon provide a way of approaching the evolution of attentional networks that certainly could not have been anticipated only a few years ago.

DEVELOPMENT

Human infants are little looking machines nearly ideal for the study of visual attention, a feature used in Chapters 24 (Colombo) and 25 (Richards) on the development of attention in infancy. Orienting is a very early developing attentional system and can be exploited from birth to separate changes in attention that accompany the early maturation of the nervous system. The development of components of attention such as inhibition of return, attention movements, and alerting can be traced week by week in infancy and efforts can be made to relate changes to specific aspects of the infants temperament (perhaps including genetic variation) and aspects of caregiving. It is quite amazing that infants of 3–4 months can be taught to orient to places in the environment in advance of presenting a stimulus at that location. We do know that different cultures emphasize different aspects of the infants' environment (Bornstein et al., 1992), but we do not yet know how influential these variations are in later development.

Although infancy is a natural time to study the development of attentional networks, it is also possible to study dramatic changes in later childhood as well. Between 3 and 7 years of age, Rueda, Posner, and Rothbart (2004) show that there is a dramatic development in the ability to resolve conflict, which appears to relate to an anterior brain network including the anterior cingulate (see Cohen et al., Chapter 6; Botvinick et al., Chapter 7). Ridderinkhof, van den Wildenberg, Wijnen, and Burle (Chapter 27) describe methods for evaluating conflict resolution and illustrate it by examining the difficulties children with ADHD have controlling their responses.

In our work we have shown how the development of the ability to resolve conflict is related to important and enduring aspects of temperament. Substantial research with children of this age has shown that the development of the executive attention network, important for resolving cognitive conflict in Stroop-like tasks, is also related to a temperamental construct of effortful measured by caregiver reports (Rothbart & Derryberry, 1981). Effortful control correlates with the ability to delay reward and to reduce negative affect and to successfully develop conscience during socialization (Kochanska, 1995; Posner & Rothbart, 2000). Studies using fMRI following instructions in adults to avoid pleasant or unpleasant emotion (Beauregard, Levesque, & Bourgouin, 2001; Ochsner, Bunge, Gross, & Gabrieli, 2002) show anterior cingulate activation is associated with carrying out the instruction. These findings show that the executive attention network is important in self-regulation of both emotion and cognition (Rueda et al., 2004).

DEFICITS OF ATTENTION

Deficits of attention are frequently found in cases of insults to the brain from stroke (Làdavas et al., Chapter 28; Swick & Turken, Chapter 29) and closed head injury and in cases of psychopathology (Pollak & Tolley-Schell, Chapter 26; Ridderinkhof et al., Chapter 27; Swanson et al., Chapter 32). A few years ago the study of lesioned patients, such as those suffering from neglect most often due to lesions of the right parietal lobe, was the only clue to how attention was organized in the human brain. Chapters 28 (Làdavas et al.) and 29 (Swick & Turken) show how productive the lesion method can be when related to animal research and human imaging studies.

In addition, it is now possible to propose rehabilitation methods based on principles arising from cognitive neuroscience studies (Chapters 28 and 30). Robertson (Chapter 30) outlines his long efforts to examine rehabilitation in patients. The ability to image patients prior to and following rehabilitation in comparison with controls provides a very strong method for testing and combining therapies that might have influence on different network or nodes within the same network. Much can be learned about brain function and plasticity from studies of rehabilitation methods.

We are also better equipped to study pathologies arising from unknown causes such as ADHD (Chapters 23, 27, and 32), autism (Rodier, 2002), schizophrenia (Frith, 1992), or borderline personality disorder (Posner et al., 2002), which may affect attention. Understanding how these disorders influence attentional networks may aid the design of behavioral or pharmacological interventions.

A number of human practices, including ingestion of drugs, meditation, and hypnotism, are known to alter attention. With the new tools it is becoming possible to specify in what ways these methods work to alter the normal processing of information by the human brain. In Chapter 31, Raz reports studies with highly hypnotizable persons who under hypnotic suggestion to view words as a meaningless string no longer show the interference of the word names on color responses (Stroop interference). It has also been reported that when such subjects are instructed to see a colored picture as black and white, the color areas of the prestriate cortex are no longer activated by the colored picture (Kosslyn, Thompson, Costantini-Ferrando, Alpert, & Spiegel, 2000). Raz shows that when the Stroop interference is lost, there is a reduction in anterior cingulate activation and also in an occipital–parietal area that might be related chunking visual letters into words (word form). These findings begin to suggest research directions for studying changes in brain processes related to special attentional states.

The last few years have been a remarkable period of rapid development for the study of attention. With the continued use of the tools currently available for its study and the likely development of new methods of probing brain activity, we should see a continuation and perhaps an acceleration of this progress in the years ahead. Understanding of attention is likely to yield progress in traditional and new approaches to education, in the study of pathologies, and in further integration of the mental and brain sciences. Ideally, this volume will make a valuable contribution to that progress.

REFERENCES

Beauregard, M., Levesque, J., & Bourgouin, P. (2001). Neural correlates of conscious self-regulation of emotion. *Journal of Neuroscience, 21*, RC165.

Bornstein, M. H., Tamis-Lamda, C. S., Tal, J., Lundemenn, P., Toda, S., Rahn, C. W., et al. (1992). Maternal responsiveness to infants in three societies the United States, France and Japan. *Child Development, 63*, 808–821.

Driver, J., & Spence, C. (1998). Crossmodal attention. *Current Opinion in Neurobiology, 8*, 245–253.

Fan, J., Fossella, J. A., Summer, T., & Posner, M. I. (2003). Mapping the genetic variation of executive attention onto brain activity. *Proceedings of the National Academy of Sciences USA, 100*, 7406–7411.

Fossella, J., Sommer, T., Fan, J., Wu, Y., Swanson, J. M., Pfaff, D. W., et al. (2002). Assessing the molecular genetics of attention networks. *BMC Neuroscience, 3*, 14.

Frith, C. D. (1992). *The cognitive neuropsychology of schizophrenia*. Hillsdale, NJ: Erlbaum.

Ito, M., & Gilbert, C. D. (1999). Attention modulates contextual influences in the primary visual cortex of alert monkey. *Neuron, 22*, 593–604.

James, W. (1890). *Principles of psychology*. New York: Holt.

Kochanska, G. (1995). Children's temperament, mothers' discipline, and security of attachment: Multiple pathways to emerging internalization. *Child Development, 66*, 597–615.

Kosslyn, S. M., Thompson, W. L., Costantini-Ferrando, M. F., Alpert, N. M., & Spiegel, D. (2000). Hypnotic visual illusion alters color processing in the brain. *American Journal of Psychiatry, 157*(8), 1279–1284.

Ochsner, K. N., Bunge, S. A., Gross, J. J., & Gabrieli, J. D. E. (2002). Rethinking feelings: An fMRI study of the cognitive regulation of emotion. *Journal of Cognitive Neuroscience, 14*, 1215–1229.

Posner, M. I., & Petersen, S. E. (1990). The attention system of the human brain. *Annual Review of Neuroscience, 13*, 25–42.

Posner, M. I., & Raichle, M. E. (1994). *Images of mind*. New York: Scientific American Library.

Posner, M. I., & Raichle, M. E. (Eds.). (1998). Overview: The neuroimaging of human brain function. *Proceedings of the National Academy of Sciences USA, 95*, 763–764.

Posner, M. I., & Rothbart, M. K. (2000). Developing mechanisms of self regulation. *Development and Psychopathology, 12*, 427–441.

Posner, M. I., Rothbart, M. K., Vizueta, N., Levy, K., Thomas, K. M., & Clarkin, J. (2002). Attentional mechanisms of borderline personality disorder. *Proceedings of the National Academy of Sciences USA, 99*, 16366–16370.

Rodier, P. M. (2002). Converging evidence for brain stem injury during autism. *Development and Psychopathology, 14,* 537–559.

Rothbart, M. K., & Derryberry, D. (1981). Development of individual differences in temperament. In M. E. Lamb & A. L. Brown (Eds.), *Advances in developmental psychology* (Vol. 1, pp. 37–86). Hillsdale, NJ: Erlbaum

Rueda, M. R., Posner, M. I., & Rothbart, M. K. (2004). Attentional control and self-regulation. In R. F. Baumeister & K. D. Vohs (Eds.), *Handbook of self-regulation* (pp. 283–300). New York: Guilford Press.

Swanson, J., Oosterlaan, J., Murias, M., Moyzis, R., Schuck, S., Mann, M., et al. (2000). ADHD children with 7-repeat allele of the DRD4 gene have extreme behavior but normal performance on critical neuropsychological tests of attention. *Proceedings of the National Academy of Sciences USA, 97,* 4754–4759.

II

COGNITIVE MODELS
OF ATTENTION

2

Attention Routines
and the Architecture of Selection

Patrick Cavanagh

Although we might all know what attention is (James, 1890), we do not all agree on what it does, except that it only does a limited amount of it. This limit, as described by Broadbent (1958), restricts the amount of the available information that can be passed on to higher processing. However, I show that this capacity limit is only one of three independent limits on the information available to higher processing. There is as well an acuity limit: a restriction on the density of items that still permits access to individual items. This resolution of selection is unexpectedly coarse in both space and time. In addition, there is a third bottleneck that I call the coding singularity. I argue that the information available from a selection is neither the raw image detail nor, when there is more than one item in the selection, the set of identities of the items. It is, instead, a single label for the entire pattern. These last two limits, acuity and singularity, may appear to be redescriptions of the same limit but they are not, as I describe later.[1] The three limits—capacity, acuity, and singularity—are part of a framework for attention that I describe in this chapter. In this framework, attention is not one thing but a set of routines that are called on to perform specific functions during a task (cf. Shimamura, 2000; Ullman, 1984). The set of attention routines is identified by one defining characteristic: the initial and final states are reportable but intermediate states are not. I briefly outline this proposal and then I focus on the details of one of these functions, selection.

ATTENTION ROUTINES

The idea of attention routines is an extension of Shimon Ullman's proposal of visual routines (1984, 1996). It is also related to Shimamura's (2000) proposals concerning executive attention and working memory where the building blocks of metacognitive control are the functions of selection, maintenance, updating, and rerouting of information. Following the work of Newell and Simon (1972) and others of the early era of cognitive psychology and computer metaphor, Ullman pointed out that many visual tasks could be solved with an explicit, serially executed algorithm. What differentiated Ullman's proposal from those of Newell and Simon and others was that the steps of Ullman's visual routines were not obvious, nor were they always available to introspection. In the earlier work (e.g., Newell & Simon, 1972), problems like the arithmetic word puzzle DONALD + GERALD = ROBERT (solve for the numerical value of each letter given only that D = 5) could be studied by asking subjects to describe their steps out loud as they solved the problem. The subject could report goals, subgoals, and intermediate steps with sufficient detail to allow the experimenters to construct a computer model of the logic of the mental operations involved and infer their reliance on, for example, short-term memory and problem space representation.

In the tasks that Ullman examined (e.g., Figure 2.1), the subject responded rapidly, often within a second or less (Jolicoeur, Ullman, & Mackay, 1986, 1991; Ullman, 1984). The answer appeared with little conscious thought, or with few deliberations that could be reported. Is the X in Figure 2.1 inside or outside the contour? We certainly have to set ourselves to the task, but the steps along the way to the answer seem to leave few traces that we can describe explicitly. Unlike the local, hardwired processing of, say, the retina, the processing underlying the analysis of the X and its surrounding contours might well be some serial set of steps that could be captured by an algorithm.

Ullman offered no particular organization for the different types of routines that could be called on and attention was just one of a variety of operators that were available. However, if we organize the routines into three groups, as depicted in Figure 2.2, we can remove attention as an agent or resource of any kind and leave it as just the name of a particular level in the hierarchy of routines. This is similar to the way in which, say, a trial by jury is a particular part of the legal system where certain functions take place. We could think of a trial as a resource or an agent but really it is a grouping of functions. In the case of attention routines, we wish to identify what functions these might be and understand how they work. What Ullman had called attention in his 1984 paper now becomes principally one routine, selection, in a larger set that is distinguished by having reportable initial and final states and no reportable intermediate steps.

The hierarchy in Figure 2.2 has three levels: vision routines, attention routines, and cognition routines. They are differentiated by the number of reportable steps each has. Vision routines are inaccessible to awareness. They are implemented outside conscious control and have no reportable features. Some of these might be hardwired from birth (e.g., computation of opponent color responses), others might emerge with early visual experience (e.g., effectiveness of pictorial cues), and still others may be dependent on extensive practice (e.g.,

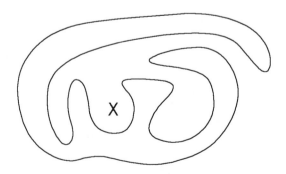

FIGURE 2.1. Does the X lie within a closed contour? Ullman (1984, 1996) proposed a set of visual routines that would compute the response.

1. Vision Routines

    Automatic, no introspection
    Examples: Grouping, light constancy, shape recognition, pictorial cues

2. Attention Routines

    Voluntary initiation, reportable output
    No intermediate, accessible states
    Examples: set selection criteria, spatial and temporal relations, tracking

3. Cognition Routines

    Multiple steps
    Intermediate steps are accessible to introspection
    Examples: Counting, cooking, surgery

FIGURE 2.2. Three levels of visual routines.

text recognition). Attention routines are consciously initiated by setting a goal or a filter or a selection target and have a reportable outcome but no reportable intermediate steps. Their intermediate steps are vision routines. Finally, cognition routines are, like the classic cases of Newell and Simon, multistep routines with several reportable intermediate states, where each individual step is a call to one attention routine.

What have we gained by reshuffling the bits and pieces of a computer metaphor for visual functions? The goal is to produce a list of the specific functions that fall in the attention group and then to find out how these work. This provides an alternative framework for sorting and interpreting the results of the attention literature (cf. Pashler, 1998; Posner, 1994; Posner & Driver, 1992). Attention routines that begin and end with a reportable state divide the flow of mental activity at its boundaries where the content of awareness changes: New goals are set, new outcomes are computed, and these enter and exit awareness as the principal working buffer of these mental tasks. By using reportable states as the syntax to carve up the flow, we identify sets of processes that are bracketed by changes in the content of awareness. For example, if we are asked to report the middle letter of the following three-letter word *any*, we are aware of the task goals and the word itself to begin with. We can also report the outcome, "n." The initial and final states are reportable but the intermediate states are less accessible. How did we segment the letters, find the middle one, and extract it from the word? These steps are highly automated and execute with little or no conscious guidance.

Classically, attention has been characterized by its limited capacity. Here, however, that limit is taken to be a consequence of representing the initial and final states of the attention routine in awareness. The suggestion is that the capacity limit is imposed by the constraints of awareness not by attention or attention routines themselves. I discuss this in more detail at the end of this chapter.

What is a possible list of functions of the attention group? Following is an incomplete, rough set: setting a selection filter, selection itself, binding multiple selections into a compound description, composing descriptions of visual events (Cavanagh, 2003), sending these descriptions to other cortical modules, receiving, decoding, and acting on "requests" from other modules (Logan & Zbrodoff, 1999). This is far from even a working list of candidates, but it suggests what a list might be like. The purpose of this chapter is not to generate and test routines on this list but to propose that attention is such a group of routines and to pick one particular routine, selection, and describe its function in more detail.

THE ARCHITECTURE OF SELECTION

Attention has been described as the selection of stimuli for higher-level processing. I outline the spatial and temporal constraints on the selection mechanisms and provide a description of the type of information that is picked up by selection and what can be done with it. I start with the constraints on selection and the evidence for multiple, independent selection operators.

When visual items are selected from a predefined or cued location, many suggest that the effect is like shining a spotlight on that region. Details in the illuminated region are then well defined and can be scrutinized or picked off for further processing. This spotlight metaphor is only a metaphor, of course, but it has been very influential. It has three critical aspects: There is only one "spotlight"; the details within the spotlight can be scrutinized; and selection is limited to this spotlight region. Despite the durable influence of this metaphor, evidence now shows that the first two of its properties, indivisibility and scrutiny, do not hold.

More Than One Spotlight

We know from studies of multiple item tracking (Pylyshyn & Storm, 1988; Yantis, 1992), flanker interference (Driver & Baylis, 1989), and multiple target selection (Awh & Pashler, 2000; Castiello & Umilta, 1992; Kramer & Hahn, 1995) that more than one region can be selected at the same time and that this is not accomplished with simply a larger selection area that encompasses the multiple items. Awh and Pashler (2000), for example, show that the cueing advantage that is seen at both target locations is not seen for targets occasionally presented midway between the two cued locations. These results indicate that there can be more than one selection region. Evidence from multiple item tracking experiments suggests that it may be possible to deploy and control as many as four or five independent selection regions.

How big or small are these selection regions? Many authors have proposed that the selection region can be quite large or quite small depending on the task requirements (e.g., the zoom-lens concept; Eriksen & St. James, 1986; Klein & McCormick, 1989; LaBerge, 1983). However, it does appear that there is a minimum size for the selection region and that this smallest size is quite a bit larger than the smallest detail we can see. Our studies of the crowding effect give us some idea of the minimum spacing of objects that still allows selection. If we think of the smallest size of the selection region as the acuity of selection, it varies from 5 times worse than the acuity of vision at the fovea to 30 times worse at only 15 degrees eccentricity (Intriligator & Cavanagh, 2001) and continues this steep downward trend to the limit of the visual field. If our vision were limited to the acuity of selection, we would be legally blind.

Crowding and Acuity of Selection

While looking at the plus sign in Figure 2.3, we can clearly see the lines to the right but cannot individuate or count through them, at least not easily beyond the first two. They are within the resolution limit of vision but beyond the limits of selection. This is a demonstration of the crowding phenomenon, more typically explored with letters as in Figure 2.4.

The traditional view of crowding was that lateral interactions suppress or mask features early in visual processing. This view changed recently when a study in our lab (He,

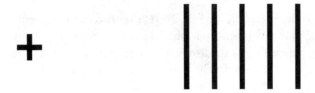

FIGURE 2.3. When fixating the plus sign, the vertical bars can be seen. They are thin, parallel, and all of equal length. But it is very hard to count them, indicating that at least the middle bars cannot be easily individuated.

Cavanagh, & Intriligator, 1996) showed that crowded grating patches could induce orientation specific aftereffects even though observers were unable to report the orientation of the patches. The stimuli are clearly registered up to at least a level where orientation analysis emerges, level V1 in the visual cortex. Even more recently, Parkes, Lund, Angelucci, Solomon, and Morgan (2001) showed that the orientation of a target in a crowded array of gabor patches could not be reported, but, nevertheless, the estimate of the average orientation of the gabors in the array was directly influenced by the orientation of the target. The authors conclude that even though the individual identities in a crowded array are blocked from awareness, they nonetheless do get through to higher levels, albeit in the form of a contribution to the array's overall texture.

These results suggest that the features of a crowded item are not suppressed or masked at an early level. What then accounts for the inability to report the item? We have claimed

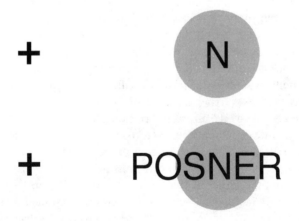

FIGURE 2.4. When fixating the plus sign on the top left, the N to the right is easily identified. When fixating the plus sign just below, the N seems to meld into a jumbled texture of letters. This is the crowding effect of the surrounding items on the availability of an individual item. Notice that this is not just a function of eccentricity as the letter R, even further in the periphery, can be identified. The N is not in fact lost but contributes efficiently to our judgments of the texture itself (Parkes et al., 2001). The circular gray region depicts a hypothetical, smallest region of selection possible at the eccentricity of the letter N. It enables the selection of the N as an individual letter. When the N is embedded within the string, the same selection region no longer retrieves a single letter but several letters. If the selection were like a spotlight enabling scrutiny within the region of interest, the N would be available as would the S and E. This does not happen. We appear to have access only to a texture-like description within the selection region. This coding singularity prevents access to the raw image and provides only a single description of the entire selection.

(He et al., 1996; Intriligator & Cavanagh, 2001) that this crowding effect is due to limits on the spatial resolution of attentional selection. In severe crowding like that in Figure 2.4, a target embedded in a dense array of distractors cannot be selected alone and thus cannot be consciously identified or reported. The target is seen only as part of an indivisible, fuzzy grouping that ties together all items within the selection region.

A second experiment showed that the grain of selection is inhomogeneous across the visual field. The task required subjects to mentally step through a set of discs arrayed around a circle while they fixated the center of the circle. Stepping started with one disc that briefly flashed red and then subjects mentally stepped back and forth under computer instruction. After six or seven steps, a probe disc turned red and the subject reported whether or not it was the disc they had stepped to. By varying the number of discs arrayed around the circumference, we measured the density at which the subject could no longer individuate the discs. The results showed that the acuity of selection gets rapidly worse with increasing eccentricity and is coarser in the upper visual field than in the lower field. Moreover, at locations outside the fovea, acuity is coarser in the radial direction—the direction along the radius from the fovea through the location—than it is in the tangential direction. These were the first measures of the resolution of selection to assess purely the selection of location with no identification required for the target. Our stepping tasks tracked location in dense arrays of identical items and so were unaffected by any preattentive feature interactions that might degrade the recognition measures used in crowding and flanker tasks. The pattern of results for the access to location closely matched those for letter identification in the standard crowding task (e.g., Toet & Levi, 1992). This suggests that the errors of identification in crowding tasks can be attributed to the inability to select the item at the target location. The determining factor is therefore the loss of access to the location and not the loss of the feature information at that location. Sharma, Levi, and Klein (2000) have proposed that this acuity of selection is even more restricted in the amblyopic eye.

Could the resolution of selection depend on attentional load? As a first attempt to address this question we compared the critical radius for crowding with single items (stepping experiment) against the critical radius for crowding estimated from data in the multiple item tracking when four items were being tracked (Intriligator & Cavanagh, 2001). The two estimates matched fairly well. Nevertheless, the critical radius might vary as a function of the number of items being tracked. We addressed this question (Intriligator & Cavanagh, 2001) by varying the number of targets to be tracked from one to four in the multiple-item tracking task. Fewer resources are required to track a single target than four targets. As a result, when only a single target is tracked, the surplus resources may be applied to further shrink the selection field around the target. If this is true, there may be no fixed acuity limit for selection, only a size that depends inversely on the resources applied to its maintenance (cf. Lavie, 1995). In the limit, according to this view, attentional selection for single targets might be limited only by visual resolution.

The experiment showed that this did not happen. Tracking was indeed more accurate at moderately small display sizes when tracking only a single target, but the display size at which tracking became impossible was ultimately the same, no matter how many targets were being tracked. At this point, the moving items could be seen clearly, their spacing was about a factor of 10 above the visual resolution limit. Nevertheless, they could not be tracked. This evidence suggests that the spatial limit to selection is an absolute one: It cannot change elastically as more resources become available. It is the same size whether one or four of the regions of selection are being deployed.

In a recent experiment on crowding, we (Tripathy & Cavanagh, 2002) were also able to show that the spatial extent of crowding was fixed, having the same size for large and small targets as well as for luminance-defined and color-defined targets. Local interactions at early levels in the cortex might be expected to scale with the size of the targets and might also be expected to differ in range for color stimuli and luminance stimuli. Because neither effect was observed, we argue that the spatial extent of crowding is set by the physiological process that accesses the early cortical representation in order to select information. In this case, the size of the region of access would be dependent on the connections from higher levels but independent of target properties.

What Is Selected: The Coding Singularity

What can be encoded from each selection region? Clearly, not all features within the region can be picked up as if a piece of the visual image were cut out and passed along for detailed analysis. Many studies have shown that only the features of the target object are selected initially (Egly, Driver, & Rafal, 1994) and not the features of other objects even though they are at the same location (Duncan, 1984). More recently, Blaser, Pylyshyn, and Holcombe (2000) superimposed two gabor patches at the same location and asked subjects to track the features of one or both patches as they smoothly changed their orientations, colors, and bar widths over time. Subjects could keep track of the features of one of the two objects, accurately reporting the direction of any abrupt changes in two properties, say, the target's orientation and color. However, they could not track the properties of both objects at the same location even though they still had to report only the changes in two features, say, the orientation of one and the color of the other.

These results suggest not only that the information available at a location is limited to the features of the target object but also that only one object can be selected at a given location. This remains to be examined in a wider range of situations. Whether or not two objects can be selected at the same location, studies of crowding show that the information available in a single selection is highly constrained.

In the phenomenon of crowding, the inability to identify or even access the location of crowded items implies a fundamental property for the information available for selection. If the selection region were just like a spotlight where details could be scrutinized, a minimum selection region would not create any significant problem. If we could simply select the visual image within the region and scrutinize it (like the gray region in the lower set of letters in Figure 2.4), we could read out the letters or items within. We cannot do that.

This result suggests that the information available for selection is some highly processed description or label of the contents of the selection region. If a single, familiar item is within the region, the result of selection is to acquire the label of that item, say, an object such as a "face," or "shoe," or a letter "B," or number "5," and so on. If more than one item lies within the selection region, there may be no description of the combination available from early vision that allows us to then break it down to access each constituent item individually. If two letters are in the selection region, for example, the result might be a description such as "letters," or "some letters," or "some lines," depending on what is available. None of these allows us to recover the identities of the letters.

I have used the crowding results to argue for two separate limits: acuity—the minimum spacing of items that allows access to individuals—and singularity—the sparse nature of the description available within the selection. These two limits are closely intertwined. Specifically, if there were no coding singularity, we could scrutinize the details of a selection region and access components down to the limit of visual resolution. The acuity limit of selection would be no coarser than visual acuity. Thus the acuity limit exists only because of the coding singularity; however, the singularity does not set the value of the acuity limit. The example of pixellated images makes this point clear. The coding singularity is analogous to the effect of pixellation on a photograph. Within each region, each pixel, there is only one value and no further scrutiny of the photograph is possible at finer scales. The acuity limit of selection described in this chapter is equivalent to the smallest possible size of the pixels. Interestingly, the selection pixels are larger than the available pixels of visual detail. The selection pixels can be scaled up as the regions of interest expand to cover larger areas (as in the zoom-lens models, Eriksen & St. James, 1986; Klein & McCormick, 1989; LaBerge, 1983). However, as these pixels scale up, they do not preserve the new detail they capture; they lose it by giving access to only the single label of the larger area. The singularity limit is equivalent to the claim that the information in one pixel has no internal detail even when the pixel size is scaled up above the minimum size. Selecting a region larger than the minimum size does not provide access to the details of the region at the finest grain but gives a single label for the whole region, no matter how large (see the iconic bottleneck of Nakayama, 1990, for a related proposal).

The support for this claim comes from visual search experiments. A number of studies show that it is the highest-level descriptions of the items that are initially available and not the underlying features of each item even though the items are not crowded. For example, when searching for an upward curved arc among downward arcs, the search is significantly slower when the arcs are arranged to make mouths and eyebrows of schematic faces (Suzuki & Cavanagh, 1995). We argued that the initial descriptions available for selection are at the face level, not at the constituent feature level. Similarly, He and Nakayama (1992) used test items where one square overlaps another producing an L-shaped region as the only visible part of the square in the back. They showed that subjects could not perform a search for the L shape of the partial occlusion, suggesting that the subjects had access only to the completed square shapes and not the image features. This is also the same point that Hochstein and Ahissar (2002) make in their reverse hierarchy theory. Attention can select initially only at the highest level of description, even when the selection region is much larger than its minimum size. The singularity of coding is not seen only in crowding experiments. It is not a consequence of the small size of the selection region demanded by the crowding paradigm; it is a basic property of selection.

If no scrutiny is available for the information within a single selection, how is compound or complex information selected, bound, and identified. The suggestion here is simply that the four or so independent selection operators pick up local, identifiable pieces and, with some further analysis, construct a combined description (Figure 2.5). This suggestion repositions scrutiny and binding from actions operating within a region of selection to actions of an attention routine (bind, group) acting over multiple selections where each individual selection is quite limited in what it can pick up.

Temporal Limits of Selection

The acuity limits of selection in time mirror those of selection in space. In particular, the selection and individuation of events in a rapid stream show very coarse temporal resolution. A spot flickering at slow rates can be perceived as the succession of light and dark phases, but when flickering at a high rate, only flicker is perceived. At even higher rates, the light and dark phases fuse and no flicker is seen. The range of rates over which flicker is visible but the individual light and dark phases are no longer accessible is equivalent to the spatial

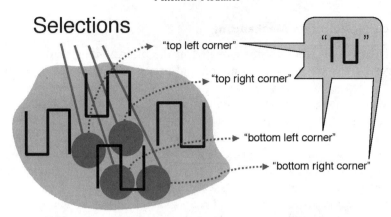

FIGURE 2.5. Multiple, simultaneous selections can combine the separate parts of an unfamiliar shape. An unfamiliar shape would have no distinctive label or description if it were selected as a whole, other than the equivalent of "some lines." When the four familiar parts (corners) are individually selected and identified they can then be packaged together with their spatial relations as a distinctive description. This new description can be used to distinguish this shape from, say, the shape to its left.

resolution example in Figure 2.1 where the spatial pattern of the bars can be clearly seen but individual bars cannot accessed or counted. Many phenomena that involve selection or tracking of sequential events show this low temporal limit of about 4–8 Hz (see Verstraten, Cavanagh, & LaBianca, 2000, for a summary). This rate is 8–16 frames per second, consistent with the highest rates at which target scenes or words can be identified in rapid serial visual presentation experiments (Potter, 1993).

Even more important and demanding than selecting disparate bits of a changing scene or object is to integrate and recognize a familiar motion pattern. Many objects and activities have characteristic motions easily revealed in a moment spent imagining the trajectories of butterflies, bike riders, joggers, frisbees, or flapjacks in flight. The recognition of characteristic motions is so robust that a human form is rapidly recognized from the motions of a set of lights attached to a person filmed while walking, running, or performing pushups in the dark (Johansson, 1973; Neri, Morrone, & Burr, 1998). Although the immediacy of Johansson's point-light walkers suggested that the construction of these motion percepts is effortless, our visual search study (Cavanagh, Labianca, & Thornton, 2001) showed that they are not.

The internal modeling of trajectories and speed can underlie the perception of simple motions as well as complex. A tracked object in smooth (Verstraten et al., 2000) or random motion (Pylyshyn & Storm, 1988) may be supported by the internal representation of its current and expected trajectory. The case of an ambiguous motion (Wertheimer, 1912) is the most compelling example. Wertheimer presented a cross alternating with an X, the 45-degree rotation of the cross. Clockwise or counterclockwise motion could be seen depending on the "set and posture" of attention (Wertheimer, 1912, translated in Shipley, 1961, p. 1070). Only one direction is seen at a time and the path seen depends necessarily on the choice of an internal model because the stimulus itself is ambiguous. We have proposed that the high-level motion system (cf. Anstis, 1980; Braddick, 1980) is anchored by this type of model-based attention tracking. In other words, it relies on set of attention routines that acquire and track targets (Cavanagh, 1992) and it is limited by the very slow temporal acuity constraints of attention routines (Verstraten et al., 2000).

Cortical Locus of Selection Mechanisms

Where are the attention routines implemented in the brain? Many studies have suggested that the parietal areas are involved in attentional processing (Corbetta & Shulman, 2002; Gazzaniga & Ladavas, 1987; Posner, Walker, Friedrich, & Rafal, 1984, 1987). Our own imaging and neuropathology studies (Battelli et al., 2001; Battelli, Cavanagh, Martini, & Barton, 2003; Culham et al., 1998; Culham, Cavanagh, & Kanwisher, 2001) indicate that at least the selection routines are strongly represented in the parietal lobes. Our evidence for the parietal locus of selection mechanisms begins with the coarseness and inhomogeneity of the acuity of selection. It is too coarse to be based in cortical area V1 and its variations are more similar to those we would expect for the parietal regions.

The smallest region of selection might be, for example, a hypercolumn as it is not possible to select a smaller unit and represent all the possible features that might occur within the region. We know that there are at least a few thousand hypercolumns in human area V1, but we found evidence for only about 60 independently accessible regions of the central 30 degrees of visual space (Intriligator & Cavanagh, 2001). Moreover, in our study of adaptation and crowding (He et al., 1996), we found that information can be registered in area V1 (as shown by orientation-specific aftereffects) but impossible to select and report. Selection, then, would appear to occur later than area V1.

We also found that the lower visual field has better selection resolution than the upper (He et al., 1996; Intriligator & Cavanagh, 2001). The lower visual field is overrepresented in the occipital–parietal regions. This result again suggests that the locus of the selection lies beyond the early retinotopic areas that have relatively similar representations of the upper and lower visual fields. This parietal locus is also supported by our studies of attentive tracking tasks (Culham et al., 1998, 2001). The areas that are involved in eye movements for tracking and pursuit seem closely linked to those for attentional selection.

Recent results in a study of tracking in our lab (G. A. Alvarez, personal communication, 2003) also suggest that these selection routines may be strongly lateralized in that they operate independently in the left and right hemifields. Tested with the displays shown in Figure 2.6, the eight subjects could track four items with high accuracy if two of the targets

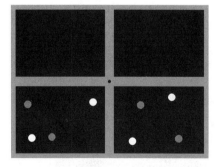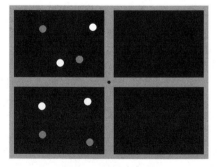

FIGURE 2.6. Paired multiple item tracking tasks. On the left, two of the four panels centered at the fixation point have two targets and two distractors each. All items start to move and the white items, which the subject is meant to track, change to gray, indistinguishable from the distractors. On the right is the display where the two tracking tasks are both in the same hemifield. The items bounce off the walls of their respective regions, never crossing the gray separators. Preliminary data (Alvarez, 2003) show that tracking with the two regions in separate hemifields (example on the left) is much easier than when the two regions are in the same hemifield (example on the right).

were in the left field and two were in the right field. In fact, they were no less accurate track-ing two in each field than when tracking just two alone, either in the left or right field. This suggested that the targets in the separate hemifields did not draw on the same capacity. More important, when the four targets were placed in the same field, either left or right, per-formance plummeted. This implies that the capacity for tracking and the number of inde-pendent selection operators is limited within hemifields to about two per field. This result places interesting constraints on the physiological site where selection operators are con-trolled (it must have independent representations of the two hemifields) and on the process of tracking an object as it crosses the midline where some handoff may be required between fields. Note that if this result holds up and generalizes to other relevant tasks, the claim of independent tracking capacity in the two hemifields is, in the framework of the attention routines here, a claim about awareness. Specifically, the capacity of awareness must be, to some extent, independently limited for stimuli from the two hemifields. This would not be surprising for split-brain patients, but the suggestion that this holds for some tasks in nor-mals calls for further testing.

Finally, patients who have lesions to the parietal areas show profound deficits in attentive tracking and object enumeration in the hemifield contralateral to the parietal damage (Battelli et al., 2001). In addition to this contralateral loss in spatial selection, we have recently identi-fied a separate loss in temporal selection. Specifically, patients with right parietal damage have a *bilateral* deficit in differentiating onsets and offsets (Battelli et al., 2003). In contrast, left pa-rietal patients show no loss in distinguishing onsets and offsets in either field suggesting that this distinction is a function of the right parietal area alone. Because the right parietal patients can detect flickering targets normally, we argued that the deficit occurs at a high level of pro-cessing where attention routines sort out which transients belong together. For example, an in-crease in brightness can be due to the appearance of a bright object or the disappearance of a dark object. The assignment of on and off transients to the appearance and disappearance of objects is contingent upon the representation of the objects and their properties. We suggest that this object-based labeling of events is the function of the right parietal lobe. The parietal area is therefore both the site of control for spatial attention routines, where the left and right parietal areas each deal with the contralateral field, and of the temporal aspects of selection, where the right parietal area alone analyzes both hemifields. In this function, the right parietal area could be seen as part of a "When" pathway marking the appearance and disappearance of objects and the beginning and end of events.

CONCLUSIONS

The role of attention is now a topic of research in almost all corners of cognitive neurosci-ence (Figure 2.7). Despite the recent burst of activity, the basic elements of attention were identified many hundreds of years ago. It was already noted in the 4th century B.C. that at-tention appears to have a single focus (Aristotle, trans. 1984), and, in the 1st century B.C., that attended items are experienced with more detail and vividness (Lucretius, trans. 1951). Attention could be voluntary (Aristotle, trans. 1984) or involuntary (Augustine, 6th century A.D., trans. 1993). In the 11th century A.D., Alhazen (trans. 1989) pointed out that some fea-tures in vision are apprehended rapidly, in a single glance whereas others require scrutiny. Wolff (1745) proposed a feature integration theory where attention to the parts of an object is required to integrate them into a whole. A number of these points continue to be debated and refined, but the aspects of selection, binding, and limited capacity remain the defining

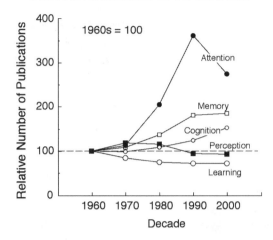

FIGURE 2.7. Relative numbers of publications for each of five key words, normalized to their relative frequencies in the 1960–1969 decade. The 2000 data span only the years 2000–2003.

characteristics of attention. Indeed, they are still pretty much all we have (cf. Hatfield, 1998). As Fodor (2001) said, "That's what so nice about cognitive science, you can drop out for a couple of centuries and not miss a thing" (p. 49).

Despite the development of more sophisticated models (cf. Logan, 1996), there are widely divergent opinions concerning the basic nature of attention. For some authors, attention is an active agent that does things—selects or binds, for example (e.g., Treisman, 1988). For others, it is a resource that must be shared among competing processes (e.g., Kahneman, 1973; Norman & Bobrow, 1975) or a factor that amplifies signals and improves sensitivity (e.g., Lu & Dosher, 1998; Yeshurun & Carrasco, 1998). More recently, some have noted that it is perhaps just a catchall grouping of widely diverse mental functions and phenomena. Driver (2001) has called attention an umbrella term that groups a broad area of research. Walsh (2003) has argued that attention has unrestrained explanatory range; it is freely used for any side of any argument. Like the cosmological ether of pre-20th-century physics, says Walsh, it is everywhere, but in the end, nowhere.

The first proposal in this chapter was to divide visual processes according to the availability of reportable states. Attention is then the set of routines that have reportable initial and final states but no accessible intermediate states. Visual routines, the components of these attention routines, have no properties that are accessible to awareness. Cognition routines, processes that comprise sequences of attention routines, have multiple, reportable steps, each one a call to an attention routine. These three levels correspond loosely to the categories of early or preattentive vision (vision routines), to mid- and high-level vision (attention routines), and to cognition or, at least, visual cognition.

The second part of the chapter laid out three processing limits of attention routines. First, there is a capacity limit that is set by the constraints of representing the initial and final states of the routines in awareness. The limit on the number of items simultaneously in awareness appears to be four or five although it may be further constrained as a separate limit of about two for each hemifield. Second, the evidence from crowding experiments suggests the acuity of selection is disturbingly coarse, an order of magnitude or more below spatial and temporal visual acuity. Finally, crowding also revealed a coding singularity. The information available within a single selection is limited to a single, high-level label, affording no opportunity for scrutiny of details within a selection.

One of the two classic characteristics of attention has been its limited capacity. In the definition of attention routines given here, there is no mention of capacity, only of reportability. The initial and final states of an attention routine are consciously registered and reportable. This, of course, entails a limit in the ability to simultaneously register multiple items in consciousness. The suggestion is that this is the capacity limit affecting attention. The routines themselves may execute without interference, but when initial states or output values must be posted in awareness, interference arises because of the limited ability to hold multiple items in awareness.

The dependence on awareness and reportability to define attention routines may appear restrictive. We are now comfortable with the notion of reporting our mental states either verbally to others or by motor responses to a computer, or just by introspection to ourselves. But does this criterion put animal research out of reach? I do not believe it does. Alert monkey experiments deal regularly with motor responses that are used to report mental states whether the detection or discriminations of motions, the recognition of target objects, or the enumeration of arbitrary items. These are not reflexes or automated responses, although they can become automated with practice.

This very simple criterion raises many questions and I can only note a few here. Reportability, for example, will always underrepresent the actual information that entered and exited awareness. Moreover, some of the limits of attention, attributed here to the capacity of awareness, may be due to limits of working memory, not just limits of visual awareness. The reportability criterion limit might appear to limit this framework to human research. Clearly, many in the alert animal research area allow that responses can be contingent on the mental states of their test animals. In the case of arbitrary responses that are not highly overlearned, the responses should be as valid an index of reportability as a button push is in human psychophysics experiments. However, this view is not without controversy. Finally, the capacity limits of awareness and working memory may not be defined in terms of the number of items that can be held (Luck & Vogel, 1997) but may be more accurately described in terms of the overall amount of detail to be held (for memory, Alvarez & Cavanagh, 2004; for attention, Davis, Welsh, Holmes, & Shepherd, 2001).

The second defining characteristic is that with increased attention, performance improves. This property is of course trivially true in a context of consciously guided task responses. Without selection, there is no awareness of the target, and thus no explicit response is possible. Any number of implicit measures may reflect the processing of the target by vision routines whose output does not reach awareness but has other effects (e.g., orientation adaptation; He et al., 1996). Manipulations of selection, like cueing, that affect performance will affect the efficiency of selection in a variety of ways. For example, a nonvalid cue may cause selection operators to arrive at the real target location later than they would for a valid cue. Alternatively, the presence of nonvalid cues in a session might lead the subject to set one focused selection region at the cued location and one diffuse selection to cover all the remaining locations, reducing the efficiency of selection and therefore the quality of information retrieved from a miscued target.

Beyond the routines of selection discussed here are many other routines that we would consider part of the attention-based level of processes. Attention routines undoubtedly include feature-based and object-based selection, the packaging and description of selected items, as well as the setting of goals for selection perhaps in response to requests from other modules in the brain. The output of the attention routines must likely be some description of visual events that is shipped off to the other modules of the brain to keep them up to date on the visual world.

ACKNOWLEDGMENTS

This research was supported by National Institutes of Health grants to Patrick Cavanagh. Thanks to Mike Posner, George Alvarez, Wonmok Shim, Steven Franconeri, and Ramakrishna Chakravarthi for comments on earlier versions of the manuscript.

NOTE

1. To preview that discussion, clearly there would be no selection acuity limit without the coding singularity, as we could just scrutinize the internal details of a selection down to the limit of visual resolution. However, the existence of a coding singularity does not set the smallest size of the selection region, that smallest size is the acuity limit. Nor is the coding singularity only seen for the smallest selection regions, at the acuity limit in crowded displays. It is revealed on its own in visual search experiments with item spacing much broader than the acuity limit. See page 19 for an expanded discussion.

REFERENCES

Alhazen. (1989). *The optics of Ibn al-Haytham* (A. I. Sabra, Trans.). London: Warburg Institute.

Alvarez, G. A., & Cavanagh, P. (2004). The capacity of visual short-term memory is set both by visual information load and by number of objects. *Psychological Science, 15,* 106–111.

Anstis, S. M. (1980). The perception of apparent movement. *Philosophical Transactions of the Royal Society of London B* (Biological Sciences), *290,* 153–168.

Aristotle. (1984). Sense and sensibilia (J. I. Beare, Trans.). In J. Barnes (Ed.), *Complete works of Aristotle* (pp. 693–713). Princeton, NJ: Bollingen.

Augustine. (1993). *Confessions* (F. J. Sheed, Trans.). Indianapolis, IN: Hackett.

Awh, E., & Pashler, H. (2000). Evidence for split attentional foci. *Journal of Experimental Psychology: Human Perception and Performance, 26,* 834–846.

Battelli, L., Cavanagh, P., Intriligator, J., Tramo, M. J., Hénaff, M.-A., Michèl, F., & Barton, J. J. S. (2001). Unilateral right parietal damage leads to bilateral deficit for high-level motion. *Neuron, 32,* 985–995.

Battelli, L., Cavanagh, P., Martini, P., & Barton, J. S. S. (2003). Bilateral deficits of transient visual attention in right parietal patients. *Brain, 126,* 2164–2174.

Blaser, E., Pylyshyn, Z. W., & Holcombe, A. O. (2000). Tracking an object through feature space. *Nature, 408,* 196–199.

Braddick, O. J. (1980). Low-level and high-level processes in apparent motion. *Philosophical Transactions of the Royal Society of London B, 290,* 137–151.

Broadbent, D. E. (1958). *Perception and communication.* New York: Pergamon Press.

Castiello, U., & Umilta, C. (1992) Splitting focal attention. *Journal of Experimental Psychology: Human Perception and Performance, 18,* 837–848.

Cavanagh, P. (1992). Attention-based motion perception. *Science, 257,* 1563–1565.

Cavanagh, P. (2003). The language of vision. The *perception* lecture. *Perception, 32*(Suppl. 1).

Cavanagh, P., Labianca, A. T., & Thornton, I. M. (2001). Attention-based visual routines: Sprites. *Cognition, 80,* 47–60.

Corbetta, M., & Shulman, G. L. (2002). Control of goal-directed and stimulus-driven attention in the brain. *Nature Review of Neuroscience, 3,* 201–215.

Culham, J. C., Brandt, S. A., Cavanagh, P., Kanwisher, N. G., Dale, A. M., & Tootell, R. B. H. (1998). Cortical fMRI activation produced by attentive tracking of moving targets. *Journal of Neurophysiology, 80,* 2657–2670.

Culham, J. C., Cavanagh, P., & Kanwisher, N. G. (2001). Attention response functions: Characterizing brain areas with fMRI activation during parametric variations of attentional load. *Neuron*, *32*, 737–745.

Davis, G., Welch, V. L., Holmes, A., & Shepherd A. (2001). Can attention select only a fixed number of objects at a time? *Perception*, *30*, 1227–1248.

Driver, J. (2001). A selective review of selective attention research from the past century. *British Journal of Psychology*, *92*, 53–78.

Driver, J., & Baylis, G. C. (1989). Movement and visual attention: The spotlight metaphor breaks down. *Journal of Experimental Psychology: Human Perception and Performance*, *15*, 448–456.

Duncan, J. (1984). Selective attention and the organization of visual information. *Journal of Experimental Psychology: General*, *113*, 501–517.

Egly, R., Driver, J., & Rafal, R. D. (1994). Shifting visual attention between objects and locations: Evidence from normal and parietal lesion subjects. *Journal of Experimental Psychology: General*, *123*, 161–177.

Eriksen, C. W., & St. James, J. D. (1986). Visual attention within and around the field of focal attention: A zoom lens model. *Perception and Psychophysics*, *40*, 225–240.

Fodor, J. (2001). *The mind doesn't work that way.* Cambridge, MA: MIT Press.

Gazzaniga, M. S., & Ladavas, E. (1987). Disturbances in spatial attention following lesion or disconnection of the right parietal lobe. In M. Jeannerod (Ed.), *Neurophysiological and neuropsychological aspects of spatial neglect* (Vol. 45, pp. 203–213). Amsterdam, Netherlands: Elsevier.

Hatfield, G. (1998). Attention in early scientific psychology. In R. D. Wright (Ed.), *Vancouver studies in cognitive science: Vol. 8. Visual attention* (pp. 3–25). New York: Oxford University Press.

He, S., Cavanagh, P., & Intriligator, J. (1996). Attentional resolution and the locus of visual awareness. *Nature*, *383*, 334–337.

He, Z. J., & Nakayama, K. (1992). Surfaces versus features in visual search. *Nature*, *359*, 231–233.

Hochstein, S., & Ahissar, M. (2002). View from the top: Hierarchies and reverse hierarchies in the visual system. *Neuron*, *36*, 791–804.

Intriligator, J., & Cavanagh, P. (2001). The spatial resolution of visual attention. *Cognitive Psychology*, *43*, 171–216.

James, W. (1890). *The principles of psychology.* New York: Holt.

Johansson, G. (1973). Visual perception of biological motion and a model for its analysis. *Perception and Psychophysics*, *14*, 201–211.

Jolicoeur, P., Ullman, S., & Mackay, M. (1986). Curve tracing:Aa possible basic operation in the perception of spatial relations. *Memory and Cognition*, *14*, 129–140.

Jolicoeur, P., Ullman, S., & Mackay, M. (1991). Visual curve tracing properties. *Journal of Experimental Psychology: Human Perception and Performance*, *17*, 997–1022.

Kahneman, D. (1973). *Attention and effort.* Englewood Cliffs, NJ: Prentice-Hall.

Klein, R., & McCormick, P. (1989). Covert visual orienting: Hemifield-activation can be mimicked by zoom lens and midlocation placement strategies. *Acta Psychologica*, *70*, 235–250.

Kramer, A. F., & Hahn, S. (1995). Splitting the beam: Distribution of attention over noncontiguous regions of the visual field. *Psychological Science*, *6*, 381–386.

LaBerge, D. (1983). Spatial extent of attention to letters and words. *Journal of Experimental Psychology: Human Perception and Performance*, *9*, 371–379.

Lavie, N. (1995). Perceptual load as a necessary condition for selective attention. *Journal of Experimental Psychology: Human Perception and Performance*, *21*, 451–468.

Logan, G. D. (1996). The CODE theory of visual attention: an integration of space-based and object-based attention. *Psychological Review*, *103*, 603–649.

Logan, G. D., & Zbrodoff, N. J. (1999). Selection for cognition: Cognitive constraints on visual spatial attention. *Visual Cognition*, *6*, 55–81.

Lu, Z.- L., & Dosher, B. A. (1998). External noise distinguishes attention mechanisms. *Vision Research*, *38*, 1183–1198.

Luck, S. J., & Vogel, E. K. (1997). The capacity of visual working memory for features and conjunctions. *Nature*, *390*, 279–281.

Lucretius. (1951). *On the nature of the universe* (R. Latham, Trans.). London: Penguin Books.

Nakayama, K. (1990). The iconic bottleneck and the tenuous link between early processing and perception. In C. Blakemore (Ed.), *Vision: Coding and efficiency* (pp. 411–422). Cambridge, UK: Cambridge University Press.

Neri, P., Morrone M. C., & Burr, D. C. (1998). Seeing biological motion. *Nature, 395,* 894–896.

Newell, A., & Simon, H. A. (1972). *Human problem solving.* Englewood Cliffs, NJ: Prentice-Hall.

Norman, D. A., & Bobrow, D. G. (1975). On data-limited and resource-limited processes. *Cognitive Psychology, 7,* 44–64.

Parkes, L., Lund, J., Angelucci, A., Solomon, J. A., & Morgan, M. (2001). Compulsory averaging of crowded orientation signals in human vision. *Nature Neuroscience, 4,* 739–744.

Pashler, H.(1998). *The psychology of attention.* Cambridge, MA: MIT Press.

Posner, M. I. (1994). Attention: the mechanisms of consciousness. *Processes of the National Academy of Sciences USA, 91,* 7398–7403.

Posner, M. I., & Driver, J. (1992). The neurobiology of selective attention. *Current Opinions in Neurobiology, 2,* 165–169.

Posner, M. I., Walker, J. A., Friedrich, F. J., & Rafal, R. D. (1984). Effects of parietal injury on covert orienting of attention. *Journal of Neuroscience, 4,* 1863–1874.

Posner, M. I., Walker, J. A., Friedrich, F. A., & Rafal, R. D. (1987). How do the parietal lobes direct covert attention? Special Issue: Selective visual attention. *Neuropsychologia, 25,* 135–145.

Potter, M. C. (1993). Very short-term conceptual memory. *Memory and Cognition, 21,* 156–161.

Pylyshyn, Z. W., & Storm, R. W. (1988). Tracking multiple independent targets: Evidence for a parallel tracking mechanism. *Spatial Vision, 3,* 179–197.

Sharma, V., Levi, D. M., & Klein, S. A. (2000). Undercounting features and missing features: Evidence for a high-level deficit in strabismic amblyopia. *Nature Neuroscience, 3,* 496–501.

Shimamura, A. P. (2000). Toward a cognitive neuroscience of metacognition. *Consciousness and Cognition, 9,* 313–323.

Shipley, T. (Ed.). (1961). *Classics in psychology.* New York: Philosophical Library.

Suzuki, S., & Cavanagh, P. (1995). Facial organization blocks access to low-level features: An object inferiority effect. *Journal of Experimental Psychology: Human Perception and Performance, 21,* 901–913.

Toet, A., & Levi, D. M. (1992). The two-dimensional shape of spatial interaction zones in the parafovea. *Vision Research, 32,* 1349–1357.

Treisman, A. (1988). Features and objects: the fourteenth Bartlett memorial lecture. *Quarterly Journal of Experimental Psychology A, 40,* 201–237.

Tripathy, S. P., & Cavanagh, P. (2002). The extent of crowding in peripheral vision does not scale with target size. *Vision Research, 42,* 2357.

Ullman, S. (1984). Visual routines. *Cognition, 18,* 97–159.

Ullman, S. (1996). *High-level vision.* Cambridge, MA: MIT Press.

Verstraten, F. A. J., Cavanagh, P., & Labianca, A. T. (2000). Limits of attentive tracking reveal temporal properties of attention. *Vision Research, 40,* 3651–3664.

Walsh, V. (2003). A theory of magnitude: Common cortical metrics of time, space and quantity. *Trends in Cognitive Science, 7,* 483–488.

Wertheimer, M. (1912). Experimentelle Studien über das Sehen von Bewegung. *Zeitschrift für Psychologie, 61,* 161–165.

Wolff, C. (1745). *Psychologie ou traité sur l'âme.* Hildesheim: Georg Olms Verlag.

Yantis, S. (1992). Multi-element visual tracking: Attention and perceptual organization. *Cognitive Psychology, 3,* 295–340.

Yeshurun, Y., & Carrasco, M. (1998). Attention improves or impairs visual performance by enhancing spatial resolution. *Nature, 396,* 72–75.

3

On the Control of Visual Orienting

Raymond M. Klein

Processing of the visual environment is characterized by selectivity: Some locations or objects may be given priority over others. Spatial selectivity can be accomplished by a shift in gaze direction to control which region of visual space is processed by the sensitive fovea or by an internal assignment of processing resources: a shift of attention. Shifts in gaze direction are referred to here as *overt orienting* because these shifts (in the form of eye or head movements, or both) can be seen by an external observer. Adjustments in the absence of an overt movement are referred to here as *covert orienting* because these shifts cannot be directly observed and, therefore, must be inferred from performance. Whether overt or covert, visual orienting can be controlled reflexively by external stimulation or voluntarily by internally generated signals. Following Posner (1980), the terms *exogenous* and *endogenous*, respectively, are used here to label these two kinds of control of orienting. Seeking to characterize the modes of orienting that are illustrated in Figure 3.1, to illuminate their neural implementation, and to understand the nature of their interactions, we have developed or borrowed experimental paradigms that strip away unwanted variables while honing in on those under consideration. Purely behavioral evidence converges with neuroscientific evidence to reveal that (1) when the fixation stimulus is removed prior to the presentation of a target, a dramatic decrease in saccadic reaction time (SRT) is found; (2) neural machinery in the superior colliculus (SC) is resposible for this effect; (3) endogenous and exogenous signals for control of eye movements converge on the intermediate layer of the SC; (4) covert attention has different effects on the processing of targets when it is controlled endogenously versus exogenously; and (5) despite the anatomical overlap in the control of overt and covert orienting, there is considerable independence between the two systems.

OVERT ORIENTING

When we consider overt orienting it is clear that regardless of the control mechanism(s) involved, it is the direction of gaze that is being controlled. Normally overt orienting is accomplished by a collaborative effort of the eyes and head. But in most behavioral and

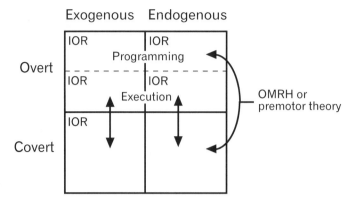

FIGURE 3.1. The research surveyed in this chapter is aimed at understanding relations among the four kinds of orienting entailed in the orthogonal combination of the exogenous and endogenous control over overt and covert orienting. The boxes representing exogenously and endogenously controlled overt orienting have been split to recognize the fact that some studies have explored separately the preparation and execution of eye movements (overt orienting). The vertical arrows represent the linkage between the execution of eye movements under exogenous and endogenous control and consequent shifts of attention. The arrow connecting endogenous programming of overt orienting and endogenous covert orienting represents the assumption of the oculomotor readiness hypothesis (and premotor theory) that preparing a saccade generates a shift of attention. The occurrence of inhibition of return following some modes of orienting is indicated by the initials IOR.

neuroscientific studies the situation is simplified by keeping the head still. There are three isolable eye movement systems (Robinson, 1968). Saccades are quasi-ballistic jumps in the position of the eye in the orbit. They are referred to as voluntary eye movements, but this is a misnomer. Like breathing, we can make or withhold saccades on purpose and under instruction; but normally as we inspect a scene or navigate our environment we make several saccades per second of which we are little aware. The vestibulo-ocular reflex allows gaze direction to remain stationary in space while the head moves. It is an important component of the collaboration referred to previously. The pursuit system follows, with a matched velocity, a smoothly moving stimulus. Here we focus on saccadic eye movements as might be made during scene perception and reading.

Endogenous and Exogenous Control

The extraocular muscles and the neural machinery in the brain stem which controls them, collectively are the "oculomotor plant," which is the final common path for the different kinds of eye movements. Upstream from here are a multitude of brain structures with different roles in the control of gaze direction. Notable among these are the SC and frontal eye field (FEF). Stimulation of specific regions of these structures elicits topographically consistent saccades, and saccadic eye movements are possible when either but not both structures are lesioned (Schiller, True, & Conway, 1980). From these findings and others it is often assumed that the SC is primarily involved in exogenous control of saccades while the FEF is primarily involved in endogenous control. Even if such a division of labor were as clear-cut as this common belief, it is hardly informative about how the two modes of control are implemented. We should not conclude, however, that because geographical knowledge is not particularly revealing about mechanism, it is not useful. Quite the contrary, it tells us where to focus our tools to reveal how neural assemblies and circuitry control behavior. Of the variety of model tasks that have been used to explore the complex interplay between exogenous and endogenous control of saccadic eye movements, only a few are mentioned here.

As illustrated in Figure 3.2a, when observers are asked to execute saccades to a peripheral target, the latency of these saccades can be dramatically reduced if the fixation point is turned off some time (200 msec) before the target appears (e.g., Fischer & Ramsperger, 1984; Kingstone & Klein, 1993b; Saslow, 1967; Schiller, Sandell, & Maunsell, 1987). This reduction has been called the "gap effect" because it is most robustly generated when there is a 100- to 200-msec gap between the removal of fixation and the appearance of the target. Why do such gaps reduce SRTs?

Borrowing from Posner's framework for covert visual orienting, in which a shift of attention involves disengaging from its current focus, then moving to a new location, and finally engaging on the object there, Fischer and Breitmeyer (1987) proposed that when covert visual attention is engaged the saccadic system is inhibited and that when attention is disengaged the saccadic system is enabled. By removing an attended or unattended *peripheral* stimulus Kingstone and Klein (1993a) demonstrated that SRT benefited equally whether the attended or unattended stimulus was removed, and that removing fixation produced a much greater reaction time reduction than removing a peripheral object. This pattern of results, which was observed with both endogenous and exogenous covert orienting, demonstrates that the locus and/or disengagement of covert visual attention plays no role in the gap effect. To explain our overall pattern of results we proposed a two-process model (see also Klein & Kingstone, 1993; Reuter-Lorenz, Hughes, & Fendrich, 1991) in which:

1. Any offset serves as a warning signal and results in generalized *alertness*, and
2. Fixation offsets produce added facilitation by *exogenously disengaging the oculomotor system from fixation.*

If the engagement of the oculomotor system upon a stimulus at fixation inhibits saccades, then in the real world—where objects rarely disappear—how could we ever make an eye movement? It is, thus, logically necessary to add a third component to our proposal (Taylor, Kingstone, & Klein, 1998):

3. The observer may *endogenously disengage the oculomotor system from fixation* in preparation for making an eye movement.

That these three components might additively combine to yield the gap effect is illustrated by the arrows in Figure 3.2a. Taylor and colleagues (1998) generated empirical support for the three-component model by combining the removal of fixation or of a peripheral stimulus with the presence or absence of a tone that reliably predicted when the target would appear. The data from this experiment are shown in Figure 3.2c and our derivation, from these data, of the three isolable components of the gap effect is illustrated in Figure 3.2b. The presence of a temporally predictive tone allows the observer to become alert and to endogenously disengage the oculomotor system from fixation. In this context the additional (temporally nonpredictive) disappearance of a peripheral item has no effect on SRT compared to the overlap condition (no visual stimuli are removed). In contrast, removal of fixation results in a further 40- to 45-msec decrease in SRT around 100 msec after its disappearance. We take this decrease (represented by the gray arrow in Figure 3.2b) to be due to the exogenous disengagement of the oculomotor system. In the absence of the temporally predictive tone, any nonpredictive visual event serves as an alerting signal resulting in a

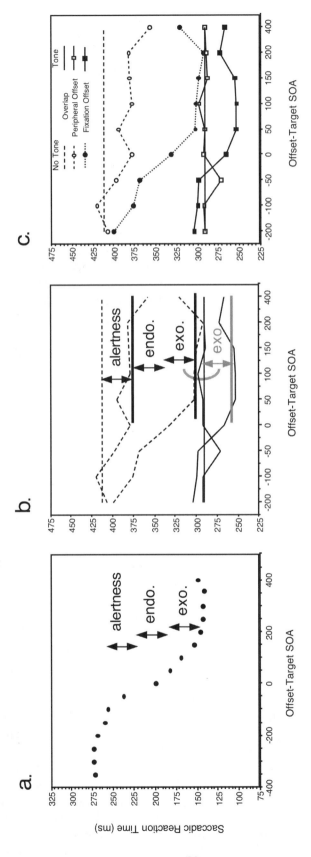

FIGURE 3.2. Components of the gap effect. (a) Saccadic reaction time (SRT) as a function of the interval between removal of fixation and the appearance of a target (negative means the target appears before fixation removal) calling for a choice saccadic response (redrawn from Saslow, 1967, blocked data). (b) Vertical arrows represent the hypothetical contributions to this "gap effect" from the three components proposed by Taylor et al. (1998) and derived from their data. (c) Redrawn from Taylor et al. See text for explanation.

32

small decrease in SRT (as reflected in the difference between the overlap condition and a peripheral offset). Assuming alertness to be roughly equivalent following a central or peripheral visual event, the difference in performance between these conditions in the no tone condition is taken to reflect oculomotor disengagement. Subtracting from this difference the 40- to 45-msec *exogenous* disengagement component (gray curve) as measured in the presence of the tone provides an estimate (about 30 msec) of the *endogenous* disengagement component.

Converging evidence for some of these ideas comes from neurophysiological studies of "fixation cells" in the middle layers of the rostral pole of the monkey superior colliculus, by Munoz and Wurtz (1993, 1995). They have shown that these cells are involved in the active maintenance of visual fixation. For example, chemical activation (bicuculine) or electrical stimulation of this region can delay saccadic initiation, and the latter can abruptly cancel a saccade in midflight. Following reversible deactivation of this region of the SC (by injection of muscimol), animals that had previously been trained to withhold execution of a saccade to the appearance of a visual target until the disappearance of fixation were unable to do so making large numbers of very rapid (incorrect) responses to the appearance of the target. It is as if deactivation of the rostral pole of the SC is functionally equivalent to removal of or disengagement from the fixation point.

Whereas fixation removal is often used to boost the exogenous control of overt orienting, the antisaccade task, wherein the observer must saccade away from the target rather than toward it, has been frequently used to explore endogenous control (Guitton, Buchtel, & Douglas, 1985; Roberts, 1994). The antisaccade task is a powerful but also somewhat messy tool. Not only must the observer endogenously compute and endogenously execute the correct saccade, but in addition it is essential that the reflexive machinery in the SC be prevented from executing an exogenously controlled saccade to the target when it appears. When used clinically (Everling & Fischer, 1998) a group showing a deficit might do so because of a difficulty with the endogenous computation and execution or with the endogenous suppression of exogenous orienting. Forbes and Klein (1996) tested this idea by using a manipulation of fixation removal in three different overt orienting tasks: prosaccades, antisaccades, and purely endogenous saccades made in response to verbal commands (presented auditorily). We predicted that the gap effect (reduction in SRT due to the prior removal of fixation) would be similar with prosaccades and in the purely endogenous condition and would be reduced with antisaccades because of the hypothetical suppression of the SC, which is necessary to avoid errors in the antisaccade task. This is precisely what we found (Figure 3.3).

The "oculomotor capture" paradigm developed by Theeuwes, Kramer, Han, and Irwin (1998) is one of the most powerful tools for exploring the interaction between exogenous and endogenous control of overt orienting. In one version, six gray disks were placed around fixation and when five of the objects changed to red, subjects were instructed to orient to the remaining gray object. On some of the trials, an irrelevant red item was added to the array around the time that the singleton target was revealed by the color change. Responses were slowed by the appearance of this new object, but more important, about 30% of the time, observers made erroneous eye movements toward this irrelevant distracter in spite of their intention to move to the target. These errors, of which the observers were usually unaware, were rapidly corrected—sometimes even in "midflight."

All these studies are consistent with the idea that endogenous and exogenous signals compete for control of the oculomotor system (see also Godijn & Theeuwes, 2002). Following the lead of Kopecz (1995; Kopecz & Schöner, 1995), Trappenberg, Dorris, Munoz, and

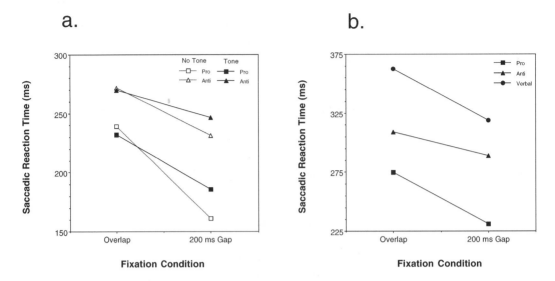

FIGURE 3.3. The gap effect with prosaccades, antisaccades, and purely endogenous saccades. a) Results from studies comparing the gap effect with pro- and antisaccades. No-tone data are from Fischer and Weber (1992) and Reuter-Lorenz, Oonk, Barnes, and Hughes (1995). Tone data are from Reuter-Lorenz et al. (1991, 1995), and Forbes and Klein (1996, E1). (b) Results from Forbes and Klein (1996, E2) using pro-, anti- and verbally instructed saccades. (Note: As illustrated in Figure 3.2, tones speed SRT in the one study that used both tones and no tones. This effect is not seen in the present graph because the data using tones and no tones are not drawn from the same studies.)

Klein (2001) developed a neural field model in which endogenous and exogenous signals converge upon the intermediate layer of the SC where overt orienting is determined by a process of competitive integration. This model simulates a variety of behavioral effects (of distractors, fixation removal, target probability effect, and antisaccades). In addition, our model was designed so that its pseudoneurons behave much as real neurons do during the administration of these paradigms (Dorris & Munoz, 1995, 1997; Dorris, Paré, & Munoz, 1997; Everling, Dorris, Klein, & Munoz, 1999).

COVERT ORIENTING

Helmholtz and Wundt provided early demonstrations that gaze direction could be dissociated from attention. But it was not until the pioneering work of Broadbent, Sperling, Eriksen, and Posner that paradigms for gaining objective control over the allocation of attention took hold and the concept yielded to scientific exploration. The spatial cueing paradigm developed by Posner has been the most widely used and some of its variants are described in the next section. It is a critical feature of covert orienting that there be no overt orienting.

Endogenous and Exogenous Control

When we consider covert orienting it is an empirical question whether an identical system is being oriented in two different ways under endogenous and exogenous control, or whether different, perhaps overlapping, mechanisms are involved. Using central arrow cues that were informative about the upcoming target's location, long delays, and monitoring of eye position to ensure that fixation was maintained, Posner and colleagues established the powerful cost/benefit method for exploring *endogenous covert orienting* and popularized the metaphor (James, 1890) of attention as a beam or spotlight (Posner, Snyder, & Davidson, 1980). Many investigators, hoping to illuminate properties of this "spotlight," chose to use uninformative peripheral cues (that elicit attention shifts exogenously) with cue–target stimulus-onset asynchronies short enough to prevent the observer from foveating the target with the help of the cue.

Jonides (1981) provided some of the earliest data comparing visual orienting under endogenous (central) and exogenous (peripheral) control. Among the differences he reported were that visual orienting is more rapid with exogenous cueing (see also Müller & Rabbitt, 1989), and that endogenous but not exogenous orienting was affected by a memory load and the likelihood of a central versus peripheral cue. Jonides attributed these differences to "transportation"; he assumed that the two control systems were carrying the same attentional resources to the cued location but that one "vehicle" was fast and automatic while the other was slow and voluntary.

There are, however, sufficient differences in the effects of covert orienting when controlled endogenously versus exogenously that this assumption must be questioned (see Table 3.1). Klein and Shore (2000) review a double dissociation in normal human performance (shown in bold in the last two lines of Table 3.1) that was uncovered in my laboratory and is highlighted here. When the target task involves the possibility of illusory conjunctions, the presence versus absence of this possibility is additive with covert orienting (valid vs. invalid cue condition) under endogenous control while it interacts with covert orienting under ex-

TABLE 3.1. Dissociations between Covert Orienting under Endogenous and Exogenous Controls

	Control	
Behavior	Endogenous	Exogenous
Speed[a]	Slow	Fast
Memory load effect[a]	Yes	No
Probability of endogenous versus exogenous cues[a]	Yes	No
Spreads on objects[b]	Not necessarily	Yes
Meridian crossing cost[c]	Yes	No
Disengage deficit with parietal damage[d]	No (or small)	Big
Inhibition of return[e]	No	Yes
Stimulus enhancement[f]	No	Yes
Interacts with illusory conjunctions[g]	**No**	**Yes**
Interacts with nonspatial expectancies[h]	**Yes**	**No**

[a] Each of these differences was first noted by Jonides (1981; see also Müller & Rabbitt, 1989).
[b] This dissociation can be seen in the findings of Egly, Driver, and Rafal (1994); Maquistan (1997); and Arrington, Dagenbach, McCartan, and Carr (2000) (but see Abrams & Law, 2000). Recent work, however, of Goldsmith and Yeari (2003) suggests a different explanation for the different findings.
[c] Reuter-Lorenz and Fendrich (1992); for a review, see Klein and Pontefract (1994).
[d] For a review, see Losier and Klein (2001).
[e] See Posner and Cohen (1984) and Rafal et al. (1989).
[f] Lu and Dosher (2000) demonstrated that external noise reduction accompanied both types of orienting, while stimulus enhancement was only elicited by exogenous orienting.
[g] Briand and Klein (1987) and Briand (1998).
[h] Klein and Hansen (1990), Klein (1994), and Kingstone and Egly (2003).

ogenous control (Briand, 1998; Briand & Klein, 1987). Conversely, when the task involves the manipulation of the probability of a relevant, nonspatial feature of the target (e.g., in a size discrimination task, large targets may be more likely than small ones) the nonspatial expectancy interacts with covert orienting under endogenous control but is additive with covert orienting under exogenous control (Klein, 1994). This latter pattern (single dissociation) is shown in the upper panels of Figure 3.4.

The interaction seen in reaction time when endogenous orienting is combined with manipulation of the probability of a task-relevant nonspatial feature seemed to challenge the spotlight metaphor, suggesting that only targets containing the likely feature were benefiting from attention (Klein & Hansen, 1990). However, the pattern of errors allowed for the possibility that attention was operating on targets containing the likely and unlikely feature but that a later pigeon-holing mechanism associated with the decision might be overshadowing an attention-related benefit at earlier stages of processing. We (Handy, Green, Klein, & Mangun, 2001) tested this possibility by recording event-related potentials during an endogenous cueing paradigm in which the observer's task was to decide whether the orientation of the target was horizontal or vertical, with one of these much more likely than the other. While replicating the behavioral pattern shown by Klein (1994) (see Figure 3.3c), we found that the early amplification of the brain's response to targets at the attended location was similar for targets with the likely and unlikely feature (Figure 3.3d). Thus, when attention is endogenously allocated to a location in space, the early effects upon stimulus processing accrue equally for objects with the expected and unexpected feature. The reduced (Figure 3.4a) or absent (Figure 3.4c) effect of location cueing upon reaction time to the unlikely objects must, therefore, be due to postperceptual stages of processing.

Klein and Shore (2000) noted that there are several forms of orienting whose underlying control mechanism is ambiguous. Orienting in the direction of the gaze of another person shares properties with both endogenous (the stimulus is centrally presented; its location is not the location toward which orienting occurs) and exogenous (orienting occurs even when the gaze is uninformative; indeed, even when it is counterinformative, attention is initially shifted in the direction of the gaze) orienting. We recommended that the double dissociation identified at the bottom of Table 3.1 be used to provide converging evidence for the kind of orienting involved. In a partial application of this strategy, Ivanoff and Klein (in press) have demonstrated that inhibition of return (see later) interacts with a nonspatial expectancy. Thus, even though inhibition of return is the aftermath of exogenous orienting (see Table 3.1) it has a partially endogenous signature. It is an open question whether IOR will add or interact with the possibility of illusory conjunctions.

OVERT–COVERT LINKAGES

When a salient peripheral event occurs it tends to attract both overt and covert orienting reflexively. When volitional control prevents the overt orienting, covert orienting may nevertheless take place. Under some circumstances (e.g., an attentional control setting may be put in place that effectively filters out the salient peripheral event [see, e.g., Theeuwes, 1991]) covert orienting may also be suppressed. When overt orienting actually occurs there is a relatively tight coupling with covert orienting. Whether controlled exogenously (Posner, 1980; Remington, 1980) or endogenously (Hoffman & Subramaniam, 1995; Shepard, Findlay, & Hockey, 1986) covert attention tends to precede the eyes to the target location (see vertical arrows in Figure 3.1). Whereas some view this linkage as obligatory, there are a few excep-

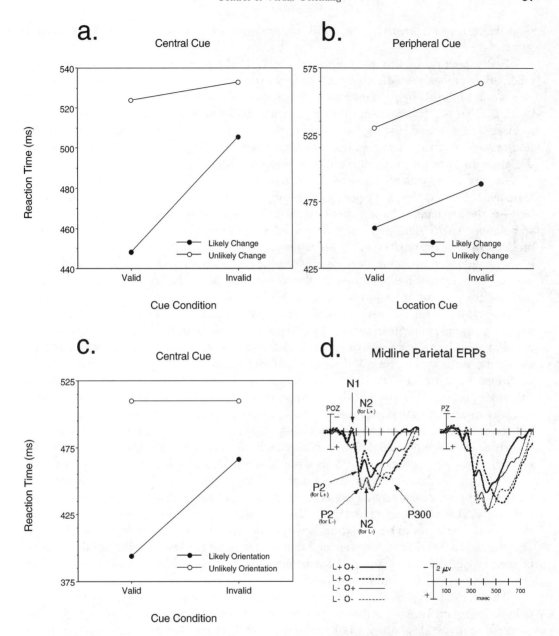

FIGURE 3.4. (a) Endogenous covert orienting interacts with a nonspatial expectancy (whether the target will increase or decrease in size) from Klein (1994). (b) Exogenous covert orienting is additive with the same nonspatial expectancy as in (a) also from Klein. (c) Endogenous covert orienting interacts with a nonspatial expectancy (whether the target is horizontal or vertical) from Handy et al. (2001). (d) ERPs to targets in the four conditions from panel (c). L+/– refers to whether the target's location was expected (+) or unexpected (–) (covert orienting); O+/– refers to whether the target's orientation was expected or unexpected.

tions (Fischer, 1999; Stelmach, Campsall, & Herdman, 1997) that suggest the linkage can be gated.

Partly because of this tight linkage, Klein (1980) proposed an explicit oculomotor readiness hypothesis (OMRH), which suggests that endogenous covert orienting of attention is accomplished by *preparing* to move the eyes to the to-be-attended location (see Figure 3.1). That is, "When attention to a particular location is desired, the observer prepares to make an eye movement to that location; the oculomotor readiness, via as yet unknown feedforward pathways, has the effect of enhancing processing in or from sensory pathways dealing with information from the target location" (Klein, 1980, p. 262).

In this view, which is shared by Rizzolatti's premotor theory (Rizzolatti, Riggio, Dascola, & Umilta, 1987), the process of getting ready to move the eyes—oculomotor readiness—*is* the mechanism by which visual attention is endogenously oriented in advance of stimulation. The finding that attention precedes an eye movement to the target location is often taken as evidence in favor of this proposal, but by definition it cannot be. The hypothesis is about covert orienting—orienting when the eyes do not move. Hence, the kind of preparatory activity that the hypothesis is about must not merely be prior to an eye movement but possible without an eye movement being executed.

The OMRH proposal makes two distinct predictions. First, if the subject is attending to a location, eye movements to that location should be facilitated. Second, if the subject is prepared to move his or her eyes to a particular location, the detection of events presented there should be facilitated. Using a dual-task paradigm, each of these predictions was disconfirmed by Klein (1980), Klein and Pontefract (1994), and, most recently, Hunt and Kingstone (in press). Endogenously attending to a location in space did not result in faster saccades toward the attended location, and preparing a saccade to a location in space did not result in more efficient target processing. A unique feature of the study by Hunt and Kingstone is its use of a dual task in which saccades were always speeded while attention was assessed using an unspeeded orientation discrimination task with accuracy as the dependent variable. Because of the large number of participants tested, Hunt and Kingstone's study might provide converging evidence for or against independence of covert endogenous orienting and oculomotor preparation. The OMRH (and premotor theory) predicts that there should be a positive correlation between the size of the cueing effect for one kind of orienting when it is the primary task and that for the other kind when it is secondary. As can be seen in Figure 3.5, in Hunt and Kingstone's study the correlation, while not significant ($r = -.229$, $p > .1$), is certainly not positive.

Thus direct tests provide no support for the OMRH as proposed by Klein (1980) and entailed in Rizzolatti's premotor theory.[1] On the contrary, the findings provide strong support for the conclusion (see also Posner, 1980; Remington, 1980) that endogenous covert orienting and endogenous overt orienting are accomplished by isolable subsystems. One might wonder, then, why neuroimaging studies have tended to find so much overlap between the brain structures activated when overt and covert orienting are activated endogenously (see Corbetta et al., 1998). Three issues must be considered. First, in order to attend without looking, there will be inhibition of the overt orienting machinery. Present neuroimaging methods may be unable to distinguish between neural activity whose objective is disabling from neural activity whose objective is enabling. Second, there is considerable nonoverlap. The fact that we normally move our attention and our eyes together may be partly responsible for the overlap, while the ability to move them independently may be mediated by the structures that appear to be activated separately. Finally, different neural circuits in the same neural structures may, via different projection patterns, control covert and overt orienting endogenously.

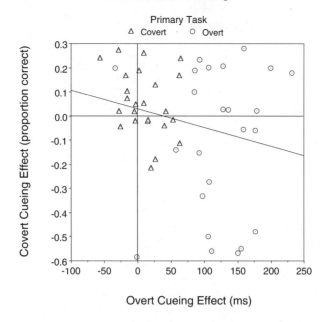

FIGURE 3.5. Each symbol represents the data from one of the participants in Hunt and Kingstone's (in press) two dual-task conditions. Cueing effects (computed so that a positive value means that performance in the cued direction was superior) from the nonspeeded orientation discrimination task and from the speeded, endogenous saccade task are plotted on the y and x axes, respectively. For 24 participants (triangles) the primary task, which involved covert endogenous orienting, revealed a significant cueing effect: For the orientation discrimination, valid accuracy minus invalid accuracy was greater than zero which is seen in the fact that most triangles are above the horizontal line. Yet for these participants, when an eye movement was occasionally required (consider x-axis values for the triangles), there was no tendency for saccades to be faster in the attended direction (if this were the case, most triangles above the horizontal line would be to the right of the vertical line). For another 24 participants (circles) the primary task, which involved endogenous preparation of overt orienting, revealed a significant preparation effect: For saccadic performance, prepared eye movements were faster than unprepared movements which is seen in the fact that most circles are to the right of the vertical line. Yet when the locus of attention was occasionally probed (consider y-axis values for the circles) there was no tendency for performance to be better in the direction of the prepared eye movement (if this were the case, most circles to the right of the vertical line would be above the horizontal line). I gratefully acknowledge the cooperation of Amelia Hunt in providing the data that made this graphic presentation possible. (Note: The results from one participant have been omitted from this analysis because his/her overt cueing effect was more than 4 standard deviations greater than the mean. When this participant is included, the negative correlation is significant.)

Together with our findings, the literature points to the following conclusions:

1. There is a tight linkage between saccade *execution* and covert visual orienting: Shifts of attention precede eye movements whether the saccades are elicited endogenously (Shepherd et al., 1986; Hoffman & Subramaniam, 1995) or exogenously (Posner, 1980). In other words, overt orienting is preceded by covert orienting.
2. Stimulus events that normally elicit eye movements may also attract attention even when the saccadic responses are suppressed. In other words, overt and covert orienting are exogenously activated by similar stimulus conditions.
3. Endogenous covert orienting of attention is not mediated by endogenously generated saccadic programming.

INHIBITION OF ORIENTING

Using a variant of the spatial cueing paradigm, Posner and Cohen (1984) discovered an inhibitory aftermath of orienting: For about 200 msec after an uninformative peripheral cue, target detection time was faster at the cued location, but after 300 msec, target detection was slower at the cued location. Posner and Cohen forwarded the idea that the function of this inhibitory aftereffect (later called inhibition of return [IOR]) was to encourage orienting toward novelty. Directly supporting this proposal, inhibitory tags have been observed following inefficient but not following popout search (Klein, 1988; Müller & von Mühlenen, 2000; Takeda & Yagi, 2000) and during oculomotor search for a camouflaged target (Klein & MacInnes, 1999; see also MacInnes & Klein, 2003). IOR is not generated by all forms of orienting (for a review, see Taylor & Klein, 1998). Rafal, Calabresi, Brennan, and Sciolto (1989) used exogenous or endogenous control to elicit an eye movement, to prepare an eye movement, or to shift attention covertly. Then, when the eyes had returned to fixation or the oculomotor preparation or shift of attention was canceled by a signal at fixation, a target calling for a simple detection response was presented. Responses to this target when it was presented at the previously cued location were delayed unless orienting had been covert and under endogenous control (see Table 3.1). Because each of the other five conditions involves activation of the oculomotor system, it is reasonable to conclude that it is this activation (whether or not an eye movement is made) that generates the inhibitory tag called IOR.

Once generated, what kinds of processing does IOR affect? There is excellent evidence that IOR slows response to targets, and that this effect is mediated, at least in part, by a reluctance to respond in the originally cued direction (Ivanoff & Klein, 2001). Although perceptual arrival times do not appear to be delayed by IOR (Klein, Schmidt, & Müller, 1998), exogenous orienting toward the target would appear to be one such inhibited response. Because IOR is not caused by endogenous covert orienting it would be interesting to know if one of its effects is to delay such orienting. As far as I know, there are no direct tests of this possibility, which would require generating IOR and then measuring the time course of endogenous covert orienting by varying the interval between a central informative cue and the target.

It is generally accepted that an intact SC is necessary for the generation of IOR (e.g., Sapir, Soroker, Berger, & Henik, 1999). This is compatible with the critical causal role attributed to oculomotor activation that has been inferred from purely behavioral studies. Reflecting IOR at the single-unit level, Dorris, Klein, Everling, and Munoz (2002) have shown that the sensory responses of SC neurons are markedly suppressed to visual stimuli presented at the cued location. Yet, in this same study we demonstrated that saccades toward the cued region of space elicited by electrical stimulation are not delayed, suggesting that the SC itself is not inhibited but rather is receiving signals that have already been reduced in amplitude. IOR can be maintained at environmental locations when an eye movement intervenes between a cue and target (Maylor & Hockey, 1985; Posner & Cohen, 1984), and IOR can be tagged to objects and move with them through space (Tipper, Driver, & Weaver, 1991). These behavioral findings strongly implicate cortical mechanisms in the maintenance of IOR, but precisely which ones are involved and how the tagging by the SC is transferred to these cortical structures remains to be demonstrated (for a review of the cognitive neuroscience of IOR, see Klein, 2004).

IOR, then, is a consequence of the activation of overt orienting that results in the inhibition of subsequent orienting—both overt and covert. By inhibiting orienting toward previously inspected locations and objects, IOR serves as a foraging facilitator (Klein, 1988; Klein & MacInnes, 1999).

NOTE

1. In one of the most promising tests of OMRH, Kustov and Robinson (1996) used electrical stimulation of the SC to elicit a saccade while their monkey observers were supposed to have been covertly orienting in response to endogenous cues or while the monkeys were endogenously preparing to make a saccade. From the similar vector deviations in these two conditions the authors concluded that preparing a saccade and attending covertly activate the same oculomotor circuitry in the SC in the same manner. As pointed out by Klein and Shore (2000) and others, this conclusion is fatally compromised by the fact that the monkeys' task was to localize the upcoming target. Thus, the endogenous cue not only informed the monkey where to expect a stimulus to appear (covert orienting) but also permitted the monkey to prepare the localizing response. It is impossible to know, then, whether performance benefit on validly cued trials was due to covert attention or to motor preparation. The effects on saccade deviation suffer from the same confound. The task used to measure whether the monkey was attending must be orthogonal to the spatial nature of the cue (cf. Spence & Driver, 1997).

REFERENCES

Abrams, R. A., & Law, M. B. (2000). Object-based visual attention with endogenous orienting. *Perception and Psychophysics*, 62, 818–833.

Arrington, C. M., Dagenbach, D., McCartan, M. K., & Carr, T. H. (2000, November). *The reliability of object-based attention following peripheral and central cues*. Poster presented at the annual meeting of the Psychonomic Society, New Orleans, LA.

Briand, K. A. (1998). Feature integration and spatial attention: More evidence of a dissociation between endogenous and exogenous orienting. *Journal of Experimental Psychology: Human Perception and Performance*, 24, 1243–1256.

Briand, K. A., & Klein, R. M. (1987). Is Posner's "beam" the same as Treisman's "glue"?: On the relation between visual orienting and feature integration theory. *Journal of Experimental Psychology: Human Perception and Performance*, 13, 228–241.

Corbetta, M., Akbudak, E., Conturo, T. E., Snyder, A. Z., Ollinger, J. M., Drury, H. A., et al. (1998). A common network of functional areas for attention and eye movements. *Neuron*, 21, 761–773.

Dorris, M. C., Klein, R. M., Everling, S., & Munoz, D. P. (2002). Contribution of the primate superior colliculus to inhibition of return. *Journal of Cognitive Neuroscience*, 14(8), 1256–1263.

Dorris, M. C., & Munoz, D. P. (1995). A neural correlate for the gap effect on saccadic reaction times in monkey. *Journal of Neurophysiology*, 73, 2558–2562.

Dorris, M. C., & Munoz, D. P. (1997). Neural activity in monkey superior colliculus related to the initiation of saccadic eye movements. *Journal of Neuroscience*, 18, 7015–7026.

Dorris, M. C., Paré, M., & Munoz, D. P. (1997). Neural activity in the monkey superior colliculus related to the initiation of saccadic eye movements. *Journal of Neuroscience*, 17, 8566–8579.

Egly, R., Driver, J., & Rafal, R. D. (1994). Shifting visual attention between objects and locations: Evidence from normal and parietal lesion subjects. *Journal of Experimental Psychology: General*, 123, 161–177.

Everling, S., Dorris, M. C., Klein, R. M., & Munoz, D. P. (1999). Role of primate superior colliculus in preparation and execution of anti- and pro-saccades, *Journal of Neuroscience*, 19(7), 2740–2754

Everling, S., & Fischer, B. (1998) The antisaccade: A review of basic research and clinical studies. *Neuropsychologia*, 36, 885–899.

Fischer, B., & Ramsperger, E. (1984). Human express saccades: Extremely short reaction times of goal directed eye movements. *Experimental Brain Research*, 57, 191–195.

Fischer, B., & Breitmeyer, B. (1987). Mechanisms of visual attention revealed by saccadic eye movements. *Neuropsychologia*, 25, 73–83.

Fisher, B., & Weber, H. (1993). Express saccades and visual attention. *Behavioural and Brain Sciences*, 16, 553–610.

Fischer, M. H. (1999). An investigation of attention allocation during sequential eye movement tasks. *Quarterly Journal of Experimental Psychology, 52A*, 649–677.

Forbes, K., & Klein, R. M. (1996). The magnitude of the fixation offset effect with endogenously and exogenously controlled saccades. *Journal of Cognitive Neuroscience, 8*, 344–352.

Godijn, R., & Theeuwes, J. (2002). Programming of endogenous and exogenous saccades: Evidence for a competitive integration model. *Journal of Experimental Psychology: Human Perception and Performance, 28*, 1039–1054.

Goldsmith, M., & Yeari, M. (2003). Modulation of object-based attention by spatial focus under endogenous and exogenous orienting. *Journal of Experimental Psychology: Human Perception and Performance, 29*, 897–918.

Guitton, D., Buchtel, H. A., & Douglas, R. M. (1985). Frontal lobe lesions in man cause difficulties in suppressing reflexive glances and in generating goal-directed saccades. *Experimental Brain Research, 58*, 455–472.

Handy, T., Green, V., Klein, R. M., & Mangun, G. R. (2001). Combined expectancies: ERPs reveal early benefits of spatial attention that are absent in reaction time. *Journal of Experimental Psychology: Human Perception and Performance, 27*, 303–317.

Hoffman, J. E., & Subramaniam, B. (1995). The role of visual attention in saccadic eye movements. *Perception and Psychophysics, 57*, 787–795.

Hunt, A., & Kingstone, A. (2003). Covert and overt voluntary attention: Linked or independent? *Cognitive Brain Research, 18*, 102–105.

Ivanoff, J., & Klein, R. M. (in press). Stimulus-response expectancies and inhibition of return. *Psychonomic Bulletin and Review.*

James, W. (1890). *The principles of psychology.* New York: Dover.

Jonides, J. (1981). Voluntary versus automatic control over the mind's eye's movement. In J. B. Long & A. D. Baddeley (Eds.), *Attention and performance* (Vol. 9, pp. 187–203). Hillsdale, NJ: Erlbaum.

Kingstone, A., & Egly, R. (2003). *Endogenous and exogenous orienting during the maintenance of a form expectancy.* Manuscript under review.

Kingstone, A., & Klein, R. M. (1993a). Visual offsets facilitate saccadic latency: Does predisengagement of visuospatial attention mediate this gap effect? *Journal of Experimental Psychology: Human Perception and Performance, 19*, 1251–1265.

Kingstone, A., & Klein, R. M. (1993b). What are human express saccades? *Perception and Psychophysics, 54*, 260–273.

Klein, R. M. (1980). Does oculomotor readiness mediate cognitive control of visualattention? In R. Nickerson (Ed.), *Attention and performance* (Vol. 8, pp. 259–276). New York: Academic Press.

Klein, R. M. (1988). Inhibitory tagging system facilitates visual search. *Nature, 334*, 430–431.

Klein, R. M. (1994). Perceptual-motor expectancies interact with covert visual orienting under endogenous but not exogenous control. *Canadian Journal of Experimental Psychology, 48*, 151–166.

Klein, R. M. (2004). Orienting and inhibition of return. In M. S. Gazzaniga (Ed.), *The handbook of cognitive neuroscience* (3rd ed.). Cambridge, MA: MIT Press

Klein, R. M., & Hansen, E. (1990). Chronometric analysis of spotlight failure in endogenous visual orienting. *Journal of Experimental Psychology: Human Perception and Performance, 16*, 790–801.

Klein, R. M., & Kingstone, R. M. (1993). Why do visual offsets reduce saccadic latencies? *Behavioral and Brain Sciences, 16*, 583–584.

Klein, R. M., & MacInnes, W. J. (1999). Inhibition of return is a foraging facilitator in visual search. *Psychological Science, 10*, 347–352.

Klein, R. M., & Pontefract, A. (1994). Does oculomotor readiness mediate cognitive control of visual attention? Revisited! In R. Nickerson (Ed.), *Attention and performance. Vol. XV: Conscious and nonconscious information processing* (pp. 333–350). Hillsdale, NJ: Erlbaum.

Klein, R. M., Schmidt, W. C., & Müller, H. K. (1998). Disinhibition of return: Unnecessary and unlikely. *Perception and Psychophysics, 60*, 862–872.

Klein, R. M., & Shore, D. I. (2000). Relations among modes of visual orienting. In S. Monsell & J.

Driver (Eds.), *Attention and performance XVIII: Control of cognitive processes* (pp. 195–208). Cambridge: MIT Press.

Kopecz, K. (1995). Saccadic reaction time in gap/overlap paradigm: A model Based on integration of intentional and visual information on neural, dynamic fields. *Vision Research, 35,* 2911–2925.

Kopecz, K., & Schöner, G. (1995). Saccadic motor planning by integrating visual information and expectation on neural dynamic fields. *Biological Cybernetics, 73,* 49–60.

Kustov, A. A., & Robinson, D. L. (1996). Shared neural control of attention shifts and eye movements. *Nature, 384,* 74–77.

Losier, B. J. W., & Klein, R. M. (2001). A review of the evidence for a disengage deficit following parietal lobe damage. *Neuroscience and Biobehavioral Reviews, 25,* 1–13.

Lu, Z. L., & Dosher, B. A. (2000). Spatial attention: Different mechanisms for central and peripheral temporal precues? *Journal of Experimental Psychology: Human Perception and Performance, 26,* 1534–1548.

MacInnes, W. J., & Klein, R. M. (2003). Inhibition of return biases orienting during the search of complex scenes. *Scientific World Journal, 3,* 75–86.

Macquistan, A. D. (1997). Object-based allocation of visual attention in response to exogenous, but not endogenous, spatial precues. *Psychonomic Bulletin and Review, 4,* 512–515.

Maylor, E., & Hockey, R. (1985). Inhibitory component of externally controlled covert orienting in visual space. In M. I. Posner & O. S. M. Marin (Eds.), *Attention and performance XI* (pp. 189–203). Hillsdale, NJ: Erlbaum.

Müller, H. J., & Rabbitt, P. M. A. (1989). Reflexive and voluntary orienting of visual attention: Time course of activation and resistance to interruption. *Journal of Experimental Psychology: Human Perception and Performance, 15,* 315–330.

Müller, H., & von Mühlenen, A. (2000). Probing distractor inhibition in visual search. *Journal of Experimental Psychology: Human Perception and Performance, 26,* 1591–1605.

Munoz, D. P., & Wurtz, R. H. (1993). Fixation cells in monkey superior colliculus. II. Reversible activation and deactivation. *Journal of Neurophysiology, 70,* 2313–2333.

Munoz, D. P., & Wurtz, R. H. (1995). Saccade-related activity in monkey superior colliculus: I. Characteristics of burst and buildup cells. *Journal of Neurophysiology, 73,* 559–575.

Posner, M. I. (1980). Orienting of attention. *Quarterly Journal of Experimental Psychology, 32,* 3–25.

Posner, M. I., & Cohen, Y. (1984). Components of visual orienting. In H. Bouma & D. Bonwhuis (Eds.), *Attention and performance X: Control of language processes* (pp. 551–556). Hillsdale, NJ: Erlbaum.

Posner, M. I., Snyder, C. R., & Davidson, B. J. (1980). Attention and the detection of signals. *Journal of Experimental Psychology: General, 109,* 160–174.

Rafal, R. D., Calabresi, P. A., Brennan, C. W., & Sciolto, T. K. (1989). Saccade preparation inhibits reorienting to recently attended locations. *Journal of Experimental Psychology: Human Perception and Performance, 15,* 673–685.

Remington, R. W. (1980). Attention and saccadic eye movements, *Journal of Experimental Psychology: Human Perception and Performance, 6,* 726–744.

Reuter-Lorenz, P. A., & Fendrich, R. (1992). Oculomotor readiness and covert orienting: Differences between central and peripheral precues. *Perception and Psychophysics, 52*(3), 336–344.

Reuter-Lorenz, P. A., Hughes, H. C., & Fendrich, R. (1991). The reduction of saccadic latency by prior offset of the fixation point: An analysis of the gap effect. *Perception and Psychophysics, 49*(2), 167–175.

Reuter-Lorenz, P. A., Oonk, H. M., Barnes, L., & Hughes, H. C. (1995). Effects of warning signals and fixation point offsets on the latencies of pro- vs. anti- saccades: Implications for an interpretation of the gap effect. *Experimental Brain Research, 103,* 287–293.

Rizzolatti, G., Riggio, L., Dascola, I., & Umilta, C. (1987). Reorienting attention across the horizontal and vertical meridians: Evidence in favor of a premotor theory of attention. *Neuropsychologia, 25,* 31–40.

Roberts, R. J., Hager, L. D., & Heron, C. (1994). Prefrontal cognitive processes: Working memory and inhibition in the antisaccade task. *Journal of Experimental Psychology: General, 123,* 374–393.

Robinson, D. A. (1968). Eye movement control in primates. *Science, 161*, 1219–1224

Sapir, A., Soroker, N., Berger, A., & Henik, A. (1999). Inhibition of return in spatial attention: Direct evidence for collicular generation. *Nature Neuroscience, 2*, 1053–1054 .

Saslow, M. G. (1967). Effects of components of displacement-step stimuli upon latency of saccadic eye movement. *Journal of the Optical Society of America, 57*, 1024–1029.

Schiller, P. H., Sandell, J. H., & Maunsell, H. R. (1987). The effect of frontal eye field and superior colliculus lesions on saccadic latencies in the rhesus monkey. *Journal of Neurophysiology, 57*(4), 1033–1049.

Schiller, P. H., True, S. D., & Conway, J. L. (1980). Deficits in eye movements following frontal eye-field and superior colliculus ablations. *Journal of Neurophysiology, 44*, 1175–1189.

Shepherd, M., Findlay, J. M., & Hockey, R. J. (1986). The relationship between eye movements and spatial attention. *Quarterly Journal of Experimental Psychology, 38A*, 475–491.

Spence, C., & Driver, J. (1997). On measuring selective attention to a specific sensory modality. *Perception and Psychophysics, 59*, 389–403.

Stelmach, L. B., Campsall, J. M., & Herdman, C. M. (1997). Attentional and ocular movements. *Journal of Experimental Psychology: Human Perception and Performance, 23*, 823–844.

Takeda, Y., & Yagi, A. (2000). Inhibitory tagging in visual search can be found if search stimuli remain visible. *Perception and Psychophysics, 62*, 927–934.

Taylor, T., Kingstone, A. F., & Klein, R. M. (1998). Visual offsets and oculomotor disinhibition: Endogenous and exogenous contributions to the gap effect. *Canadian Journal of Experimental Psychology, 52*, 192–200.

Taylor, T. L., & Klein. R. M. (1998). On the causes and effects of inhibition of return. *Psychonomic Bulletin and Review, 5*, 625–643.

Theeuwes, J. (1991). Exogenous and endogenous control of attention: The effect of visual onsets and offsets. *Perception and Psychophysics, 49*, 83–90.

Theeuwes, J., Kramer, A. F., Han, S., & Irwin, D. E. (1998). Our eyes do not always go where want them to go: Capture of the eyes by new objects. *Psychological Science, 9*, 379–385.

Tipper, S. P., Driver, J., & Weaver, B. (1991). Object-centred inhibition of return of visual attention. *Quarterly Journal of Experimental Psychology [A], 43*, 289–298.

Trappenberg, T. P., Dorris, M. C., Munoz, D. P., & Klein, R. M. (2001). A model of saccade initiation based on the competitive integration of exogenous and endogenous signals in the superior colliculus. *Journal of Cognitive Neuroscience, 13*, 256–271.

4

Inhibitory Processing
in the Attentional Networks

Luis J. Fuentes

Attention has been recently thought of as a brain system composed of several anatomical networks that perform specific computations. Within this cognitive neuroscience framework of attention, one of the most elaborated proposal is that put forward by Michael Posner and his collaborators in the last two decades (Posner, 1988; Posner & Petersen, 1990; Posner & Raichle, 1994): several attention networks seem to coordinate to accomplish the important function of selecting relevant objects and/or locations according to task demands.

One network is involved in locating relevant objects in space, orienting sensory organs to those locations, and filtering out irrelevant information that might compete for attention. Such a network is the *orienting network*. Single-cell recording studies with alert primates, careful assessment of patients with rather well-localized brain lesions, and recordings of larger-scale brain areas through neuroimaging (e.g., functional magnetic resonance imaging [fMRI]) and/or electrophysiological techniques (e.g., event-related potentials [ERPs]) converge to reveal important areas in the brain very much involved in orienting attention in a rather orchestrated way. Orienting attention has been illustrated in multiple variations of the visual spatial orienting task (Posner, 1980). In such a task, a cue signals the most likely location where the target will be presented (see Figure 4.1a), and portions of the posterior parietal lobe, midbrain, and thalamus seem to play a role. For instance, the lateral intraparietal area activates following cue presentation (Corbetta, Kincade, Ollinger, McAvoy, & Shulman, 2000), whereas the temporal–parietal junction is involved when the target occurs at an uncued location and attention must be disengaged from the cued location (Corbetta et al., 2000; Friedrich, Egly, Rafal, & Beck, 1998). The parietal lobe is also involved in creating a map of salient spatial representations where potential targets might appear (for a review, see Colby & Goldberg [1999]), allowing the superior colliculus to control shifts of attention and/or eye movements to the location of the cue. Targets appearing in that location will be focused by the pulvinar nucleus of the thalamus, by filtering out any other

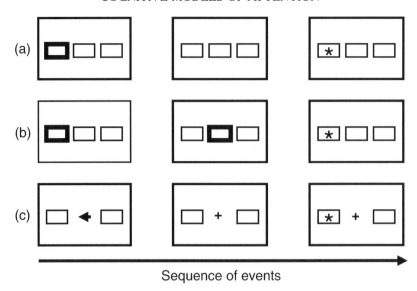

Sequence of events

FIGURE 4.1. Displays used in a visual orienting task. Cues are represented by thick squares (peripheral cueing, a and b) or by an arrow (central cueing, c). Subjects are told to detect target (asterisk) onset.

irrelevant information that might appear along with the target (LaBerge & Buchsbaum, 1990).

The *executive network* plays its main role when processing and/or responding requires any kind of control. For example, control is necessary when response conflict occurs because a well-learned task (reading) has to be overridden in favor of a less practiced task (naming the color of a color word); when a short-term memory task requires any kind of manipulation of information in retrieval (say a string of digits in reverse order); when a wrong response has been emitted and the subject has noticed it; when activation in the memory system is strategically maintained, as in semantic priming tasks, either because the prime-target interval is long (Fuentes, Carmona, Agis, & Catena, 1994; Fuentes & Tudela, 1992; Neely, 1991) or because expectations about the target are also manipulated (Neely, 1977); or even when attention is selectively addressed to a determined characteristic (e.g., shape) of a multidimensional target (Corbetta, Mienzi, Dobmeyer, Shulman, & Petersen, 1990). Importantly, the executive network is also involved in controlling the orienting network, as in those cases in which the cue is presented in the center and has to be interpreted (e.g., a central arrow pointing to left or right, see Figure 4.1c). Anatomy comprises a rather complex circuitry involving the frontal lobe (mainly the dorsolateral and ventromedial prefrontal cortex) and the anterior cingulate cortex, brain regions that activate together when executive control is necessary (Duncan & Owen, 2000). Other cortical (e.g., the supplementary motor area) and subcortical (some portions of the basal ganglia, which supply dopamine to the network) areas are also relevant parts of the network. Different areas also play different functions in the executive network (Botvinick, Nystrom, Fissell, Carter, & Cohen, 1999; Casey et al., 2000). For instance, the prefrontal cortex seems to play its main role in representing and maintaining active task demands (Kane & Engel, 2002), whereas the anterior cingulate is involved in monitoring of conflict, as in the incongruent condition of the Stroop task (MacDonald, Cohen, Stenger, & Carter, 2000; van Veen & Carter, 2002).

In this chapter I provide evidence from my own work that inhibitory mechanisms are crucial in understanding the functional properties of the aforementioned attentional networks. It is worth noting here that inhibition at the behavioral level is usually inferred from a slowing of reaction and/or a decrease in response accuracy to target stimuli in a condition supposed to involve inhibitory processing (the inhibition condition), in comparison with a condition in which inhibitory processing is assumed not to occur (the control condition). In neuroimaging, the system causing the slowing in reaction times may show increased activation in comparison with the control condition.

The aim of this review is threefold: (1) to illustrate inhibitory functioning of both the orienting and the executive networks; (2) to show how this function is affected differentially in patients with pathology involving the orienting or the executive network, respectively; and (3) to present a model of how inhibitory mechanisms of both networks cooperate in accomplishing the function of fostering detection and processing of new compared with old objects in the environment.

INHIBITION IN THE ORIENTING NETWORK

In a task such as that illustrated in Figure 4.1a, subjects will respond faster (shorter reaction times [RTs]) and more accurately to a target presented at the previously cued location than if it appears in the uncued location. This advantage of valid (target at cued locations) compared with invalid (target at uncued locations) trials is the *validity effect* (Posner, 1980) and illustrates the facilitatory function of the orienting attention network.

That facilitatory function is complemented with an inhibitory one. If the interval between the peripheral cue and the target is longer than 300 msec and the cue is not informative with respect to the target location, the facilitatory effect becomes inhibitory. That is, now RTs and/or accuracy show a disadvantage of valid compared with invalid trials. Posner and Cohen (1984) called this inhibitory effect *inhibition of return* (IOR).

Inhibition of Return in Visual Orienting Tasks

Figure 4.1a shows a standard procedure in which a single peripheral cue (e.g., one of the peripheral boxes brightening) is used to summon attention to that location. I refer to this version of the orienting task as the *single-cue procedure* for IOR. In Figure 4.1b, a central cue (the central box brightening) is included between the peripheral cue and the target. This central cue plays a role in helping subjects to allocate attention to the middle in waiting for the target to come up, assuming that the movement of attention to the middle is a necessary condition to observe IOR. I refer to this version of the orienting task as the *double-cue procedure* for IOR. Although IOR is easily obtained with both procedures, there is a crucial difference that has important repercussions for some patients (e.g., Faust & Balota, 1997, found that Alzheimer patients failed to show IOR with the single- but not with the double-cue procedure). In the single-cue procedure, subjects have to voluntarily move their attention to the middle before the target comes up, whereas in the double-cue procedure, attention is moved to the middle reflexively triggered by the central cue onset. It is assumed that cortical areas (e.g., the eye frontal fields) are involved in the former but not in the latter procedure.

Inhibition of return serves an important adaptive mission: to avoid reexamination of already explored locations in searching for relevant targets (Klein, 2000).

Inhibitory Tagging in Inhibition of Return

Previous findings showed that it takes longer to detect (Posner & Cohen, 1984), make a saccade (Abrams & Dobkin, 1994), discriminate (Lupiáñez, Milán, Tornay, Madrid, & Tudela, 1997), or even make lexical decisions (Chasteen & Pratt, 1999; Fuentes, Vivas, & Humphreys, 1999a) regarding targets appearing at cued compared with uncued locations. All these results suggest that IOR is a rather complex phenomenon. Fuentes, Vivas, and Humphreys (1999b) went further to investigate the fate of stimuli that are presented to a location subject to IOR. Taking the early- versus late-selection controversy as a framework, they combined an IOR procedure with several tasks that were assumed to tap different levels of processing. Thus, if the access of inhibited stimuli to the memory system is compromised in IOR, it is expected that semantic priming from primes presented at cued (inhibited) locations will be affected, compared with semantic priming from primes at uncued (noninhibited) locations. To assess whether access of inhibited stimuli to the response system was compromised, instead, we combined the IOR procedure with the flanker task. Fuentes and colleagues (1999b) found a striking pattern of results. Positive semantic priming became negative (longer RTs with related targets) when primes were at locations subject to IOR (cued locations). That is, semantic processing was not compromised, but for any reason the access of related targets to the response was inhibited. Such an inhibition effect did not last in time because it vanished with prime-target intervals longer than 250 msec. The combination of a flanker task with IOR produced also an interesting reversal of the standard compatibility effect when flankers occupied the cued location. Compatible flankers produced longer RTs than did incompatible ones. Again, these results seemed to fit with the idea that something was blocking (inhibiting) the access of flankers at cued locations to the response system. Fuentes and colleagues (1999b) concluded that a kind of *"inhibitory* tagging" (IT) mechanism was acting in IOR. This mechanism would act inhibiting temporally the links between the activated representations of inhibited stimuli and their appropriate response.

Inhibition of Return and Inhibitory Tagging in Parietal Patients

Previous studies associated IOR with the function of the superior colliculus (Sapir, Soreker, Berger, & Henik, 1999). Patients with progressive supranuclear palsy, a degenerative disease that affects the midbrain, did not show the typical IOR effect when cues and targets were presented in a vertical arrangement (Posner, Rafal, Choate, & Vaughan, 1985). This effect is also stronger with stimuli presented at the temporal than at the nasal hemifield (Rafal, Calabresi, Brennan, & Sciolto, 1989). All these findings suggest a major role of the superior colliculus in IOR. However, recently, other brain areas have been also involved in IOR.

In a recent study, Vivas, Humphreys, and Fuentes (2003) assessed both IOR and IT in a group of parietal patients. Patients showed preserved IOR when targets were presented at the contralesional field, but no effect was observed when presented at the ipsilesional field. This pattern agrees with other lesion (Bartolomeo, Sieroff, Decaix, & Chokron, 2001) and fMRI (Lepsien & Pollmann, 2002; Rosen et al., 1999) studies that also implicated the parietal lobe in IOR, suggesting parietal modulation of this effect. Vivas and colleagues (2003) also combined an IOR procedure with the Stroop task. Stroop interference reduced when stimuli were presented at the cued compared with the uncued location, a result compatible with IT acting in a location subject to IOR (an explanation of this result is offered later, when the networks interactive model is presented). However, that was true for contralesional but not for ipsilesional stimuli. In the latter case, Stroop interference was similar for both visual fields. These results suggest that IT requires intact IOR and the parietal lobe affects IOR but not IT.

Inhibition of Return and Inhibitory Tagging in Schizophrenia

A different pattern of IOR and IT interactive effects emerged when we combined the IOR paradigm and the Stroop task in patients diagnosed with schizophrenia (for a review, see Fuentes, 2001). The results showed relatively preserved IOR in both hemifields (Fuentes, Boucart, Vivas, Alvarez, & Zimmerman, 2000; Fuentes & Santiago, 1999), and the effect was similar irrespective of whether the single- or double-cue procedure (see Figure 4.1a and 4.1b) was used (Fuentes, Boucart, Alvarez, Vivas, & Zimmerman, 1999).[1] However, schizophrenic patients did not show any reduction in the Stroop interference effect when stimuli were presented at locations subject to IOR (Fuentes et al., 2000), which suggests a deficit in IT associated with schizophrenia.

Taken together, data from parietal and schizophrenic patients suggest that both IOR and IT are two distinct inhibitory mechanisms acting at already explored locations, in orienting tasks. IOR seems to depend on intact midbrain, although other cortical areas, such as the parietal lobe, modulate it. IT needs intact IOR to act, although the aforementioned dissociations suggest a different neural circuitry, perhaps involving the frontal lobe.

INHIBITION IN THE EXECUTIVE NETWORK

One of the executive functions of attention is the control of language processing. Neely's (1977) seminal study nicely illustrates how inhibition plays a fundamental role in strategy-based semantic priming. In one condition, subjects were told to expect, say, an exemplar of the category *bird* as target when, say, *body* category label was presented as prime. Compared to a neutral condition (X's as prime), unexpected related targets (exemplars of the prime category label *body*) produced positive semantic priming with the short interval but negative semantic priming with the long interval. That is, according to the instructions, subjects had effectively inhibited a well-learned association (a category label with its associates) in favor of an association created ad hoc for the experiment (a category label with exemplars of a different category), a function that has been clearly associated with the executive network (see Posner & Raichle, 1994, for further evidence).

Semantic Inhibition

In a recent study, Fuentes and colleagues (1999a) asked whether the executive network exhibits inhibitory functions that mimic in the semantic domain what IOR makes in the spatial domain. Note that this is an important question because if evidence is found for a kind of inhibition or return to the "semantic space," we would be entitled to conclude that bias in favor of novelty is a pervasive property of the attention system. In our semantic priming study (see Experiment 2) we presented an intervening stimulus between the prime and the target (see Figure 4.2 for illustration). The target could be related or unrelated to the prime, and the intervening stimulus could be a word of a different category to that of prime and target, or a string of X's. With the string of X's as the intervening stimulus, related targets produced shorter RTs than unrelated targets, although the effect was not statistically significant (see Fuentes et al., 1999a, for further explanation of this result). Interestingly, the facilitatory ef-

(a)   (b)

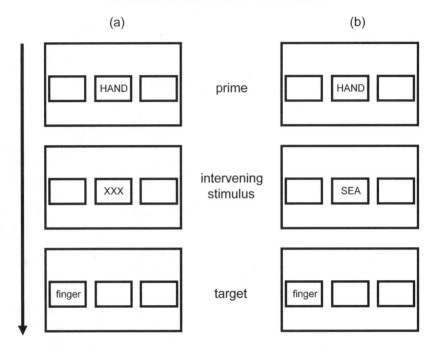

FIGURE 4.2. Displays used in a semantic inhibition task. Primes are presented within the central rectangle followed by a string of X's (a) or by a word (b) as the intervening stimulus. The lowercase word is the target. Subjects are told to make a lexical decision on the target.

fect became inhibitory (longer RTs with related targets) when the intervening stimulus was a word. We argued that the intervening word had the effect of addressing attention to a different category to that of the prime, similarly to the role of the central cue in the IOR double-cue procedure. Thus, attention should be returned to the category of the previous prime when a related target was presented, whereas that did not occur when the target was unrelated to the prime. We called this kind of semantic inhibition of return *semantic inhibition*, and attributed the effect to the executive attention network.

Semantic Inhibition in Schizophrenia

If semantic inhibition is an inhibitory function of the executive network, patients with damage to this network should show a sort of deficit in this function. Fuentes and Santiago (1999) replicated the semantic priming task with the intervening stimulus procedure of Fuentes and colleagues' (1999a) with a group of inpatients diagnosed with schizophrenia. When targets were presented to the left visual field, involving mainly the right hemisphere, a normal pattern of semantic inhibition effect was found (longer RTs with related targets). However, when targets were presented to the right visual field, involving mainly the left hemisphere, semantic facilitation instead of inhibition was then observed. These results suggest that semantic processing is not altered in these patients but the inhibitory function of the executive network is. However, this deficit appears only when the left hemisphere is involved, a lateralized deficit that agrees with a bulk of evidence in the schizophrenia literature (for a review, see Posner & DiGirolamo [1998]).

RELATIONS BETWEEN THE ORIENTING
AND THE EXECUTIVE ATTENTION NETWORKS

Although there is evidence that both the orienting and the executive networks are independent pieces of the attention system, under certain circumstances they might interact (Fan, McCandliss, Sommer, Raz, & Posner, 2002). Interactions take the form of mutual interference, and the expression of such influence might depend on differential attentional processing demands of tasks tapping one network or the other. Accordingly, the executive network modulates the orienting network when processing demands are greater for the executive (e.g., counting backward from a three-digit number) than for the orienting task (Posner, Inhoff, Friedrich, & Cohen, 1987); the orienting network modulates executive attention functioning when detection of target location has priority (see report of Fuentes et al.'s, 1999a, study); and modulation goes in both directions when both tasks (e.g., prime-target category matching and IOR tasks) might have similar priority (Langley, Fuentes, Overmier, Bastin de Jong, & Prod'Homme, 2001). Here, I further illustrate interactive inhibitory functioning of the networks in a series of studies that combined procedures supposed to tap the orienting network (e.g., IOR) or the executive network (e.g., semantic inhibition/facilitation and Stroop interference).

Fuentes and colleagues (1999a) combined IOR and lexical decision procedures.[2] They showed IOR for both target words and nonwords, but both attention-dependent semantic inhibition (Experiment 3) and attention-dependent semantic facilitation (Experiment 4) vanished when target words were presented at the previously cued location. This suggests that the executive network could not maintain prime activation when targets were presented at a location inhibited by the orienting network.

Vivas and Fuentes (2001) combined IOR and Stroop procedures.[3] Again, IOR was observed, but Stroop interference was greatly reduced when stimuli were located at the cued location. Vivas and Fuentes attributed such a reduction in interference to the action of the IT mechanism acting at locations subject to IOR. There is now evidence that IT might depend on some areas of the executive network because it has been found IT deficits in patients diagnosed with schizophrenia (Fuentes et al., 2000), a disease that has been associated with a dysregulation of the anterior cingulate cortex (DiGirolamo & Posner, 1996).

Finally, I illustrate how interactive functioning of the two networks takes the form of cooperation to prevent the subject from reexploring already attended locations. Figure 4.3 shows a model of how mechanisms involved in a situation that requires orienting attention (visual orienting task) and conflict solving (Stroop task) interact. When the incongruent stimulus (the word *blue* in red color) is presented at the uncued location, the executive network has to resolve the conflict between the task-relevant dimension, the color, and the task-irrelevant but prepotent dimension of the stimulus, the word. The prefrontal cortex and the anterior cingulate, among others, coordinate to resolve the conflict and organize the correct response. The net result is a weak response to the color expressed in longer RTs and/or more errors (Stroop interference). When the incongruent stimulus is presented at the cued location, the orienting network had already tagged that location with inhibition. The parietal lobe might contain a map of locations where the cued location might have been inhibited. Thus, via inhibitory links with the superior colliculus, neither attention nor the eyes are facilitated to move in that direction. The net result is longer manual and/or saccades responses to the cued location (IOR effect). Concurrently, the parietal cortex might translate the attention/oculomotor bias in subcortical structures into a signal to those areas concerned

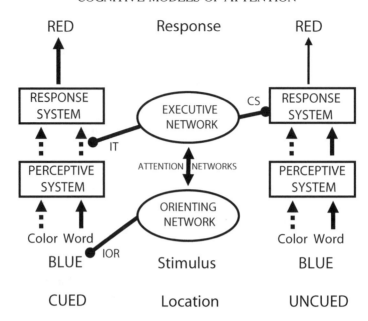

FIGURE 4.3. Model of how inhibitory mechanisms involved in the attention networks interact. Arrows connecting the stimulus with the perceptive and response systems indicate coding of Stroop stimulus dimensions, color and word, being the former weaker (dotted lines) than the latter (solid lines). Arrows connecting the response system with the response RED indicate color response in the Stroop task. At this level, the thicker arrow (left) indicates shorter latencies and/or more accuracy than the thinner arrow (right). Arrows departing from the attention networks represent the effects of inhibitory mechanisms functioning (IOR, inhibition of return; IT, inhibitory tagging; CS, conflict solving). The arrow connecting the networks represents the anatomical and functional links between them.

with response selection (the executive network). Those areas, then, would inhibit the prepotent attribute of the stimulus, the word meaning, interrupting its access to the response system. The net result is an indirect facilitation in color responses, and therefore a reduction in Stroop interference (IT effect).

Briefly, when stimuli can appear at different spatial locations, and the task requires something more than their mere detection, the orienting and the executive networks coordinate to accomplish together the relevant role of biasing the individual for novelty.

CONCLUDING REMARKS

Inhibitory mechanisms are relevant in understanding the orienting and executive networks functioning, working in isolation, competition, or coordination, according to task demands. By looking at the networks in isolation we find a main role of the networks in avoiding reexaminations, either by preventing reiterative attention to already explored locations (the orienting network) or by preventing attention from returning to the word space of an already attended word (the executive network). This property of the networks suggests a main role of attention in biasing the organism for novelty. However, to understand how attention operates to control information processing, it is necessary to understand the way in which attentional networks relate to one another. Two ways of interaction have been briefly illustrated here, one in which the networks interfere one to another and other in which they cooperate. The tasks assumed to tap each network provided relevant insights about their interactions when used in combination. Such interactions enable coherent behavior to emerge across networks concerned with selecting, via facilitation and inhibition functioning, different types of information.

Admittedly, some aspects of the present proposal about inhibitory functioning of the networks are still rather speculative. As suggested earlier, the inhibitory mechanisms revealed through the use of behavioral tasks seem to form part of a neural circuitry involving both cortical and subcortical areas. That brain circuitry might be then revealed by looking at the patterns of cerebral activation usually obtained with neuroimaging techniques, when subjects perform similar experiments to those illustrated here. I have no doubt that follow-up studies conducted at both the behavioral and the neural levels will provide new insights about *how* the networks interact to accomplish their main inhibitory (and facilitatory) functions and *where* in the brain occur such interactions.

ACKNOWLEDGMENTS

Preparation of this chapter was supported by Grant No. BSO2003-04594 from the Ministerio de Ciencia y Tecnología. The research reviewed here has largely benefited from collaboration with colleagues and friends whom I am most grateful: I. F. Agis, M. Boucart, E. Carmona, A. Catena, G. Humphreys, L. Langley, E. Santiago, P. Tudela, and A. Vivas. I thank Carmen González for helpful comments on the manuscript.

NOTES

1. Patients of Fuentes and colleagues' (1999) study were medicated outpatients. When the task was used with a nonmedicated patient (reported in Fuentes, 2001), or with a group of psychotic patients with predominant negative symptoms (Fuentes & Santiago, 2002), IOR with the single-cue procedure vanished in the former and reduced in the latter case, compared with the double-cue procedure. These results suggest that medication and severity of the disease might be important factors affecting the processes that lead to IOR rather than IOR per se.
2. The procedure was similar to that illustrated in Figure 4.2, except that the prime was presented within the left or right peripheral box to measure IOR.
3. The procedure was similar to that illustrated in Figure 4.1b, except that Stroop stimuli, instead of the asterisk, were presented as targets.

REFERENCES

Abrams, R. A., & Dobkin, R. S. (1994). Inhibition of return: Effects of attentional cueing on eyes movement latencies. *Journal of Experimental Psychology: Human Perception and Performance, 20,* 467–477.

Bartolomeo, P., Sieroff, E., Decaix, C., & Chokron, S. (2001). Modulating the attentional bias in unilateral neglect: The effects of strategic set. *Experimental Brain Research, 137,* 432–444.

Botvinick, M., Nystrom, L. E., Fissell, K., Carter, C. S., & Cohen, J. D. (1999). Conflict monitoring versus selection-for-action in anterior cingulate cortex. *Nature, 402,* 179–181.

Casey, B. J., Thomas, K. M., Welsh, T. F., Badgaiyan, R., Eccard, C. H., Jennings, J. R., et al. (2000). Dissociation of response conflict, attentional selection, and expectancy with functional magnetic resonance imaging (fMRI). *Proceedings of the National Academy of Sciences USA, 97,* 8728–8733.

Chasteen, A. L., & Pratt, J. (1999). The effect of inhibition of return on lexical access. *Psychological Science, 10,* 41–46.

Colby, C. L., & Goldberg, M. E. (1999). Space and attention in parietal cortex. *Annual Review of Neuroscience, 22,* 319–349.

Corbetta, M., Kincade, J. M., Ollinger, J. M., McAvoy, M. P., & Shulman, G. L. (2000). Voluntary orienting is dissociated from target detection in human posterior parietal cortex. *Nature Neuroscience, 3,* 292–297.

Corbetta, M., Mienzi, F. M., Dobmeyer, S., Shulman, G. L., & Petersen, S. E. (1990). Attentional modulation of neural processing of shape, color, and velocity in humans. *Science, 248,* 1556–1559.

DiGirolamo, G. J., & Posner, M. I. (1996). Attention and schizophrenia: A view from cognitive neuroscience. *Cognitive Neuropsychiatry, 1,* 95–102.

Duncan, J., & Owen, A. M. (2000). Common regions of the human frontal lobe recruited by diverse cognitive demands. *Trends in Neuroscience, 23,* 475–482.

Fan, J., McCandliss, B. D., Sommer, T., Raz, A., & Posner, M. I. (2002). Testing the efficiency and independence of the attentional networks. *Journal of Cognitive Neuroscience, 14,* 340–347.

Faust, M. E., & Balota, D. A. (1997). Inhibition of return and visuospatial attention in healthy older adults and individuals with dementia of the Alzheimer type. *Neuropsychology, 11,* 13–29.

Friedrich, F. J., Egly, R., Rafal, R. D., & Beck, D. (1998). Spatial attention deficits in humans: A comparison of superior parietal and temporal-parietal junction lesions. *Neuropsychology, 12,* 193–207.

Fuentes, L. J. (2001). A cognitive neuroscience framework to study the attentional deficits associated with schizophrenia. In F. Columbus (Ed.), *Advances in psychology research* (Vol. 3, pp. 1–23). New York: Nova.

Fuentes, L. J., Boucart, M., Álvarez, R., Vivas, A. B., & Zimmerman, M. A. (1999). Inhibitory processing in visuospatial attention in healthy adults and schizophrenic patients. *Schizophrenia Research, 40,* 75–80.

Fuentes, L. J., Boucart, M., Vivas, A. B., Álvarez, R., & Zimmerman, M. A. (2000). Inhibitory tagging in inhibition of return is affected in schizophrenia: Evidence from the Stroop task. *Neuropsychology, 14,* 134–140.

Fuentes, L. J., Carmona, E., Agis, I. F., & Catena, A. (1994). The role of the anterior attention system in semantic processing of both foveal and parafoveal words. *Journal of Cognitive Neuroscience, 6,* 17–25.

Fuentes, L. J., & Santiago, E. (1999). Spatial and semantic inhibitory processing in schizophrenia. *Neuropsychology, 13,* 259–270.

Fuentes, L. J., & Santiago, E. (2002, April). *Deficits in inhibitory mechanisms of attention in schizophrenic and psychotic patients with predominant negative symptoms.* Paper presented at the fourth Congress of the Spanish Experimental Psychology Society, Oviedo, Spain.

Fuentes, L. J., & Tudela, P. (1992). Semantic processing of foveally and parafoveally presented words in a lexical decision task. *Quarterly Journal of Experimental Psychology, 45A,* 299–322.

Fuentes, L. J., Vivas, A. B. & Humphreys, G. W. (1999a). Inhibitory mechanisms of attentional networks: Spatial and semantic inhibitory processing. *Journal of Experimental Psychology: Human Perception and Performance, 25,* 1114–1126.

Fuentes, L. J., Vivas, A. B., & Humphreys, G. W. (1999b). Inhibitory tagging of stimulus properties in inhibition of return: Effects on semantic priming and flanker interference. *Quarterly Journal of Experimental Psychology: Human Experimental Psychology, 52,* 149–164.

Kane, M. J., & Engle, R. W. (2002). The role of prefrontal cortex in working-memory capacity, executive attention, and general fluid intelligence. *Psychonomic Bulletin and Review, 9,* 637–671.

Klein, R. M. (2000). Inhibition of return. *Trends in Cognitive Sciences, 4,* 138–147.

LaBerge, D., & Buchsbaum, M. S. (1990). Positron emission tomographic measurements of pulvinar activity during an attention task. *Journal of Neuroscience, 10,* 613–619.

Langley, L. K., Fuentes, L. J., Overmier, J. B., Bastin de Jong, C., & Prod'Homme, M. M. (2001). Attention to semantic and spatial information in aging and Alzheimer's disease. *Psicológica, 22,* 293–324.

Lepsien, J., & Pollman, S. (2002). Covert reorienting and inhibition of return: An event-related fMRI study. *Journal of Cognitive Neuroscience, 14,* 127–144.

Lupiáñez, J., Milán, E. G., Tornay, F. J., Madrid, E., & Tudela, P. (1997). Does IOR occur in discrimination task? Yes, it does, but later. *Perception and Psychophysics, 59,* 1241–1254.

MacDonald, A. W., Cohen, J. D., Stenger, V. A., & Carter, C. S. (2000). Dissociating the role of the dorsolateral prefrontal and anterior cingulate cortex in cognitive control. *Science, 288,* 1835–1838.

Neely, J. H. (1977). Semantic priming and retrieval from lexical memory: Roles of inhibitionless spreading activation and limited-capacity attention. *Journal of Experimental Psychology: General, 106,* 226–254.

Neely, J. H. (1991). Semantic priming effects in visual word recognition: A selective review of current findings and theories. In D. Besner & G. W. Humphreys (Eds.), *Basic processes in reading: Visual word recognition* (pp. 264–336). Hillsdale, NJ: Erlbaum.

Posner, M. I. (1980). Orienting of attention. *Quarterly Journal of Experimental Psychology, 32,* 3–25.

Posner, M. I. (1988). Structures and functions of selective attention. In T. Boll & B. K. Bryant (Eds.), *Clinical neuropsychology and brain functions: Research, measurement, and practice* (pp. 173–202). Washington, DC: American Psychological Association.

Posner, M. I., & Cohen, Y. A. (1984). Components of visual orienting. In H. Bouma & D. G. Bouwhuis (Eds.), *Attention and performance X* (pp. 513–556). Hillsdale, NJ: Erlbaum.

Posner, M. I., & DiGirolamo, G. J. (1998). Executive attention: Conflict, target detection and cognitive control. In R. Parasuraman (Ed.), *The attentive brain* (pp. 401–423). Cambridge, MA: MIT Press.

Posner, M. I., Inhoff, A. W., Friedrich, F. J., & Cohen, A. (1987). Isolating attentional systems: A cognitive-anatomical analysis. *Psychobiology, 15,* 107–121.

Posner, M. I., & Petersen, S. E. (1990). The attention system of the human brain. *Annual Review of Neuroscience, 13,* 25–42.

Posner, M. I., Rafal, R. D., Choate, L., & Vaughan, J. (1985). Inhibition of return: Neural basis and function. *Cognitive Neuropsychology, 2,* 211–228.

Posner, M. I., & Raichle, M. E. (1994). *Images of mind.* New York: Scientific American Library.

Rafal, R. D., Calabresi, P. A., Brennan, C. W., & Sciolto, T. K. (1989). Saccade preparation inhibits reorienting to recently attended locations. *Journal of Experimental Psychology: Human Perception and Performance, 15,* 673–685.

Rosen, A. C., Rao, S. M., Caffarra, P., Scaglioni, A., Bobholz, J. A., Woodley, S. J., et al. (1999). Neural basis of endogenous and exogenous spatial orienting: A functional MRI study. *Journal of Cognitive Neuroscience, 11,* 135–152.

Sapir, A., Soroker, N., Berger, A., & Henik, A. (1999). "Inhibition of return" in spatial attention: Direct evidence for collicular generation. *Nature Neuroscience, 2,* 1053–1054.

van Veen, V., & Carter, C. S. (2002). The timing of action-monitoring processes in the anterior cingulate cortex. *Journal of Cognitive Neuroscience, 14,* 593–602.

Vivas, A. B., & Fuentes, L. J. (2001). Stroop interference is affected in inhibition of return. *Psychonomic Bulletin and Review, 8,* 315–323.

Vivas, A. B., Humphreys, G. W., & Fuentes, L. J. (2003). Inhibitory processing following damage to the parietal lobe. *Neuropsychologia, 41,* 1531–1540.

5

A Multilevel Approach to Selective Attention

Monitoring Environmental Space, Choosing Stimuli for Deep Processing, and Retrieving Information from Memory

Thomas H. Carr

Just about everyone takes for granted that when there are several things to do at once, speed and accuracy of performance will suffer compared to the luxury of dealing with one thing at a time. Enter *selective attention*, a system of cognitive processes that manages the burden of having too much to do at once by prioritizing among stimuli to be processed, information to be retrieved from memory, decisions to be made, and responses to be produced. Benefits of exercising attentional selectivity are well documented, but costs accrue as well. After all, there is no such thing as a "free lunch." Work in my laboratory has addressed the balance between attentional benefits and "the cost of the attentional lunch" in the sequence of stages of information processing that mediate between visual stimulus events in the external environment and task-appropriate action. These stages include (1) selecting a region of the environment to monitor for an important visual input, (2) selecting among visual inputs for access to "deep" processing (identification, semantic interpretation, and computation of response potential), and (3) selecting among activated representations in memory during the process of semantic interpretation. Emphasis is on the operating characteristics of the mechanisms underlying the selectivity that is observed, in an attempt to show commonalities between selection of visual inputs from the environment and selection of activated semantic representations from memory.

SELECTING A REGION OF SPACE TO MONITOR FOR AN IMPORTANT VISUAL INPUT: LOCATION-BASED VERSUS OBJECT-BASED ATTENTIONAL PROCESSES DURING VISUAL ENCODING

Theories of visual attention once took for granted that visual attention selects a region of space defined on environmental coordinates, which is then inspected for the presence of interesting or useful information. Such theories are "location-based" (Eriksen & Yeh, 1985; Henderson, 1991; LaBerge & Brown, 1989; Posner, 1980). Strong evidence for such a purely spatial mode of selection comes from studies in which the visual field is blank, leaving nothing but environmental coordinates for guiding the deployment of attention, yet a cue such as an arrow presented at fixation still facilitates detection of a target occurring in the locale toward which the arrow points. Furthermore, comparisons pitting spatial location against a nonspatial property of the stimulus being sought, such as color, suggest that attention is first moved to a location in space at which a stimulus is present, after which the nonspatial property becomes the criterion for whether to stay and fully process the stimulus or move on to a new location (Moore & Egeth, 1998). Finally, there is evidence from Steinman, Steinman, and Lehmkuhle (1995) that a penumbra of inhibition may surround the region of facilitation, forming a kind of "Mexican hat" pattern of input modulation centered on the selected location, at least when there are other stimuli close by that might produce interference. Steinman and colleagues defined this region of inhibition in terms of an impact on behavioral judgments that indicated slower entrance to processing for stimulus information arising near the focus of attention than for stimulus information arising further away—a surprising result. Such a pattern of "center–surround organization" protects extraction of the selected region's stimulus information from competition created by other streams of input processing driven by nearby stimuli and calls to mind the discoveries of Desimone and colleagues on the ability of visual attention to bias competition between nearby stimuli falling into the receptive fields of the same sets of neurons in visual cortex (Desimone & Duncan, 1995).

Thus the idea of location-based selection is well established. During the last 20 years, however, a major development in attention theory has been the emergence of evidence for an additional process of object-based selection, in which object boundaries rather than environmental coordinates are used to guide the deployment of visual attention (Egly, Driver, & Rafal, 1994), or objects themselves are selected, unmediated by spatial location and abstracted from environmental coordinates per se (Duncan, 1984; Kanwisher & Driver, 1992; Vecera & Farah, 1994).

In an attempt to explore the neural substrate of object-based selection and discover how it differs from that of location-based selection, Arrington, Mayer, Carr, and Rao (2000) used event-related functional magnetic resonance imaging (fMRI) to measure brain activity during a cued forced-choice discrimination task that required perceivers to orient visual attention in anticipation of an upcoming target letter. The target could appear at various locations arrayed around a central fixation cross. On every trial, a cue display appeared 1 second before the target. The cue display contained a shape (the object cue) that enclosed two adjacent target locations as well as an arrow that replaced the fixation cross and pointed halfway between two locations. Each cue suggested a region of space—one bounded by the object shape, the other unbounded and defined only on environmental coordinates—in which the target letter was likely to occur. In one block of imaging trials perceivers were instructed to orient to the region bounded by the object shape, ignoring the direction of the arrow. In another block, perceivers oriented in the direction of the arrow, ignoring the object shape. The two cues were uncorrelated, and in each block the relevant cue was 80% valid, making it worthwhile to try to use it.

Both cues produced faster and more accurate letter identification when the target letter occurred in the cued region (valid trials) than when it occurred elsewhere in the visual field (invalid trials). Analysis of blood-oxygenation-level-dependent (BOLD) evidence of neuronal activity on valid trials revealed greater neuronal activation when attention selected a region bounded by an object shape than when attention selected an unbounded region indicated by an arrow. This activation was strongly lateralized to the left hemisphere and formed a widely distributed network including (1) structures in parietal and temporal cortex and thalamus previously implicated in visual attention; (2) ventral-stream object processing structures in occipital, inferior temporal, and parahippocampal cortex; and (3) medial and dorsolateral prefrontal structures previously implicated in executive control.

These imaging results suggest that object-guided deployment of visual attention is achieved by imposing additional constraints, supported by additional neuronal activation, over and above those already operating to achieve selection of an unbounded region defined on environmental coordinates. Thus, as indicated by BOLD evidence, it is costly to focus specifically on an object. However, the perceiver receives a return on this investment in that the behavioral impact of the object cue, in terms of increased speed and accuracy of letter identification on valid as opposed to invalid trials, was greater than that of the directional arrow cue. This increased facilitation may result from the increased concentration of attentional resources inside the object's boundary, relative to a possibly more diffuse deployment to an unbounded region of the environment.

The event-related fMRI design used in this study allowed a direct comparison of activation on invalid versus valid trials within each cue condition, thereby delineating brain structures involved in the reorientation of attention after its initial deployment proved incorrect. All areas of activation that differentiated invalid from valid trials showed greater activity on the invalid trials and were approximately the same regardless of whether attention was initially deployed in response to the object cue or the location cue. This outcome suggests that additional brain regions over and above those already activated in response to the cue are recruited in order to reorient attention to a target appearing at an uncued location.

Thus in addition to the BOLD-related physiological cost of focusing attention on an object rather than an unbounded region of space observed on valid trials, there is an additional cost imposed by being wrong in this guess about where to devote resources. The areas of increased neuronal activation specific to attentional reorientation were strongly right-lateralized and included posterior temporal, temporoparietal, and inferior parietal regions previously implicated in visual attention, as well as prefrontal regions that likely subserve control processes, particularly related to inhibition of inappropriate responding. Thus stimuli occurring in selected regions of the visual world are processed all the way through to a response more easily than stimuli occurring in ignored regions.

To summarize, visual attention can select an unbounded region of environmental space and in so doing increase the efficiency of processing a stimulus event that might occur there. It can gain greater benefit by focusing more specifically on the space defined by an object, but at a physiological cost indicated by changes in blood oxygenation levels. And if it picks the wrong space on which to focus, an additional cost is incurred, both behaviorally and physiologically.

What if the object itself, rather than the space it defines, is the intended target of selection? This is perhaps the more usual case during human beings' perceptually guided interactions with the world, and hence it may be the more important case to understand.

SELECTING OBJECTS TO PROCESS DEEPLY: MANAGING INTERFERENCE FROM MULTIPLE STIMULI THAT HAVE BEEN IDENTIFIED AND INTERPRETED

Whenever there are many stimuli in the environment—which in the real world is most of the time—a critical decision for the human information processing system, given its limited capacity for perception, short-term storage, and control of action, is how much analysis to give the sensory input from each stimulus. The issue is basically one of depth of process-ing—how much to learn about each stimulus that happens to be present in the environment at any given time. We have just seen that visual attention alters the speed, accuracy, and physiological demands of processing, making selected stimuli easier to carry through to a task-relevant response and making ignored stimuli harder. The question naturally arises as to when and how this differential preference is imposed in the course of processing selected and ignored stimuli.

In principle, selection for deep analysis could be temporally *early* in the stream of pro-cessing, based on rather easily computed sensory properties and supported by interactions between posterior sensory processing structures and temporal, temporoparietal, and parietal attentional structures. One or more stimuli with a particular value of such a property could be given priority to be admitted to the more complex and demanding processes of identifica-tion, activation and retrieval of meaning, and computation of task relevance and response potential, with other stimuli attenuated or excluded from deep processing. "Early selection" would be a good strategy when easily computed sensory properties do in fact distinguish task-relevant from irrelevant-stimulli (e.g., the location and simple shape cues described in the previous section) and—perhaps more important—task-irrelevant stimuli can safely go unidentified and uninterpreted.

However, early selection would be disadvantageous or even dangerous if unexpected stimuli could turn out to be important but would go unnoticed if their identitites, meanings, and response potentials were not computed because attention was occupied elsewhere. Fur-thermore, early selection would be an impossible strategy whenever task relevance cannot be defined on easily computed sensory features or when the specific properties of potentially relevant stimuli are not known in advance but must be recognized and related to task de-mands after deep processing.

Under the latter kinds of conditions, temporally *late* selection, supported by prefrontal control structures, would become the strategy of choice—or of necessity—with as many en-vironmental stimuli as possible being analyzed for identity, meaning, and response potential before selective priorities are imposed among them. Shifting the locus of selection toward deeper processing would confer some benefits that would be lost under early selection. However, "late selection" also carries some disadvantages.

One problem arises from interference that is created by many streams of deep stimulus processing going on simultaneously. Crosstalk among parallel streams of processing is known to degrade information, with degradation increasing as a function of the similarity of the information being handled in the various streams (Brown, Roos-Gilbert, & Carr, 1995; Desimone & Duncan, 1995; Navon & Miller, 1987). One function of visual attention is to focus on the environmental source of one stream of processing at the expense of others in order to reduce crosstalk (Brown, Gore, & Carr, 2002). However, such "biasing of competi-tion" (Desimone & Duncan, 1995) requires that spatial location, or some other easily com-putable sensory feature, be available to guide the focusing of attention prior to deep stimu-lus processing. That is, protection from crosstalk requires the conditions that support early selection.

A second problem accompanying late selection has been called by many names in many different literatures—*response competition, decision competition, monitoring of response conflict, selection for action, inhibitory control,* and *interference control* in the literatures on attention, cognitive aging, cognitive development, and attention-deficit/hyperactivity disor-der (Allport, 1989; Barch, Braver, Sabb, & Noll, 2000; Barkley, 1997; Botella, 1996; Dagenbach & Carr, 1994; Dempster, 1993; Eriksen & Hoffman, 1973; Hasher & Zacks,

1988; Henik & Carr, 2002; Nigg, 2001; Zacks & Hasher, 1994). Underlying the diversity of nomenclature is a simple but important idea. The more stimuli in addition to the task-appropriate target stimulus that are processed for identity, meaning, and response potential, the greater the chance that one or more of the nontarget stimuli will distract or capture the mechanisms of decision, response selection, and motor programming that ought to be focused on choosing and executing the action appropriate to the target. The cognitive system must avoid or recover from being "garden-pathed" by the response potential of irrelevant stimuli and ensure that the proper task-relevant target stimulus is in fact controlling action. If interference control succeeds, the correct action will be produced, but more slowly than if response competition had not occurred. If it fails, the wrong action will be produced.

Eriksen's well-known "flanker paradigm" (Eriksen & Hoffman, 1972, 1973) is a model system for studying the difficulties created by response competition and the resulting need for effective interference control. If "flankers"—irrelevant stimuli that might elicit an incorrect response if processed by mistake—are located close enough to a relevant stimulus to which a response must be made, interference occurs, showing that the logically irrelevant stimulus is nevertheless processed to sufficient depth to activate its potential responses. This paradigm illustrates quite clearly that processing multiple stimuli to depth can impose a cost on effective and efficient primary task performance. It also suggests limits on how tightly visual attention can be focused and on the efficacy of the penumbra of inhibition or center-surround selection identified by Steinman and colleagues (1995). If visual attention could be focused completely accurately, on a small enough region, and surrounded by a sufficiently impenetrable inhibitory surround, then the flanker should never get processed deeply enough to produce response competition. Complete elimination of flanker processing is rarely observed, with a greater likelihood when the stimulus–response mappings required by the task being performed are relatively new and unpracticed than when they are familiar and well learned (Brown et al., 2002). In a moment we consider a general proposal regarding what determines how much flanker processing is alllowed to happen.

Given that neither strategy—early versus late selection—is perfect and cost-free, the question becomes how a choice is made between them. Recent investigations combining a visual search task with the Eriksen flanker paradigm suggest a dynamic solution in which the locus of selection (early vs. late in the stream of information processing) varies from situation to situation as a function of a theoretical construct called perceptual load (Lavie, 1995).

Suppose there is a circular search array surrounding fixation that contains one or the other of two target letters, plus one to five distractor letters. The task is to indicate as rapidly and accurately as possible which target letter is present. "Perceptual load" is defined by the amount of task-relevant information within the visual search array based on the total number of items and their complexity. Thus a search array with a target and five distractors imposes a greater perceptual load than a search array with a target and one distractor (Lavie, 1995; Lavie & Cox, 1997; Lavie & Fox, 2000; Lavie & Tsal, 1994).

Now suppose there is also a task-irrelevant letter at another location in the visual field, outside the search array (a stimulus that *should* be ignored if possible, to limit the potential for crosstalk and response competition, and that *can* be ignored with impunity, because it is defined from the outset as task-irrelevant). This letter is presented at a more eccentric location flanking the array, and it is bigger than the letters in the search array. The differences in location and size provide two easily computed sensory properties that could be used to implement early selection by focusing visual attention on the region occupied by the search array to the exclusion of the irrelevant flanker. However, the added size makes the flanking letter visually resolvable despite its greater eccentricity. If early selection is implemented to exclude the flanker, it will not be processed to depth, but if early selection is relaxed, the quality of sensory input is sufficient for the flanker to be processed through to computing its response potential. Once the representation of a response to the flanker is activated, it can interfere with computing, selecting, and executing the task-appropriate response actually called for by the target in the search array.

Following Eriksen and Hoffman's original logic, the depth of processing of the flanker is measured by the occurrence of response competition. The flanker can be a neutral letter that would elicit no response were it in the search array—just another distractor—but it can also be one of the target letters. When the flanker is a target letter and it is response incompatible—if processed to depth, it will elicit the opposite response to that required by the actual target in the search array—then if attention does not exclude it from deep processing, response competition will occur. This competition can be observed as longer response time or increased error rate in the flanker-incompatible condition.

Results show that response competition varies with the size of the search array—that is, it depends on perceptual load. Small arrays are accompanied by a relatively large amount of response competition, which decreases as array size increases. Lavie and colleagues interpret these results as showing that if the perceptual load imposed by the task-relevant information in the search array is too small to consume the perceiver's available perceptual capacity, then all stimuli are processed *automatically*, regardless of task relevance, until perceptual capacity is exhausted. Under such "low-load" circumstances, selection occurs in the later stages of information processing. As perceptual load increases and begins to exhaust perceptual capacity, selection shifts from late to early and comes under the control of processes that respond to sensory and perceptual features rather than identity, meaning, and afforded actions. As early selection comes to dominate input selection, the flanker receives less processing, reducing its impact on performance. In essence, then, the cognitive system implements a selection strategy dynamically and adaptively, relying on the trading relation between early and late selection to balance the benefits of processing many environmental stimuli to depth against the costs of having too many deeply processed stimuli competing for control of action.

This evidence for a trading relation raises questions about cognitive development, individual differences, and psychopathology. The "visual search plus flanker" paradigm developed by Lavie and her colleagues can be used as a model system in which to explore such questions. If any of the factors that determine the locus of selection in this paradigm—perceptual capacity, interference control, or the ability to react to increasing perceptual load by implementing the shift from late to early selection—changes developmentally, then perceivers at different stages of development will demonstrate different patterns of performance. Similarly, if these factors are vulnerable to psychopathology, then patterns of performance will differ between abnormal and normal perceivers with other developmental and demographic variables held constant.

Maylor and Lavie (1998) applied this logic in a comparison of older and younger adults. They found that older adults suffer greater response competition with small array sizes than do younger adults. This suggests that interference control decreases with cognitive aging. Furthermore, older adults showed reductions in response competition with increasing load at smaller absolute array sizes than did younger adults. Shifting toward early selection at a lower perceptual load suggests that older adults exhaust their perceptual capacity at lower loads, and hence that they have less perceptual capacity available for encoding and processing environmental stimuli. Thus the visual search plus flanker paradigm exposes changes with cognitive aging of two types: decreasing interference control or increasing susceptibility to response competition from processed stimuli, accompanied by reduced capacity for processing stimuli to begin with. While both of these changes can be troublesome to task performance, note that the fundamentally adaptive character of the selective attention system appears to remain intact, as the two factors trade off against one another to produce a shift toward early selection at smaller perceptual loads than one would expect based on the performance of younger adults. This works to some degree to shield older adults from the full impact of their compromised interference control.

Huang-Pollack, Carr, and Nigg (2002) have applied the same logic to development during childhood, testing second-graders, fourth-graders, sixth-graders, and college students in the visual search plus flanker paradigm. Again, developmental changes were found, and the pattern was the mirror image of that observed for cognitive aging by Maylor and Lavie. Perceivers of all ages showed a reduction in flanker-induced response competition with increasing visual-search array size. However, younger children showed the onset of these reductions at smaller array sizes than did older children or young adults. Furthermore, younger children suffered larger response competition effects at the smallest perceptual load, indicating greater susceptibility to the impact of response competition under conditions of late selection. Thus cognitive development is marked by increases in perceptual capacity and interference control, whereas cognitive aging is marked by decreases.

Huang-Pollack, Nigg, and Carr (2004) extended this use of the visual search plus flanker paradigm to the analysis of attention deficits in attention-deficit/hyperactivity disorder (ADHD). Despite the name of the syndrome, it is a matter of considerable debate whether there actually is any attention deficit per se in ADHD. Indeed, theories of the combined subtype of ADHD, whose directly observable behavioral phenotype includes both hyperactivity and inattention to environmental signals, have moved away from hypothesizing attention deficits, focusing instead on executive control and inhibition of inappropriate behavioral choices (Barkley, 1997; Nigg, 2001). Theories of the primarily inattentive subtype of ADHD, whose behavioral phenotype includes mainly a certain "spaciness" based on inattention to environmental signals, still maintain a place for attentional deficits per se (Milich, Balentine, & Lynam, 2001).

A crucial part of the problem in settling this debate hinges on the fact that multiple definitions of "attention" are mixed together in the literature on ADHD, sometimes without being explicit about which definition appies in any given discussion or in crafting any given experimental test. Here taxonomies of the varieties of attention taken from the cognitive–psychological and cognitive–neuroscientific literature can be helpful (Carr, 1979; Carr & Bacharach, 1976; Posner & Snyder, 1975; Posner & Petersen, 1990). These taxonomies make four major distinctions. Two of them fall under the rubric of selective attention as it is being used in the present chapter. The first is selective attention to environmental stimuli as sources of sensory information—"input regulation" in the general case and "visual attention" in the more specfic cases of visual information processing considered here. The second is selective attention to memory representations activated either by environmental stimuli or by internally generated expectations and retrieval operations. A third type of attention involves staying "on task"—attending to one goal-directed task performance and not being distracted by other goals. This type of attention involves the executive control processes of working memory and includes the processes of inhibition of inappropriate behavioral choices emphasized by Barkley (1997). The fourth type of attention is arousal, referring to a generalized readiness to respond to any environmental input or task goal, independently of the specifics of information content that underlie the selectivity among inputs and goals represented by the first three types of attention. At present, there is little doubt in the ADHD literature that staying aroused and staying on task are problems for people diagnosable as ADHD. The debate surrounds whether there may be an additional deficit in "selective attention."

Available empirical evidence regarding a deficit in selective attention is quite mixed (Nigg, 2001). This is largely because the sorts of tasks used to provide measures of selective attention have not been very diagnostic, either failing to present a large enough stimulus load to stress the system or failing to include stimuli capable of causing competition with task responses, or both.

The visual search plus flanker paradigm is well suited to solving these problems. In a comparison of 8- to 12-year-old children with ADHD-combined, those with ADHD primarily inattentive, and those who were normally developing, Huang-Pollack and her colleagues found no differences among the three groups in any of the aspects of selective attention diagnosable from performance in this task. Both groups of ADHD children showed normal amounts of flanker-induced response competition at low loads, both groups showed reductions in response competition as load increased, and both groups showed the onset of this reduction at about the same array size as the normal children. While null results are never entirely satisfying, the study was conducted with sufficient power to find small effect sizes in these between-group comparisons. Hence, as indicated by the visual-search-plus-flanker paradigm used as a diagnostic instrument, selective attention appears to be substantially intact among children with ADHD. These findings converge on the trend toward emphasizing executive control, inhibition of inappropriate behavior, and deficits in maintaining arousal as the primary locus of disability in ADHD.

SELECTING CODES TO BE RETRIEVED FROM SEMANTIC MEMORY: MANAGING INTERFERENCE WHEN SEMANTIC INTERPRETATION IS DIFFICULT

Selective attention is often thought of as a set of processes that operate at the sensory and perceptual levels, providing a gateway for incoming information from the environment. Once environmental information enters the cognitive system, however, additional selection problems arise. Constructs already discussed from the study of selective attention to incoming information from the environment can be extended to the selection and retrieval of activated information from memory during the interpretation processes by which encoded perceptual stimuli are identified, processed for meaning, and their interpreted codes entered into working memory for use in task performance.

The basic idea in drawing this analogy between the role of attention in "retrieving" information from the environment and a possible role for attention in retrieving information from semantic memory is a spatial one, facilitated by thinking of the semantic memory system as a network of distinct local representations arrayed in a multidimensional semantic space (Anderson, 1983; Besner, 1999; Collins & Loftus, 1975; McNamara, 1992; Neely, 1991). In this conceptualization, semantic representations reside at different distances from one another, much as objects are arrayed in environmental space, and interact with one another in both facilitatory and inhibitory ways as a function of their strength and distance. Facilitation among near neighbors in semantic space occurs via spreading activation. As a representation becomes active, it "spreads the message" to related representations, creating a region of activation that corresponds to something like the superordinate category membership or "meaning neighborhood" of the originally activated representation. If a general idea of the meaning of a stimulus is sufficient to guide task performance, this region of coactivated representations can do the job—much as when, during visually guided action, it is sufficient to know that there is a crowd of objects at a particular location or in a particular direction, without being able to discriminate one object from another. That is, sometimes localization of a "blob" in space is sufficient, without further determination of its composition.

But if the specific meaning of an individuated stimulus is needed, more must be done to differentiate among the representations in the activated region of semantic space. In some cases the originally activated representation will be sufficiently more active than any of the others in the region that it will "pop out," exceeding threshold for retrieval into working memory much as a very intense, salient, or distinctive visual stimulus will "pop out" of the visual field during visual encoding and search (Miller, 2000; Wolfe, 1998; Yantis, 2000). In other cases, however, the differences in activation among representations within the activated region will not be sufficient for one representation rather than another to pop out. In these cases, an attentional process may be needed to focus on one representation and facilitate its retrieval by enhancing the activation of that representation and shielding it from competitive interactions with other representations—again, much as attention works to facilitate information from one stimulus in space while shielding it from competitive interactions with near neighbors in space (Desimone & Duncan, 1995).

Furthermore, inherent differences in the strength of representations in semantic memory may make some of them much easier to activate and much easier to retrieve, allowing them to compete successfully with weaker representations, even if they are not the ones required for task performance. This possibility also has its analog in visual encoding of objects arrayed in environmental space, where stronger, more intense, and more salient stimuli tend to mask weaker stimuli, especially when they occur close together in space and time. It is well established that stronger (better learned, higher frequency, more familiar) semantic representations are easier to activate, reaching criterion levels of activation for retrieval into working memory faster than weaker representations (Anderson, 1983; Collins & Loftus, 1975; Dagenbach, Horst, & Carr, 1990). This might make it possible for stronger representations to mask weaker representations, again even if they are not the ones required for task performance. Such competitive interactions are likely to be greater and more bothersome in more crowded regions of semantic memory—that is, activated near neighbors in semantic space may, under some circumstances, be the most difficult to discriminate from one another and selectively retrieve, just as near neighbors in visual space can be more difficult to discriminate than objects separated by large environmental distances.

This analogy between internal representations in semantic space and external stimuli in environmental space suggests the hypothesis that retrieval from semantic memory may require the services of an attention-like process. Under circumstances conducive to competition for retrieval, this mechanism of attention might operate to select one representation and facilitate its activation while protecting the selected representation from crosstalk and competition created by other nearby representations (Carr & Dagenbach, 1990; Dagenbach & Carr, 1994; Dagenbach, Carr, & Wilhemsen, 1989). Pursuit of this hypothesis has yielded evidence that attempting to retrieve a meaning that is being driven by incoming perceptual input may require the active inhibition of related semantic codes that are better learned and therefore stronger.

The paradigm and the basic pattern of results supporting this notion can be illustrated by the vocabulary learning experiments of Dagenbach, Carr, and Barnhart (1990). People began by studying a list of unusual new vocabulary words, such as *accipiter: a hawk*, *drupe: a cherry*, and *moil: hard work*. Enough study time was provided to make the words and their meanings verifiable by all participants in a test of recognition memory (indicating that the relationship had been stored in memory). However, only about half of the meanings were explicitly retrievable by any one participant in a standard paired-associate cued recall test (indicating that the representations of some of them had gotten strong enough so that the new word presented as the stimulus could succeed in activating its associated meaning sufficiently to raise the meaning above threshold for explicit retrieval into working memory, but others had not). Even for word-meaning pairs for which cued recall succeeded, retrieval was still quite effortful. The newly learned associations were weak, leaving activation and retrieval of the newly learned meanings difficult and prone to failure.

These weakly learned new words became the "primes" for "semantically primed lexical decisions" about well-learned words. On each trial of this task, the perceiver read and tried to call to mind the meaning of a prime word—one of the weakly learned new vocabulary items, such as *accipiter* or *drupe*—then saw either a well-known word (such as *eagle*, *peach*, or *play*) or a pronounceable nonword (such as *ergle*, *deach*, or *plap*. The subject had to respond to the second stimulus, indicating as rapidly and accurately as possible whether it was a word on a nonword. In this task, a semantically related pairing of a newly learned prime word and a well-learned target word might be "accipiter–eagle." An unrelated pairing might be "drupe–eagle."

What should be expected to happen? If these weakly learned new words behave like strongly represented, well-learned words in this priming task, then we would expect to see the standard facilitatory priming effect in which lexical decisions about related target words are facilitated and decisions about unrelated target words are inhibited.

This result did emerge, but not for all primes. The newly learned primes were divided into two groups for each participant separately: those whose meaning could be successfully retrieved in the cued recall test (that is, the "stronger" of the weakly learned new words) and those whose meaning could not be retrieved (i.e., the "weaker" of the weakly learned new words—the ones whose meanings were the most difficult to activate and retrieve). The stronger newly learned words did produce the standard facilitatory priming effect. However, the newly learned primes whose meanings were the most difficult to retrieve—and in this task, did not end up reaching working memory at all, as indicated by the cued recall test—produced the opposite impact. They inhibited related targets rather than facilitating them.

Dagenbach and colleagues suggested that this pattern of inhibitory semantic priming following a prime whose meaning is extremely difficult to activate and retrieve might indicate the operation of a center–surround attentional mechanism—analogous to the center–surround attentional mechanism identified in visual perception by Steinman and colleagues (1995). If no representation is activated sufficiently in semantic memory to rise above threshold for retrieval into working memory, attention centers on the most activated of the partially activated representations. Attention then tries to raise that representation's activation above threshold for retrieval. It does this by enhancing activation in the sought-for representation on which it has been centered and simultaneously inhibiting any nearby representations that may also have become partially activated and hence are creating competition. The most activated representation is most likely to be the one actually being driven by the stimulus input, so this attentional strategy is likely to be trying to enhance the correct code. What about the neighboring codes that are being inhibited? Because semantic memory is organized according to meaning and association, the nearby representations will be semantically related. Hence, the efforts made by the center–surround attentional mechanism to aid retrieval of the newly learned but very weak code will inhibit better learned related codes. If one of these inhibited codes is needed for task performance a short time later, it will be less accessible than normal because of residual inhibition. Therefore, performance based on activating that representation will be slowed, resulting in the inhibitory priming effect that was observed.

While this pattern of results was surprising and the interpretation speculative, quite similar results were obtained in a subsequent test of the interpretation using artificial category learning (Dagenbach & Carr, 1994; see Appendix for description). Thus it appears that a center–surround attentional mechanism operates in the service of selection among activated semantic representations from memory, analogous to a similar mechanism observed to operate during selection of activated object representations from environmental space.

CONCLUSION

In each of the three rather different domains of investigation described in this chapter, we have seen a trading relation between the benefits and the costs of exercising the powers of attentional selection to aid in processing selected stimuli or representations at the expense of ignored stimuli or representations. In some cases, these costs were rather surprising, as in the case of the center–surround phenomena observed both in visual encoding of environmental stimuli by Steinman and colleagues (1995) and in semantic processing by Dagenbach and colleagues (Carr & Dagenbach, 1990; Dagenbach & Carr, 1994). How "high up" into the attentional system such center–surround-like phenomena can be observed remains to be seen. Recent work on executive control of task switching by Arrington, Altmann, and Carr (2003) indicates that similarity among tasks influences the time needed to switch from one task to another, with more similar and hence more closely related tasks easier to switch between than less similar tasks. Arrington and colleagues speculated that learning a set of tasks may behave somewhat like learning a set of word meanings—the tasks are represented in a "task space" that is organized in terms of the similarity relations among the tasks. If so, then one might wonder what would happen if after learning a set of tasks to a high criterion, one tried to add a new task to the established task space. Activating and retrieving the new task might exhibit the same sorts of facilitatory and inhibitory priming effects that have supported center–surround attentional hypotheses in visual encoding and retrieval from semantic memory. This possibility is worth pursuing in the future, in order to further develop a unified theory of selective attention that applies to selection of environmental information to process deeply, to memorial representations to retrieve into working memory, and to task goals to be pursued and achieved in overt action. Such a theory would cross boundaries between the study of attention's contributions to perception, attention's contributions to memory, and attention's contributions to task execution that have stood in the way of a clearer understanding of how all the sources of information and knowledge available to an individual are coordinated to support real-time task performance.

APPENDIX: DESCRIPTION OF ARTIFICIAL CATEGORY LEARNING EXPERIMENT

In this study, people practiced category membership judgments for two arbitrary sets of visual shapes until judgment times asymptoted. At this point, a test of primed category membership judgments revealed facilitatory priming in which exemplars of a category presented as primes speeded membership judgments about other exemplars of the same category presented as targets. Thus practice at judging category membership for these visual shapes had established an artificial "semantic memory."

Next, a few new exemplars in each category were studied just enough to make accurate category membership judgments, but these judgments were made more slowly than judgments about the original well-learned category exemplars, and with considerable variability in judgment time from one new member to the next.

Based on this variability in judgment time, the new exemplars were split into two groups based on a median split of category membership judgment times. One group of new exemplars was somewhat better learned (faster membership judgments) and the other group of new exemplars was quite weakly learned (slower membership judgments). The two groups of newly learned exemplars were then used as primes in primed category membership judgments about the old, well-learned exemplars.

The group of more slowly categorized new exemplars were the "weakest of the weakly learned" and ought to be most in need of the help of a center–surround attentional mechanism in order to be categorized correctly, whereas the group of more rapidly categorized new exemplars ought to be better able to respond to incoming stimulus information and protect themselves from competition by stronger exemplars stored nearby in semantic space. Therefore, if the center–surround attentional mechanism proposed on the basis of the earlier vocabulary learning studies could also be seen at work in this shape categorization task, then the slowly categorized new exemplars ought to produce inhibitory priming, whereas the more rapidly categorized new exemplars ought not.

The results were as predicted by the center–surround hypothesis. The more rapildly classifiable (and therefore easier to activate) primes facilitated judgments about older, better learned exemplars of the same category, but the more slowly classifiable (and hence harder to activate) primes did the opposite. They inhibited judgments about older, better learned exemplars of the same category.

REFERENCES

Allport, A. (1989). Visual attention. In M. I. Posner (Ed.), *Foundations of cognitive science* (pp. 631–682). Cambridge, MA: MIT Press.

Anderson, J. R. (1983). *The architecture of cognition.* Cambridge, MA: Harvard University Press.

Arrington, C. M., Altmann, E. M., & Carr, T. H. (2003). Tasks of a feather flock together: Similarity effects in task switching. *Memory and Cognition, 31,* 781–789.

Arrington, C. M., & Carr, T. H. (2003). Attention. In B. S. Fogel, R. B. Schiffer, & S. M. Rao (Eds.), *Neuropsychiatry* (2nd ed., pp. 405–425). Baltimore: Lippincott, Williams & Wilkins.

Arrington, C. M., Mayer, A. R., Carr, T. H., & Rao, S. M. (2000). Neural mechanisms of spatial attention: Object-based versus location-based selection. *Journal of Cognitive Neuroscience, 12*(Suppl. 2), 106–117.

Barch, D. M., Braver, T. S., Sabb, F. W., & Noll, D. C. (2000). Anterior cingulate and the monitoring of response conflict: Evidence from an fMRI study of overt verb generation. *Journal of Cognitive Neuroscience, 12,* 298–311.

Barkley, R. (1997). Behavioral inhibition, sustained attention, and executive functions: Constructing a unifying theory of ADHD. *Psychological Bulletin, 121,* 65–94.

Besner, D. (1999). Basic processes in reading: Multiple routines in localist and connectionist models. In R. Klein & P. McMullen (Eds.), *Converging methods for understanding reading and dyslexia* (pp. 413–458). Cambridge, MA: MIT Press.

Botella, J. (1996). Decision competition and response competition: Two main factors in the flanker compatibility effect. In A. F. Kramer, M. G. H. Coles, & G. D. Logan (Eds.), *Converging operations in the study of visual selective attention* (pp. 503–518). Washington, DC: American Psychological Association.

Brown, T. L., Gore, C., & Carr, T. H. (2002). Visual attention and word recognition in Stroop color naming: Is word recognition "automatic"? *Journal of Experimental Psychology: General, 131,* 220–240.

Brown, T. L., Roos-Gilbert, L., & Carr, T. H. (1995). Automaticity and word perception: Evidence from Stroop and Stroop dilution effects. *Journal of Experimental Psychology: Learning, Memory, and Cognition, 21,* 1395–1411.

Carr, T. H. (1979). Consciousness in models of human information processing: Primary memory, executive control, and input regulation. In G. underwood & R. Stevens (Eds.), *Aspects of consciousness: Vol. 1. Psychological issues* (pp. 123–153). London: Academic Press.

Carr, T. H., & Bacharach, V. R. (1976). Perceptual tuning and conscious attention: Mechanisms of input regulation in visual information processing. *Cognition, 4,* 281–302.

Carr, T. H., & Dagenbach, D. (1990). Semantic priming and repetition priming from masked words: Evidence for a center-surround attentional mechanism in perceptual recognition. *Journal of Experimental Psychology: Learning, Memory, and Cognition, 16,* 341–350.

Collins, A. M., & Loftus, E. F. (1975). A spreading-activation theory of semantic processing. *Psychological Review, 82,* 407–428.

Dagenbach, D., & Carr, T. H. (1994). Inhibitory semantic priming due to retrieval failures. In D. Dagenbach & T. H. Carr (Eds.), *Inhibitory processes in attention, memory, and language* (pp. 327–357). San Diego, CA: Academic Press.

Dagenbach, D., & Carr, T. H. (Eds.). (1994). *Inhibitory processes in attention, memory, and language.* San Diego, CA: Academic Press.

Dagenbach, D., Carr, T. H., & Barnhardt, T. (1990). Inhibitory semantic priming of lexical decisions is caused by failure to retrieve weakly activated codes. *Journal of Experimental Psychology: Learning, Memory, and Cognition, 16,* 328–340.

Dagenbach, D., Carr, T. H., & Wilhelmsen, A. (1989). Task-induced strategies and near-threshold priming: Conscious influences on unconscious perception. *Journal of Memory and Language, 28,* 412–443.

Dagenbach, D., Horst, S., & Carr, T. H. (1990). Priming studies of learning in semantic memory. *Journal of Experimental Psychology: Learning, Memory, and Cognition, 16,* 581–591.

Dempster, F. (1993). Resistance to interference: Developmental changes in basic processing mechanisms. In M. L. Howe & R. Pasnak (Eds.), *Emerging themes in cognitive development* (Vol. 1, pp. 3–27). New York: Springer-Verlag.

Desimone, R., & Duncan, J. (1995). Neural mechanisms of selective visual attention. *Annual Review of Neuroscience, 18,* 193–222.

Duncan, J. (1984). Selective attention and the organization of visual information. *Journal of Experimental Psychology: General, 87,* 272–300.

Egly, R., Driver, J., & Rafal, R. D. (1994). Shifting visual attention between objects and locations: Evidence from normal and parietal lesion subjects. *Journal of Experimental Psychology: General, 123,* 161–177.

Eriksen, C. W., & Hoffman, J. E. (1972). Temporal and spatial characteristics of selective encoding from visual displays. *Perception and Psychophysics, 12,* 201–204.

Eriksen, C. W., & Hoffman, J. E. (1973). The extent of processing noise elements during selective encoding from visual displays. *Perception and Psychophysics, 14,* 155–160.

Eriksen, C. W., & Yeh, Y. Y. (1985). Allocation of attention in the visual field. *Journal of Experimental Psychology: Human Perception and Performance, 11,* 583–597.

Hasher, L., & Zacks, R. T. (1988). Working memory, comprehension, and aging: A review and a new view. *Psychology of Learning and Motivation, 22,* 122–149.

Henderson, J. M. (1991). Stimulus discrimination following covert attentional orienting to an exogenous cue. *Journal of Experimental Psychology: Human Perception and Performance, 17,* 91–106.

Henik, A., & Carr, T. H. (2002). Inhibition. In V. S. Ramachandran (Ed.), *Encyclopedia of the human brain.* San Diego, CA: Academic Press

Huang-Pollock, C. L., Carr, T. H., & Nigg, J. T. (2002). Development of selective attention: Perceptual load influences early versus late selection in children and adults. *Developmental Psychology, 38,* 363–375.

Huang-Pollack, C. L., Nigg, J. T., & Carr, T. H. (2004). *Deficient attention is hard to find: Applying the perceptual load model of selective attention to attention deficit hyperactivity disorder subtypes.* Manuscript under review.

Kanwisher, N., & Driver, J. (1992). Objects, attributes, and visual attention: Which, what, and where. *Current Directions in Psychological Science, 1,* 26–31.

LaBerge, D., & Brown, V. (1989). Theory of attentional operations in shape identification. *Psychological Review, 96,* 101–124.

Lavie, N. (1995). Perceptual load as a necessary condition for selective attention. *Journal of Experimental Psychology: Human Perception and Performance, 21,* 451–468.

Lavie, N., & Cox, S. (1997). On the efficiency of attentional selection: Efficient visual search results in inefficient rejection of distraction. *Psychological Science, 8,* 395–398.

Lavie, N., & Fox, E. (2000). The role of perceptual load in negative priming. *Journal of Experimental Psychology: Human Perception and Performance, 26,* 1038–1052.

Lavie, N., & Tsal, Y. (1994). Perceptual load as a major determinant of the locus of selection in visual attention. *Perception and Psychophysics, 56,* 183–197.

Maylor, E., & Lavie, N. (1998). The influence of perceptual load on age differences in selective attention. *Psychology and Aging, 13,* 563–573.

McNamara, T. P. (1992). Priming and constraints it places on theories of memory and retrieval. *Psychological Review, 99,* 650–662.

Milich, R., Balentine, A., & Lynam, D. (2001). ADHD combined type and ADHD predominantly inattentive type are distinct and unrelated disorders. *Clinical Psychology Science and Practice, 8,* 463–488.

Miller, E. K. (2000). The neural basis of top-down control of visual attention in the prefrontal cortex. In S. Monsell & J. Driver (Eds.), *Control of cognitive processes: Attention and performance* (Vol. 18, pp. 512–534). Cambridge, MA: MIT Press.

Moore, C. M., & Egeth, H. (1998). How does feature-based attention affect visual processing? *Journal of Experimental Psychology: Human Perception and Performance, 24,* 1296–1310.

Navon, D., & Miller, J. (1987). Role of outcome conflict in dual-task interference. *Journal of Experimental Psychology: Human Perception and Performance, 13,* 435–448.

Neely, J. H. (1991). Semantic priming effects in visual word recognition: A selective review of current findings and theories. In D. Besner & G. Humphreys (Eds.), *Basic processes in reading: visual word recognition* (pp. 264–336). Hillsdale, NJ: Erlbaum.

Nigg, J. (2001). Is ADHD an inhibitory disorder? *Psychological Bulletin, 5,* 571–598.

Posner, M. I. (1980). Orienting of attention. *Quarterly Journal of Experimental Psychology, 32,* 3–25.

Posner, M. I., & Petersen, S. (1990). The attention system of the human brain. *Annual Review of Neuroscience, 13,* 25–42.

Poser, M. I., & Synder, C. R. R. (1975). Attention and cognitive control. In R. L. Solso (Ed.), *Information processing and cognition* (pp. 55–85). Hillsdale, NJ: Erlbaum.

Steinman, B. A., Steinman, S. B., & Lehmkuhle, S. (1995). Visual attention mechanisms show a center–surround organization. *Vision Research, 35,* 1859–1869.

Vecera, S. P., & Farah, M. J. (1994). Does visual attention select objects or locations? *Journal of Experimental Psychology: General, 123,* 146–160.

Wolfe, J. M. (1998). Visual search. In H. Pashler (Ed.), *Attention* (pp. 13–73). London: Psychology Press.

Yantis, S. (2000). Goal-directed and stimulus-driven determinants of attentional control. In S. Monsell & J. Driver (Eds.), *Control of cognitive processes: Attention and performance* (Vol. 18, pp. 73–103). Cambridge, MA: MIT Press.

Zacks, R. T., & Hasher, L. (1994). Directed ignoring: Inhibitory regulation of working memory. In D. Dagenbach & T. H. Carr (Eds.), *Inhibitory processes in attention, memory, and language* (pp. 241–264). San Diego, CA: Academic Press.

6

A Systems-Level Perspective on Attention and Cognitive Control

Guided Activation, Adaptive Gating, Conflict Monitoring, and Exploitation versus Exploration

Jonathan D. Cohen, Gary Aston-Jones, and Mark S. Gilzenrat

THE SCOPE OF ATTENTION

An understanding of attention is arguably one of the most important goals of the cognitive sciences and yet also has proven to be one of the most elusive. Most attention researchers will agree that a major problem has been agreeing on a definition of the term and the scope of the phenomena to which it applies. There are no doubt as many explanations for this state of affairs as there are those who consider themselves "attention researchers." However, most will probably agree that, in large measure, this is because attention is not a unitary phenomenon—at least not in the sense that it reflects the operation of a single mechanism, or a single function of one or a set of mechanisms. Rather, attention is the emergent property of the cognitive system that allows it to successfully process some sources of information to the exclusion of others, in the service of achieving some goals to the exclusion of others. This begs an important question: If attention is so varied a phenomenon, how can we make progress in understanding it? There are two simple answers to this question: Be precise about the specific (aspects of the) phenomena to be studied, and be precise about the mechanisms thought to explain them.

In this chapter, we address a particular type of attentional phenomenon—that associated with cognitive control. Furthermore, we focus on an account that addresses not only the functional characteristics of this form of attention but also how it is implemented in neural machinery. This neurally oriented approach is attractive not only because it is intrinsically interesting to understand how the mechanisms of the brain give rise to the processes of the mind but more specifically because this exercise has proven useful in generating insights into how controlled attention operates at the systems level. By assuming that information is

71

represented as patterns of activity, and information processing occurs as the flow of activity, it becomes possible to understand how information represented in one part of the system can influence the processing of information in other parts of the system—that is, how attention and control operate at the systems level. The sections that follow develop this idea in greater detail, first by providing a particular example of controlled attention and how it can be modeled in terms of explicit processing mechanisms, then by showing how it can explain some of the most important observations that have been made about attention and control, and finally by reviewing recent elaborations of the basic model that have begun to address broader questions about the psychological and neural mechanisms that underlie cognitive control.

AN EXAMPLE

To see how attentional effects can be understood in terms of specific processing mechanisms, it is useful to consider an example of a model of a specific task. There are now models of a variety of tasks that could serve this purpose well. Here, we focus on a model of the Stroop task (Cohen, Dunbar, & McClelland, 1990), because this task has occupied such a central role in studies of attention (both basic and clinical), because the model illustrates in a relatively straightforward manner the principles of interest, and because this model has been used to explain a wide array of findings using the Stroop task. This model was developed within the connectionist or parallel distributed processing (PDP) framework, which has been described and elaborated in great detail elsewhere (e.g., McClelland, 1993; O'Reilly & Munakata, 2000; Rumelhart, McClelland, & PDP Research Group, 1986), and therefore we assume it is familiar (or accessible) to the reader.

In the Stroop task (Stroop, 1935), subjects must attend to one dimension of a stimulus (e.g., the color in which a word is displayed) and ignore a competing but prepotent dimension (e.g., the word itself). For example, subjects are asked to name the color of an incongruent stimulus, such as the word *green* displayed in red. In our model, units are arranged into two pathways (Figure 6.1). Stimulus units representing the color project to associative units in the color-naming pathway, which project in turn to verbal response units. The word pathway converges on the same set of verbal response units. Furthermore, connections are stronger in the word pathway, capturing the assumption that written words are more frequently and consistently mapped to their pronunciations than are visual color stimuli to the utterance of their names. As a result, with no additions to the model, it will respond to the incongruent Stroop stimulus above by "reading" the word (i.e., activating the "green" response unit). In fact, this is how human subjects respond if not instructed otherwise. That is, they produce the strongest (e.g., most familiar or salient) response to a stimulus. Critically, however, they can respond to the weaker dimension of a stimulus when asked to do so (i.e., name the color in the Stroop task). This an elementary—and perhaps the most studied— form of controlled, or voluntary, attention.

To explain this ability, we make the following set of modifications to the model. First, we assume that at-rest units have relatively low activity. This corresponds well with the properties of neurons (especially those in cortical areas), which typically exhibit relatively low firing rates at rest. This can be seen in Figure 6.2a, by noting that for an input of zero, the activity of the unit is also near zero.[1] Second, we include an additional set of task demand units,[2] each of which corresponds to one of the tasks subjects are asked to perform (color naming and word reading). We assume that each of these units is connected to all of the associative units in the corresponding pathway. Thus, the color-naming unit is connected to the associative units in the color-naming pathway, and similarly for the word-reading unit. When one of these task demand units is activated, it sends activity to all the associative units in the corresponding pathway. This has the effect of sensitizing these units to input from the stimulus units. Because this effect sits at the core of how attention operates in this model, it is important to consider this in greater detail.

Figure 6.2a illustrates the activation function for a unit—that is, the function that determines its activity based on the summed input it receives from other units. Note that this function is nonlinear.[3] This is central to our account of attentional effects. Recall that units have low activity at rest (that is, when their input is zero). In this range the activation function is relatively flat. In other words, even if one of the stimulus units were to be activated and pass activity to the corresponding associative unit, this would have limited impact on the activity of that associative unit. Now assume that one of the task-demand units is activated. This passes activity to the associative units in that pathway. Let us assume further that the amount of activity is sufficient to move these units to the midpoint of their activation function, where this is steepest. Note that this does not provide any specific information to that pathway. That is, all the units in that pathway have been equally activated, so none drive one response more than the others. However, now any input to these units from the stimulus units will have a large impact on their activity. Even a small excitatory input to one of these associative units will quickly drive its activity up, while inhibitory input to the other will drive its activity down. In other words, the effect of activating the task-demand unit is

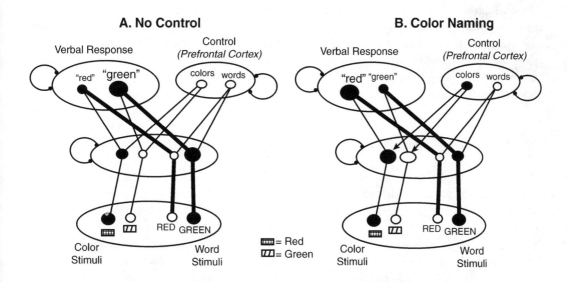

FIGURE 6.1. Model of the Stroop task. Circles represent processing units and line weights the strength of connections between units. Active units are filled (larger = more active). Looped connections with small black circles indicate mutual inhibition among units within that layer. (A) No control. Activation of conflicting inputs in the two pathways (green word input and red color input) produces a response associated with the word, due to the stronger connections in the word reading pathway. (B) Control present. The color task-demand unit is activated, representing the current intent to name the color. This passes activation to the associative units in the color naming pathway, which primes those units (indicated by larger size), and biases processing in favor of activity flowing along this pathway. This biasing effect favors activation of the response unit corresponding to the color input, even though the connection weights in this pathway are weaker than those in the word pathway.

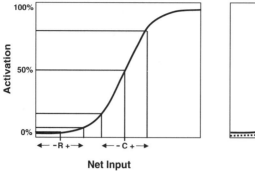
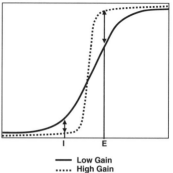

FIGURE 6.2. Activation function (see note 1 for the equation for this function). (A) Units are inhibited at rest (point labeled "R"), so that a change in the net input has relatively little effect on the unit's activity. Top-down input (from the task-demand, or control layer) places the unit near the midpoint of its activation function (point labeled "C"), where a change in the net input (+ = excitatory; − = inhibitory) has a considerably larger impact on the unit's activity. (B) An increase in gain (dotted line) increases the activity of units receiving excitatory input (E), and decreases the activity of units receiving inhibitory input (I), thus increasing the contrast between activated and inhibited units.

to bias the associative units in that pathway, placing them in the sensitive range of their activation function. This serves to modulate the responsivity of those units, making them more sensitive to the inputs.[4] This, in turn, allows the system to respond selectively to one source of information while ignoring another. For example, by activating the color-naming task-demand unit, the model can now respond to the color of the stimulus even when a conflicting word stimulus is present. That is, the model exhibits attention. This attentional effect derives from the ability of the task-demand units to guide the flow of activity along one pathway, while attenuating the flow along another. For this reason, we have come to refer to this as the guided activation theory of cognitive control (Miller & Cohen, 2001).

ATTENTION AND RELATED CONSTRUCTS

Models that implement the guided activation theory provide a quantitative account of attentional effects in a wide range of tasks (e.g., Braver, Barch, & Cohen, 1999; Braver & Cohen, 2001; Cohen, Servan-Schreiber, & McClelland, 1992; Cohen, Romero, Serven-Schreiber, & Farah, 1994; Dehaene & Changeux, 1989, 1991; Mozer, 1988; O'Reilly, Noelle, Braver, & Cohen, 2002; O'Reilly & Munakata, 2000; Phaff, van der Heijden, & Hudson, 1990; Servan-Schreiber, Bruno, Carter, & Cohen, 1998; Schneider & Detweiler, 1988). Equally important, it provides a unifying account of a constellation of processes and constructs related to attention. These are considered in the remainder of this section.

Controlled versus Automatic Processing

This is one of the oldest, and most fundamental constructs in cognitive psychology (Posner & Snyder, 1975; Shiffrin & Schneider, 1977). This distinction is cast largely in terms of the reliance on attention. Controlled processes are defined as those that rely on attention for execution, while automatic processes are defined as those that can be carried out without attention. One of the earliest applications of this construct was to the Stroop task (Posner & Snyder, 1975). Color naming was considered to be controlled because it relies on attention. Without attention to the color, subjects will read the word. Furthermore, the color has no impact on word reading, even when it conflicts with the word being read. Conversely, word reading is automatic because it does not appear to rely on attention. Even when asked to name the color, if a conflicting word is present it slows the response to the color (the classic Stroop effect; MacLeod, 1991; Stroop, 1935). This is thought to reflect the fact that the word is processed even without the allocation of attention. However, there are problems with a simple dichotomous distinction between color naming and word reading in terms of controlled versus automatic processing.

First, it is not clear that any cognitive process can occur entirely independently of attention. For example, although an individual is reading the words on this page, presumably he or she is not doing so out loud. Thus word reading, at least as it is practiced in the Stroop task, is not entirely independent of attention and control. Second, it is not clear that color naming is always dependent on attention and control. In a clever experiment, MacLeod and Dunbar (1988) had participants learn associations between arbitrary shapes (displayed in black and white) and names for them that happened to be color words. At various points during training, they tested their participants' ability to name shapes that were displayed in colors that conflicted with their names. As might be guessed, they found that early in training a shape's color interfered with the ability to provide its name. In other words, in this task, color naming behaved as if it were the automatic process, contradicting the traditional suggestion that it is controlled. Kahneman and Treisman (1984) reviewed a number of other attentional findings, concluding that all processes rely on attention to some degree, and that this may vary in a graded fashion. This is consistent with MacLeod and Dunbar's findings (which also demonstrated that, as subjects became more proficient at shape naming, the color of the shape came to influence this less, while the shape's name came to interfere with color naming). Our model offers a mechanistically explicit account of these findings.

As noted earlier, in the absence of any input from the task-demand units, neither color naming nor word reading can be carried out. This is because the associative units in both pathways rest in too unresponsive a region of their activation function. Thus, even word reading requires attention. At the same time, connections in the word-reading pathway are stronger. Thus, the amount of activity of the task-demand unit needed to support word reading is less than that needed for color naming. In other words, word reading relies less on attention or control than does color naming. It is critical to note, however, that even in the absence of task-demand unit activity *some* information can flow along a pathway. Although this may not be enough to elicit an overt response, it may be enough to influence processing. Thus color naming can be influenced by information in the word pathway and therefore demands more attention when the word conflicts with the color name than when it is congruent. However, this effect is relative. For example, when color naming competes with a *weaker* process, the reverse will be true. This was the situation in MacLeod and Dunbar's (1998) shape-naming experiment, in which the association of a shape with a color word is weaker than a color with a color word. Thus, different processes vary in the degree to which they rely on attention, and this also varies for a given process based on the context in which it is carried out. From this perspective, the distinction between controlled and automatic processing is not dichotomous and absolute but, rather, graded and relative: Some processes are more automatic than others, and processes vary in their automaticity based on the context in which they occur. While this demands quantitative rather than qualitative characterization of processes, our model offers a framework in which such quantification can be carried out in terms of the connection strengths in the relevant pathways.

Types of Attention

We began the previous section by defining controlled processes as those that rely on attention. But how do we define attention? In our model, attention can be defined as the influence that activity in the task-demand units has on processing in the color and word pathways. Note that this does not rely on any qualitatively distinct mechanisms. Attention arises from the flow of activity between units and over connections that are qualitatively identical to those used to actually perform the task. This suggests that we can define attention, in the most general way, as the modulatory influence that representations of one type have on selecting which (or to what degree) representations of other types are processed, that is, how representations of one type guide the flow of activity among other types. Thus, the representation of an object may influence which sensory features are processed, just as in our model the representation of a task demand influenced which dimensions of the stimulus were processed. The representation of a strong stimulus may even have a "bottom-up" influence on representations of task demands.[5] This idea accords well with a theory of attention that has emerged from the neurophysiological literature—the biased competition theory proposed by Desimone and Duncan (1995). This theory assumes that in the brain, different representations compete for expression, and that the role of attention is to bias this competition in favor of some competitors over others. The source of the bias can be bottom up (e.g., driven by a stimulus) or top down (driven by a higher level "template"). In our model, the top-down flow of activity from the task-demand units literally biased the associative units in each pathway, modulating their responsivity and thereby influencing the competition between information in each pathway and guiding its flow along one relative to the other.

As appealing as the generality of this perspective on attention is, it raises an important issue. On the one hand, the guided activation theory and the biased competition theory emphasize the general nature of attention and the broad range of circumstances in which attentional interactions can occur. This provides a general framework for thinking about attention and, in our case, explicitly modeling attentional interactions. On the other hand, the very breadth of this range invites the following, as yet unanswered question: Are there meaningful distinctions to be made between attentional interactions that occur in different domains, at different levels of processing, or in different "directions" (e.g., top down vs. bottom up). For example, are there systematic differences in the dynamics or scope of modulatory interactions? One answer to this question was implicit in the introduction to this chapter, in the choice to focus on "controlled attention," suggesting that attentional interactions related to "control" exhibit a cohesive set of properties that distinguish them from other types of attentional interactions. This choice is motivated both by functional and neurobiological considerations and bears a close similarity to a highly influential taxonomy proposed by Posner and Petersen (1990; see also Posner, 1980). These authors distinguished between three attentional systems in the brain: an anterior attentional system (housed in the frontal lobes) associated with cognitive control and action selection, a posterior attentional system (housed in the parietal and occiptal lobes) associated with orienting and perceptual attention, and an arousal system (subserved by brainstem neuromodulatory systems) associated with sustained attention and vigilance. Work building on our model of attention and its relationship to neural mechanisms has reached a largely convergent perspective that makes complementary contributions to our understanding of how attention and cognitive control operate and are implemented in the brain.

Functional Requirements for Cognitive Control

The modeling efforts previously discussed have focused on a specific set of mechanisms that explain how cognitive control gives rise to attentional effects. However, a more general consideration of cognitive control suggests that additional mechanisms are required for its operation. To see this, let us first consider the function of the task-demand units in the Stroop model. So far, we have focused on their attentional effects—that is, their ability to select one source of information for processing over another. However, more generally, they can be viewed as implementing a mapping from a particular set of inputs to a particular set of outputs. For example, the color task-demand unit represents the relationship between color stimuli and their names. From this vantage point, the task-demand units can be seen as carrying out the function of rules, intentions, or goal representations in other theoretical frameworks. All these specify a relationship between existing states (determined by external sensory inputs or internal influences such as memories, emotions, etc.) and desired outcomes that demand particular behaviors in order to be achieved.

Two critical requirements for the representation of task demands, rules, intentions, or goals are that these be actively maintained while the relevant behaviors are performed and then adaptively updated when behavior has achieved the desired outcome or is no longer appropriate: the task is complete, the rule has changed, or the intention or goal has been achieved. This suggests that the apparatus responsible for cognitive control include mechanisms responsible for active maintenance and adaptive updating. Interestingly, these functions are just those for which the prefrontal cortex (PFC) appears to be specialized. This has led us to propose that the PFC subserves the function carried out by the task-demand units in our model: The active and sustained representation of task demands, such as rules and goals—what we have sometimes referred to more broadly as internal representations of context (Cohen, Braver, & O'Reilly, 1996; Cohen & Servan-Schreiber, 1992)—that bias, or guide, the flow of activity along task-relevant pathways, in accord with the guided activation theory. However, the original model lacks critical features, such as the ability to determine on its own which task-demand representation should be active, just how active this should be, for how long, and how this should be updated when a new one is required—that is, it lacks mechanisms for adaptive updating.

Work over the past decade has directly addressed these issues by augmenting the basic model, constrained by neuroscientific data. Although a detailed consideration of these developments is beyond the scope of this chapter, a brief review illustrates how cognitive control can be implemented in a neural system that is self-organized and self-regulated, without recourse to unexplained mechanisms or intelligence (i.e., without the need for a "homunculus").

A NEURAL SYSTEM FOR CONTROLLED ATTENTION

Active Maintenance

The first requirement for a system of control is that it be able to actively maintain representations of task demand, rules, or goals over temporally extended periods (e.g., during performance of the task), in the absence of external support. For example, subjects do not need to be reminded, trial after trial, to name the color of the Stroop stimulus in a block of trials. Models of sustained activity in PFC have implemented this property using recurrent connectivity (Braver, Cohen, & Servan-Schreiber, 1995; Durstewizt, Seamans, & Sejnowski, 2000; Wang, 1999; Zipser, 1991). This gives rise to attractor dynamics, allowing sets of units with mutually excitatory connections to actively maintain themselves in the absence of input (i.e., as an "attractor state"; Hopfield & Tank, 1986). Recently, biophysically more detailed explorations have suggested that intracellular mechanisms may also contribute to active maintenance, allowing individual units to be "latched" into an on or an off state (Frank, Louhry, & O'Reilly, 2001). However, the importance that this has for models at the systems level remains to be explored.

Adaptive Updating

A second critical property is that the system must be able not only to maintain task representations but also to update these appropriately. This requires that representations in PFC resist perturbation by task-irrelevant inputs (i.e., avoid distraction), while responding to inputs that signal the need for a change (i.e., avoid perseveration). The ability for appropriate updating is central to the flexibility of cognitive control, and disturbances of PFC are known to be associated with distractibility, perseveration, or both. There is growing evidence to support the hypothesis that updating relies on a dopamine-mediated adaptive gating mechanism subserved by the ventral tegmental area (VTA), a dopaminergic nucleus in the brainstem that projects widely to prefrontal areas. In initial work (Braver & Cohen, 2000; O'Reilly, Braver, & Cohen, 1999), we evaluated the plausibility of a simple version of this hypothesis, by implementing a transient gating signal in the task-demand (PFC) layer, that rendered these units temporarily responsive to input from posterior structures (see Figure 6.3). In the absence of this gating signal, representations in the task-demand layer were insensitive to exogenous input, allowing them to maintain the current task demand representation against impinging sources of interference. However, when a gating signal occurred, inputs from other parts of the system could drive activity in the task-demand layer, activating a new representation in that layer. More recently, we have begun to explore the possibility that a more powerful system involving dopaminergic projections to the basal ganglia subserves this gating function (e.g., Frank et al., 2001). This elaboration allows more focused forms of gating that can support hierarchical updating of goals, subgoals, and so on. Nevertheless, the proposal that a dopaminergic, brainstem-mediated gating mechanism regulates the updating of goal representations in PFC raises a critical question: How does this system know when to produce a gating signal, and what new state to produce in the PFC?

The answer to this question comes from important new discoveries regarding the effects of dopamine. Once thought to mediate the hedonic value of a reward, recent work suggests that dopamine release may function as a learning signal, reinforcing associations that provide better predictions of reward (Shultz, Dayan, & Montague, 1997). Importantly, the parameter used to implement this function in computational models (Montague, Dayan, & Sejnowski, 1996) bears a remarkable similarity to the parameter we have used in models to implement a dopamine-based gating signal (Braver & Cohen, 2000). In a series of models, we have illustrated that implementing concurrent effects of the dopamine signal on reinforcement learning and gating allows the system to associate stimuli with the gating signal that predict reward, and thus learn how to update representations in the PFC appropriately (e.g., Braver & Cohen, 2000; Rougier & O'Reilly, 2002). We have used these mechanisms to account for detailed behavioral and neurobiological data regarding the function of the

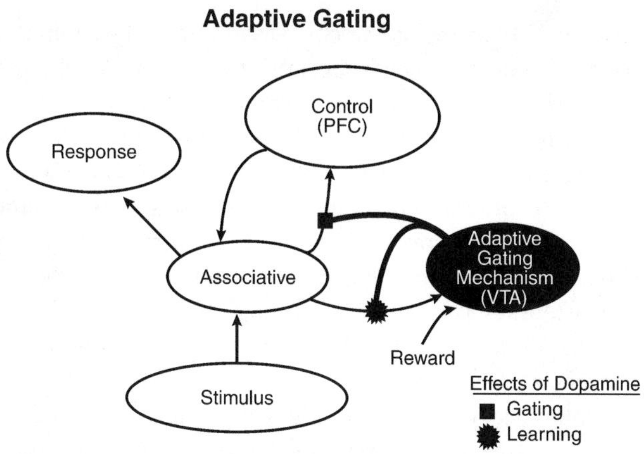

Adaptive Gating

FIGURE 6.3. Model with an adaptive gating mechanism (VTA). Activity of the VTA regulates input to the PFC layer from the associative layer, at the same time training connections from the associative layer back to the VTA. Training occurs according to the temporal differences (predictive Hebbian) learning algorithm (Sutton, 1988). This compares inputs from the associative layer with reward signals, and strengthens connections from the associative layer to the VTA for cues that successfully predict reward. This interacts synergistically with the gating mechanism, because cues that are associated with PFC representations that lead to the procurement of reward thereby predict reward. This strengthens their connections to the VTA, so that in the future they will be more likely to generate a gating signal, activate their associated PFC representation, better predict reward, and therefore receive greater strengthening, and so on.

PFC (O'Reilly et al., 2002; Reynolds & Braver, 2002) in tasks that rely on the flexible deployment of control.

Conflict Monitoring and Regulation of the Degree of Control

The mechanisms described thus far address the ability to represent task-demand information, maintain it, and update it as needed. However, they do not address a different set of questions, which is how the system knows when top-down control is needed in the first place, and just how much is needed to achieve a goal? The need for such mechanisms becomes apparent if we assume that, as in the rest of the brain, representations within the PFC compete for expression. Such competition might provide a partial explanation for the capacity limitations of cognitive control. Such capacity limitations are readily apparent to anyone who has tried to attend to e-mail and talk on the phone at the same time or to talk to a passenger while driving under adverse conditions. These limitations are also fundamental to the distinction between controlled and automatic processing, which assumes that controlled processing relies on a capacity-limited attentional system (e.g., the use of dual-task designs to identify reliance on controlled processing rests on this assumption). Given competition within the PFC, it becomes important for the system to determine whether PFC representation is needed to perform a given task, and if so, how active the representation must be to support adequate performance. Insofar as a weakly active PFC representation leaves room for others to also be active (and thereby other goals to be simultaneously pursued), it is advantageous for the system to titrate the activity of PFC representations to current task needs. In our work with the original Stroop model, we examined the requirements that different processes had for top-down control. As discussed earlier, weaker pathways (e.g., for color naming) required stronger activation of the corresponding task-demand unit to achieve the same level of performance, and this was especially true when conflicting information was present in competing pathways. Conversely, stronger pathways needed less (but always some) top-down support. Recently we have begun to consider what mechanisms might support the adaptive regulation of task demand activity to meet current task needs.

Our approach to this problem was inspired by the observations about attention with which we began: The primary function of attention is to support the processing of task-appropriate sources of information against competition from interfering sources. Put another way, the role of attention is to reduce *conflicts* in processing. Therefore, the occurrence of conflict provides a natural signal of the need for attentional control We have proposed that monitoring for conflicts in processing is subserved by a specific neural system: the anterior cingulate cortex (ACC). This hypothesis is more fully elaborated in Botvinick, Braver, Yeung, Ullsperger, Carter, and Cohen (Chapter 7, this volume). In brief, the conflict monitoring hypothesis argues that the ACC is responsive to conflict in processing pathways—in particular those that are subject to attentional control by the PFC (i.e., mappings from inputs to outputs)—and that activity in the ACC signals the need to more strongly activate representations in the PFC, in order to better support processing in the task-relevant pathway(s). For example, if the color-naming unit is not sufficiently activated in the Stroop model, then information flowing along this pathway will not compete effectively with interfering information arriving from the word pathway (in the case of an incongruent stimulus). Both response alternatives will become activated, and conflict will ensue. The conflict-monitoring hypothesis asserts that such conflict will engage the ACC, signaling the need to increase activity of the color-naming unit (see Figure 6.4). This hypothesis, and predictions that derive from it, have now received considerable support from behavioral and neuroscientific findings (for a review, see Botvinick et al., Chapter 7, this volume).[6]

The conflict-monitoring hypothesis makes the strong claim that while the ACC plays a role in conflict monitoring and the recruitment of attentional control, it is not responsible for the *allocation* of control. This function is ascribed to the PFC. This assertion contrasts with specific claims about the role of the ACC made by Posner and Petersen (1990) in their original formulation of the anterior attentional system (see also Posner & Dehaene, 1994; Posner & DiGirolamo, 1998). However, it does not violate the more general spirit of their proposal that top-down attentional control is subserved by a frontal system involving the ACC. The primary thrust of the conflict-monitoring hypothesis is to add further specification to one component of this system and suggest a modified set of structure–function relationships. One limitation of the conflict-monitoring hypothesis, however, is that in its present form it does not precisely characterize the mechanisms by which ACC conflict monitoring engages PFC control. The models that have been developed to date implement this as a direct influence of the ACC on the PFC. More recently, we have begun to explore alternative mechanisms that may mediate this influence. One hypothesis is that this involves the locus coeruleus.

The locus coeruleus (LC) is the brainstem neuromodulatory nucleus responsible for most of the norepinephrine (NE) released in the brain (Berridge & Waterhouse, 2003; Foote, Bloom, & Aston-Jones, 1983). It has widespread projections throughout the neocortex. Previous work (Servan-Schreiber, Printz, & Cohen, 1990) has suggested that the effects of NE release can be modeled as a change in the gain (steepness) of the activation function of connectionist units (see Figure 6.2b). This has the effect of augmenting the activity of

A. Detection of Conflict

B. Recruitment of Control

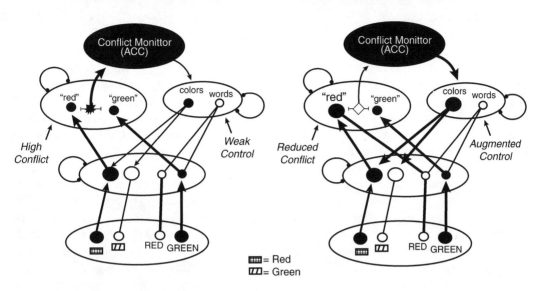

FIGURE 6.4. Model with conflict-monitoring mechanism (ACC). (A) Weak control allows conflict to develop at the response layer as a result of competing inputs from different pathways. This is detected by the ACC. (B) Detection of conflict within the ACC augments activated units in the PFC layer, producing additional top-down control and a reduction of conflict.

units that are already activated and further suppressing the activity units that are already being inhibited. That is, an increase in gain increases the contrast of the current pattern of activity. This produces precisely the effect within the PFC that is needed in response to conflict. In fact, such contrast enhancement of PFC representations is how adjustments in control have been implemented in our simulations of the conflict-monitoring hypothesis to date (Botvinick, Braver, Carter, Barch, & Cohen, 2001; Yeung, Botvinick, & Cohen, in press). However, in these models, contrast enhancement in the PFC was assumed to be produced directly by ACC activity. While this remains a possibility, we have begun to consider the possibility that this effect is actually mediated by NE release from the LC.

LC-mediated modulation of the PFC is consistent with several lines of evidence, including modeling work that specifies a role for the LC in attentional modulation (e.g., Gilzenrat et al., 2002; Holmes, Nieuwenhuis, & Gilzenrat, & Cohen, 2002; Robertson, Mattingley, Rorden, & Driver, 1998; Usher, Cohen, Servan-Schreiber, Rajkowski, & Aston-Jones, 1999; Yu & Dayan, 2002), as well as recent neuroanatomic evidence suggesting that the ACC is a primary source of cortical projections to the LC (Rajkowski, Lu, Zhu, Cohen, & Aston-Jones, 2000). The appeal of this hypothesis is that it provides a mechanism by which conflict detection within the ACC can augment control without specific knowledge about which particular representations in PFC require augmentation: A global signal can have specific effects. Although details concerning the dynamics of LC-mediated modulation of the PFC are beyond what can be considered here, it is important to note that our hypothesis is that transient (phasic) rather than sustained (tonic) release of NE mediates the modulation of PFC. This forms part of a more general theory about the role of the LC in regulating attention, that we briefly review next.

Exploration versus Exploitation and Regulation of the Focus of Attention and Control

The control mechanisms described previously explain how behavior can be guided by representations of task demands, rules, intentions, or goals in the PFC, adaptively modulating their activity as needed to support task performance. According to the conflict-monitoring hypothesis, when performance degrades and conflict increases, control should increase. However, what about situations in which behavior continues to fall short, despite compensatory adjustments in control? For example, in a Stroop experiment, what if the color stimulus is progressively degraded? The gradual increase in conflict should lead to concomitant increases in control. However, at some point, if the color is degraded beyond recognizability, it makes no sense to further augment control. Rather, control should be withdrawn from this task and some other goal should be pursued. Or, consider the following situation that is perhaps more ecologically valid: An animal is picking berries from a tree. At first berries are everywhere, and the task may not require much effort or attention, but as berries become more scarce, more attention is needed. After some point, however, increasing attention will not help; there are just too few berries left to make the effort worthwhile. At this point, some other behavior should be pursued. These situations suggest that as conflict increases and reward diminishes, at some point the relationship between conflict and control should reverse. This tension between optimizing control to reap the benefits of the current behavioral program and abandoning the current program when it may be more advantageous to sample alternative behavioral programs is well recognized in machine learning, where it is referred to as the trade-off between exploitation and exploration.

We have hypothesized that interactions between the ACC and the LC may regulate the balance in this trade-off (Usher et al., 1999). This builds on observations made by Aston-Jones, Rajkowski, Kubiak, and Alexinsky (1994), indicating that in the awake behaving monkey, the LC shifts between two operating modes that correspond closely with behavioral performance in a simple target detection task. In the "phasic mode," when the animal is performing optimally, the LC shows only moderate levels of tonic discharge, while it exhibits a phasic response selectively to target stimuli but not to distractors. In the "tonic mode," the tonic level of discharge is higher, but there are no phasic responses to target stimuli, reaction time to targets is slower, and the animal commits a greater number of false alarms to distractors.[7] Usher and colleagues (1999) developed a biophysically plausible model of LC function that accounted for transitions between phasic and tonic modes in terms of a single physiological variable (coupling between LC cells) and at the same time explained the impact of these shifts on task performance.[8] In brief, the model suggests that in the phasic mode, the strong LC response to target stimuli facilitates their processing by transiently increasing gain which, at the response layer, has the effect of lowering response threshold. Because this effect is selective to targets, it improves both target detection performance and reaction time. In contrast, in the tonic mode, the absence of a phasic response accounts for the increase in response time to target stimuli, while the increased but indiscriminant release of NE lowers the system's response threshold to other stimuli (e.g., distractors), accounting for the increase in false alarms.

The specificity of the LC phasic response to the target (in the phasic mode) has been demonstrated in a number of additional studies, including reversal experiments in which LC has been shown to reliably acquire the new target before the animal's overt behavior has done so (e.g., Aston-Jones, Rajkowski, & Kubiak, 1997). These characteristics suggest that in the phasic mode, the LC functions as an attentional filter that selects for the occurrence (i.e., *timing*) of task-relevant stimuli, much as cortical attentional systems filter the *content* of a stimulus. The existence of such a temporal filter is consistent with several recent psychophysical studies (e.g., Coull & Nobre, 1998). At the same time, by increasing the gain of cortical representations, the LC phasic response can also enhance the effects of cortical selection by content (e.g., the top-down effects of the PFC). Together, these effects allow the LC phasic response to selectively facilitate responses to task-relevant stimuli when they occur. One immediate question, however, is, What is the adaptive value of the tonic mode, which seems to deteriorate performance? We have argued that the tonic mode may support exploratory behavior. By reducing phasic responses to target stimuli, and increasing tonic NE release, the system is more effectively driven by task-irrelevant stimuli. Such responsiveness is not adaptive with respect to the specified experimental task, because it permits the processing of task-irrelevant stimuli and the sampling of other behavioral programs. However, it may be highly adaptive if either the current task is no longer remunerative, or if the environment changes and more valuable opportunities for reward or new behavioral imperatives have appeared. From this perspective, a shift from the LC phasic to the tonic mode may shift the behavioral strategy from exploitation (when this is no longer adaptive) to exploration (when a new goal should be sought). Loosely speaking, this "throws the ball up in the air, so another team can take it." Viewed from the perspective of attentional control, the LC phasic mode supports the current control state (exploitation), while the LC tonic mode provokes a withdrawal of control from the current task, favoring the sampling of other behavioral goals (exploration), which raises one more important question: What information can the system use to determine whether it should exploit (LC phasic mode) or explore (LC tonic mode)? The answer to this question closes the loop, both in the control system and in our discussion.

We hypothesize that ACC conflict monitoring can provide the necessary information. This hypothesis requires only one additional assumption: that the ACC is able to integrate conflict over two time frames—a short one (seconds) and a long one (minutes). Consider the following two circumstances. In one, performance is good and there are still rewards to be accrued from the current task, but there are occasional lapses in performance producing transient increases in conflict (e.g., on single trials). Under these conditions, control should be increased each time there is a lapse, to restore performance. That is, control should be increased when long-term conflict is low but there is a momentary increase in short-term conflict. In contrast, consider a different situation in which performance has been poor and conflict has been *persistently* high. At some point, this situation should encourage the withdrawal of control, irrespective of short-term changes in conflict. A similar situation should arise when, irrespective of performance, opportunities for reward diminish. A relatively simple equation can capture these relationships,[9] which indexes the need for control as a function of short-term conflict and reward, discounted by the accumulation of long-term conflict and dimunition of reward (see Figure 6.5). This computation can be used to drive shifts between LC phasic and tonic modes by influencing simple physiological parameters (Brown et al., 2004; Usher et al., 1999). Taken together, these mechanisms would constitute a self-regulating system that is responsive to demands for control over different time scales and is sensitive to the current value of exploration versus exploitation (Figure 6.6). These mechanisms are consistent with known properties of the LC, ACC, and their anatomic connectivity; however, their validation presents a challenge to further neurophysiological investigation.[10]

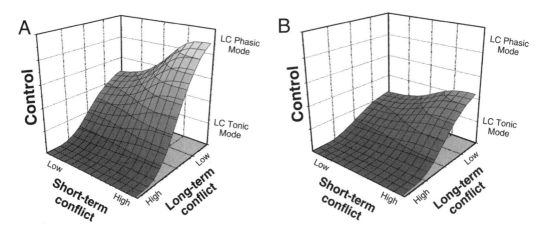

FIGURE 6.5. Relationship of control to conflict and reward (see note 9 for the equation defining this relationship). (A) Under conditions of high reward and low long-term conflict, transient increases in conflict (short-term conflict) produce greater control, by driving LC into the phasic mode. This effect is diminished as long-term conflict increases, driving LC into tonic mode. (B) Low reward damps the effect of short-term conflict, driving the LC into the tonic mode irrespective of conflict.

Neural System for Adaptive Regulation of Control

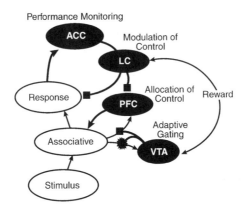

FIGURE 6.6. Integrated neural system for the adaptive regulation of control. This system is able to adaptively update control representations in PFC, learn how to do so, and modulate the strength of top-down control in response to prevailing balance between reward and short-term and long-term degradations in performance (as indexed by conflict).

CONCLUSIONS AND FUTURE CHALLENGES

This chapter has reviewed recent theoretical work, pursued within the connectionist framework, that addresses the nature of controlled attention and its neural implementation. The goal of this work is to provide a mechanistically explicit account of how processes that give rise to the phenomena of attention and control are implemented in the brain. The hypotheses reviewed suggest that control relies on the activation of appropriate representations in the PFC. These representations can be thought of as task demands, rules, intentions, or goals that direct behavior to produce desired outcomes by biasing processing and guiding the flow of activity along pathways responsible for mapping inputs to desired outputs. As summarized in Figure 6.6, PFC representations are regulated by several mechanisms, including a dopamine-mediated system for updating PFC representations in specific task contexts, and learning how to do so; an ACC-mediated system for assessing the demand for control; and an LC-mediated system for modulating PFC representations in response to these demands. These hypotheses define a mechanistically explicit, self-regulating system of control that is responsive to adaptive needs at different time scales and of fundamentally different types (e.g., exploration vs. exploitation). One important feature of these hypotheses is their suggestion that brainstem neuromodulatory systems—once thought to be responsible for the regulation of nonspecific aspects of psychological function, such as motivation (dopamine) and arousal (NE)—may play a significantly more central and specific role in information processing.

Of course, these mechanisms represent only a first step toward a more complete understanding of the neural mechanisms that underlie attention and control. First, they address only controlled attention, and not the many other forms and levels of attentional effects. However, even within the scope of controlled attention, many challenges remain. For example, it is possible to register a goal or intention for the future and then to dispatch this for pursuit sometime (hours, days or even years) in the future. These forms of control cannot be explained by active maintenance of representations in PFC alone, but they are likely to involve interactions between the PFC and medial temporal lobe structures that subserve episodic memory (Cohen & O'Reilly, 1996). There are also critical interactions between control and motivation, most likely involving interactions between the PFC and limbic structures. Perhaps the most perplexing puzzle that remains concerns the nature of representations in the PFC. Our models to date have stipulated the presence of representations in the PFC required to perform a given task. However, it seems unlikely that without infinite capacity, the PFC can house all the possible representations needed to meet the arbitrarily large set of potential task demands. A characteristic feature of human behavior is the flexibility of control, manifest as the ability to perform novel tasks, or to creatively structure new forms of behavior in a novel task environment. How then, with a large but finite set of resources, can the system exhibit the flexibility we witness in our everyday behavior? This question is closely related to an equally important one: How do representations develop in PFC?

Recent work has begun to address many of the questions raised here (for reviews, see Miller & Cohen, 2001; O'Reilly et al., 1999, 2002; Rougier, Noelle, Braver, Cohen, & O'Reilly, 2004). Nevertheless, the human ability to flexibly deploy attention and control, navigating the vast repositories of information available both from the environment and the system's stored knowledge, to respond appropriately under familiar circumstances and creatively under unfamiliar ones, remains one of the most fundamental and interesting mysteries of science. We hope to have illustrated in this chapter that this mystery need not remain intractable to theoretical analysis.

ACKNOWLEDGMENTS

The work reviewed in this chapter has been conducted under the generous and ongoing support of the National Institute of Mental Health and the National Alliance for Research on Schizophrenia and Depression. The authors would also like to note that most of the ideas and findings described in this chapter have emerged from longstanding collaborations with Deanna Barch, Matthew Botvinick, Todd Braver, Cameron Carter, Sander Nieuwenhuis, David Noelle, Randy O'Reilly, and Nick Yeung, as well as Eric Brown and Philip Holmes.

NOTES

1. This reflects the assumption that units are negatively biased. This can be seen from the expression for the activation function: activity $= 1/(1 + e^{-(net\ input)})$. For a net input of 0, this evaluates to an activity of 0.5. However, by assuming that a constant negative bias value is added to the net input (e.g., −4 as was used in Cohen et al., 1990), the unit will have a low activity value for a zero net input.

2. Task-demand units have, in different papers—both our own and those of others—variously been referred to as attention units, context units (designating the "task context"), mapping units, and goal units, which reflects the various perspectives that can be taken on their function (to which we return at the end of the chapter). It also highlights the perils of pursuing scientific research using natural language and the value of explicit, formal models. Ultimately, our theory of attention and its relationship to cognitive control is expressed in the form of the model and *not* in the words that are used to describe it. Thus, where any ambiguity or disagreement may arise about what is claimed by our theory, the model itself (and whatever elaboration of it is required to address the issue) is the final arbiter and not any words used to describe it.

3. The assumption of nonlinearity is justified on both theoretical and empirical grounds. Theoretically, it has been shown that using nonlinear rather than linear units confers considerably greater computational power on the system (e.g., Rumelhart, Hinton, & Williams, 1986). Empirically, it is clear that neurons (whether considered individually or in populations) have finite upper and lower bounds on their activity levels.

4. Two points are worth noting about this effect. First, the term "modulation" often implies a multiplicative effect. Here, however, modulation is produced by adding (biasing) activity from the task-demand unit to the associative units. Nevertheless, because this addition occurs to the net input, which appears in the exponent of the activation function, the effect is in fact multiplicative. Second, note that the effect of this modulation is to place units in the linear range of their activation function, which provides a justification for mathematical models that assume linear response properties (e.g., Brown & Holmes, 2001), by suggesting that those units primarily responsible for processing (i.e., those that are in the "focus of attention") reside in the linear range of an otherwise nonlinear response function.

5. This assumes that there are bottom-up connections to the task-demand units in the model. Although these were not included in the original Cohen et al. (1990) model, variants have included such connections (e.g., Cohen & Huston, 1994; O'Reilly & Munakata, 2000).

6. While this hypothesis proposes that conflict monitoring is subserved by the ACC, it does not claim that this is the *only* function of this structure. Rather, we view conflict monitoring as one of a family of functions subserved by the ACC, that monitor internal processing states for breakdowns in performance, much as the amygdala is thought to monitor the environment for external signs of threat.

7. At present, it is not clear whether these represent dichotomous modes, or ends of a continuum of states that the LC can occupy.

8. Recently, Brown and colleagues (2004) have proposed that changes in baseline firing rate may also serve to drive transitions between LC phasic and tonic modes. Which of these mechanisms (electrotonic coupling, baseline firing rate, or both) is actually operative in the LC remains an area of inquiry. However, what is relevant for present purposes is that LC mode can be determined by one or two easily regulated physiological parameters.

9. Control = reward / [f(conflict$_{long-term}$)*(1 − f(conflict$_{short-term}$))], where f(conflict) = 1/(1 + $e^{-conflict}$)

10. The LC receives extensive projections from both the ACC and the orbitofrontal cortex (Aston-Jones et al., 2002; Rajkowski et al., 2000), which may provide evaluative information regarding both performance and rewards (e.g., Bush et al., 2002; Rolls, 2000). We should also note that the LC has extensive projections throughout the brain (except the hypothalamus and striatum, which it does not innervate). We propose that while NE release in PFC directly modulates control representations, simultaneous release of NE in areas outside the PFC serves to reinforce this effect in other sensory, motor, and associative areas.

REFERENCES

Aston-Jones, G., Rajkowski, J., & Kubiak, P. (1997). Conditioned responses of monkey locus coeruleus neurons anticipate acquisition of discriminative behavior in a vigilance task. *Neuroscience, 80,* 697–715.

Aston-Jones, G., Rajkowski, J., Kubiak, P., & Alexinsky, T. (1994). Locus coeruleus neurons in monkey are selectively activated by attended cues in a vigilance task. *Journal of Neuroscience, 14*(7), 4467–4480.

Aston-Jones, G., Rajkowski, J., Lu, W., Zhu, Y., Cohen, J. D., & Morecraft, R.J. (2002). Prominent projections from the orbital prefrontal cortex to the locus coeruleus in monkey. *Society for Neuroscience Abstracts, 28,* 86–89.

Berridge, C. W., & Waterhouse, B. D. (2003). The locus coeruleus-noradrenergic system: modulation of behavioral state and state-dependent cognitive processes. *Brain Research: Brain Research Review, 42,* 33–84.

Botvinick, M. M., Braver, T. S., Carter, C. S., Barch, D. M., & Cohen, J. D. (2001). Conflict monitoring and cognitive control. *Psychological Review, 108*(3), 624–652.

Braver, T. S., Barch, D. M., & Cohen, J. D. (1999). Cognition and control in schizophrenia: A computational model of dopamine and prefrontal function. *Biological Psychiatry, 46*(3), 312–328.

Braver, T. S., & Cohen, J. D. (2000). On the control of control: The role of dopamine in regulating prefrontal function and working memory. In S. Monsell & J. Driver (Eds.), *Attention and performance XVIII: Control of cognitive processes* (pp. 713–737). Cambridge, MA: MIT Press.

Braver, T. S., & Cohen, J. D. (2001). Working memory, cognitive control, and the prefrontal cortex: Computational and empirical studies. *Cognitive Processing, 2,* 25–55.

Braver, T. S., Cohen, J. D., & Servan-Schreiber, D. (1995). A computational model of prefrontal cortex function. In D. S. Touretzky, G. Tesauro, & T. K. Leen (Eds.), *Advances in neural information processing systems* (Vol. 7, pp. 141–148). Cambridge, MA: MIT Press.

Brown, E., & Holmes, P. (2001). Modeling a simple choice task: Stochastic dynamics of mutually inhibitory neural groups. *Stochastics and Dynamics, 1*(2), 159–191.

Brown, E., Moehlis, J., Holmes, P., Clayton, E., Rajkowski, J., & Aston-Jones, G. (2004). *The influence of spike rate and stimulus duration on noradrenergic neurons.* Manuscript submitted for publication.

Bush, G., Vogt, B. A., Holmes, J., Dale, A. M., Greve, D., Jenike, M. A., et al. (2002). Dorsal anterior cingulate cortex: a role in reward-based decision making. *Proceedings of the National Academy Science USA, 99*(1), 523–528.

Cohen, J. D., Braver, T. S., & O'Reilly, R. C. (1996). A computational approach to prefrontal cortex, cognitive control, and schizophrenia: Recent developments and current challenges. *Philosophical Transactions of the Royal Society of London B, (Biological Sciences), 351,* 1515–1527.

Cohen, J. D., Dunbar, K., & McClelland, J. L. (1990). On the control of automatic processes: A parallel distributed processing model of the Stroop effect. *Psychological Review, 97*(3), 332–361.

Cohen, J. D., & Huston, T. A. (1994). Progress in the use of parallel distributed processing models for understanding attention and performance. In C. Umiltà & M. Moscovitch (Eds.), *Attention and performance XV: Conscious and nonconscious information processing* (pp. 453–476). Cambridge, MA: MIT Press.

Cohen, J. D., & O'Reilly, R. C. (1996). A preliminary theory of the interactions between prefrontal cortex and hippocampus that contribute to planning and prospective memory. In M. Brandimonte, G. O. Einstein, & M. A. McDaniel (Eds.), *Prospective memory: Theory and applications* (pp. 267–295). Hillsdale, NJ: Erlbaum.

Cohen, J. D., Romero, R. D., Servan-Schreiber, D., & Farah, M. J. (1994). Mechanisms of spatial attention: The relation of macrostructure to microstructure in parietal neglect. *Journal of Cognitive Neuroscience, 6*(4), 377–387.

Cohen, J. D., & Servan-Schreiber, D. (1992). Context, cortex and dopamine: A connectionist approach to behavior and biology in schizophrenia. *Psychological Review, 99*, 45–77.

Cohen, J. D., Servan-Schreiber, D., & McClelland, J. L. (1992). A parallel distributed processing approach to automaticity. *American Journal of Psychology, 105*, 239–269.

Coull, J. T., & Nobre, A. C. (1998). Where and when to pay attention: The neural systems for directing attention to spatial locations and to time intervals as revealed by both PET and fMRI. *Journal of Neuroscience, 18*, 7426–7435.

Dehaene, S., & Changeux, J. P. (1989). A simple model of prefrontal cortex function in delayed-response tasks. *Journal of Cognitive Neuroscience, 1*(3), 244–261.

Dehaene, S., & Changeux, J. P. (1991). The Wisconsin card sorting test: Theoretical analysis and modeling in a neuronal network. *Cerebral Cortex, 1*(1), 62–79.

Desimone, R., & Duncan, J. (1995). Neural mechanisms of selective visual attention. *Annual Review of Neuroscience, 18*, 193–222.

Durstewitz, D., Seamans, J. K., & Sejnowski, T. J. (2000). Dopamine-mediated stabilization of delay-period activity in a network model of prefrontal cortex. *Journal of Neurophysiology, 83*(3), 1733–1750.

Foote, S. L., Bloom, F. E., & Aston-Jones, G. (1983). Nucleus locus ceruleus: New evidence of anatomical and physiological specificity. *Physiology Review, 63*, 844–914.

Frank, M. J., Loughry, B., & O'Reilly, C. (2001). Interactions between frontal cortex and basal ganglia in working memory: A computational model. *Cognitive, Affective, and Behavioral Neuroscience, 1*(2), 137–160.

Gilzenrat, M. S., Holmes, B. D., Holmes, P. J., Rajkowski, J., Aston-Jones, G., & Cohen, J. D. (2002). A modified Fitzhugh-Nagumo system simulates locus coeruleus-mediated regulation of cognitive performance. *Neural Networks, 15*, 647–663.

Holmes, B. D., Nieuwenhuis, S., Gilzenrat, M. S., & Cohen, J. D. (2002). *The role of locus coeruleus in mediating the attentional blink: A neurocomputational model.* Poster presented at the annual meeting of the Psychonomic Society, Kansas City, MO.

Hopfield, J. J., & Tank, D. W. (1986). Computing with neural circuits: A model. *Science, 233*, 625–633.

Kahneman, D., & Treisman, A. (1984). Changing views of attention and automaticity. In R. Parasuranam & D. R. Davies (Eds.), *Varieties of attention* (pp. 29–59). New York: Academic Press.

MacLeod, C. M. (1991). Half a century of research on the Stroop effect: An integrative review. *Psychological Bulletin, 109*(2), 163–203.

MacLeod, C. M., & Dunbar, K. (1988). Training and Stroop-like interference: Evidence for a continuum of automaticity. *Journal of Experimental Psychology: Learning, Memory and Cognition, 14*(1), 126–135.

McClelland, J. L. (1993). Toward a theory of information processing in graded, random, and interactive networks. In D. E. Meyer & S. Kornblum (Eds.), *Attention and performance XIV: Synergies in experimental psychology, artificial intelligence, and cognitive neuroscience* (pp. 655–688). Cambridge, MA, MIT Press.

Miller, E. K., & Cohen, J. D. (2001). An integrative theory of prefrontal cortex function. *Annual Review of Neuroscience, 24*, 167–202.

Montague, P. R., Dayan, P., & Sejnowski, T. J. (1996). A framework for mesencephalic dopamine systems based on predictive Hebbian learning. *Journal of Neuroscience, 16*(5), 1936–1947.

Mozer, M. (1988). A connectionist model of selective attention in visual perception. In *Proceedings of the tenth annual conference of the Cognitive Science Society* (pp. 195–201). Hillsdale, NJ: Erlbaum.

O'Reilly, R. C., Braver, T. S., & Cohen, J. D. (1999). A biologically-based neural network model of working memory. In P. Shah & A. Miyake (Eds.), *Models of working memory* (pp. 375–411). Cambridge, UK: Cambridge University Press.

O'Reilly, R. C., & Munakata, Y. (2000). *Computational explorations in cognitive neuroscience: Understanding the mind by simulating the brain.* Cambridge, MA: MIT Press.

O'Reilly, R. C., Noelle, D. C., Braver, T. S., & Cohen, J. D. (2002). Prefrontal cortex in dynamic categorization tasks: Representational organization and neuromodulatory control. *Cerebral Cortex, 12*, 246–257.

Phaf, R. H., Van der Heijden, A. H. C., & Hudson, P. T. (1990). SLAM: A connectionist model for attention in visual selection tasks. *Cognitive Psychology, 22*(3), 273–341.

Posner, M. I. (1980). Orienting of attention. *Quarterly Journal of Experimental Psychology, 32*(1), 3–25.

Posner, M. I., & Dehaene, S. (1994). Attentional networks. *Trends in Neuroscience, 17*, 75–79.

Posner, M. I., & DiGirolamo, G. J. (1998). Executive Attention: Conflict, target detection and cognitive control. In R. Parasuraman (Ed.), *The attentive brain* (pp. 401–423). Cambridge: MIT Press.

Posner, M. I., & Petersen, S. E. (1990). The attention system of the human brain. *Annual Review of Neuroscience, 13*, 25–42.

Posner, M. I., & Snyder, C. R. R. (1975). Attention and cognitive control. In R. L. Solso (Ed.), *Information processing and cognition* (pp. 55–85). Hillsdale, NJ: Erlbaum.

Rajkowski, J., Lu, W., Zhu, Y., Cohen, J., & Aston-Jones, G. (2000). Prominent projections from the anterior cingulate cortex to the locus coeruleus (LC) in rhesus monkey. *Society of Neuroscience Abstracts, 26*, 838.15.

Reynolds, J. R., & Braver, T. S. (2002, April). *Computational and neural mechanisms of task-switching.* Paper presented at the ninth annual meeting of the Cognitive Neuroscience Society, San Francisco.

Robertson, I. H., Mattingley, J. B., Rorden, C., & Driver, J. (1998). Phasic alerting of neglect patients overcomes their spatial deficit in visual awareness. *Nature, 395*, 169–172.

Rolls, E. T. (2000). The orbitofrontal cortex and reward. *Cerebral Cortex, 10*(3), 284–294.

Rougier, N. P., Noelle, D. C., Braver, T. S., Cohen, J. D., & O'Reilly, R. C. (2004). *Prefrontal cortex and the flexibility of cognitive control: Rules without symbols.* Manuscript in submission.

Rumelhart, D. E., Hinton, G. E., & Williams, R. J. (1986). Learning internal representations by error propagation. In D. E. Rumelhart, J. L. McClelland, & PDP Research Group (Eds.), *Parallel distributed processing: Explorations in the microstructure of cognition* (Vol. 1, pp. 318–362). Cambridge, MA: MIT Press.

Rumelhart, D. E., McClelland, J. L., & PDP Research Group. (Eds.). (1986). *Parallel distributed processing: Explorations in the microstructure of cognition.* Cambridge, MA: MIT Press.

Schneider, W., & Detweiler, M. (1988). The role of practice in dual-task performance: toward workload modeling in a connectionist/control architecture. *Human Factors, 30*(5), 539–566.

Schultz, W., Dayan, P., & Montague, P. R. (1997). A neural substrate of prediction and reward. *Science, 275*, 1593–1599.

Servan-Schreiber, D., Bruno, R., Carter, C., & Cohen, J. D. (1998). Dopamine and the mechanisms of cognition. Part I: A neural network model predicting dopamine effects on selective attention. *Biological Psychiatry, 43*, 713–722.

Servan-Schreiber, D., Printz, H., & Cohen, J. D. (1990). A network model of catecholamine effects: Gain, signal-to-noise ratio, and behavior. *Science, 249*, 892–895.

Shiffrin, R. M., & Schneider, W. (1977). Controlled and automatic human information processing: II. Perceptual learning automaticity, attending and a general theory. *Psychological Review, 84*(2), 127–190.

Stroop, J. R. (1935). Studies of interference in serial verbal reactions. *Journal of Experimental Psychology, 18,* 643–662.

Sutton, R. (1988). Learning to predict by the method of temporal difference. *Machine Learning, 3,* 9.

Usher, M., Cohen, J. D., Servan-Schreiber, D., Rajkowski, J., & Aston-Jones, G. (1999). The role of locus coeruleus in the regulation of cognitive performance. *Science, 283,* 549–554.

Wang, X. J. (1999). Synaptic basis of cortical persistent activity: The importance of NMDA receptors to working memory. *Journal of Neuroscience, 19,* 9587–9603.

Yeung, N., Botvinick, M. M., & Cohen, J. D. (in press). The neural basis of error detection: Conflict monitoring and the error-related negativity. *Psychologial Review.*

Yu, A. J., & Dayan, P. (2002). Acetylcholie in cortical inference. *Neural Networks, 15,* 719–730.

Zipser, D. (1991). Recurrent network model of the neural mechanism of short-term active memory. *Neural Computation, 3*(2), 179–193.

7

Conflict Monitoring

Computational and Empirical Studies

Matthew Botvinick, Todd S. Braver, Nick Yeung, Markus Ullsperger,
Cameron S. Carter, and Jonathan D. Cohen

One of the most remarkable aspects of the human brain is its capacity to process tremendous amounts of information in parallel. As powerful as this capacity is, it comes at a price: a susceptibility to interference or conflict. Indeed, many "attentional" limitations on processing capacity can be viewed as stemming from conflict or competition between or within processing pathways (see, e.g., Allport, 1987; Cohen, Dunbar, & McClelland, 1990; Duncan, 1996; Navon & Miller, 1987). From this perspective, conflict prevention may be viewed as a central function of attentional or control systems (Allport, 1980).

If attention is viewed as a conflict prevention mechanism, one important question that arises is, How does the processing system "know" when attention is required? On what basis do attentional mechanisms detect situations in which there is a risk of conflict, or where conflict is already occurring? It seems reasonable to assume that there are numerous sources of information that attentional systems might exploit to this end. In the laboratory setting these might include task instructions, explicit feedback concerning performance, or previous experience with similar task settings.

A series of studies across our several labs has suggested another possibility: Attentional systems may evaluate for conflict directly, through a process we have called *conflict monitoring*. The overall proposal here can be stated in terms of the *conflict-monitoring hypothesis*, which has two parts:

1. Specific subsystems of the human brain respond to the occurrence of conflicts in information processing, and in particular response competition.
2. The detection of conflict triggers compensatory adjustments in attention or control, which have the effect of preventing or reducing conflict in subsequent performance.

Over the past 5 years, considerable evidence has emerged in support of this two-part hypothesis. In our own work, empirical support has come from two general sources: behavioral studies, using chronometric techniques to probe attentional function, and studies using methods from cognitive neuroscience, focusing, in particular on the anterior cingulate cortex. In addition, a special, integrative role has been played by a third research modality, computational modeling. Modeling has served the overall research program in several ways. First, implementing the conflict-monitoring hypothesis in the form of explicit neural network simulations has allowed, indeed required, us to be as explicit as possible about what the theory proposes (and, equally importantly, what it leaves open). Second, it has provided a means to validate the internal consistency of the theory, and to demonstrate its sufficiency in accounting for available data. Third, it has provided a language for bridging between neuroscientific and behavioral data. Finally, and perhaps most important, it has given rise to numerous predictions, many of which we have successfully confirmed through empirical studies.

In what follows, we review some of the central results from our work on the conflict-monitoring hypothesis, with a focus on the synergistic relationship between computational modeling and empirical work. In addition, we present results from new two studies, which were conducted in response to a recent challenge to the conflict-monitoring hypothesis.

CONFLICT DETECTION AND ANTERIOR CINGULATE CORTEX

One of the original motivations for the conflict-monitoring hypothesis came from a review of neuroimaging and electrophysiology studies reporting activation of a particular area of the frontal lobe, the anterior cingulate cortex (ACC). Botvinick, Braver, Barch, Carter, and Cohen (2001) noted that most such studies could be seen as falling into one of three categories: (1) studies involving tasks in which the subject needed to override a prepotent response tendency (e.g., the Stroop task); (2) studies involving tasks in which the subject selected among several, equally correct responses, a circumstance referred to as underdetermined responding (e.g., stem completion); and (3) studies in which ACC activation was associated with error commission.

The conflict-monitoring hypothesis arose out of an attempt to find a common feature among these three task settings, which might explain the presence in each of ACC engagement. According to the theory, ACC activation in all three settings can be understood as a response to the occurrence of conflict, and in particular response competition.

Botvinick and colleagues (2001) sought to articulate this interpretation, and to evaluate its sufficiency to account for some benchmark empirical findings, through a series of three computational models. The approach, in each case, was to start with an existing neural network model of a relevant task, adding only a single "conflict-monitoring unit." This took input from the output or response units in the base model, computing a measure of response competition or conflict (Figure 7.1). With this additional element in place, the underlying models were used, otherwise unaltered from their original form, to simulate tasks studied in pivotal ACC activation studies, with the prediction that the conflict-monitoring unit would show a profile of activity matching that of the ACC in corresponding task contexts.

A first model focused on a classic response override task, the Stroop color-naming task. Neuroimaging studies had revealed greater ACC activation on incongruent trials in this task than congruent or neutral ones (e.g., Carter, Mintun, & Cohen, 1995). To simulate this finding, we implemented a model of the Stroop task originally described by Cohen and colleagues (1990) and modified by Cohen and Huston (1994), adding to the latter the conflict-

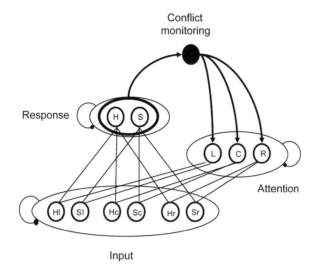

Conflict
monitoring

Response

Attention

Input

FIGURE 7.1. Illustration of the model employed by Botvinick et al. (2001) to simulate ACC activation in the setting of error commission and to simulate the Gratton effect. Connections from conflict monitoring to attention were included only in the latter simulation. Labels for attention units denote left, right, and center. Labels for input units denote position-specific letter inputs (e.g., Hl —letter H in lefthand position). The same model was employed by Yeung et al. (in press) to simulate detailed aspects of the error-related negativity (see Figure 7.2).

monitoring unit described earlier. Activity in this unit was recorded as the base model was used to simulate congruent, neutral, and incongruent trials. The conflict-monitoring unit showed greater activation on incongruent trials, matching the profile of ACC activation in the empirical studies.

A second model focused on an underdetermined responding task, stem completion. Empirical work had shown ACC activation in association with this task, as compared with baseline tasks involving more highly constrained responding (e.g., Buckner et al., 1995). To show how the conflict-monitoring hypothesis might account for this finding, we again adopted a preexisting model of the task of interest (McClelland & Rumelhart, 1981), adding only a conflict-monitoring unit. The base model was used to simulate stem completion and, for comparison, word reading. As in the first simulation, activation in the conflict-monitoring unit paralleled ACC activation, rising higher on the underdetermined responding task (here due to transient competition among candidate responses). The same mechanism that had been used to account for ACC activation in response override tasks thus appeared adequate to account for ACC activation in the setting of underdetermined responding.

The third area in which ACC activation had been repeatedly demonstrated was in association with errors. Rather than neuroimaging data, the relevant findings here came from human electrophysiology studies, where a midline frontal evoked potential, the error-related negativity (ERN) had been reported to follow error commission (Gehring, Coles, Meyer, & Donchin, 1990), and had been traced to the vicinity of the ACC. It had been proposed that the ERN might reflect the detection of a mismatch between actual and intended responses (Coles, Sheffers, & Fournier, 1995). However, the conflict-monitoring hypothesis offered an alternative explanation, namely, that the ERN might reflect response conflict associated with errors. A range of empirical data pointed to the idea that, even as erroneous responses are executed, central stimulus-identification and response-selection processes can continue to evolve, often causing belated activation of the correct response. Even though this covert response reversal comes too late, it may nonetheless give rise to a brief interval during which representations for correct and incorrect responses are simultaneously active, in other words, a period of response conflict. According to the conflict-monitoring hypothesis, it is this period of conflict that triggers the ERN. To test the sufficiency of this account, we adopted a model of the well-known flanker task (the task most frequently employed in ERN studies), adding, as in our previous simulations, a single conflict-monitoring unit. Once again, the conflict-monitoring unit behaved like the ACC, its activity rising higher on error trials than correct ones (see Figure 7.2, top, for similar results from a later study). In line with the motivating hypothesis, this difference was due to continued processing and a belated activation of the correct response on error trials, leading to a brief period of response conflict, usually just following initiation of the error response. Subsequent work with this model has shown that it accounts for many aspects of the ERN, including the temporal profile of this scalp potential and its dependence on stimulus congruency, stimulus frequency, response force, and speed–accuracy trade-off conditions (Yeung, Botvinick, & Cohen, in press).

Together, these three foundational models showed how a single mechanism or process, conflict monitoring, could account for ACC activation in a wide range of behavioral con-

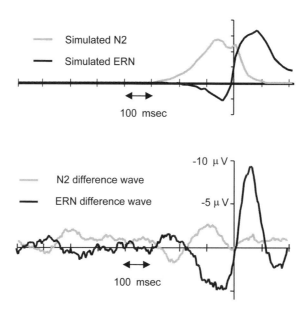

FIGURE 7.2. Computational modeling results (top) and electrophysiological data (bottom) from Yeung et al. (in press). In the upper plot, each trace reflects the response-aligned, average activity of the conflict-monitoring unit over time, in the model illustrated in Figure 7.1. Cycles of processing were converted to time intervals, expressed in milliseconds, based on a linear regression onto behavioral data. The location of the *y* axis corresponds to the point at which the response threshold was crossed. The trace labeled *ERN* shows activation on error trials; *N2*, activation on correct trials. As the plot indicates, the model predicts that ACC activation in association with errors should peak following error commission, consistent with preexisting data concerning the ERN. A novel prediction, reflected in the N2 trace, was that there should also be transient ACC activation just *prior* to responding on high-conflict trials. As shown in the lower panel, the accompanying empirical study confirmed this prediction.

texts. Importantly, each phase of the modeling work described so far resulted in specific predictions, many of which have subsequently been investigated and confirmed. For example, the ERN simulations just mentioned led to the prediction that a potential similar to the ERN should be observed in association with correct responses on high-conflict trials, but rather than following responding (like the ERN), this potential should precede the response. This prediction was confirmed in an electroencephalographic (EEG) experiment (Yeung et al., in press; Figure 7.2). The conflict-monitoring hypothesis also predicted that error-related activity should localize to the same location within the ACC as activation on response override tasks such as the Stroop task, a prediction that was confirmed using functional magnetic resonance imaging (fMRI; Carter, Braver, Barch, et al., 1998). These empirical findings concerning error-related activity in the ACC provided an alternative to the idea that the ERN reflects the operation of a comparator, supporting instead the idea that ACC activation reflects conflict monitoring.

Another competing account of ACC activation interprets it as directly reflecting the operation of attentional or control mechanisms (Posner & DiGirolamo, 1998). A series of empirical studies tested between this view of ACC function and the one articulated in our computational modeling work, according to which the ACC serves a monitoring function rather than an executive or regulative one. Two studies took advantage of tasks containing both high-control/low-conflict trials and low-control/high-conflict trials. In these task domains, the regulative account expressed by Posner and DiGirolamo (1998) and others predicted greater ACC activation on high-control/low-conflict trials; the conflict-monitoring hypothesis predicted precisely the reverse. Botvinick, Nystrom, Fissell, Carter, and Cohen (1999) tested between these predictions, leveraging a sequential effect observed in performance of the flanker task, described in the next section. As predicted by the conflict-monitoring hypothesis, ACC activation varied in proportion to the degree of response conflict rather than the degree of top-down control, rising higher in the setting of high conflict and low control than on trials involving low conflict and high control. Carter and colleagues (2000) pursued the same strategy in a different task domain, manipulating both conflict and control by varying trial-type frequency in the Stroop task. Once again, ACC activation was found to be higher on low-control/high-conflict trials than on high-control/low-conflict trials. This result has recently been replicated and extended by Braver and colleagues (Hoyer, Braver, & Brown, 2003).

In yet another study, McDonald, Cohen, Stenger, and Carter (2000) examined brain activity in a task-switching Stroop paradigm, in which an instructional task cue indicated whether subjects were to perform color naming (high conflict) or word reading (low conflict) in the upcoming trial. Greater ACC activation was observed on high-conflict color-naming trials, but, importantly, this activation was present only after stimulus onset. Preparation for control-intensive color-naming trials, as reflected in the relatively greater activity following the task cue for color naming (as opposed to word reading), was observed in prefrontal cortex but not the ACC. Once again, ACC activation appeared to be tied more closely to conflict than to control.

In addition to predictions concerning response override and error commission, predictions stemming from the simulation of underdetermined responding have also been tested. Specifically, Barch and colleagues studied ACC activation in the verb-generation task, a classic underdetermined responding task, finding it to be largest on trials where response selection was least constrained (Barch, Braver, Sabb, & Noll, 2000), precisely as predicted by the conflict-monitoring hypothesis.

CONFLICT MONITORING AND COGNITIVE CONTROL

The work reviewed thus far was intended to address the first part of the conflict-monitoring hypothesis, the idea that response conflicts are detected and, more specifically, that they trigger ACC activation. The second part of the conflict-monitoring hypothesis suggests that conflict detection is causally related to compensatory adjustments in attention or control. Whereas evidence for the first part of the conflict-monitoring hypothesis has come primarily from neuroscientific data, this second half of the hypothesis has rested mainly on behavioral findings. A key impetus for the theory comes from a group of findings that appear to reflect reactive, performance-based adjustments in control.

A particularly interesting example, which we refer to as the Gratton effect, was originally reported by Gratton, Coles, and Donchin (1992). This study focused on the flanker task originally reported by Eriksen and Eriksen (1974). Here, subjects are asked to identify a centrally presented item (typically one of two letters, e.g., S or H, or a left- or right-facing arrow), with a corresponding keypress. Distracter items appear on both sides of the target, and these can either map to the same response as the target (compatible trials, e.g., SSSSS) or the opposite response (incompatible trials, e.g., HHSHH). Numerous studies have shown incompatible trials to be associated with response competition, as reflected in longer response times. What Gratton and colleagues showed, in addition, was that this interference effect varies depending on what kind of stimulus was presented on the preceding trial. Specifically, responses on incompatible trials were found to be faster and more accurate if the preceding trial was incompatible than if it was compatible. For compatible trials, in contrast, responses were slower if the preceding trial was incompatible than if it was compatible (Figure 7.3, left). That is, the influence of the flankers on response selection appeared to be attenuated following incompatible trials, arguably reflecting more focused attention or stronger input from top-down control.

Another behavioral finding that seems to reflect reactive adjustments in control comes from the Stroop task. Here, it has been found that the classic Stroop interference effect varies in magnitude depending on the frequency of incongruent trials. Specifically, Stroop interference is larger when incongruent trials are infrequent than when they are frequent (see, e.g., Tzelgov, Henik, & Berger, 1992).

A third and final example of reactive adjustments in control comes from work on behavior following errors. Laming (1968) observed that in forced-choice decision tasks, responses tend to be relatively slow just following errors. Here, as in the preceding two cases, attention or control seems to adjust dynamically to an ongoing evaluation of performance or of task demands.

Botvinick and colleagues (2001) suggested that conflict monitoring might be partly responsible for strategic adjustments in control such as those just described. In each case, it was noted, shifts toward more focused attention or tighter top-down control follow events associated with response conflict (incompatible flanker trials, incongruent Stroop trials, and errors). Conflict monitoring thus appeared to provide a possible mechanism for the observed variations in behavior.

This hypothesis was examined through a new set of three neural network models (Botvinick et al., 2001). The first model addressed the Gratton effect and was based on the model of the flanker task described earlier. The new simulation made only one change to the earlier model, which was to link the conflict-monitoring unit to a set of "attention" units in the base model, which served to bias processing to specific items in the input array (see Figure 7.1). The new connections were arranged such that high activity in the conflict-monitor-

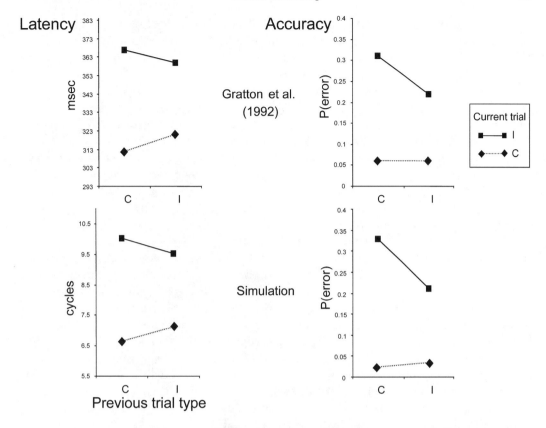

FIGURE 7.3. Top: Data from Gratton et al. (1992). I, incompatible; C, compatible. Bottom: Results from the simulation of the Gratton effect reported by Botvinick et al. (2001; see Figure 7.1). Both adapted with permission from the American Psychological Association.

ing unit would lead to a shift, on the next trial, toward more focus on the central target item in the input array, and low activity to a broader distribution of spatial attention. Setting in place this simple feedback loop led to behavior (response latencies and error rates) closely matching those reported by Gratton and colleagues (1992; Figure 7.3). In this particular case, conflict monitoring appeared sufficient to account for empirically observed reactive adjustments in control.

A second simulation model demonstrated how the conflict-monitoring hypothesis might also provide an explanation for the effects of trial-type frequency that had been observed in the Stroop task. The approach was essentially identical to that taken in addressing the Gratton effect. The model of conflict monitoring in the Stroop task developed earlier, and described in the previous section, was modified to allow activity in the conflict-monitoring unit to influence "attentional" units within the model (here, units biasing the model toward the word-reading or color-naming task) on the next trial. High activity in the conflict-monitoring unit led to stronger activation of the color-naming task unit, whereas low conflict-monitoring activity led to a decrease in this unit's activation. This simple arrangement gave rise to response latencies closely matching those reported in the empirical literature, showing again, but in a different domain, how conflict monitoring might account for reactive adjustments in control.

The slowing Laming (1968) had reported following errors is also compatible with an explanation based on the conflict monitoring hypothesis. Our earlier simulation of the ERN lent weight to the idea that errors are associated with response conflict, giving rise to the possibility that the slowdown Laming reported might be based on conflict monitoring. A third computational model made this proposal explicit. Here, a preexisting model of forced-choice decision (Usher & McClelland, 2001) was supplemented with a conflict-monitoring unit, and this unit was linked back to a unit in the base model whose activity level influenced the trade-off between speed and accuracy in the generation of responses. It was assumed that in this task, increasing control meant adopting a more conservative position along this trade-off, favoring accuracy over speed. Thus, in the model, error-related conflict activated the control unit, which in turn increased the threshold for responding. Establishment of this simple feedback loop gave rise to overt behavior closely resembling that reported by Laming.

Like the first series of computational models, this second series gave rise to a set of testable predictions. For example, based on further work with the forced-choice model just discussed, Braver and colleagues (Jones, Cho, Nystrom, Cohen, & Braver, 2002) predicted that responses should be slower and more accurate following correct responses that were slow (marking the presence of response conflict) than after fast correct responses, reflecting a shift along the speed–accuracy trade-off curve akin to those that follow errors. A behavioral study yielded results closely resembling those predicted by the simulations.

In addition to such predictions about behavior, the second set of simulations has also given rise to predictions about ACC activation. The Stroop model, for example, predicts that Stroop interference should be larger after trials with low ACC activation than after trials involving high activation. Kerns and colleagues (2003) have recently confirmed this prediction, through a correlation of fMRI and behavioral data.

A RECENT CHALLENGE

In a recent article, Mayr, Awh, and Laurey (2003) proposed that at least some of the phenomena we had attributed to conflict monitoring might actually have a less interesting explanation: priming. They focused, in particular, on the Gratton effect. Note that one way of describing this effect is as a speeding of response times on trials where the stimulus type (compatible vs. incompatible) is the same as on the preceding trial (see Figure 7.3). Note, also, that, in the usual version of the task, such trial-type repeats also frequently involve a repetition of the entire stimulus (e.g., SSHSS → SSHSS). Taking both of these points into account, Mayr and colleagues suggested that stimulus repetition itself might be responsible for the faster response times seen with trial-type repeats, simply as a consequence of repetition priming. They presented evidence for this account from two experiments. In the first, subjects performed a version of the flanker task using left- and right-facing arrowheads. Although their performance displayed a Gratton effect, the effect was isolated to stimulus-repeat trials. Other trials, where there was no stimulus repeat, showed no Gratton effect. A second experiment, in which stimulus elements never repeated from one trial to the next, also failed to show a Gratton effect.

By focusing on priming, Mayr and colleagues (2003) pointed out a methodologically important aspect of the flanker task (extending earlier work by Stadler & Hogan, 1996). However, our own subsequent research suggests that the attribution of the Gratton effect to priming alone may be premature. In two separate experiments, we have observed a Gratton effect that cannot be attributed entirely to priming (Ullsperger, Botvinick, Bylsma, & von Cramon, 2003). Each experiment used a version of the flanker task only slightly different from those employed by Mayr and colleagues. In the first study, target and flanker items were chosen from among the numerals 1 through 9 (e.g., 33733), an approach that served to minimize repetitions of stimulus elements from one trial to the next. Subjects identified the central target number using the numeric keypad on the computer keyboard. Reaction time results showed a clear Gratton effect, in the form of an interaction between current and previous trial types. Importantly, this effect remained statistically significant even when analysis was limited to stimuli for which no component digit had appeared on the preceding trial, making it impossible to attribute the effect to repetition priming.

Our second experiment employed the same arrowhead version of the flanker task that Mayr and colleagues (2003) had used in their first experiment, but with minor changes to stimulus timing (shorter stimulus exposure and a longer intertrial interval). Unlike the Mayr study, this experiment produced a Gratton effect, present in both reaction times and error rates. This effect remained significant even when target repeat trials were excluded from the analysis. Thus, once again, the effect could not be attributed entirely to priming.

Of course, it is an interesting question why the specific task implementations we employed yielded a priming-independent Gratton effect, while those used by Mayr and colleagues (2003) did not. Two potentially important differences between their task design and ours relate to stimulus duration (shorter in our experiments) and intertrial interval (quite long in our second experiment). We speculate elsewhere (Botvinick et al., 2003) on why these parameters may affect behavioral outcomes, and experiments are under way to clarify the relevant issues. The results already in hand, however, are enough to indicate that the results of Mayr and colleagues fail to generalize, a fact that undermines the theoretical challenge their findings initially seemed to present to the conflict-monitoring hypothesis.

Another point in favor of the conflict-monitoring hypothesis, and against the argument of Mayr and colleagues (2003), is that shifts in performance analogous to the Gratton effect can be observed in tasks other than the flanker task, and under circumstances that rule out a priming account. For example, in a study of the Stroop task, Kerns and colleagues (2003) found less influence of word identity on color naming following incompatible than compatible trials, consistent with the idea that subjects focused more exclusively on the task-relevant color dimension following high-conflict incongruent trials. Sohn and Carter (2003) obtained parallel results in the Simon task. Here, subjects respond with a right or left keypress, based on the color of a circle appearing to their right or left. Trials where the stimulus appears opposite to the correct response are labeled incongruent and tend to be associated with slower response times than do congruent trials, where the stimulus appears on the same side as the correct response. Sohn and Carter found that this interference effect was attenuated on trials following incongruent trials, again consistent with the idea that subjects focused more on the task-relevant stimulus dimension following high-conflict responses. Analogous results have been obtained in the setting of a two-alternative forced-choice decision. Here, Jones and colleagues (2002) found shifts toward slower, more accurate responding following trials associated with high levels of response conflict (as inferred from their large reaction times).

In each of these studies, a shift toward more focused or conservative behavior was observed following high-conflict responses. Importantly, in every study, measures were taken to exclude an explanation based on repetition priming, either by avoiding stimulus repeats or by excluding such repeats from analysis. Thus, the explanation proposed by Mayr and colleagues (2003) does not apply. Contrary to their argument, the conflict-monitoring account appears to provide the best available explanation for the current set of findings.

EMERGING ISSUES AND FUTURE DIRECTIONS

Over the 5 years or so since its original proposal, the conflict-monitoring hypothesis has garnered considerable support from both behavioral and neuroscientific investigations. The studies we have reviewed, along with numerous others, provide convergent support for both parts of the theory: (1) that conflict is detected and that its occurrence engages the ACC; and (2) that the detection of conflict drives reactive adjustments in attention or cognitive control.

Not surprisingly, even as empirical support has accrued for conflict monitoring, other findings have posed new questions. One particularly pressing issue relates to how conflict monitoring fits into the broader functional role of the ACC. A number of findings suggest that the ACC may serve an evaluative function that goes beyond conflict monitoring, perhaps involving an evaluation of the degree to which events predict eventual reward (Gehring & Willoughby, 2002; Holroyd & Coles, 2002). If this view turns out to be correct, it will be necessary to determine how conflict monitoring relates to this larger function. One possibility is that conflict is one among many kinds of event to which the ACC responds in carrying out a single evaluative function. Another, increasingly compelling possibility is that different types of evaluative (or affective) functions may be carried out in different subregions of the ACC (Kiehl, Liddle, & Hopfinger, 2000; Picard & Strick, 2001). Nevertheless, these may still reflect a cohesive family of functions, all of which serve to monitor for breakdowns in processing or behavior, that indicate the need to recruit control.

Another current question pertains to the relations between conflict monitoring and control systems. While there are clear functional links between ACC and prefrontal cortex, we have proposed that the connectivity of the ACC might also allow conflict monitoring to modulate activity in other centers with a role in attention and control, in particular brainstem dopaminergic and adrenergic nuclei (Botvinick et al., 2001). Available data support this view, indicating, for example, that the ACC interacts significantly with the locus ceruleus (Jodo, Chiang, & Aston-Jones, 1998). Further work is needed to clarify the functional relations between conflict monitoring, as evidently implemented in the ACC, and the mechanisms responsible for attention and control.

As research on conflict monitoring continues to move forward, we anticipate that computational modeling will continue to play an important role. The research we have conducted so far demonstrates how computational work can be leveraged to make explicit the implications of initially broad hypotheses, and how it can enter into a synergistic relationship with empirical work.

REFERENCES

Allport, A. (1980). Attention and performance. In G. Claxton (Ed.), *Cognitive psychology: New directions* (pp. 112–153). London: Routledge & Kegan Paul.

Allport, A. (1987). Selection for action: Some behavioral and neurophysiological considerations of attention and action. In H. Heuer & A. F. Sanders (Eds.), *Perspectives on perception and action* (pp. 395–419). Hillsdale, NJ: Erlbaum.

Barch, C. M., Braver, T. S., Sabb, F. W., & Noll, D. C. (2000). Anterior cingulate and the monitoring of response conflict: Evidence from an fMRI study of verb generation. *Journal of Cognitive Neuroscience, 12*(2), 298–309.

Botvinick, M. M., Braver, T. S., Barch, D. M., Carter, C. S., & Cohen, J. D. (2001). Conflict monitoring and cognitive control. *Psychological Review, 108,* 624–652.

Botvinick, M., Braver, T. S., Yeung, N., Ullsperger, M., Carter, C. S., & Cohen, J. D. (2003). *A conflict over conflict monitoring.* Manuscript submitted for publication.

Botvinick, M. M., Nystrom, L., Fissell, K., Carter, C. S., & Cohen, J. D. (1999). Conflict monitoring vs. selection-for-action in anterior cingulated cortex. *Nature, 402,* 179–181.

Buckner, R. L., Petersen, S. E., Ojemann, J. G., Miezin, F. M., Squire, L. R., & Raichle, M. E. (1995). Functional anatomical studies of explicit and implicit memory retrieval tasks. *Journal of Neuroscience, 15,* 12–29.

Carter, C. S., Braver, T. S., Barch, D. M., Botvinick, M. M., Noll, D., & Cohen, J. D. (1998). Anterior cingulate cortex, error detection, and the on-line monitoring of performance. *Science, 280,* 747–749.

Carter, C. S., MacDonald, A. M., Botvinick, M., Ross, L. L., Stenger, A., Noll, D., et al. (2000). Parsing executive processes: strategic versus evaluative functions of the anterior cingulate cortex. *Proceedings of the National Academy of Sciences USA, 97*(4), 1944–1948

Carter, C. S., Mintun, M., & Cohen, J. D. (1995). Interference and facilitation effects during selective attention: An $H_2{}^{15}O$ PET study of Stroop task performance. *Neuroimage, 2,* 264–272.

Cohen, J. D., Dunbar, K., & McClelland, J. L. (1990). On the control of automatic processes: A parallel distributed processing account of the Stroop effect. *Psychological Review, 97,* 332–361.

Cohen, J. D., & Huston, T. A. (1994). Progress in the use of interactive models for understanding attention and performance. In C. Umilta & M. Moscovitch (Eds.), *Attention and performance* (Vol. 15, pp. 453–456). Cambridge, MA: MIT Press.

Coles, M. G. H., Sheffers, M. K., & Fournier, L. (1995). "Where did you go wrong?": Errors partial errors, and the nature of human information processing. *Acta Psychologica, 90,* 129–144.

Duncan, J. (1996). Cooperating brain systems in selective perception and action. In T. Inui & J. L. McClelland (Eds.), *Attention and performance* (Vol. 16, pp. 549–578). Cambridge, MA: MIT Press.

Eriksen, B. A., & Eriksen, C. W. (1974). Effects of noise letters on the identification of a target letter in a nonsearch task. *Perception and Psychophysics, 16,* 143–149.

Gehring, W. J., Coles, M. G. H., Meyer, D. E., & Donchin, E. (1990). The error-related negativity: An event-related potential accompanying errors. *Psychophysiology, 27,* S34.

Gehring, W. J., & Willoughby, A. R. (2002). The medial frontal cortex and the rapid processing of monetary gains and losses. *Science, 295,* 2279–2282.

Gratton, G., Coles, M. G. H., & Donchin, E. (1992). Optimizing the use of information: Strategic control of activation and responses. *Journal of Experimental Psychology: General, 121,* 480–506.

Holroyd, C. B., & Coles, M. G. H. (2002). The neural basis of human error processing: Reinforcement learning, dopamine, and the error-related negativity. *Psychological Review, 109*(4), 679–709.

Hoyer, C., Braver, T., & Brown, J. (2003). *Cognitive control in the Stroop task: A sustained effect?* Poster presented at the annual meeting of the Cognitive Neuroscience Society, New York.

Jodo, E., Chiang, C., & Aston-Jones, G. (1998). Potent excitatory influence of prefrontal cortex activity on noradrenergic locus coeruleus neurons, *Neuroscience, 83,* 63–80.

Jones, A. D., Cho, R. Y., Nystrom, L. E., Cohen, J. D., & Braver, T. S. (2002). A computational model of anterior cingulate function in speeded response tasks: Effects of frequency, sequence and conflict. *Cognitive, Affective, and Behavioral Neuroscience 2*(4), 300–317.

Kerns, J. G., Cohen, J. D., MacDonald, A. W. III, Cho, R. Y., Stenger, V. A., & Carter C. S. (2004). Anterior cingulate conflict monitoring and adjustments in control. *Science, 303,* 1023–1026.

Kiehl, K. A., Liddle, P. F., & Hopfinger, J. B. (2000). Error processing and the rostral anterior cingulate: an event-related fMRI study. *Psychophysiology, 37,* 216–223.

Laming, D. R. J. (1968). *Information theory of choice-reaction times.* London: Academic Press.

Mayr, U., Awh, E., & Laurey, P. (2003). Conflict adaptation effects in the absence of executive control. *Nature Neuroscience 6*(5), 450–452.

McDonald, A. W., Cohen, J. D., Stenger, V. A., & Carter, C. S. (2000). Dissociating the role of the dorsolateral prefrontal cortex and anterior cingulate cortex in cognitive control. *Science, 288,* 1835–1838.

McClelland, J. L., & Rumelhart, D. E. (1981). An interactive activation model of context effects in letter perception: Part 1. An account of basic findings. *Psychological Review*, *88*, 375–407.

Navon, D., & Miller, J. (1987). Role of outcome conflict in dual-task interference. *Journal of Experimental Psychology*, *3*, 435–448.

Picard, N., & Strick, P. L. (2001). Imaging the premotor areas. *Current Opinion in Neurobiology*, *11*(6), 663–672.

Posner, M. I., & DiGirolamo, G. J. (1998). Executive attention: Conflict, target detection and cognitive control. In R. Parasuraman (Ed.), *The attentive brain* (pp. 401–423). Cambridge, MA: MIT Press.

Sohn, M. H., & Carter, C. S. (2003). *Conflict adaptation is independent of stimulus repetition: Evidence for the conflict monitoring model.* Manuscript submitted.

Stadler, M. A., & Hogan, M. E. (1996). Varieties of positive and negative priming. *Psychonomic Bulletin and Review*, *3*, 87–90.

Tzelgov, J., Henik, A., & Berger, J. (1992). Controlling Stroop effects by manipulating expectations for color words. *Memory and Cognition*, *20*, 727–735.

Ullsperger, M., Botvinick, M., Bylsma, L., & von Cramon, D. Y. (2003). *The conflict–adaptation effect: It's not just priming.* Manuscript submitted for publication.

Ullsperger, M., & Szymanowski, F. (in press). ERP correlates of error relevance. In M. Ullsperger & M. Falkenstein (Eds.), *Errors, conflicts and the brain: Current opinions on performance monitoring.* Leipzig, Germany: Max Planck Institute of Cognitive Neuroscience.

Usher, M., & McClelland, J. L. (2001). On the time course of perceptual choice: A leaky competing accumulator model. *Psychological Review*, *108*, 550–592.

Yeung, N., Botvinick, M. M., & Cohen, J. D. (in press). The neural basis of error-detection: Conflict monitoring and the error-related negativity. *Psychological Review*.

III

IMAGING ATTENTION

8

Selective Attention in Distributed Brain Systems

John Duncan

What is "attention"? As Wittgenstein (1953) pointed out, many concepts cannot be given a formal definition. It would be hard to give a rule, for example, specifying exactly what does and does not count as a "game"; instead the many things we call games share a number of family resemblances (i.e., features in common, though perhaps no single defining feature shared by all). The same applies to concepts such as "attention." In experimental psychology and neuroscience, many phenomena have been studied as examples of attention. Again, these are a family of individuals, some perhaps very similar, some very different.

To illustrate, when Broadbent wrote *Perception and Communication* (1958), it was sensible to propose a single "limited capacity system" that was responsible for many processing limitations—inability to listen to two simultaneous speech streams, tendency to drift off task with the passage of time, different processing styles of extraverts and introverts, and so on. Systematic study of dual-task performance—of limitations in "divided attention"— soon showed a more complex picture. As in Broadbent's dichotic listening experiments, it is often very difficult to identify two simultaneous inputs in the same sensory modality. The problem can be much less for inputs in different modalities (Duncan, Martens, & Ward, 1997; Treisman & Davies, 1973). Evidently there is not one limit in "divided attention", but somewhat separate limits in separate, modality-specific systems. Similarly, much evidence suggests that rather different limitations affect identification of simultaneous stimuli and selection of simultaneous responses (Arnell & Duncan, 2002; Pashler, 1989), though these limitations are not completely separate (see Jolicoeur, 1998). Along with many other results, such data show that processing conflicts—limitations in "divided attention"—occur separately in many different ways and many separate cognitive systems (Allport, 1980). These different processing limits may share important family resemblances, but they cannot be understood in terms of a single limited attentional capacity.

In this chapter I focus on one family member—selective visual attention. Many aspects of visual attention have been well specified at the behavioral level. At the same time, physiological results suggest how these functions might be implemented at the neural level. Here I present an account based on three general principles: (1) competitive processing in the multiple brain regions responding to visual input, (2) bias by task relevance, and (3) between-system integration. Together these make up the *integrated competition* model (Desimone & Duncan, 1995; Duncan, 1996). To conclude, I consider relations between visual attention and the broader family of biased competition in many different processing systems.

COMPETITION

Multiple cortical and subcortical systems respond to visual input (Desimone & Ungerleider, 1989). These include the multiple "visual areas" in occipital, parietal, and temporal cortex; frontal lobe regions including the frontal eye fields, premotor cortex, and prefrontal cortex; and subcortical regions including the superior colliculus and multiple thalamic nuclei. Though onset latencies differ from one region to another, thereafter there is concurrent processing throughout this network. Our first proposal is that, in many and perhaps all of these regions, processing is competitive—a stronger response to one object in a visual scene means weaker responses to others.

In behavioral experiments, such competition is reflected in the limited attentional capacity described previously: As attention is directed to one object, so others are processed less effectively. Not only object shapes but also simple features such as color and size are identified less well; in the extreme, even the presence of an unattended stimulus may pass unnoticed (Rock, Linnett, Grant, & Mack, 1992). Behavioral experiments have detailed many properties of this limited attentional capacity.

One important question is dependence on spatial separation between attended and unattended inputs. Commonly, different objects occur at different spatial locations; attention directed to the left visual field, for example, impairs processing on the right (Posner, Snyder, & Davidson, 1980). Competition is much the same, however, even if separate objects overlap at the same spatial location (Duncan, 1984; Rock & Gutman, 1981). The most compelling examples use transparent motion displays (e.g., two overlapping fields of dots rotating in opposite directions). Such a display produces a strong percept of two separate surfaces moving past one another. Though the two have complete spatial overlap, still attending to one suppresses processing of the other (Valdes-Sosa, Cobo, & Pinilla, 1998).

Experiments have also detailed the time course of competition. In a typical study, a brief target object (e.g., a letter to be identified) is followed by a second at either the same (Raymond, Shapiro, & Arnell, 1992) or a different (Duncan, Ward, & Shapiro, 1994) location. Though each target may be presented very briefly, still attending to the first produces sustained interference with the second, resolving only after a few hundred milliseconds.

In physiological studies, competition is reflected in strong responses to attended inputs, and weak or suppressed responses to inputs that are ignored. Single-unit studies in the monkey (Figure 8.1) show this relative enhancement of responses to the attended stimulus, or relative suppression of responses to the ignored stimulus, throughout the visual areas of occipital, parietal, temporal, and frontal cortex (Desimone & Duncan, 1995). The strength of the effect tends to increase from earlier to later areas (Mehta, Ulbert, & Schroeder, 2000; O'Connor, Fukui, Pinsk, & Kastner, 2002). In early visual areas, the strongest effect is spatially local, when attended and unattended inputs lie in the same cell's receptive field (Figure ...e Luck, Chelazzi, Hillyard, & Desimone, 1997; Moran & Desimone, 1985; Treue & ...ll, 1996). In later areas, the effect is more global (Moran & Desimone, 1985). Effec-

(a) V4 (Luck et al., 1997)

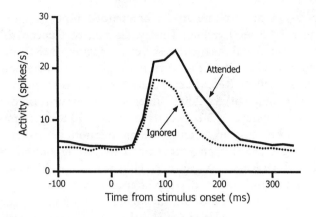

(b) IT (Chelazzi et al., 1998)

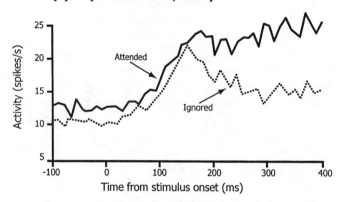

(c) PF (Everling et al., 2002)

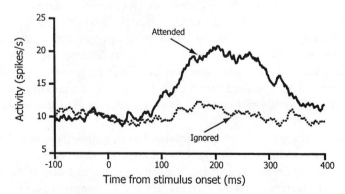

FIGURE 8.1. Single-unit recording studies of attention in the behaving monkey. For recordings from each cell, responses to a preferred visual input are measured when that input is attended (solid line) or ignored (dotted line). Each histogram shows mean response in a selected cell population. (a) Occipital area V4. Attentional selection based on cued spatial location (data from Luck et al., 1997). (b) Inferotemporal cortex (IT). Attentional selection based on object identity (data from Chelazzi et al., 1998). (c) Prefrontal cortex (PF). Attentional selection based on cued spatial location (data from Everling et al., 2002).

tively complete suppression of response to an unattended input has been observed in prefrontal cortex (Figure 8.1c; see Everling, Tinsley, Gaffan, & Duncan, 2002).

In the human brain, functional magnetic resonance imaging (fMRI) shows stronger responses to attended inputs over much of the cortical visual system, including primary visual cortex or V1 (Tootell et al., 1998). Recent data, indeed, show this result even at the level of the lateral geniculate (O'Connor et al., 2002). Interestingly, event-related potential (ERP) data suggest that the first response of V1, occurring around 50 msec from stimulus onset, is not sensitive to attention. Instead, attentional modulation begins around 100 msec (Hillyard, Munte, & Neville, 1985), then affecting activity throughout much of the cortical visual system, V1 included (Di Russo, Martínez, & Hillyard, 2003). Monkey data also commonly show that attentional modulations develop after an initial visual response, both in V1 (Roelfsema, Lamme, & Spekreijse, 1998) and in higher visual areas (Figures 8.1a, 8.1b). These data suggest a first, feedforward wave of visual processing that is rather independent of attention, followed by later competitive processing leading to relevant object selection (Dehaene, Sergent, & Changeux, 2003)—a conclusion consistent with the extended time course of competition shown in behavioral studies.

Returning to the single-unit level, recent data show more to the story than simple spike rate or response strength. In extrastriate cortex, cells responding to an attended stimulus show increased synchrony between spikes and local cortical field potentials, reflecting net local synaptic activity. Attentional modulation of synchrony, indeed, may be more robust than spike rate effects (Fries, Reynolds, Rorie, & Desimone, 2001). In all probability, synchrony-based mechanisms as well as simple response strength play an important role in processing competition.

BIAS

Different behavior requires attention to different objects. Depending on task requirements, relevant objects can be of any kind, of any size, in any location, and so on. Thus if objects compete for representation across the sensorimotor network, it must be possible to bias this competition to those specific objects of relevance to current concerns.

Behavioral experiments show the expected flexible attentional selection. For example, even if a letter display is too brief for eye movements, people can read just the letters in a certain row (selection by location), just those with a certain color (selection by object properties), just letters and not numbers (selection by object category), and so on. In all these cases, attention favors the specified targets; the experience is that they stand out from the display, with little information extracted from nontargets (Duncan, 1980; von Wright, 1970).

Competitive advantage for targets is measured in experiments manipulating the number of targets and/or the number of nontargets (Bundesen, Shibuya, & Larsen, 1985). A simple example is the "visual search" experiment, measuring the time taken to find a specified target in a display of nontargets. If nontargets are weak competitors, then the number of nontargets in a display should have little effect. This happens in easy search tasks (e.g., search for a red target among green nontargets), when the target appears to "pop out" from the display (Egeth, Jonides, & Wall, 1972). If nontargets are strong competitors, then target detection slows down for every nontarget added. In the worst cases, the effect of each nontarget can be 200 msec or more (Bricolo, Gianesini, Fanini, Bundesen, & Chelazzi, 2002). Search efficiency varies continuously between these extremes, suggesting continuous variation in the ability to bias processing competition by task context (Bundesen, 1990; Duncan & Humphreys, 1989). Not surprisingly, the single most important factor is similarity between targets and nontargets (Duncan & Humphreys, 1989).

At the neural level, one obvious way to bias competition might be to preactivate or prime those neurons responding to behaviorally relevant objects (Desimone & Duncan, 1995). Two contrasting cases are space and object selection. In a spatial selection study, the animal is cued to pay attention to a certain location. In occipital areas V2 and V4, the cue sometimes results in sustained activation of cells whose receptive field encompasses the attended location (Luck et al., 1997). In an object selection study, the animal is cued to attend to a certain object. Here priming is unlikely early in the visual system, where object identification is incomplete. Indeed, object cues have little effect in V4 (Chelazzi, Miller, Duncan, & Desimone, 2001), but produce sustained activity in inferotemporal cells selective for the cued object (Chelazzi, Duncan, Miller, & Desimone, 1998).

Despite the Luck and colleagues (1997) results, spatial cues do not always affect V4 response rates in the postcue interval (e.g., McAdams & Maunsell, 1999). In fMRI, priming should be reflected in signals following the instruction cue (e.g., a cue to pay attention to the left) but preceding actual stimulus presentation (Kastner, Pinsk, De Weerd, Desimone, & Ungerleider, 1999). For spatial selection, such experiments suggest some activation in occipital areas V1, V2, and V4, but stronger effects in parietal cortex, including the intraparietal sulcus and superior parietal lobule, as well as the frontal eye field (Corbetta, Kincade, Ollinger, McAvoy, & Shulman, 2000; Kastner et al., 1999). These may be especially important regions in establishing a spatial attentional focus.

INTEGRATION

Our third proposal is that competition must be integrated between the different parts of the sensorimotor network. As an object becomes dominant in one region, it gains a competitive advantage elsewhere. For the network as a whole, the tendency is to converge on the same dominant object, different regions coding its different properties and implications for action. As outlined previously, this convergence may be reflected in gradual development of attentional modulations following a first, feedforward processing phase.

Behavioral results require integration of this sort. While different objects in the visual input compete to be processed, different properties of the same object do not (Duncan, 1984, 1993a, 1993b). Instead, multiple properties of the same object can be identified simultaneously, without loss of accuracy. Again, competition between but not within objects occurs either when objects are spatially separate or when they overlap as in the transparent motion display (Valdes-Sosa et al., 1998).

Physiological evidence for integration is also beginning to appear. According to the integration principle, dominance for an attended object should apply to all of its features, even those irrelevant to the current task. In a recent fMRI study, O'Craven, Downing, and Kanwisher (1999) used a display of two objects (a face and a house) transparently overlaid. Even regions responding to task-irrelevant features gave stronger activity when those features belonged to the attended object. A recent ERP study using the transparent motion display showed that attentional modulation of irrelevant features occurred rather late, around 200 msec after stimulus onset (Schoenfeld et al., 2003). Such data are strongly in line with a gradual convergence of different cortical regions to work on the different properties of the same selected object.

One important aspect of integration may be feedback from higher to lower levels of the visual system (Dehaene et al., 2003; Schneider, 1995). In this way, a competitive advantage established at a higher level can distribute its effects, modulating earlier levels and hence all those other systems to which they project.

THE BROADER PICTURE

Certainly biased competition is not restricted to vision. Instead it seems likely that many systems have their own competitive processing limits. When two operations (e.g., identification of two visual targets) call on much the same systems, competition is strong and "divided attention" difficult. When systems are more separate (e.g., target identification in different modalities, or concurrent target identification and response selection), there is less basis for competition and more evidence for parallel processing.

A degree of separation, however, should not be taken to mean that different systems typically work independently. Effective behavior requires selective focus on particular sensory inputs, on suitable actions and goals, on information retrieved from semantic memory, and so on; usually, we "attend" to all these related things as a coherent whole. In vision, we have seen how different parts of the sensorimotor network integrate to select the same, dominant object from the visual input. More broadly, a general principle may be that a dominant processing focus in any one cognitive system supports processing of related material elsewhere. Thus many cognitive systems will usually integrate to produce processing with a common or related focus.

When inputs are spatially separate, common location is certainly one strong influence on integration. It is easier, for example, to process simultaneous inputs in different sensory modalities if they arise from the same location (Driver & Spence, 1994). Orienting the eyes, head, or trunk to one side can bias sensory processing toward that side, even for auditory or tactile inputs (Driver & Grossenbacher, 1996; Morais, 1978). Spatial bias can also occur after damage to one side of the brain. In spatial extinction (Bender, 1952), impaired processing on the side opposite to a lesion is especially strong if there is simultaneous, competing input on the ipsilesional side. Such data suggest a competitive imbalance favoring ipsilesional input. Spatial extinction can follow many unilateral lesions, both cortical and subcortical (Vallar, Rusconi, Bignamini, Geminiani, & Peroni, 1994). Through spatial integration, any weakening of processing on one side may tend to produce a global competitive imbalance against that side (Duncan, 1996).

One strong force toward cognitive integration may be provided by prefrontal cortex. Through inputs from many parts of the cerebral cortex, and strong connections between one frontal region and another, prefrontal neurons have access to many kinds of information. Potentially, therefore, many different inputs might compete for prefrontal representation. Correspondingly, recordings from prefrontal units show a distributed representation of many different kinds of information—stimuli in different modalities, movements of the eyes or limbs, delay activity carrying information between its presentation and use, information concerning task rules, rewards, and so on (Duncan, 2001; Miller & Cohen, 2001).

Prefrontal neurons, furthermore, show high specificity for information of current relevance (Rainer, Asaad, & Miller, 1998; Sakagami & Niki, 1994). Even when neurons are randomly selected, many are found to code the specific information required by the particular, arbitrary task the monkey has been trained to perform. Having trained monkeys to categorize stimuli as cats or dogs, for example, Freedman, Riesenhuber, Poggio, and Miller

(2001) found over 20% of randomly selected neurons categorizing stimuli in this way. Changing the categorization rule changed the information that prefrontal neurons carried (Freedman et al., 2001). As described earlier, a similar focus on task-relevant information is found with manipulation of spatial attention. If attention is focused on a specific location, visual inputs from that location produce strong responses in prefrontal cortex, beginning around 100 msec from stimulus onset. Meanwhile, there is little or no response to inputs from ignored locations (Everling et al., 2002). This strong prefrontal focus on task-relevant information may support related processing in many other regions of the brain (Miller & Cohen, 2001), providing one strong source of cognitive coherence.

William James (1890) wrote:

> Every one knows what attention is. It is the taking possession by the mind, in clear and vivid form, of one out of what seem several simultaneously possible objects or trains of thought. Focalization, concentration, of consciousness are of its essence. It implies withdrawal from some things in order to deal effectively with others. . . . (pp. 403–404)

Modern work suggests that there is no one "attention" underlying the experience of "focalization, concentration, of consciousness." Instead, the experience arises as multiple sources of biased competition converge to work on the same coherent line of thought and behavior.

REFERENCES

Allport, D. A. (1980). Attention and performance. In G. Claxton (Ed.), *Cognitive psychology: New directions* (pp. 112–153). London: Routledge & Kegan Paul.

Arnell, K., & Duncan, J. (2002). Separate and shared sources of dual-task cost in stimulus identification and response selection. *Cognitive Psychology, 44,* 105–147.

Bender, M. B. (1952). *Disorders in perception.* Springfield, IL: Charles C. Thomas.

Bricolo E., Gianesini T., Fanini A., Bundesen, C., & Chelazzi L. (2002). Serial attention mechanisms in visual search: A direct behavioral demonstration. *Journal of Cognitive Neuroscience, 14,* 980–993.

Broadbent, D. E. (1958). *Perception and communication.* London: Pergamon Press.

Bundesen, C. (1990). A theory of visual attention. *Psychological Review, 97,* 523–547.

Bundesen, C., Shibuya, H., & Larsen, A. (1985). Visual selection from multielement displays: A model for partial report. In M. I. Posner & O. Marin (Eds.), *Attention and performance* (Vol. 11, pp. 631–649). Hillsdale, NJ: Erlbaum.

Chelazzi, L., Duncan, J., Miller, E. K., & Desimone, R. (1998). Responses of neurons in inferior temporal cortex during memory-guided visual search. *Journal of Neurophysiology, 80,* 2918–2940.

Chelazzi, L., Miller, E. K., Duncan, J., & Desimone, R. (2001). Responses of neurons in macaque area V4 during memory-guided visual search. *Cerebral Cortex, 11,* 761–772.

Corbetta, M., Kincade, J. M., Ollinger, J. M., McAvoy, M. P., & Shulman, G. L. (2000). Voluntary orienting is dissociated from target detection in human posterior parietal cortex. *Nature Neuroscience, 3,* 292–297.

Dehaene, S., Sergent, C., & Changeux, J.-P. (2003). A neuronal network model linking subjective reports and objective physiological data during conscious perception. *Proceedings of the National Academy of Sciences USA, 100,* 8520–8525.

Desimone, R., & Duncan, J. (1995). Neural mechanisms of selective visual attention. *Annual Review of Neuroscience, 18,* 193–222.

Desimone, R., & Ungerleider, L. G. (1989) Neural mechanisms of visual processing in monkeys. In F. Boller & J. Grafman (Eds.), *Handbook of neuropsychology* (Vol. 2, pp. 267–299). Amsterdam: Elsevier.

Di Russo, F., Martínez, A., & Hillyard, S. A. (2003). Source analysis of event-related cortical activity during visuo-spatial attention. *Cerebral Cortex*, *13*, 486–499.

Driver, J., & Grossenbacher, P. G. (1996). Multimodal spatial constraints on tactile selective attention. In T. Inui & J. L. McClelland (Eds.), *Attention and performance* (Vol. 16, pp. 209–235). Cambridge, MA: MIT Press.

Driver, J., & Spence, C. J. (1994). Spatial synergies between auditory and visual attention. In C. Umiltà & M. Moscovitch (Eds.), *Attention and performance* (Vol. 15, pp. 311–331). Cambridge, MA: MIT Press.

Duncan, J. (1980). The locus of interference in the perception of simultaneous stimuli. *Psychological Review*, *87*, 272–300.

Duncan, J. (1984). Selective attention and the organization of visual information. *Journal of Experimental Psychology: General*, *113*, 501–517.

Duncan, J. (1993a). Coordination of what and where in visual attention. *Perception*, *22*, 1261–1270.

Duncan, J. (1993b). Similarity between concurrent visual discriminations: Dimensions and objects. *Perception and Psychophysics*, *54*, 425–430.

Duncan, J. (1996). Cooperating brain systems in selective perception and action. In T. Inui & J. L. McClelland (Eds.), *Attention and performance* (Vol. 16, pp. 549–578). Cambridge, MA: MIT Press.

Duncan, J. (2001). An adaptive coding model of neural function in prefrontal cortex. *Nature Reviews Neuroscience*, *2*, 820–829.

Duncan, J., & Humphreys, G. W. (1989). Visual search and stimulus similarity. *Psychological Review*, *96*, 433–458.

Duncan, J., Martens, S., & Ward, R. (1997). Restricted attentional capacity within but not between sensory modalities. *Nature*, *387*, 808–810.

Duncan, J., Ward, R., & Shapiro, K. (1994). Direct measurement of attentional dwell time in human vision. *Nature*, *369*, 313–315.

Egeth, H., Jonides, J., & Wall, S. (1972). Parallel processing of multielement displays. *Cognitive Psychology*, *3*, 674–698.

Everling, S., Tinsley, C. J., Gaffan, D., & Duncan, J. (2002). Filtering of neural signals by focused attention in the monkey prefrontal cortex. *Nature Neuroscience*, *5*, 671–676.

Freedman, D. J., Riesenhuber, M., Poggio, T., & Miller, E. K. (2001). Categorical representation of visual stimuli in the primate prefrontal cortex. *Science*, *291*, 312–316.

Fries, P., Reynolds, J. H., Rorie, A. E., & Desimone, R. (2001). Modulation of oscillatory neural synchronization by selective visual attention. *Science*, *291*, 1560–1563.

Hillyard, S. A., Münte, T. F., & Neville, H. J. (1985). Visual-spatial attention, orienting, and brain physiology. In M. I. Posner & O. S. M. Marin (Eds.), *Attention and performance* (Vol. 11, pp. 63–84). Hillsdale, NJ: Erlbaum.

James, W. (1890). *The principles of psychology*. New York: Holt.

Jolicoeur, P. (1998). Modulation of the attentional blink by on-line response selection: Evidence from speeded and unspeeded Task 1 decisions. *Memory and Cognition*, *26*, 1014–1032.

Kastner, S., Pinsk, M. A., De Weerd, P., Desimone, R., & Ungerleider, L. G. (1999). Increased activity in human visual cortex during directed attention in the absence of visual stimulation. *Neuron*, *22*, 751–761.

Luck, S. J., Chelazzi, L., Hillyard, S. A., & Desimone, R. (1997). Mechanisms of spatial selective attention in areas V1, V2, and V4 of macaque visual cortex. *Journal of Neurophysiology*, *77*, 24–42.

McAdams, C. J., & Maunsell, J. H. R. (1999). Effects of attention on the orientation tuning functions of single neurons in macaque area V4. *Journal of Neuroscience*, *19*, 431–441.

Mehta, A. D., Ulbert, I., & Schroeder, C. E. (2000). Intermodal selective attention in monkeys. I: Distribution and timing of effects across visual areas. *Cerebral Cortex*, *10*, 343–358.

Morais, J. (1978). Spatial constraints on attention to speech. In J. Requin (Ed.), *Attention and performance* (Vol. 7, pp. 245–260). Hillsdale, NJ: Erlbaum.

Moran, J., & Desimone, R. (1985). Selective attention gates visual processing in the extrastriate cortex. *Science*, *229*, 782–784.

Miller, E. K., & Cohen, J. D. (2001). An integrative theory of prefrontal function. *Annual Review of Neuroscience, 24*, 167–202.

O'Connor, D. H., Fukui, M. M., Pinsk, M. A., & Kastner, S. (2002). Attention modulates responses in the human lateral geniculate nucleus. *Nature Neuroscience, 5*, 1203–1209.

O'Craven, K. M., Downing, P. E., & Kanwisher, K. (1999). fMRI evidence for objects as the units of attentional selection. *Nature, 401*, 584–587.

Pashler, H. (1989). Dissociations and dependencies between speed and accuracy: Evidence for a two-component theory of divided attention in simple tasks. *Cognitive Psychology, 21*, 529–574.

Posner, M. I., Snyder, C. R. R., & Davidson, B. J. (1980). Attention and the detection of signals. *Journal of Experimental Psychology: General, 109*, 160–174.

Rainer, G., Asaad, W. F., & Miller, E. K. (1998). Selective representation of relevant information by neurons in the primate prefrontal cortex. *Nature, 393*, 577–579.

Raymond, J. E., Shapiro, K. L., & Arnell, K. M. (1992). Temporary suppression of visual processing in an RSVP task: An attentional blink? *Journal of Experimental Psychology: Human Perception and Performance, 18*, 849–860.

Rock, I., & Gutman, D. (1981). The effect of inattention on form perception. *Journal of Experimental Psychology: Human Perception and Performance, 7*, 275–285.

Rock, I., Linnett, C. M., Grant, P., & Mack, A. (1992). Perception without attention: Results of a new method. *Cognitive Psychology, 24*, 502–534.

Roelfsema, P. R., Lamme, V. A. F., & Spekreijse, H. (1998). Object-based attention in the primary visual cortex of the macaque monkey. *Nature, 395*, 376–381.

Sakagami, M., & Niki, H. (1994). Encoding of behavioral significance of visual stimuli by primate prefrontal neurons: Relation to relevant task conditions. *Experimental Brain Research, 97*, 423–436.

Schneider, W. X. (1995). VAM: A neuro-cognitive model for visual attention control of segmentation, object recognition and space-based motor actions. *Visual Cognition, 2*, 331–376.

Schoenfeld, M. A., Tempelmann, C., Martínez, A., Hopf, J.-M., Sattler, C., Heinze, H. J., & Hillyard, S. A. (2003). Dynamics of feature binding during object-selective attention. *Proceedings of the National Academy of Sciences USA, 100*, 11806–11811.

Tootell, R. B., Hadjikhani, N., Hall, E. K., Marrett, S., Vanduffel, W., Vaughan, J. T., et al. (1998). The retinotopy of visual spatial attention. *Neuron, 21*, 1409–1422.

Treisman, A. M., & Davies, A. (1973). Divided attention to ear and eye. In S. Kornblum (Ed.), *Attention and performance* (Vol. 4, pp. 101–117). London: Academic Press.

Treue, S., & Maunsell, J. H. R. (1996). Attentional modulation of visual motion processing in cortical areas MT and MST. *Nature, 382*, 539–541.

Valdes-Sosa, M., Cobo, A., & Pinilla, T. (1998). Transparent motion and object-based attention. *Cognition, 66*, B13–B23.

Vallar, G., Rusconi, M. L., Bignamini, L., Geminiani, G., & Perani, D. (1994). Anatomical correlates of visual and tactile extinction in humans: A clinical CT scan study. *Journal of Neurology, Neurosurgery, and Psychiatry, 57*, 464–470.

von Wright, J. M. (1970). On selection in visual immediate memory. In A. F. Sanders (Ed.), *Attention and performance* (Vol. 3, pp. 280–292). Amsterdam: North-Holland.

Wittgenstein, L. (1953). *Philosophical investigations.* Oxford, UK: Blackwell.

9

Two Cortical Systems
for the Selection of Visual Stimuli

Gordon L. Shulman, Serguei V. Astafiev, and Maurizio Corbetta

Attention is broadly concerned with how people selectively process information in the environment that is relevant to their behavioral goals. We have used neuroimaging techniques in order to understand how this selectivity is related to neural activity in different brain regions.

Selective processing occurs at the service of the organism's goals. Although selectivity can be induced in a purely stimulus-driven fashion, as when our attention is drawn to an abruptly occurring stimulus (Jonides, 1981; Yantis & Jonides, 1990), the most important and common forms of selectivity occur in response to voluntary commands. We control whether we search in the refrigerator for an orange or for the milk. The perceptual set corresponding to these two situations are quite different. The milk may be kept in a different part of the refrigerator than the orange and has different visual features. The motor movements for grasping an orange are also different than for grasping a milk carton. Before the refrigerator door is even opened, signals reflecting the appropriate perceptual and motor sets may be implemented. When the door is opened, these preexisting signals modulate the incoming activity in sensory and associative areas produced by the objects in the refrigerator, and it is these modulations that ultimately result in the selective behavior that satisfies the person's goal (grasping the milk carton).

From this perspective, it is critical to separate the neural signals that reflect perceptual and motor sets from the effects of those signals on the sensory and motor activity induced by subsequent events. When we first began to study the neuroimaging of human attention using positron emission tomography (PET), this separation was not possible (Corbetta, Miezin, Dobmeyer, Shulman, & Petersen, 1991; Corbetta, Miezin, Shulman, & Petersen, 1993). However, functional magnetic resonance imaging (fMRI) has an increased temporal resolution that allows the analysis of the neural signals on individual trials of an experiment, a technique called event-related fMRI. Moreover, these analyses are even possible with fast-paced trials, in which the hemodynamic responses on successive trials overlap. Using fast-paced event-related fMRI, we have developed methods that separate the top-down signals from a cue that implements a voluntary perceptual or motor set from the modulations of subsequent activity in a target stimulus produced by that set (Corbetta, Kincade, Ollinger, McAvoy, & Shulman, 2000; Ollinger, Corbetta, & Shulman, 2001; Ollinger, Shulman, & Corbetta, 2001; Shulman et al., 1999).

These methods were based on two innovations. First, in addition to presenting standard trials, in which a cue stimulus was followed by a target stimulus, we randomly interspersed cue trials, in which the trial ended following the cue. Second, we estimated the time course of the blood-oxygenation-level-dependent (BOLD) response for the cue and target events using a linear model that made no assumptions about the shape of the hemodynamic response. Many fast-paced event-related fMRI studies assume a shape for the expected hemodynamic response on a trial. This assumed hemodynamic shape is generated by convolving an impulse function with an assumed waveform of the neural activity during the task. The assumed shape may deviate from the actual shape because of errors in the impulse function or in the assumed neural activity during the task, which is often modeled as a rectangle function that lasts for the duration of the trial. Unfortunately, on any trial the neural activity at a brain region may reflect several different processes, particularly if the task is complex and the trial duration is long. For example, during visual search for a target, regions in the intraparietal sulcus (IPs) are affected by sensory stimulation, by search through nontargets, and by target detection (Shulman et al., 2003). Because these processes can come online at different timepoints and last for different periods of time, the overall neural activity in a region may be very different from a rectangle function, resulting in a BOLD time course with a complex shape (see d'Avossa, Shulman, & Corbetta, 2003, for a discussion). Therefore, methods that do not assume a shape for the hemodynamic response, including those based on linear models and related methods based on "selective averaging" of responses (Burock, Buckner, Woldorff, Rosen, & Dale, 1998; Dale & Buckner, 1997), have certain advantages. However, almost all published studies using fast-paced event-related fMRI, irrespective of whether they make shape assumptions, do assume the linearity of the BOLD response. Existing work indicates that linearity is fairly good, but more studies on this topic are needed (Boynton, Engel, Glover, & Heeger, 1996; Dale & Buckner, 1997; Huettel & McCarthy, 2000; Miezin, Maccotta, Ollinger, Petersen, & Buckner, 2000; Ollinger et al., 2001; Pollmann, Dove, Von Cramon, & Wiggins, 2000).

TOP-DOWN SIGNALS ASSOCIATED WITH PERCEPTUAL AND MOTOR SETS

These techniques have been used to image the signals that implement perceptual sets for spatial location (Corbetta et al., 2000; Corbetta, Kincade, & Shulman, 2002) and visual features such as motion direction (Shulman, d'Avossa, Tansy, & Corbetta, 2002; Shulman et al., 1999). In the spatial attention experiment, subjects saw an arrow cue that pointed left or right and indicated with high probability the location in which a subsequent target stimulus would occur. Previous work has shown that subjects use the arrow cue to shift attention to the predicted target location (Posner, Snyder, & Davidson, 1980). These shifts of attention are indexed by faster reaction times to targets that occur at the cued than noncued locations.

The arrow cue was presented for 2.3 seconds and was followed by a target stimulus that could occur between 1.5 and 3 seconds from the offset of the arrow. On delay trials, no target was presented and subjects maintained their attention at a particular location for a sustained period in the absence of new sensory input.

The results showed that spatial cues activated regions along the intraparietal sulcus/superior parietal lobule (IPs/SPL) and in the precentral sulcus (see the horizontal black crosshatchings in Figure 9.1A, left panel for a summary of dorsal frontoparietal areas activated by cues to attend to visual locations and features). These latter activations included the putative human homologue of the frontal eye field (FEF) at the intersection of the precentral sulcus and superior frontal sulcus. These activations were time-locked to the presentation of the cue, as shown in Figure 9.1B. Moreover, the time course of the signal was sustained during delay trials as subjects maintained their attention at the cued location. It is therefore likely that they were related to the shift and maintenance of attention. However, imaging research is correlational in nature. To relate these activations more firmly to the spatial shift of attention, we have begun to investigate whether the magnitude of the BOLD signal during the cue period predicts the behavioral and neural response to subsequent targets at the cued and noncued locations (Sapir et al., 2003).

An important question is whether these cortical regions contain spatial maps for directing attention to particular locations. The parietal and frontal activations during the cue period were largely bilateral, both for leftward and rightward cues, although the FEF and the ventral IPs showed modest field asymmetries. While rightward cues activated these regions equally well in both hemispheres, leftward cues activated the right hemisphere more strongly than the left hemisphere. Sereno, Pitzalis, and Martinez (2001) have recently reported a spatial map in IPs during the monitoring of peripheral locations for a target, with each hemisphere holding a half-field representation. The spatial relationship between this map and the regions activated by spatial cues is currently under investigation.

Sustained preparatory signals were not observed in occipital regions, although these have been reported in other studies (Kastner, Pinsk, De Weerd, Desimone, & Ungerleider, 1999). The fact that spatial cues invariably produce dorsal frontoparietal activity but only produce occipital activations under certain circumstances suggests that the former regions are the source of the selective set. Increasing the difficulty of the upcoming perceptual discrimination, either because the object must be discriminated from distracters (Kastner et al., 1999) or because it is presented at contrast threshold (Ress, Backus, & Heeger, 2000), may determine whether this set is expressed during task preparation in lower-level occipital regions.

Selection of task-relevant information is often based on visual features as well as spatial location. Top-down signals that bias the processing of particular features, such as color, motion, or shape, are a basic component of models of visual search (Wolfe, 1994). We have observed preparatory activity for motion direction in IPs and SPL (Shulman et al., 1999, 2002). These motion-selective activations correspond with both anatomical and physiological evidence in macaque (Colby, Duhamel, & Goldberg, 1993; Eskandar & Assad, 1999; Maunsell & Van Essen, 1983; Ungerleider & Desimone, 1986; Williams, Elfar, Eskandar, Toth, & Assad, 2003) as well as lesion-behavior studies in humans (Battelli et al., 2001) for parietal involvement in the perception of motion. In a recent study (Shulman et al., 2002), subjects indicated whether the hue or motion direction of a centrally presented, colored random-dot pattern matched a memorized standard feature. Each subject memorized two standard hues (a specific shade of red or green) and two standard directions (left-oblique, right-oblique). A visual word cue, prior to the onset of the random dots, indicated which standard

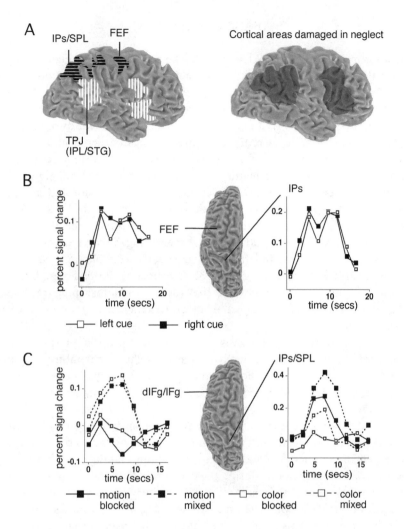

FIGURE 9.1. (A) The left panel shows a surface rendering of the right hemisphere. The black horizontal cross-hatching shows dorsal frontoparietal areas that are involved in the voluntary control of attention. These regions were determined from a meta-analysis of studies that have measured the activations following a cue to direct attention to a visual location or feature (see Corbetta & Shulman, 2002, for details). The white horizontal cross-hatching shows ventral areas that are activated when subjects respond to unexpected target stimuli. These regions were determined from a meta-analysis of studies that have measured the activations to invalidly cued stimuli or to low-frequency stimuli that have been presented in a train of stimuli (see Corbetta & Shulman, 2002, for details). The right panel shows the regions associated with spatial neglect. (B) A surface rendering of a dorsal view of the left hemisphere. The graph shows the time course of the response in the left frontal eye field (FEF) and intraparietal sulcus (IPs) on delay trials following a central arrow cue to shift attention to a location in the left or right visual field. The *x* axis shows the time following the onset of the cue, with time zero indicating the onset of the cue, while the *y* axis shows the magnitude of the measured BOLD signal. (C) A surface rendering of a dorsal view of the left hemisphere. The graph shows the time course of the response in the left dorsal inferior frontal gyrus/inferior frontal sulcus (dIFg/IFs) and the left intraparietal sulcus/superior parietal lobule (IPs/SPL) following word cues to attend to a particular direction of motion (filled symbols) or hue (open symbols) in a subsequent display of moving, colored random dots. Time zero indicates the onset of the cue word. Solid lines refer to scans in which motion and color cues were randomly mixed, while dashed lines refer to scans in which only motion or only color cues were presented. The time courses reflect only the BOLD signals generated during the cue period, not the BOLD signals generated by the subsequent target display. Figure 9.1A is from Corbetta and Shulman (2002). Copyright 2002 by Nature Publishing Group. Reprinted by permission. Figure 9.1C is from Shulman, D'Avossa, Tansy, and Corbetta (2002). Copyright 2002 by Oxford University Press. Reprinted by permission.

feature was appropriate (red, green, left, right). The time courses in Figure 9.1C show that regions in left IPs/SPL were significantly more activated following motion word cues than color word cues.

We also varied whether trials in a block involved only motion or color word cues (e.g., only "left" or "right" cues occurred in a block), or whether both kinds of cues occurred unpredictably (i.e., "left," "right," "red," and "green" cues occurred in a block). This was done to indicate whether signals for task preparation were related to specifying the relevant dimension as well as the relevant feature. Activations in left parietal (Figure 9.1C, right graph) and prefrontal cortex (Figure 9.1C, left graph) for both color and motion cues were increased when the cues for different dimensions were mixed rather than blocked. Therefore, preparatory signals for specifying the task-relevant dimension generalized over the color and motion tasks. Several studies of task switching, involving very different tasks, have reported similar activations in left parietal cortex (Dove, Pollmann, Schubert, Wiggins, & Von Cramon, 2000; Kimberg, Aguirre, & D'Esposito, 2000; Sohn, Ursu, Anderson, Stenger, & Carter, 2000). Our results show that these general task preparation signals partially overlap parietal regions in which dimension-specific (i.e., motion-selective) preparatory signals are found.

Finally, task preparation also involves setting up an appropriate response to a stimulus (e.g., reaching for the milk carton). Behavioral studies show that motor responses can be speeded by advance information, indicating that preparatory signals can prime or bias motor structures (Abrams & Jonides, 1988; Rosenbaum, 1980). Astafiev et al. examined preparatory activations for eye movements and limb movements (Astafiev et al., 2003). Subjects were shown an arrow cue indicating the direction in which a target stimulus would occur, as in our original study. In different scans, subjects pointed to the target, moved their eyes to the target, or covertly detected the target without making a response. Although activity was observed in some regions during the cue period that was common to all three conditions, some parietal regions showed greater preparatory activity for pointing movements than saccades or covert detection. The time course in Figure 9.2A shows this differential activity in the left precuneus. This region is medial to the IPs regions that showed common activity across conditions, consistent with evidence for a reach-related area in macaques that is more medial than the lateral intraparietal region (LIP), which is involved in the control of eye movements and attention (Colby & Goldberg, 1999; Snyder, Batista, & Andersen, 1997).

These studies show that preparatory activity for both perceptual and motor sets is present in dorsal frontoparietal regions (see also Connolly, Goodale, Menon, & Munoz, 2002; Hopfinger, Buonocore, & Mangun, 2000; Kastner et al., 1999). Other studies have reported signals that specify the mapping between stimuli and responses (Iacoboni, Woods, & Mazziotta, 1996; Rushworth, Paus, & Sipila, 2001), although it is not clear whether these signals are preparatory in nature. However, while preparatory signals for different functions have been observed, the anatomical relationship between them is currently unclear. For example, are motion-selective signals separate from those for spatial selection or for specifying a stimulus–response mapping? Can these signals be localized to different spatial maps? Building a map of preparatory signals in parietal cortex will require intensive investigation of multiple paradigms in single subjects. Single-subject analyses will also be critical for relating BOLD activity to behavior, as discussed earlier, which we believe will be a critical part of assessing the functional significance of these preparatory signals. Therefore, while prior studies have examined activity averaged across a group of subjects, future work will concentrate on more extensive testing of single subjects.

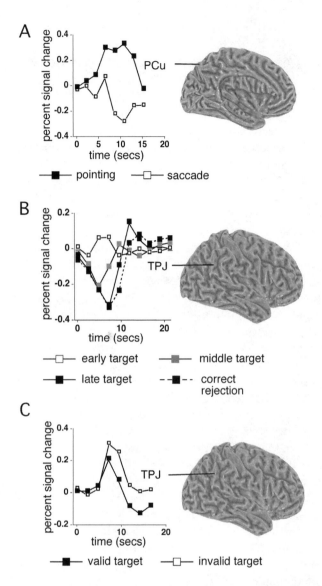

FIGURE 9.2. (A) A surface rendering of a medial view of the left hemisphere The graph shows the time course of the response in the left precuneus (PCu) as subjects prepared a pointing movement or an eye movement to a location indicated by a central arrow cue. Time zero indicates the onset of the cue. The time courses reflect only the BOLD signals generated during the cue period, not the responses generated by the subsequent motor movement to the target. (B) A surface rendering of a lateral view of the right hemisphere. The graph shows the time course of the response in the right TPJ during an RSVP search task. Time zero indicates the onset of the RSVP display. The three functions with solid lines reflect the time course on trials in which a target was presented early, middle, or late in the RSVP sequence and was detected, resulting in short, medium, or long search durations. The function with the dashed line reflects the time course on correct rejection trials in which no target was presented and search was sustained for the duration of the RSVP sequence. Right TPJ is deactivated during search but is then activated by target detection or detection of the end of the trial. The exact shape of the time courses can be accurately modeled on the assumption of additive stimulus, search, and detection processes (see Shulman et al., 2003, for details). (C) A surface rendering of a lateral view of the right hemisphere. The graph shows the BOLD response in the TPJ to targets that have been validly or invalidly cued. Time zero indicates the onset of the target period. The time course reflects only the BOLD response during the target period, not the response to the preceding cue. Figure 9.2A is from Astafiev et al. (2003). Copyright 2003 by the Society for Neuroscience. Reprinted by permission. Figure 9.2B is from Shulman et al. (2003). Copyright 2003 by the American Physiological Society. Reprinted by permission.

MODULATION OF SENSORY INPUT BY TOP-DOWN SIGNALS
FOR PERCEPTUAL SET

When target and nontarget stimuli are presented following a cue, the preparatory signals discussed previously interact with the sensory signals evoked by these stimuli. This interaction yields the selective effects associated with attention; signals for targets are enhanced relative to the signals for nontargets.

Interestingly, this interaction is observed in the visual system. Some years ago, we reported modulations in feature-specific extrastriate regions when the task-relevant feature of an object was attended. For example, MT+, an extrastriate region involved in motion processing, was modulated when subjects attended to the motion rather than the color or shape of the sample and test objects in a match-to-sample paradigm (Corbetta et al., 1991). This study involved a blocked paradigm, in which activations were summed over an entire block of trials. Therefore, it was not possible to determine whether the MT+ modulation affected sensory signals evoked by the moving sample and/or target objects, memory-related signals for maintaining the sample motion in working memory, or tonic signals that reflected the set for a motion task. However, the match-to-sample study discussed in the previous section was conducted as an event-related design, which means that all measured activity was time-locked to the onset of individual events during the scan. We have already discussed the activity time-locked to the onset of the motion and color word cues. We also isolated the activity time-locked to the onset of the target stimulus, which consisted of a colored, moving random-dot pattern. We found that the BOLD signal evoked by this target in MT+ was greater when the preceding cue word specified a motion direction rather than a hue. Presumably, the preparatory signals generated by the motion cue in parietal regions directly or indirectly increased processing in MT+ of the motion of the target object.

Other work has shown similar modulations for spatial selection rather than selection of features, even in early visual areas such as V1 (Brefczynski & DeYoe, 1999; Gandhi, Heeger, & Boynton, 1999; Martinez et al., 1999). For example, Tootell and colleagues (1998) reported that attending to a peripheral stimulus in a quadrant increased the activation at the corresponding retinotopic location in V1, relative to passive viewing, while signals to peripheral stimuli in nonattended quadrants were decreased, relative to passive viewing. Moreover, deactivations (decreases in the BOLD signal relative to a nonstimulated or no-task baseline) were observed in nonstimulated and unattended foveal locations, relative to the signals in those locations during passive viewing of either the peripheral stimuli or even a uniform gray field. These deactivations may reflect the attenuation of signals from unattended and nonstimulated locations (Shmuel et al., 2002), similar to the relative signal decreases seen at unattended but stimulated locations.

The relative enhancement of attended locations/attenuation of nonattended locations in occipital cortex may underlie the increased efficiency of perceptual processing at attended locations that has been noted in behavioral studies (Carrasco & McElree, 2001; Carrasco, Penpeci-Talgar, & Eckstein, 2000; Dosher & Lu, 2000; Posner et al., 1980; Yeshurun & Carrasco, 1999). It may also ensure that stimuli at task-relevant locations are selectively processed by higher-order associative regions that are strongly capacity-limited (Broadbent, 1958) or that can generate conflicting signals to multiple stimuli (Allport, 1989). Conversely, the occipital modulations might be a consequence of selective processing of targets in higher-order regions. Measurements of the time course of these activations from studies that integrate fMRI with magnetic encephalographic or event-related potentials (ERPs) may help separate the relative contributions of feedforward and feedback modulations (Martinez et al., 1999; Noesselt et al., 2002).

In recent work, we have studied how top-down signals interact with sensory-evoked signals to produce differential responses to targets and nontargets during visual search tasks in higher-order associative areas as well as in sensory areas. In one experiment subjects searched for a digit target among letter nontargets in four rapid serial visual presentation (RSVP) streams presented within a virtual circle at an eccentricity of 1.5 degrees (Shulman et al., 2003). Deactivations were observed in anterior medial occipital regions that presumably subserve nonstimulated peripheral regions of the visual field, analogous to the results noted earlier (Shmuel et al., 2002; Tootell et al., 1998). However, during search through letter nontargets we also observed deactivations in associative regions such as the temporal–parietal junction (TPJ, which is broadly defined here as including both the inferior parietal lobule and superior temporal gyrus and sulcus) and to a lesser extent in parts of lateral prefrontal cortex. Figure 9.2B shows the time courses in a region of the TPJ as a detected target was presented further into the RSVP sequence and therefore the duration of search was extended. The deactivation was sustained for the duration of search, but was terminated by an activation when the digit target was detected.

We have speculated that the deactivation in the TPJ reflects a restriction of the sensory input to this region to stimuli that are consistent with the task set. This restriction is implemented by signals from dorsal frontoparietal regions and results in deactivations during search through nontargets (which are filtered) and activations to targets (which pass the filter). The input to the TPJ may be filtered for several reasons. First, the TPJ could be part of a workspace of limited capacity, which underlies the interference from multiple targets in behavioral studies (Duncan, 1980; Marois, Chun, & Gore, 2000a). Filtering prevents this workspace from being overloaded with irrelevant information. Studies by Duncan and colleagues indicate that damage over broad regions of the right TPJ and parietal cortex decreases capacity during partial and whole report tasks in both visual fields (Duncan et al., 1999). Moreover, imaging studies indicate that the inferior parietal lobule is activated during working-memory tasks, although its exact role is unclear (Chein & Fiez, 2001; Jonides et al., 1993; Smith et al., 1995). A second reason for filtering the input to the TPJ, discussed in more detail in the next section, is that the TPJ appears to be involved in the reorienting of attention to unexpected stimuli. Filtering prevents salient but irrelevant stimuli from generating shifts of attention that interfere with the current task.

STIMULUS-DRIVEN CHANGES IN SELECTION

While preparatory signals in dorsal frontoparietal regions enable prespecified tasks to be performed, selection must be sufficiently flexible to handle unexpected contingencies. While searching the refrigerator for the milk carton, the phone may ring. Therefore, behavioral events can require changes in selectivity. The TPJ may signal when these changes are necessary.

We have studied this issue by comparing responses to expected and unexpected target stimuli, as an unexpected stimulus generally requires a change in the prepared task set. In the spatial cueing experiment discussed earlier (Corbetta et al., 2000), while targets usually occurred at the cued location, they sometimes occurred at the noncued location. The time course in Figure 9.2C shows that these unexpected targets generated larger BOLD signals than expected targets in the right TPJ. Similar results have been reported in location "oddball" experiments in which subjects monitor a stream of standard stimuli in one location for a target that may occur with low frequency at a different location (Marois, Leung, & Gore, 2000). The white vertical cross-hatching in Figure 9.1A shows the regions activated by unexpected stimuli in cueing experiments or oddball experiments, as determined in a meta-analysis (see Corbetta & Shulman, 2002, for details). These results suggest that the TPJ may be involved in reorienting attention to the unexpected stimulus. Interestingly, damage to the right TPJ in humans is most frequently associated with spatial neglect (Figure 9.1A, left panel shows the regions associated with neglect), in which patients fail to orient or respond to stimuli in the left visual field. Several studies have shown (Friedrich, Egly, Rafal, & Beck, 1998; Posner, Walker, Friedrich, & Rafal, 1984) that right parietal lesions result in a failure of unattended but behaviorally important stimuli in the neglected visual field to disengage attention from the current focus so that it can be reoriented. Moreover, in the single-unit literature, cells in area 7a, on the gyral surface inferior to IPs, respond better to salient stimuli at unattended locations than at attended locations (Constantinidis & Steinmetz, 2001; Robinson, Bowman, & Kertzman, 1995; Steinmetz & Constantinidis, 1995), again suggestive of a role in reorienting attention to new contingencies. As in the case of IPs, an important question that is currently under investigation is whether the TPJ contains a spatial map that might guide the reorienting of attention.

In the absence of a task set that enforces selective processing of particular stimuli, attention may be oriented to any highly salient stimulus. Correspondingly, under passive viewing conditions, the TPJ is strongly activated by salient sensory stimuli (Downar, Crawley, Mikulis, & Davis, 2000). However, in the presence of a task set, reorienting to new contingencies must be carefully regulated to ensure that salient but irrelevant stimuli do not interfere with the current task. As noted previously, the TPJ is deactivated during search through nontarget RSVP displays (Shulman et al., 2003), consistent with a filtering of the input to prevent responses to distracting information. Correspondingly, the deactivated regions in the right TPJ overlap extensively with regions that show increased responses to invalid targets (Shulman et al., 2003). Similarly, TPJ responses to stimulus changes in one modality (e.g., a change in a continuous "buzzing" sound) are decreased if subjects are attending to stimulus changes in a different modality (e.g., a change in the orientation of a repeatedly flashed object) (Downar, Crawley, Mikulis, & Davis, 2001). Finally, Serences, Shomstein, Leber, Yantis, and Egeth (2001) reported that a distracter color singleton only produced behavioral interference with target detection and a large TPJ response when it matched the color of the target that subjects had to detect. Therefore, TPJ activation in the presence of a task set is heavily dependent on signals reflecting the behavioral relevance of the stimulus. Future work will need to consider the TPJ activations produced by stimuli that are of enduring biological significance or are associated with highly learned responses (e.g., a ringing telephone).

Although we have discussed a possible role of the TPJ in initiating reorienting of spatial attention to visual stimuli, TPJ activity is observed even when an unexpected target stimulus does not require a shift of spatial attention. For example, an oddball target (e.g., a low-frequency shape) appearing at the currently attended location can generate a TPJ response (Linden et al., 1999; Marois et al., 2000; McCarthy, Luby, Gore, & Goldman-Rakic, 1997). Moreover, TPJ activation is multimodal. The TPJ is activated by tactile stimuli at noncued locations (Macaluso, Frith, & Driver, 2002) and by auditory oddballs (e.g., tones of infrequent frequency) (Kiehl, Laurens, Duty, Forster, & Liddle, 2001; Linden et al., 1999). Therefore, the putative function of this region in signaling a change in selectivity is not limited to spatial reorienting to visual stimuli (see Corbetta & Shulman, 2002, for a review).

This selective review, centered on our recent work, has focused on three topics. First we considered the dorsal frontoparietal regions that generate the top-down signals that bias the selection of subsequent sensory stimuli. We then briefly examined the interaction of these top-down signals with sensory signals in occipital and associative cortex, producing a relative enhancement of attended features and locations that may underlie the selection and analysis of task-relevant input. Finally, we discussed how sensory events may require a change in the top-down signals that bias selection, and discussed the role of the TPJ in signaling those changes.

REFERENCES

Abrams, R. A., & Jonides, J. (1988). Programming saccadic eye movements. *Journal of Experimental Psychology: Human Perception and Performance, 14*, 428–443.

Allport, A. (1989). Visual attention. In M. I. Posner (Ed.), *Foundations of cognitive science* (pp. 631–682). Cambridge, MA: MIT Press.

Astafiev, S. V., Shulman, G. L., Stanley, C. M., Snyder, A. Z., Van Essen, D. C., & Corbetta, M. (2003). Functional organization of human intraparietal and frontal cortex for attending, looking, and pointing. *Journal of Neuroscience, 23*, 4689–4699.

Battelli, L., Cavanagh, P., Intrilligator, J., Tramo, M. J., Henaff, M.-A., Michel, F., et al. (2001). Unilateral right parietal damage leads to bilateral deficit for high-level motion. *Neuron, 32*, 985–995.

Boynton, G. M., Engel, S. A., Glover, G. H., & Heeger, D. J. (1996). Linear systems analysis of functional magnetic resonance imaging in human V1. *Journal of Neuroscience, 16*, 4207–4221.

Brefczynski, J. A., & DeYoe, E. A. (1999). A physiological correlate of the "spotlight" of visual attention. *Nature Neuroscience, 2*, 370–374.

Broadbent, D. E. (1958). *Perception and communication.* London: Pergamon Press.

Burock, M., Buckner, R. L., Woldorff, M., Rosen, B. R., & Dale, A. M. (1998). Randomized event-related experimental designs allow for extremely rapid presentation rates using functional MRI. *Neuroreport, 9*, 3735–3739.

Carrasco, M., & McElree, B. (2001). Covert attention accelerates the rate of visual information processing. *Proceedings of the National Academy of Sciences USA, 9*, 5353–5367.

Carrasco, M., Penpeci-Talgar, C., & Eckstein, M. (2000). Spatial covert attention increases contrast sensitivity across the CSF: Support for signal enhancement. *Vision Research, 40*, 1203–1215.

Chein, J. M., & Fiez, J. A. (2001). Dissociation of verbal working memory system components using a delayed serial recall task. *Cerebral Cortex, 11*, 1003–1014.

Colby, C. L., Duhamel, J.-R., & Goldberg, M. E. (1993). Ventral intraparietal area of the macaque: anatomic location and visual response properties. *Journal of Neurophysiology, 69*, 902–914.

Colby, C. L., & Goldberg, M. E. (1999). Space and attention in parietal cortex. *Annual Review of Neuroscience, 22*, 319–349.

Connolly, J. D., Goodale, M. A., Menon, R. S., & Munoz, D. P. (2002). Human fMRI evidence for the neural correlates of preparatory set. *Nature Neuroscience, 5*, 1345–1352.

Constantinidis, C., & Steinmetz, M. A. (2001). Neuronal responses in area 7a to multiple stimulus displays: II. responses are suppressed at the cued location. *Cerebral Cortex, 11*, 592–597.

Corbetta, M., Kincade, J. M., Ollinger, J. M., McAvoy, M. P., & Shulman, G. L. (2000). Voluntary orienting is dissociated from target detection in human posterior parietal cortex. *Nature Neuroscience, 3*, 292–297.

Corbetta, M., Kincade, J. M., & Shulman, G. L. (2002). Neural systems for visual orienting and their relationship with working memory. *Journal of Cognitive Neuroscience, 14*, 508–523.

Corbetta, M., Miezin, F. M., Dobmeyer, S., Shulman, G. L., & Petersen, S. E. (1991). Selective and divided attention during visual discriminations of shape, color, and speed: Functional anatomy by positron emission tomography. *Journal of Neuroscience, 11*, 2383–2402.

Corbetta, M., Miezin, F. M., Shulman, G. L., & Petersen, S. E. (1993). A PET study of visuospatial attention. *Journal of Neuroscience, 13,* 1202–1226.

Corbetta, M., & Shulman, G. L. (2002). Control of goal-directed and stimulus-driven attention in the brain. *Nature Reviews Neuroscience, 3,* 201–215.

d'Avossa, G., Shulman, G. L., & Corbetta, M. (2003). Identification of cerebral networks by classification of the shape of BOLD responses. *Journal of Neurophysiology, 90,* 360–371.

Dale, A. M., & Buckner, R. L. (1997). Selective averaging of rapidly presented individual trials using fMRI. *Human Brain Mapping, 5,* 329–340.

Dosher, B. A., & Lu, Z.-L. (2000). Mechanisms of perceptual attention in precuing of location. *Vision Research, 10–12,* 1269–1292.

Dove, A., Pollmann, S., Schubert, T., Wiggins, C. J., & Von Cramon, D. (2000). Prefrontal cortex activation in task switching: An event-related fMRI study. *Cognitive Brain Research, 9,* 103–109.

Downar, J., Crawley, A. P., Mikulis, D. J., & Davis, K. D. (2000). A multimodal cortical network for the detection of changes in the sensory environment. *Nature Neuroscience, 3,* 277–283.

Downar, J., Crawley, A. P., Mikulis, D. J., & Davis, K. D. (2001). The effect of task relevance on the cortical response to changes in visual and auditory stimuli: An event-related fMRI study. *Neuroimage, 14,* 1256–1267.

Duncan, J. (1980). The locus of interference in the perception of simultaneous stimuli. *Psychological Review, 87,* 272–300.

Duncan, J., Bundesen, C., Olson, A., Humphreys, G., Chavda, S., & Shibuya, H. (1999). Systematic analysis of deficits in visual attention. *Journal of Experimemtal Psychology: General, 128,* 450–478.

Eskandar, E. N., & Assad, J. A. (1999). Dissociation of visual, motor and predictive signals in parietal cortex during visual guidance. *Nature Neuroscience, 2,* 88–93.

Friedrich, F. J., Egly, R., Rafal, R. D., & Beck, D. (1998). Spatial attention deficits in humans: A comparison of superior parietal and temporal-parietal junction lesions. *Neuropsychology, 12,* 193–207.

Gandhi, S. P., Heeger, D. J., & Boynton, G. M. (1999). Spatial attention affects brain activity in human primary visual cortex. *Proceedings of National Academy of Sciences USA, 96,* 3314–3319.

Hopfinger, J. B., Buonocore, M. H., & Mangun, G. R. (2000). The neural mechanisms of top-down attentional control. *Nature Neuroscience, 3,* 284–291.

Huettel, S. A., & McCarthy, G. (2000). Evidence for a refractory period in the hemodynamic response to visual stimuli as measured by MRI. *Neuroimage, 11,* 547–553.

Iacoboni, M., Woods, R. P., & Mazziotta, J. C. (1996). Brain–behavior relationships: evidence from practice effects in spatial stimulus–response compatibility. *Journal of Neurophysiology, 76,* 321–331.

Jonides, J. (1981). Voluntary vs. automatic control over the mind's eye's movement. In M. I. Posner & O. Marin (Eds.), *Attention and performance* (Vol. 11, pp. 187–205). Hillsdale, NJ: Erlbaum.

Jonides, J., Smith, E. E., Koeppe, R. A., Awh, E., Minoshima, S., & Mintun, M. A. (1993). Spatial working memory in humans as revealed by PET. *Nature, 363,* 623–625.

Kastner, S., Pinsk, M. A., De Weerd, P., Desimone, R., & Ungerleider, L. G. (1999). Increased activity in human visual cortex during directed attention in the absence of visual stimulation. *Neuron, 22,* 751–761.

Kiehl, K. A., Laurens, K. R., Duty, T. L., Forster, B. B., & Liddle, P. F. (2001). Neural sources involved in auditory target detection and novelty processing: An event-related fMRI study. *Psychophysiology, 38,* 133–142.

Kimberg, D. Y., Aguirre, G. K., & D'Esposito, M. (2000). Modulation of task-related neural activity in task-switching: An fMRI study. *Cognitive Brain Research, 10,* 189–196.

Linden, D. E. J., Prvulovic, D., Formisano, E., Vollinger, M., Zanella, F. E., Goebel, et al. (1999). The functional neuroanatomy of target detection: An fMRI study of visual and auditory oddball tasks. *Cerebral Cortex, 9,* 815–823.

Macaluso, E., Frith, C. D., & Driver, J. (2002). Supramodal effects of covert spatial orienting triggered by visual or tactile events. *Journal of Cognitive Neuroscience, 14,* 389–401.

Marois, R., Chun, M. M., & Gore, J. C. (2000). Neural correlates of the attentional blink. *Neuron*, 28, 299–308.

Marois, R., Leung, H. C., & Gore, J. C. (2000). A stimulus-driven approach to object identity and location processing in the human brain. *Neuron*, 25, 717–728.

Martinez, A., Anllo-Vento, L., Sereno, M. I., Frank, L. R., Buxton, R. B., Dubowitz, D. J., et al. (1999). Involvement of striate and extrastriate visual cortical areas in spatial attention. *Nature Neuroscience*, 2, 364–369.

Maunsell, J. H. R., & Van Essen, D. C. (1983). The connections of the middle temporal visual ara (MT) and their relationship to a cortical hierarchy in the macaque monkey. *Journal of Neuroscience*, 3, 2563–2586.

McCarthy, G., Luby, M., Gore, J., & Goldman-Rakic, P. (1997). Infrequent events transiently activate human prefrontal and parietal cortex as measured by functional MRI. *Journal of Neurophysiology*, 77, 1630–1634.

Miezin, F. M., Maccotta, L., Ollinger, J. M., Petersen, S. E., & Buckner, R. L. (2000). Characterizing the hemodynamic response: Effects of presentation rate, sampling procedure, and the possibility of ordering brain activity based on relative timing. *NeuroImage*, 11, 735–759.

Noesselt, T., Hillyard, S. A., Woldorff, M., Schoenfeld, A., Tempelmann, C., Hinrichs, H., et al. (2002). Delayed striate cortical activation during spatial attention. *Neuron*, 35, 575–587.

Ollinger, J. M., Corbetta, M., & Shulman, G. L. (2001). Separating processes within a trial in event-related functional MRI: II. Analysis. *NeuroImage*, 13, 218–229.

Ollinger, J. M., Shulman, G. L., & Corbetta, M. (2001). Separating processes within a trial in event-related functional MRI: I. The method. *NeuroImage*, 13, 210–217.

Pollmann, S., Dove, A., Von Cramon, D., & Wiggins, C. J. (2000). Event-related fMRI: Comparison of conditions with varying BOLD overlap. *Human Brain Mapping*, 9, 26–37.

Posner, M. I., Snyder, C. R. R., & Davidson, B. J. (1980). Attention and the detection of signals. *Journal of Experimental Psychology: General*, 109, 160–174.

Posner, M. I., Walker, J. A., Friedrich, F. J., & Rafal, R. D. (1984). Effects of parietal injury on covert orienting of attention. *Journal of Neuroscience*, 4, 1863–1874.

Ress, D., Backus, B. T., & Heeger, D. J. (2000). Activity in primary visual cortex predicts performance in a visual detection task. *Nature Neuroscience*, 3, 940–945.

Robinson, D. L., Bowman, E. M., & Kertzman, C. (1995). Covert orienting of attention in Macaques. II. Contributions of parietal cortex. *Journal of Neurophysiology*, 74, 698–721.

Rosenbaum, D. A. (1980). Human movement initiation: Specification of arm, direction and extent. *Journal of Experimental Psychology: General*, 109, 444–474.

Rushworth, M. F., Paus, T., & Sipila, P. K. (2001). Attention systems and the organization of the human parietal cortex. *Journal of Neuroscience*, 21, 5262–5271.

Sapir, A., d'Avossa, G., McAvoy, M., Young, A., Shulman, G. L., & Corbetta, M. (2003). *Trial-by-trial correlation between BOLD signals and shifts of spatial attention*. Paper presented at the annual meeting of the Society for Neuroscience, New Orleans, LA.

Serences, J., Shomstein, S., Leber, A., Yantis, S., & Egeth, H. E. (2001). *Neural mechanisms of stimulus-driven and goal-directed attentional control*. Paper presented at the annual meeting of the Psychonomic Society, Orlando, FL.

Sereno, M. I., Pitzalis, S., & Martinez, A. (2001). Mapping of contralateral space in retinotopic coordinates by a parietal cortical area in humans. *Science*, 294, 1350–1354.

Shmuel, A., Yacoub, E., Pfeuffer, J., Van de Moortele, P.-F., Adriany, G., Hu X., et al. (2002). Sustained negative BOLD, blood flow and oxygen consumption response and its coupling to the positive response in the human brain. *Neuron*, 36, 1195–1210

Shulman, G. L., D'Avossa, G., Tansy, A. P., & Corbetta, M. (2002). Two attentional processes in the parietal lobe. *Cerebral Cortex*, 12, 1124–1131.

Shulman, G. L., McAvoy, M. P., Cowan, M. C., Astafiev, S. V., Tansy, A. P., d'Avossa, G., et al. (2003). Quantitative analysis of attention and detection signals during visual search. *Journal of Neurophysiology*, 90, 3384–3397.

Shulman, G. L., Ollinger, J. M., Akbudak, E., Conturo, T. E., Snyder, A. Z., Petersen, S. E., et al.

(1999). Areas involved in encoding and applying directional expectations to moving objects. *Journal of Neuroscience*, *19*, 9480–9496.

Smith, E. E., Jonides, J., Koeppe, R. A., Awh, E., Schumacher, E. H., & Minoshima, S. (1995). Spatial versus object working memory: PET investigations. *Journal of Cognitive Neuroscience*, *7*, 337–356.

Snyder, L. H., Batista, A. P., & Andersen, R. A. (1997). Coding of intention in the posterior parietal cortex. *Nature*, *386*, 167–170.

Sohn, M.-H., Ursu, S., Anderson, J. R., Stenger, V. A., & Carter, C. S. (2000). The role of prefrontal cortex and posterior parietal cortex in task switching. *Proceedings of the National Academy of Sciences USA*, *97*, 13448–13453.

Steinmetz, M. A., & Constantinidis, C. (1995). Neurophysiological evidence for a role of posterior parietal cortex in redirecting visual attention. *Cerebral Cortex*, *5*, 448–456.

Tootell, R. B. H., Hadjikhani, N., Hall, E. K., Marrett, S., Vanduffel, W., Vaughan, J. T., et al. (1998). The retinotopy of visual spatial attention. *Neuron*, *21*, 1409–1422.

Ungerleider, L. G., & Desimone, R. (1986). Cortical connections of visual area MT in the macaque. *Journal of Comparative Neurology*, *248*, 190–222.

Williams, Z. M., Elfar, J. C., Eskandar, E. N., Toth, L. J., & Assad, J. A. (2003). Parietal activity and the perceived direction of ambiguous apparent motion. *Nature Neuroscience*, *6*, 616–623.

Wolfe, J. M. (1994). Guided search 2.0: A revised model of visual search. *Psychonomic Bulletin and Review*, *1*, 202–238.

Yantis, S., & Jonides, J. (1990). Abrupt visual onsets and selective attention: Voluntary versus automatic allocation. *Journal of Experimental Psychology: Human Perception and Performance*, *16*, 121–134.

Yeshurun, Y., & Carrasco, M. (1999). Spatial attention improves performance in spatial resolution tasks. *Vision Research*, *39*, 293–306.

10

Attention and Contrast Gain Control

John H. Reynolds

Attention has been known to play a central role in perception since the dawn of experimental psychology (James, 1890), but it has only recently become feasible to begin to describe attention in terms of its biological underpinnings. New techniques for imaging the human brain have enabled neuroscientists to map out in unprecedented detail the set of areas that mediate the allocation of attention in the human (for recent reviews, see Corbetta & Shulman, 2002; Yantis & Serences, 2003) and to examine how feedback from these areas alters neural activity in the visual cortices (reviewed by Chun & Marois, 2002; Kastner & Ungerleider, 2000). Recordings of the activity of neurons in awake behaving monkeys have made it possible to interpret these changes in activity in the context of what is known about the network of interconnected excitatory and inhibitory neurons within each cortical area. That is, it is now possible to account for attention-dependent changes in firing rate as resulting from feedback signals modulating interactions between the neurons that make up this cortical microcircuit.

In this chapter, I outline recent progress in understanding the circuits within the visual cortex that are modulated by attentional feedback, with emphasis on spatial attention, where the most detailed mechanistic understanding has been achieved. I argue that attention has co-opted the circuits that mediate contrast gain control—the dynamic calibration of neuronal responsiveness that helps align neuronal sensitivity with the prevailing strength of visual input—and that it operates by increasing the effective contrast of the attended stimulus. I then briefly describe microstimulation studies that have helped provide evidence for a causal connection between activity in one attentional control center, the frontal eye fields, and the observed increases in responsiveness in the visual cortices. I then review recent work in the slice that is helping to explain, at a biophysical level, how such changes in neuronal sensitivity arise from modulatory feedback.

SPATIAL ATTENTION: FACILITATION AND SELECTION

Psychophysical studies, event-related-potential studies, and brain-imaging studies of spatial attention have documented the phenomenon of *attentional facilitation*: the improved processing of a single stimulus appearing alone at an attended location (Posner, Snyder, & Davidson, 1980). Attention improves observers' ability to detect faint stimuli appearing at an attended location (Bashinski & Bacharach, 1980; Hawkins et al., 1990; Handy, Kingstone, & Mangun, 1996; Muller & Humphreys, 1991), and to discriminate features of the attended stimulus, such as its orientation (Downing, 1988; Lee, Itti, Koch, & Braun, 1999). Attention enhances signal strength, as measured by the contrast increment required to equate accuracy in discriminating features of stimuli appearing at an attended versus an unattended location (Carrasco, Penpeci-Talgar, & Eckstein, 2000; Lu & Dosher, 1998). This signal enhancement is reflected in stronger stimulus-evoked neuronal activity, as measured by scalp potentials (reviewed by Hillyard & Anllo-Vento, 1998; see also Anllo-Vento, Schoenfeld, & Hillyard, Chapter 13, this volume), and brain imaging (reviewed by Pessoa, Kastner, & Ungerleider, 2003; Yantis & Serences, 2003).

Single-unit recording studies in monkeys trained to perform attention-demanding tasks have found that spatial attention characteristically enhances neuronal responses evoked by a single stimulus in the receptive field, in neurons throughout the visual system (Ito & Gilbert, 1999; McAdams & Maunsell, 1999a; Motter, 1993; Mountcastle, Motter, Steinmetz, & Sestokas, 1987; Roelfsema & Spekreijse, 2001; Spitzer, Desimone, & Moran, 1988; Treue & Maunsell, 1996). Figure 10.1, which shows data recorded by Reynolds, Pasternak, and

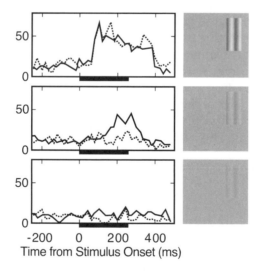

FIGURE 10.1. Responses of an example area V4 neuron as a function of attention and stimulus contrast. The contrast of the stimulus in the receptive field varied from 5% (bottom panel) to 10% (middle panel) to 80% (upper panel). On any given trial, attention was directed either to the location of the stimulus inside the receptive field (solid line) or to a location far away from the receptive field (dotted line). The animal's task was to detect a target grating at the attended location. Attention reduced the threshold level of contrast required to elicit a response without causing a measurable change in response at saturation contrast (80%). From Reynolds, Pasternak, and Desimone (2000). Copyright 2000 by Cell Press. Adapted by permission.

Desimone (2000), illustrates this idea. The dashed line in each panel shows the response evoked by a stimulus that appeared in the receptive field (RF) of a V4 neuron when the monkey was attending away from the receptive field to detect a target for juice reward. The RF stimulus appeared at different levels of luminance contrast: two of which (5%, bottom panel and 10%, middle panel) were too faint to evoke a response. That is, they were below the neuron's *contrast response threshold*. The third contrast (80%, top panel), exceeded the level of contrast at which the response saturated. Solid lines show responses under identical sensory conditions, when spatial attention was directed to the location of the RF stimulus.

Attention had no measurable effect on the response that was evoked at 5% contrast, which was well below the neuron's contrast response threshold. However, the 10% contrast stimulus, which was just below the neuron's contrast response threshold, evoked a clear response when attention was directed to its location in the receptive field. Thus, attention reduced the neuron's contrast response threshold from above 10% to a value between 5% and 10%. Attention had no effect on the neuronal response that was elicited by the stimulus when it was presented above saturating contrast.

Although attention can clearly enhance processing of a faint stimulus appearing against a blank background, an arguably more ecologically relevant purpose is served by *attentional selection*: the selection of behaviorally relevant stimuli from among distracters (Duncan & Humphreys, 1989; Treisman & Gelade, 1980; Wolfe, Cave, & Franzel, 1989). Like any information-processing system, the visual system is limited in the amount of information it is able to process at each moment in time. The visual scene typically contains much more information than we can process in a single glimpse. Therefore, it is necessary to have neural mechanisms in place to select behaviorally relevant information to guide behavior.

The operation of such selection mechanisms is revealed within the extrastriate cortex. When multiple stimuli appear within a neuron's receptive field, the firing rate is characteristically determined primarily by the task-relevant stimulus. The first study to document this notion was carried out by Moran and Desimone (1985). They presented two stimuli within the RF: one that was of the neuron's preferred color and orientation and a second that was of a nonpreferred color and orientation. The monkey performed a task that required it to report the identity of one of the stimuli to earn a juice reward. The neuron's response to the pair was greater when the monkey attended to the preferred stimulus than to the nonpreferred stimulus.

This fundamental observation has been replicated both in the ventral stream areas studied by Moran and Desimone (Chelazzi, Duncan, Miller, & Desimone, 1998; Chelazzi, Miller, Duncan, & Desimone, 1993, 2001; Luck, Chelazzi, Hillyard, & Desimone, 1997; Motter, 1993; Reynolds, Chelazzi, & Desimone, 1999; Reynolds & Desimone, 2003; Sheinberg & Logothetis, 2001) as well as in the dorsal stream (Recanzone & Wurtz, 2000; Treue & Martinez Trujillo, 1999; Treue & Maunsell, 1996; see, however, Seidemann & Newsome, 1999). Several of these studies have compared the response when attention was either directed to one of the RF stimuli or far away from the RF. Attending to the more preferred stimulus typically increases the response to the pair, but attending to the poor stimulus often *reduces* the response evoked by the pair (Chelazzi et al., 1998, 2001; Luck et al., 1997; Martinez Trujillo & Treue, 2002; Reynolds et al., 1999; Reynolds & Desimone, 2003; Treue & Martinez Trujillo, 1999; Treue & Maunsell, 1996). This has provided support for models of attention which rely on response suppression to select one stimulus and inhibit another (Desimone & Duncan, 1995; Ferrera & Lisberger, 1995; Grossberg & Raizada, 2000; Itti & Koch, 2000; Lee et al., 1999; Niebur & Koch, 1994). These models have been used to account for observations concerning a range of topics including the interplay between attentional selection and oculomotor control, the role of working memory in guiding attention during search, and the role of visual salience in guiding attentional selection. Given the broad explanatory power of these models, it is of interest to consider what studies in anesthetized animals have taught us about the role of response suppression in the visual cortex.

CONTRAST-DEPENDENT RESPONSE MODULATION IN VISUAL CORTEX

Contrast-dependent neuronal response modulation has been the focus of extensive research. The models that have been advanced to account for these modulations rely on response suppression. Here we describe four ways in which contrast has been found to modulate neuronal responses. First, cortical neuronal responses typically saturate as contrast increases, and this saturation firing rate is stimulus-dependent. This is illustrated in Figure 10.2A. Each line shows the response of a complex cell in cat area 17 evoked by single grating appearing at the neuron's preferred orientation (top line), a suboptimal but excitatory orientation (middle line) or its null orientation, which was slightly inhibitory (bottom line). The horizontal axis indicates the luminance contrast, so each curve is the neuron's *contrast response function* for one stimulus. The neuron did not respond to stimuli presented below a minimum level of luminance contrast. Above this threshold, the response increased over a range of contrasts that comprise the dynamic range of the contrast response function, before reaching a stimulus-dependent saturation response. The fact that neurons saturate at rates that depend on the stimulus driving them is thought to depend on response suppression (Albrecht & Geisler, 1991; Carandini & Heeger, 1994; Carandini, Heeger, & Movshon, 1997; Grossberg, 1973; Heeger, 1992; McLaughlin, Shapley, Shelley, & Wielaard, 2000; Murphy & Miller, 2003; Somers, Nelson, & Sur, 1995; Sperling & Sondhi, 1968; Troyer, Krukowski, Priebe, & Miller, 1998; for recent reviews, see Ferster & Miller, 2000; Geisler & Albrecht, 2000; Shapley, Hawken, & Ringach, 2003).

Second, increasing the contrast of a stimulus characteristically results in a multiplicative increase in the neuron's tuning curves for properties such as motion and orientation. This is illustrated in Figure 10.2B. Each curve in this figure shows a simple cell's orientation tuning curves at different levels of contrast. The shallowest curve (open circles) reflects the cell's responses to gratings presented at 10% luminance contrast, and each higher curve reflects a doubling of contrast. This contrast-dependent multiplicative increase in the tuning curve is also thought to result from the interplay of excitation (which endows cells with their stimulus selectivity) and response suppression (which ensures that tuning is preserved as contrast increases, by keeping the responses to nonpreferred stimuli low.)

The aforementioned phenomena reflect increases in response when a stimulus increases in contrast. Increasing contrast has qualitatively different effects when two stimuli appear within the receptive field. Increasing the contrast of one of them can result in increases or decreases in response, depending on the neuron's selectivity for the two stimuli. This is illustrated in Figure 10.2C, which shows data recorded by Carandini and colleagues (1997) from a neuron in area V1 of the anesthetized macaque, when two spatially superimposed gratings, differing in orientation, appeared simultaneously within the receptive field (see also Bonds, 1989; DeAngelis, Robson, Ohzawa, & Freeman, 1992; Morrone, Burr, & Maffei, 1982). The circles indicate mean firing rates, with shading indicating the luminance contrast of the preferred orientation grating, ranging from 0% (white) to 50% (black). Thus, the

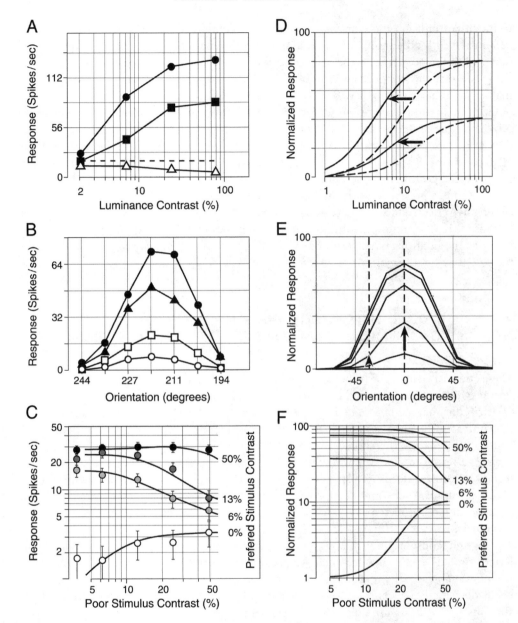

FIGURE 10.2. Contrast-dependent response modulations. (A) Contrast response functions for a stimulus of the neuron's preferred orientation (upper line), a poor but excitatory orientation (middle line) and a poor stimulus (bottom line). From Sclar and Freeman (1982). Copyright 1982 by Springer-Verlag. Adapted by permission. (B) Orientation tuning curves of a second neuron, measured using a stimulus that varied in contrast from 10% (empty circles) to 80% (filled circles). From Sclar and Freeman (1982). Copyright 1982 by Springer-Verlag. Adapted by permission. (C) Responses of an example neuron recorded in Area V1 of the anesthetized macaque. Two spatially superimposed gratings appeared within the receptive field. One grating was of the optimal orientation for the neuron, while the second grating was of a suboptimal orientation. The preferred grating varied from 0% contrast (top curve) to 50% contrast (bottom curve), and the contrast of the poor grating increased from 0% (leftmost points) to 50% (rightmost points). From Carandini, Heeger, and Movshon (1997). Copyright 1997 by the Society for Neuroscience. Adapted by permission. (D–F) The capacity of the contrast gain model to account for these contrast-dependent response modulations. See text for details.

white circles indicate the response to the poor stimulus, alone. The lines show fits to the data provided by the model of Carandini and colleagues. The contrast of the poor orientation grating is indicated on the horizontal axis.

Note that the response evoked by the poor stimulus increases with contrast, indicating that although it was poor, it was nonetheless excitatory. Despite this, increasing the contrast of the poor stimulus suppressed the response elicited by the preferred stimulus. The response evoked by the preferred stimulus presented alone at 13% contrast (~22 spikes per second, dark gray data point, left), was strongly suppressed by the addition of the poor stimulus at 50% contrast (~8 spikes per second, dark gray data point, right). Increasing the contrast of the preferred grating had the opposite effect: to increase the response to the pair. The preferred stimulus presented at the highest contrast (black circles) was virtually immune to this suppressive effect. Thus, by increasing the contrast of one of the two stimuli, it was possible to cause it to have a dominant effect on the neuronal response. Similar contrast-dependent response modulations have been observed when two stimuli appear at separate locations in the receptive field (Reynolds & Desimone, 2003).

A LINKING HYPOTHESIS: DIRECTING SPATIAL ATTENTION TO A STIMULUS INCREASES ITS *EFFECTIVE* CONTRAST

These contrast-dependent response modulations closely parallel the effect of attention when one or two stimuli appear within the receptive field, suggesting that attention modulates the same circuits that are modulated by increasing contrast. First, consider the effect of elevating the contrast of a single stimulus, as illustrated in Figures 10.2A and 10.2B. Increasing the contrast of a just subthreshold stimulus will, by definition, push it above threshold, thereby eliciting a response. For stimuli within the dynamic range of the contrast response function, increasing contrast leads to a stronger response. Thus, if attention operates by increasing the *effective contrast* of a stimulus, this would account for elevations in response that are found when attention is directed to a single stimulus—the idea of *attentional facilitation*, described previously.

Second, consider how changes in contrast alter the response when two stimuli—a preferred stimulus and a poor stimulus—appear simultaneously in the receptive field. The poor stimulus suppresses the response elicited by the preferred stimulus, and this suppression depends on the relative contrasts of the two stimuli (Figure 10.2C). At low contrast, the poor stimulus has little or no suppressive effect, but increasing its contrast drives the pair response downward. Suppression is diminished if the preferred stimulus is elevated in contrast. This is precisely what is observed when attention is directed to one of two stimuli in the RF: The attended stimulus dominates the neuronal response. An appealing linking hypothesis is that attention operates by multiplying the effective contrast of the behaviorally relevant stimulus or, equivalently, increases the neuron's contrast sensitivity.

This idea is embodied in a model of attention advanced by Reynolds and colleagues (1999), which was conceived as a way of formalizing the biased competition model of Desimone and Duncan (1995). It assumes that attention increases the effective contrast of the attended stimulus, and it is thus referred to as the *contrast gain* model of attention. It is a functional model in that it is intended to characterize the operations that are performed by the neural circuit without committing to specific biophysical or biochemical mechanisms. It is, however, mathematically related to models that have been used to account for the contrast-dependent effects described earlier. It can therefore account for the same set of contrast-dependent phenomena, as documented in Figures 10.2D–10.2F.

The model achieves orientation selectivity as a result of tuned excitatory input, which is stronger for a preferred orientation stimulus than for a nonpreferred stimulus. Both excitatory and inhibitory inputs increase in strength with contrast, and the response at high contrast is determined by the ratio of excitatory to inhibitory input. Figure 10.2D shows the model contrast response functions for an optimal (upper dashed line) and a suboptimal but excitatory stimulus (lower dashed line). Attention is assumed to lead to increases in the strength of excitatory and inhibitory inputs activated by the attended stimulus (Reynolds et al., 1999), as would occur with increasing the contrast of the stimulus. The effect of this change is to shift the model contrast response function to the left, as indicated by the arrows.

Figure 10.2E, which was obtained using the same set of parameters that yielded Figure 10.2D, documents the ability of the model to exhibit approximately multiplicative increases in the orientation tuning curve with increasing contrast. The vertical lines indicate the orientations whose contrast response functions are illustrated in Figure 10.2D. Because attention yields a shift in contrast, its effect on the tuning curve is predicted to be the same as an increase in contrast: to cause a multiplicative increase in the tuning curve. This is illustrated by the upward arrows, which show the increases in response that result from a leftward shift in the contrast response function, for the two orientations whose contrast response functions are illustrated in Figure 10.2D.

When two stimuli appear together, the effect of varying the contrast of either stimulus depends on their relative contributions of excitatory and divisive inhibitory drive. When a poor stimulus (with proportionally more inhibitory drive) is presented with a preferred stimulus, the additional inhibitory input results in a suppressed response. This response suppression can be magnified by increasing the contrast of the poor stimulus or diminished by increasing the contrast of the preferred stimulus. Figure 10.2F illustrates the model behavior when the preferred stimulus from Figure 10.2D appears together with a nonpreferred but excitatory stimulus also in the receptive field, at various levels of contrast. As is the case experimentally (Figure 10.2C), the model accounts for the finding that elevating the contrast of the poor stimulus will increase its ability to suppress a preferred stimulus. Thus, a prediction of the model is that when two stimuli appear in the receptive field, attending to the more preferred stimulus will cause an elevation in response, and attending to the poor stimulus will lead to a reduction in response.

ATTENTION-DEPENDENT MODULATIONS OF FIRING RATE MIMIC THE EFFECTS OF AN INCREASE IN CONTRAST

Recent single-unit recording and lesion studies of attention in the macaque have likened attention to increasing visual salience (Bisley & Goldberg, 2003; De Weerd, Peralta, Desimone, & Ungerleider, 1999; Gottlieb, Kusunoki, & Goldberg, 1998; Martinez Trujillo & Treue, 2002; McAdams & Maunsell, 1999a; Reynolds & Desimone, 2003; Reynolds et al., 1999, 2000; Treue, 2003). Reynolds and colleagues (2000) tested the idea that spatial attention causes a multiplicative increase in the effective contrast of a stimulus. If so, then as illustrated in Figure 10.2D, attention should cause a leftward shift in the contrast response function. Such a shift would have three effects. First, the threshold level of contrast needed to evoke a neuronal response should *diminish*. Second, the greatest elevation in firing rate should occur for stimuli that are within (or just below) the dynamic range of the cell's contrast response function. Third, attention should have little or no impact on the response elicited by a stimulus that is above the neuron's contrast saturation point.

Reynolds and colleagues (2000) tested these predictions by measuring the effect of spatial attention on responses in area V4 elicited by stimuli appearing across a range of contrasts. Monkeys performed a task that required them either to attend to the location of the gratings in the RF or else, on separate blocks, to attend to another location, far outside the RF. The task was to detect a target grating that could appear at an unpredictable time at the cued location. The luminance contrast of each target was selected at random. Thus, to perform the task reliably, the monkey had to continually attend to the cued location. The results agreed with the three predictions of the contrast gain model. This was the case for the neurons illustrated in Figure 10.1, which showed no change in firing rate with attention at saturating contrast (80%), but which exhibited a clear reduction in response threshold with attention. Figure 10.3 shows the contrast response function, averaged across the population. The response when attention was directed away from the receptive field is indicated by the thin solid line. The thick solid line indicates the response to the identical stimuli, when attention was directed to their location in the RF. The dashed and dotted lines show percent and absolute difference in firing rate across the two attention conditions, as a function of contrast. At zero contrast (stimulus absent), there was a slight increase in spontaneous activity, in agreement with previous reports (e.g., Luck et al., 1997). This observation bears on the long-standing question whether attention can be directed to an empty location in space. The elevation in spontaneous activity observed here, when no stimulus was present in the receptive field, provides direct evidence that it can.

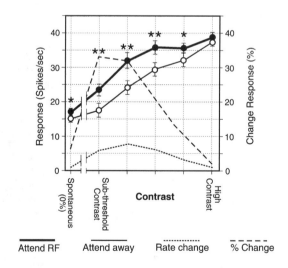

FIGURE 10.3. Attention-dependent increases in contrast sensitivity. Average responses of a population of area V4 neurons while the monkey either attended to the location of the receptive field stimulus (thick line, black circles) or else attended to a location far away from the receptive field (thin line, white circles). Luminance-modulated gratings were presented inside the receptive field at five different values of contrast which were selected to span the dynamic range of the neuron. The monkey's task was to detect a target grating that could appear at an unpredictable time at the cued location. The dashed and dotted lines show, respectively, percent and absolute difference in firing rate across the two attention conditions, as a function of contrast. From Reynolds, Pasternak, and Desimone (2000). Copyright 2000 by Cell Press. Adapted by permission.

For stimuli presented at contrasts just below each neuron's contrast response threshold ("subthreshold contrast"), there was a clear and significant response. The greatest increases in firing rate were observed at contrasts chosen to fall within the dynamic range of each neuron's contrast response function. Attention had no significant effect at the highest contrasts tested, which were chosen to be at or slightly above each neuron's contrast saturation point. Similar results were found for both preferred and poor stimuli, indicating that this failure to find attention effects at high contrast did not simply reflect an absolute firing rate limit but, instead, reflected a leftward shift in the contrast response function, consistent with the prediction illustrated in Figure 10.2D. A cell-by-cell analysis revealed that in order for a cell to detect an unattended stimulus as reliably as it could detect an attended stimulus, the unattended stimulus needed to be half again as high in contrast as the attended stimulus. That is, under the conditions of this experiment, attention was "worth" a 51% increase in contrast. This value would be expected to change as a function of task difficulty (Spitzer et al., 1988) and brain area (Cook & Maunsell, 2002; Luck et al., 1997). Nonetheless, it is in line with other studies that have also quantified spatial attention in units of luminance contrast in MT (Martinez Trujillo & Treue, 2002): 50% and V4 (Reynolds & Desimone, 2003): 56%).

McAdams and Maunsell (1999a) found results that support the conclusion that attention increases effective contrast. They held contrast constant and varied the orientation of a grating appearing alone in the receptive field. They found that, like an increase in contrast, attention causes a multiplicative increase in the orientation tuning curve. In their experiment, monkeys either attended to the stimulus in the receptive field to report whether or not two successive gratings differed in orientation or else attended to stimuli appearing at a location across the vertical meridian to report whether they differed in color. They found that attending to the receptive field caused a multiplicative increase in the neuron's orientation tuning curve. In a related study, they demonstrated that this increase in the gain of the orientation tuning curve enabled neuronal signals to better distinguish the orientation of the stimulus (McAdams & Maunsell, 1999b).

A third property that can be accounted for by the idea that spatial attention increases effective contrast is that attending to one of two stimuli appearing together in the receptive field will cause either an increase or a decrease in response, depending on the cell's relative preference for the two stimuli (see Figure 10.2F), with changes growing in proportion to the neuron's selectivity for the two stimuli. As noted previously, this prediction has been validated by several single-unit recording studies of attention (Chelazzi et al., 1998, 2001; Martinez Trujillo & Treue, 2002; Reynolds et al., 1999; Reynolds & Desimone, 2003; Treue & Martinez Trujillo, 1999; Treue & Maunsell, 1996). This prediction is illustrated in Figure 10.4, which shows responses of a single V4 neuron, which was recorded by (Reynolds et al., 1999). The upper solid black line shows the response to the preferred stimulus alone, when attention was directed away from the receptive field. The lower solid gray line shows the much weaker response that was elicited by a poor stimulus alone, again with attention away from the receptive field. The gray dotted line shows the response when the two unattended stimuli were presented together. The response to the pair falls between the responses elicited by either stimulus alone. When attention was directed to the preferred stimulus (upper dashed black line), it led to an increase in the response to the pair. When attention was directed to the poor stimulus (lower dashed gray line), it led to a substantial reduction in response, pushing the pair response down to a level similar to that which was observed when the poor stimulus appeared alone in the receptive field. This pattern is illustrative of what is observed in area V4, though the suppressive effect of directing attention to the poor stimulus is rarely this absolute. On average, we have found that attention moves the pair response

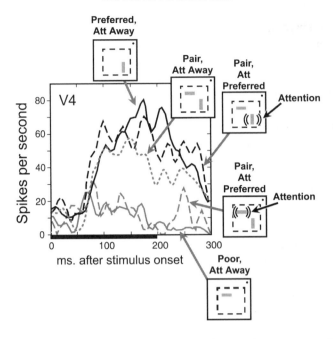

FIGURE 10.4. Effect of attention to one of two stimuli in the RF of a V4 neuron. Each line shows the response of a single V4 neuron averaged over repeated stimulus presentations, in different attentional and stimulus conditions which are indicated by each icon. The stimuli appeared for 250 milliseconds, as indicated by the thick bar on the horizontal axis. See text for details.

about 70–80% of the way to the response that would be elicited by the attended stimulus appearing alone in the receptive field.

SOURCES OF SIGNALS THAT MODULATE RESPONSES IN VISUAL CORTEX

The experiments described previously demonstrate that spatial attention causes changes in the neuronal response that are similar to the effects of increasing the effective contrast of the attended stimulus. Research from many laboratories using a variety of different techniques have identified potential sources for the feedback signals that modulate visual cortical responses during spatially directed attention (for a recent review, see Corbetta & Shulman, 2002; see also Nobre, Chapter 12; Shulman, Astafiev, & Corbetta, Chapter 9, this volume). These include the pulvinar (reviewed by Sherman, 2001), parts of the parietal cortex (Bisley & Goldberg, 2003; Colby & Goldberg, 1999; Gottlieb et al., 1998; Mountcastle et al., 1987; Steinmetz & Constantinidis, 1995; Cutrell & Marrocco, 2002), the frontal eye fields (reviewed by Schall, 1995), and the superior colliculus (Basso & Wurtz, 1998; Wurtz & Goldberg, 1972). Recently, microstimulation studies have been carried out in one of these control structures, the frontal eye field, (FEF), which also plays a prominent role in controlling eye movements (Robinson & Fuchs, 1969). These studies have found that FEF stimulation causes a spatially selective increase in contrast sensitivity at the behavioral level, as well as causing changes in the responses of V4 neurons that are similar to those which are observed with spatial attention. In addition to its role in controlling eye movements, FEF is known to play a role in the selection of stimuli during visual search (for a review, see Thompson, Bichot, & Schall, 2001). Sensitivity to stimuli has been found to increase at the location of an upcoming saccade (Hoffman & Subramaniam, 1995; Moore, Tolias, & Schiller, 1998; Rizzolatti, Matelli, & Pavesi, 1983; Shepherd, Findlay, & Hockey, 1986). FEF has direct projections to visual areas that are modulated by spatial attention, including areas V2, V3, V4, MT, MST, TE, and TEO, as well as to other potential sources of top-down attentional control such as area LIP (Stanton, Bruce, & Goldberg, 1995).

To establish a causal link between attention-dependent increases in contrast sensitivity and FEF activity, Moore and Fallah (2003) measured contrast detection thresholds while introducing electrical stimulation into FEF. Electrical stimulation of FEF neurons will cause the eyes to move from the fixation point to particular a location, which varies systematically according to the location of the microstimulating electrode. This location is referred to as the movement field of the neurons at the stimulation site. After determining the movement field, Moore and Fallah had monkeys report a brief change in the luminance of a target in the movement field to earn a juice reward. Distracter stimuli appeared randomly at locations throughout the visual field, which increased task difficulty (Figure 10.5A). On a randomly selected subset of trials, current was injected, which was calibrated to be too faint to evoke an eye movement. Using a staircase procedure, they found the minimum luminance change that the monkey could reliably detect, on trials both with and without stimulation. Microstimulating FEF reduced this contrast threshold, as illustrated in Figure 10.5B, which shows the contrasts generated by the staircase procedure. For this session, stimulation reduced the threshold luminance change from 44% to 28%. This microstimulation effect was spatially specific: The monkey only benefited when the target appeared within the movement field. Thus FEF improves contrast sensitivity at the movement field location, in much the same way as spatial attention improves contrast sensitivity in V4 neurons (Reynolds et al., 2000). In a subsequent study, Moore and Armstrong (2003) tested whether the effect of FEF stimulation increases the responsiveness of V4 neurons, by recording in area V4 while simultaneously microstimulating FEF (Figure 10.5C). They found that FEF stimulation caused the neuronal response to increase. Figure 10.5D illustrates this increase in response with FEF stimulation. The visual stimulus was present for 1 second (RF stim) and current was injected (FEF stim) 500 milliseconds after stimulus onset. The responses of one V4 neuron with and without FEF stimulation are indicated at the bottom of the figure. The response on microstimulation trials (gray) was clearly elevated, compared to the response without stimulation (black), during the period following electrical stimulation. Moore and Armstrong did not vary luminance contrast. However, consistent with an increase in effective contrast, they found that stimulation caused a greater increase in response when a preferred stimulus appeared in the receptive field, as compared to when a poor stimulus appeared in the RF. These studies thus establish that FEF microstimulation has effects at the behavioral and at the neuronal level which mimic the effect of spatial attention. These findings provide strong evidence that FEF is one of the brain areas that modulates the control of attention, along with other areas, including the pulvinar, parts of parietal cortex, and the superior colliculus, which are also believed to contribute to the allocation of attention.

MECHANISMS OF RESPONSE ENHANCEMENT

Recent intracellular recording studies using the dynamic clamp technique provide insight into how modulatory feedback from areas such as FEF might cause changes in neuronal sen-

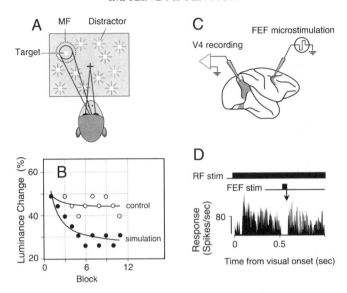

FIGURE 10.5. The effects of FEF stimulation on sensitivity. (A) During the attention task, the monkey maintained fixation while attending to a target within the movement field (MF), in order to detect a slight change in luminance. Distracters appeared throughout the visual field. On randomly selected trials, current was injected into FEF at levels too low to elicit an eye movement. From Moore and Fallah (2001). Copyright 2001 by National Academy of Sciences, USA. Adapted by permission. (B) A staircase procedure was used to determine threshold luminance changes with (black circles) and without (white circles) FEF stimulation. Thresholds were reduced by FEF stimulation. From Moore and Fallah (2001). C–D: FEF microstimulation increases neuronal responsiveness in V4. From Moore and Armstrong (2003). Copyright 2003 by Nature Publishing. Adapted by permission. (C) Subthreshold microstimulating current was injected into FEF while neuronal activity was recorded from V4. (D) The visual stimulus appeared for 1 second ("RF stim"). Five hundred milliseconds after the appearance of the visual stimulus, FEF was electrically stimulated for 50 msec ("FEF stim"). The response of a single V4 neuron with (gray) and without (black) FEF microstimulation appears below. The apparent gap in response reflects the brief period during which V4 recording was paused while current was injected into FEF. Following this interruption, recording continued, and the V4 neuron was found to have elevated responses on trials when FEF was electrically stimulated as compared to trials without FEF stimulation.

sitivity. The dynamic clamp technique enables a physiologist to simulate different patterns of conductance changes that result from the activity of a network of neurons that synapse on a recorded neuron and to measure their effect on the neuron's response to a current injection. Using this technique, Chance, Abbott, and Reyes (2002) found that they could change neuronal response gain by introducing a noisy barrage of excitation and inhibition. Excitation and inhibition were balanced so that they did not directly changing the average membrane potential of the neuron. Fellous, Rudolph, Destexhe, and Sejnowski (2003) have extended this finding, by independently varying excitatory and inhibitory modulatory inputs. Their experiments show that an increase in the variance of either inhibitory or excitatory synaptic inputs can increase neuronal gain. Such an increase in variance would be expected to result from increasing the degree of correlation between the neurons that provide the modulatory input to the cell. Thus, their experiments suggest that response synchronization among neuronal afferents could cause the increases in neuronal responsiveness that are observed with attention (see Crick & Koch, 1990; Niebur, Hsiao, & Johnson, 2002; Salinas & Sejnowski, 2001, for further discussion of this idea).

Consistent with this proposal, two recent single-unit recording studies in the macaque have documented measurable changes in synchrony with attention. Steinmetz and colleagues (2000) recorded responses in somatosensory cortex and found that when monkeys performed a tactile discrimination task, this increased the degree to which neurons fired synchronously. Fries, Reynolds, Rorie, and Desimone (2001) recorded the responses of neurons in area V4 and found evidence for an increase in high-frequency synchronization when attention was directed to the stimulus within the neuron's overlapping receptive fields. These studies, taken together with the dynamic clamp studies described earlier, suggest that response synchronization of afferent neurons may mediate the changes in response sensitivity and response gain that are observed with attention.

CONCLUSIONS

Posner and Petersen (1990) noted that the importance of attention is its role in connecting the mental level of description used in cognitive science with the anatomical level common in neuroscience. In this chapter, we have seen an example of this integration across levels of explanation. Psychophysical measures of the effects of spatial attention on performance in detection of isolated stimuli and selection of stimuli from among distracters have direct neural correlates in the extrastriate cortex, where both increases in neuronal sensitivity and selection of a stimulus that is presented with one or more distracters can be accounted for by a single cortical circuit model. These studies have found close parallels between the effect of spatial attention and increases in luminance contrast, and microstimulation of one attentional control area, the FEF, provides evidence of a causal link between feedback signals, changes in neuronal sensitivity, and changes in perceptual sensitivity. The cited studies in the cortical slice have begun to characterize, at the biophysical level, the mechanisms underlying these changes in sensitivity.

REFERENCES

Albrecht, D. G., & Geisler, W. S. (1991). Motion selectivity and the contrast-response function of simple cells in the visual cortex. *Visual Neuroscience, 7,* 531–546.

Bashinski, H. S., & Bacharach, V. R. (1980). Enhancement of perceptual sensitivity as the result of selectively attending to spatial locations. *Perception and Psychophysics, 28,* 241–248.

Basso, M. A., & Wurtz, R. H. (1998). Modulation of neuronal activity in superior colliculus by changes in target probability. *Journal of Neuroscience, 18,* 7519–7534.

Bisley, J. W., & Goldberg, M. E. (2003). Neuronal activity in the lateral intraparietal area and spatial attention. *Science, 299,* 81–86.

Bonds, A. B. (1989). Role of inhibition in the specification of orientation selectivity of cells in the cat striate cortex. *Visual Neuroscience, 2,* 41–55.

Carandini, M., & Heeger, D. J. (1994). Summation and division by neurons in primate visual cortex. *Science, 264,* 1333–1336.

Carandini, M., Heeger, D. J., & Movshon, J. A. (1997). Linearity and normalization in simple cells of the macaque primary visual cortex. *Journal of Neuroscience, 17,* 8621–8644.

Carrasco, M., Penpeci-Talgar, C., & Eckstein, M. (2000). Spatial covert attention increases contrast sensitivity across the CSF, support for signal enhancement. *Vision Research, 40,* 1203–1215.

Chance, F. S., Abbott, L. F., & Reyes, A. D. (2002). Gain modulation from background synaptic input. *Neuron, 35,* 773–872.

Chelazzi, L., Duncan, J., Miller, E. K., & Desimone, R. (1998). Responses of neurons in inferior temporal cortex during memory-guided visual search. *Journal of Neurophysiology, 80,* 2918–2940.

Chelazzi, L., Miller, E. K., Duncan, J., & Desimone, R. (1993). A neural basis for visual search in inferior temporal cortex. *Nature, 363,* 345–347.

Chelazzi, L., Miller, E. K., Duncan, J., & Desimone, R. (2001). Responses of neurons in macaque area V4 during memory-guided visual search. *Cerebral Cortex, 11,* 761–772.

Chun, M. M., & Marois, R. (2002). The dark side of visual attention. *Current Opinion in Neurobiology, 12,* 184–189.

Colby, C. L., & Goldberg, M. E. (1999). Space and attention in parietal cortex. *Annual Review of Neuroscience, 22,* 319–349.

Cook, E. P., & Maunsell, J. H. (2002). Attentional modulation of behavioral performance and neuronal responses in middle temporal and ventral intraparietal areas of macaque monkey. *Journal of Neuroscience, 22,* 1994–2004.

Corbetta, M., & Shulman, G. L. (2002). Control of goal-directed and stimulus-driven attention in the brain. *Nature Review of Neuroscience, 3,* 201–215.

Crick, F., & Koch, C. (1990). Some reflections on visual awareness. *Cold Spring Harbor Symposium on Quantum Biology, 55,* 953–962.

Cutrell, E. B., & Marrocco, R. T. (2002, May). Electrical microstimulation of primate posterior parietal cortex initiates orienting and alerting components of covert attention. *Experimental Brain Research, 144*(1), 103–113.

DeAngelis, G. C., Robson, J. G., Ohzawa, I., & Freeman, R. D. (1992). Organization of suppression in receptive fields of neurons in cat visual cortex. *Journal of Neurophysiology, 68,* 144–163.

De Weerd, P., Peralta, M. R. III, Desimone, R., & Ungerleider, L. G. (1999). Loss of attentional stimulus selection after extrastriate cortical lesions in macaques. *Nature Neuroscience, 2,* 753–758.

Desimone, R., & Duncan, J. (1995). Neural mechanisms of selective visual attention. *Annual Review of Neuroscience, 18,* 193–222.

Downing, C. J. (1988). Expectancy and visual-spatial attention: Effects on perceptual quality. *Journal of Experimental Psychology: Human Perception and Performance, 14,* 188–202.

Duncan, J., & Humphreys, G. W. (1989). Visual search and stimulus similarity. *Psychological Review, 96,* 433–458.

Fellous, J., Rudolph, M., Destexhe, A., & Sejnowski, T. J. (2003). Synaptic background noise controls the input/output characteristics of single cells in an *in vitro* model of *in vivo* activity. *Neuroscience, 122,* 811–829.

Ferrera, V. P., & Lisberger, S. G. (1995). Attention and target selection for smooth pursuit eye movements. *Journal of Neuroscience, 15,* 7472–7484.

Ferster, D., & Miller, K. D. (2000). Neural mechanisms of orientation selectivity in the visual cortex. *Annual Review of Neuroscience, 23,* 441–471.

Fries, P., Reynolds, J. H., Rorie, A. E., & Desimone, R. (2001). Modulation of oscillatory neuronal synchronization by selective visual attention. *Science, 291,* 1560–1563.

Geisler, W., & Albrecht, D. (2000). *Spatial vision* (pp. 79–128). New York: Academic Press.

Gottlieb, J. P., Kusunoki, M., & Goldberg, M. E. (1998). The representation of visual salience in monkey parietal cortex. *Nature, 391,* 481–484.

Grossberg, S. (1973). Contour enhancement, short-term memory, and constancies in reverberating neural networks. *Studies in Applied Math, 52,* 217–257.

Grossberg, S., & Raizada, R. D. (2000). Contrast-sensitive perceptual grouping and object-based attention in the laminar circuits of primary visual cortex. *Vision Research, 40,* 1413–1432.

Handy, T. C., Kingstone, A., & Mangun, G. R. (1996). Spatial distribution of visual attention: Perceptual sensitivity and response latency. *Perception and Psychophysics, 58,* 613–627.

Hawkins, H. L., Hillyard, S. A., Luck, S. J., Mouloua, M., Downing, C. J., & Woodward, D. P. (1990). Visual attention modulates signal detectability. *Journal of Experimental Psychology: Human Perception and Performance, 16,* 802–811.

Heeger, D. J. (1992). Normalization of cell responses in cat striate cortex. *Visual Neuroscience, 9,* 181–197.

Hillyard, S. A., & Anllo-Vento, L. (1998). Event-related brain potentials in the study of visual selective attention. *Proceedings of the National Academy of Sciences USA, 95,* 781–787.

Hoffman, J. E., & Subramaniam, B. (1995). The role of visual attention in saccadic eye movements. *Perception and Psychophysics*, 57, 787–795.

Ito, M., & Gilbert, C. D. (1999). Attention modulates contextual influences in the primary visual cortex of alert monkeys. *Neuron*, 22, 593–604

Itti, L., & Koch, C. (2000). A saliency-based search mechanism for overt and covert shifts of visual attention. *Vision Research*, 40, 1489–1506.

James, W. (1890). *The principles of psychology*. New York: Holt.

Kastner, S., & Ungerleider, L. G. (2000). Mechanisms of visual attention in the human cortex. *Annual Review of Neuroscience*, 23, 315–341.

Lee, D. K., Itti, L., Koch, C., & Braun, J. (1999). Attention activates winner-take-all competition among visual filters. *Nature Neuroscience*, 2, 375–381.

Lu, Z. L., & Dosher, B. A. (1998). External noise distinguishes attention mechanisms. *Vision Research*, 38, 1183–1198.

Luck, S. J., Chelazzi, L., Hillyard, S. A., & Desimone, R. (1997). Neural mechanisms of spatial selective attention in areas V1, V2, and V4 of macaque visual cortex. *Journal of Neurophysiology*, 77, 24–42.

Martinez Trujillo, J., & Treue, S. (2002). Attentional modulation strength in cortical area MT depends on stimulus contrast. *Neuron*, 35, 365–370.

McAdams, C. J., & Maunsell, J. H. (1999a). Effects of attention on orientation-tuning functions of single neurons in macaque cortical area V4. *Journal of Neuroscience*, 19, 431–441.

McAdams, C. J., & Maunsell, J. H. (1999b). Effects of attention on the reliability of individual neurons in monkey visual cortex. *Neuron*, 23, 765–773.

McLaughlin, D., Shapley, R., Shelley, M., & Wielaard, D. J. (2000). A neuronal network model of macaque primary visual cortex (V1): Orientation selectivity and dynamics in the input layer 4C alpha. *Proceedings of the National Academy of Sciences USA*, 97, 8087–8092.

Moore, T., & Armstrong, K. M. (2003). Selective gating of visual signals by microstimulation of frontal cortex. *Nature*, 421, 370–373.

Moore, T., & Fallah, M. (2001). Control of eye movements and spatial attention. *Proceedings of the National Academy of Sciences USA*, 98, 1273–1276.

Moore, T., & Fallah, M. (2004). Microstimulation of the frontal eye field and its effects on covert spatial attention. *Journal of Neurophysiology*, 91, 152–162.

Moore, T., Tolias, A. S., & Schiller, P. H. (1998). Visual representations during saccadic eye movements. *Proceedings of the National Academy of Sciences USA*, 95, 8981–8984.

Moran, J., & Desimone, R. (1985). Selective attention gates visual processing in the extrastriate cortex. *Science*, 229, 782–784.

Morrone, M. C., Burr, D. C., & Maffei, L. (1982). Functional implications of cross-orientation inhibition of cortical visual cells. I. Neurophysiological evidence. *Philosophical Transactions of the Royal Society of London B (Biological Sciences)*, 216, 335–354.

Motter, B. C. (1993). Focal attention produces spatially selective processing in visual cortical areas V1, V2, and V4 in the presence of competing stimuli. *Journal of Neurophysiology*, 70, 909–919.

Mountcastle, V. B., Motter, B. C., Steinmetz, M. A., & Sestokas, A. K. (1987). Common and differential effects of attentive fixation on the excitability of parietal and prestriate (V4) cortical visual neurons in the macaque monkey. *Journal of Neuroscience*, 7, 2239–2255.

Muller, H. J., & Humphreys, G. W. (1991). Luminance-increment detection: Capacity-limited or not? *Journal of Experimental Psychology: Human Perception and Performance*, 17, 107–124.

Murphy, B. K., & Miller, K. D. (2003). Multiplicative gain changes are induced by excitation or inhibition alone. *Journal of Neuroscience*, 23, 10040–10051.

Niebur, E., Hsiao, S. S., & Johnson, K. O. (2002). Synchrony: A neuronal mechanism for attentional selection? *Current Opinion in Neurobiology*, 12, 190–194.

Niebur, E., & Koch, C. (1994). A model for the neuronal implementation of selective visual attention based on temporal correlation among neurons. *Journal of Comparative Neurology*, 1, 141–158.

Pessoa, L., Kastner, S., & Ungerleider, L. G. (2003). Neuroimaging studies of attention: From modulation of sensory processing to top-down control. *Journal of Neuroscience*, 23, 3990–3998.

Posner, M. I., & Petersen, S. E. (1990). The attention system of the human brain. *Annual Review Neuroscience, 13*, 25–42.

Posner, M. I., Snyder, C. R., & Davidson, B. J. (1980). Attention and the detection of signals. *Journal of Experimental Psychology, 109*, 160–174.

Recanzone, G. H., & Wurtz, R. H. (2000). Effects of attention on MT and MST neuronal activity during pursuit initiation. *Journal of Neurophysiology, 83*, 777–790.

Reynolds, J. H., Chelazzi, L., & Desimone, R. (1999). Competitive mechanisms subserve attention in macaque areas V2 and V4. *Journal of Neuroscience, 19*, 1736–1753.

Reynolds, J. H., & Desimone, R. (2003). Interacting roles of attention and visual salience in V4. *Neuron, 37*, 853–863.

Reynolds, J. H., Pasternak, T., & Desimone, R. (2000). Attention increases sensitivity of V4 neurons. *Neuron, 26*, 703–714.

Rizzolatti, G., Matelli, M., & Pavesi, G. (1983). Deficits in attention and movement following the removal of postarcuate (area 6) and prearcuate (area 8) cortex in macaque monkeys. *Brain, 106*(Pt. 3), 655–673.

Robinson, D. A., & Fuchs, A. F. (1969). Eye movements evoked by stimulation of frontal eye fields. *Journal of Neurophysiology, 32*, 637–648.

Roelfsema, P. R., & Spekreijse, H. (2001). The representation of erroneously perceived stimuli in the primary visual cortex. *Neuron, 31*, 853–863.

Salinas, E., & Sejnowski, T. J. (2001). Correlated neuronal activity and the flow of neural information. *Nature Review of Neuroscience, 2*, 539–550.

Schall, J. D. (1995). Neural basis of saccade target selection. *Review of Neuroscience, 6*, 63–85.

Sclar, G., & Freeman, R. D. (1982). Orientation selectivity in the cat's striate cortex is invariant with stimulus contrast. *Experimental Brain Research, 46*, 457–461.

Seidemann, E., & Newsome, W. T. (1999). Effect of spatial attention on the responses of area MT neurons. *Journal of Neurophysiology, 81*, 1783–1794.

Shapley, R., Hawken, M., & Ringach, D. L. (2003). Dynamics of orientation selectivity in the primary visual cortex and the importance of cortical inhibition. *Neuron, 38*, 689–699.

Sheinberg, D. L., & Logothetis, N. K. (2001). Noticing familiar objects in real world scenes: The role of temporal cortical neurons in natural vision. *Journal of Neuroscience, 21*, 1340–1350.

Shepherd, M., Findlay, J. M., & Hockey, R. J. (1986). The relationship between eye movements and spatial attention. *Quarterly Journal of Experimental Psychology A, 38*, 475–491.

Sherman, S. M. (2001). Thalamic relay functions. *Progress in Brain Research, 134*, 51–69.

Somers, D. C., Nelson, S. B., & Sur, M. (1995). An emergent model of orientation selectivity in cat visual cortical simple cells. *Journal of Neuroscience, 15*, 5448–5465.

Sperling, G., & Sondhi, M. M. (1968). Model for visual luminance discrimination and flicker detection. *Journal of the Optical Society of America, 58*, 1133–1145.

Spitzer, H., Desimone, R., & Moran J. (1988). Increased attention enhances both behavioral and neuronal performance. *Science, 240*, 338–340.

Stanton, G. B., Bruce, C. J., & Goldberg, M. E. (1995). Topography of projections to posterior cortical areas from the macaque frontal eye fields. *Journal of Comparative Neurology, 353*, 291–305.

Steinmetz, M. A., & Constantinidis, C. (1995). Neurophysiological evidence for a role of posterior parietal cortex in redirecting visual attention. *Cerebral Cortex, 5*, 448–456.

Steinmetz, P. N., Roy, A., Fitzgerald, P. J., Hsiao, S. S., Johnson, K. O., & Niebur, E. (2000). Attention modulates synchronized neuronal firing in primate somatosensory cortex. *Nature, 404*, 187–190.

Thompson, K., Bichot, N. P., & Schall, J. D. (2001). From attention to action in frontal cortex. In J. Braun, C. Koch, & J. L. Davis (Eds.), *Visual attention and cortical circuits* (pp. 137–156). Cambridge, MA: MIT Press

Treisman, A. M., & Gelade, G. (1980). A feature-integration theory of attention. *Cognitive Psychology, 12*, 97–136.

Treue, S. (2003). Visual attention: The where, what, how and why of saliency. *Current Opinion in Neurobiology, 13*, 428–432.

Treue, S., & Martinez Trujillo, J. C. (1999). Feature-based attention influences motion processing gain in macaque visual cortex. *Nature, 399*, 575–579.

Treue, S., & Maunsell, J. H. (1996). Attentional modulation of visual motion processing in cortical areas MT and MST. *Nature, 382,* 539–541.

Troyer, T. W., Krukowski, A. E., Priebe, N. J., & Miller, K. D. (1998). Contrast-invariant orientation tuning in cat visual cortex: Thalamocortical input tuning and correlation-based intracortical connectivity. *Journal of Neuroscience, 18,* 5908–5927.

Wolfe, J. M., Cave, K. R., & Franzel, S. L. (1989). Guided search: An alternative to the feature integration model for visual search. *Journal of Experimental Psychology: Human Perception and Performance, 15,* 419–433.

Wurtz, R. H., & Goldberg, M. E. (1972). The primate superior colliculus and the shift of visual attention. *Investigative Ophthalmology, 11,* 441–450.

Yantis, S., & Serences, J. T. (2003). Cortical mechanisms of space-based and object-based attentional control. *Current Opinion in Neurobiology, 13,* 187–193.

11

Attentional Response Modulation in the Human Visual System

Sabine Kastner

"Selective visual attention" is a broad term that refers to a variety of different behavioral phenomena. Directing attention to a spatial location has been shown to improve the accuracy and speed of subjects' responses to target stimuli that occur in that location (Posner, 1980). Attention also increases the perceptual sensitivity for the discrimination of target stimuli (Lu & Dosher, 1998), increases contrast sensitivity (Cameron, Tai, & Carrasco, 2002), reduces the interference caused by distracters (Shiu & Pashler, 1995), and improves acuity (Yeshurun & Carrasco, 1998). What may be the neural basis underlying these and other behavioral effects of visual attention? There is converging evidence from single-cell physiology studies in nonhuman primates and functional brain-mapping studies in humans that selective attention modulates neural activity in the visual system. In this chapter, I discuss functional magnetic resonance imaging (fMRI) studies on mechanisms of selective visual attention in the human brain and how they relate to single-cell physiology studies in monkeys. In the first part, I review several attention effects that have been found at various stages of visual processing. In the second part, I ask what functions these attention effects may serve at different levels of the visual processing hierarchy. Furthermore, I describe evidence that these attention effects are not generated in the visual system but in a distributed network of higher-order areas in frontal and parietal cortex. The results of these studies may account for many of the known behavioral effects of attention, thereby providing links between systems neuroscience and cognitive psychology.

MULTIPLE EFFECTS OF SELECTIVE ATTENTION IN THE VISUAL SYSTEM

Attentional Response Enhancement

In single-cell recording studies in monkeys, neural responses to visual stimuli presented within a neuron's receptive field (RF) have been studied under conditions in which the animal covertly (i.e., without executing eye movements) directs its attention to a stimulus within the RF, or when the animal directs its attention away from the RF to another location in the visual field. Several studies have shown that neural spike rates to a single stimulus presented within the RF are enhanced when the animal directs its attention within the RF compared to when the animal attends outside the RF. This effect, which increases with task difficulty (Spitzer, Desimone, & Moran, 1988; Spitzer & Richmond, 1991), has been demonstrated in V1 (Motter, 1993), and in extrastriate areas V2 (Luck, Chelazzi, Hillyard, & Desimone, 1997; Motter, 1993), V4 (Connor, Gallant, Preddie, & Van Essen, 1996; Connor, Preddie, Gallant, & Van Essen, 1997; Haenny, Maunsell, & Schiller, 1988; Luck et al., 1997; McAdams & Maunsell, 1999; Motter, 1993; Reynolds, Chelazzi, & Desimone, 1999; Spitzer et al., 1988), and MT/MST (Cook & Maunsell, 2002; Treue & Martinez Trujillo, 1999; Treue & Maunsell, 1996). This finding suggests that mechanisms of spatial attention operate by enhancing neural responses to stimuli at attended locations, thereby facilitating information processing at the attended location.

In fMRI studies, attentional response enhancement was investigated across the human visual system by presenting checkerboard stimuli to the left or right hemifield while subjects directed attention to the stimulus (attended condition) or away from the stimulus (unattended condition) (O'Connor, Fukui, Pinsk, & Kastner, 2002). In the unattended condition, attention was directed away from the stimulus by having subjects count letters at fixation. The letter-counting task ensured proper fixation and effectively prevented subjects from covertly attending to the checkerboard stimuli. In the attended condition, subjects were instructed to covertly direct attention to the checkerboard stimulus and to detect luminance changes that occurred randomly in time at a peripheral stimulus location. Relative to the unattended condition, the mean fMRI signals evoked by a high-contrast checkerboard stimulus increased significantly in the attended condition in the lateral geniculate nucleus (LGN) and in visual cortex (Figure 11.1A). In particular, such attentional response enhancement was found in striate cortex, and in each extrastriate area along the ventral and dorsal pathways (Figure 11.2A). Similar attentional response enhancement was obtained with activity evoked by a low-contrast checkerboard stimulus (Figure 11.1A). Notably, these attention effects were shown to be spatially specific in separate studies, in which identical stimuli were presented simultaneously to the right and left of fixation, while subjects were instructed to direct attention covertly to the right or the left (O'Connor et al., 2002). Taken together, these findings suggest that selective attention facilitates visual processing in thalamic and cortical areas by enhancing neural responses to an attended stimulus relative to those evoked by the same stimulus when ignored. Attentional response enhancement may be a neural correlate for behavioral attention effects such as increased accuracy and response speed, or improved target discriminability (e.g., Lu & Dosher, 1998; Posner, 1980).

Attentional Response Suppression

Selective attention affects not only the processing of the selected information, as shown in the last section, but also the processing of the unattended information, which is typically the vast majority of incoming information. The neural fate of unattended stimuli was investigated in an fMRI experiment, in which the attentional load of a task at fixation was varied (O'Connor et al., 2002). According to attentional load theory (Lavie & Tsal, 1994), the degree to which ignored stimuli are processed is determined by the amount of attentional capacity that is not dedicated to the selection process. This account predicts that neural responses to unattended stimuli should be attenuated depending on the attentional load necessary to process the attended stimulus. This idea was tested by presenting high- and low-contrast checkerboard stimuli to the left or right hemifield while subjects performed either an easy (low load) attention task or a hard (high load) attention task at fixation and ignored the peripheral checkerboard stimuli. During the easy attention task, subjects counted infrequent, brief color changes of the fixation cross. During the hard attention task, subjects counted letters at fixation. Behavioral performance was 99% (± 1% *SEM*) correct on average in the easy attention task and 54% (± 7% *SEM*) in the hard attention task ($t(3) = 7.98$, $p < 0.01$), demonstrating the differences in attentional load.

Relative to the easy task condition, mean fMRI signals evoked by the high-contrast and by the low-contrast stimuli decreased significantly in the hard task condition in the LGN and in visual cortex (Figure 11.1B). At the cortical level, attentional response suppression was more pronounced in extrastriate than in striate cortex (Figure 11.2B). These fMRI signals reflect only activity evoked by the peripheral checkerboard stimuli when processed under conditions of different attentional load and are not confounded with activity evoked by the foveal stimuli. These results are consistent with those of Rees, Frith, and Lavie (1997), who found that fMRI responses in area MT evoked by an irrelevant motion stimulus presented peripherally were reduced during a high-load linguistic task compared to a low-load task at fixation. Taken together, these findings suggest that neural activity evoked

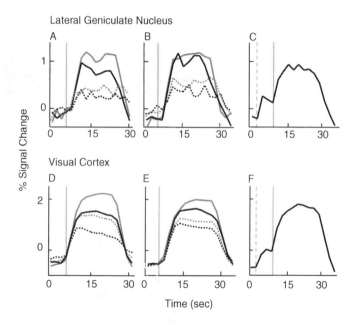

FIGURE 11.1. Time series of fMRI signals in the LGN and in visual cortex. Group analysis ($n = 4$). Data from the LGN and visual cortex were combined across left and right hemispheres. Activity in visual cortex was pooled across areas V1, V2, V3/VP, V4, TEO, V3A and MT/MST. A, D: Attentional enhancement. During directed attention to the stimuli (gray curves), responses to both the high-contrast stimulus (100%, solid curves) and low-contrast stimulus (5%, dashed curves) were enhanced relative to an unattended condition (black curves). B, E: Attentional suppression. During an attentionally demanding "hard" fixation task (black curves), responses evoked by both the high-contrast stimulus (100%, solid curves) and low-contrast stimulus (10%, dashed curves) were attenuated relative to an easy attention task at fixation (gray curves). C, F: Baseline increases. Baseline activity was elevated during directed attention to the periphery of the visual hemifield in expectation of the stimulus onset; the beginning of the expectation period is indicated by the dashed vertical line. Gray vertical lines indicate the beginning of checkerboard presentation periods. From O'Connor, Fukui, Pinsk, and Kastner (2002).

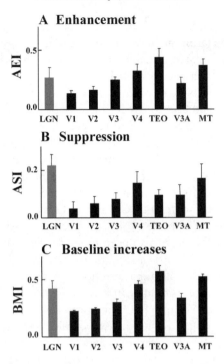

FIGURE 11.2. Attentional response modulation in the LGN and in visual cortical areas V1, V2, V3/VP, V4, TEO, V3A and MT/MST. Attentional effects that were obtained in the experiments presented in Figure 11.1 were quantified by defining several indices: (A) attentional enhancement index (AEI), (B) attentional suppression index (ASI), and (C) baseline modulation index (BMI). For all indices, larger values indicate larger effects of attention. Index values were computed for each subject based on normalized and averaged signals obtained in the different attention conditions and are presented as averaged index values from four subjects (for index definitions, see O'Connor et al., 2002). It should be noted that index scales are not identical due to differences in index definitions and attention tasks. Therefore, the magnitudes of effects cannot be easily compared across attention effects (e.g., enhancement vs. suppression). In visual cortex, attentional effects increased from early to later processing stages. Attentional effects in the LGN were larger than in V1. Vertical bars indicate *SEM* across subjects. From O'Connor, Fukui, Pinsk, and Kastner (2002).

by ignored stimuli is attenuated at several levels of visual processing as a function of the load of attentional resources engaged elsewhere. Attentional-load-dependent suppression of unattended stimuli may be a neural correlate for behavioral effects such as reduction of distracter interference (Lavie, 1995; Shiu & Pashler, 1995).

Attention-Related Increases of Baseline Activity

Selective attention not only modulates neural responses evoked by visual stimuli but also affects neural activity in the absence of visual stimulation. Single-cell recording studies have shown that spontaneous (baseline) firing rates were 30–40% higher for neurons in areas V2 and V4 when the animal was cued to attend covertly to a location within the neuron's RF before the stimulus was presented there (i.e., in the absence of visual stimulation [Luck et al., 1997; see Duncan, Chapter 8, this volume, Figure 11.1]). This increased baseline activity has been interpreted as a direct demonstration of a top-down signal that feeds back from higher-order to lower-order areas. In the latter areas, this feedback signal appears to bias neurons representing the attended location, thereby favoring stimuli that will appear there at the expense of those appearing at unattended locations.

To investigate attention-related baseline increases in the human visual system in the absence of visual stimulation (Kastner, Pinsk, De Weerd, Desimone, & Ungerleider, 1999; O'Connor et al., 2002), subjects were cued to covertly direct attention to the periphery of the left or right visual hemifield and to expect the onset of a stimulus. The expectation period, during which subjects were attending to the periphery without receiving visual input, was followed by attended presentations of a high-contrast checkerboard. During the attended presentations, subjects counted the occurrences of luminance changes. During the expectation period, fMRI signals increased relative to the preceding blank period in which subjects were fixating but not directing attention to the periphery in the LGN, in striate cortex, and in extrastriate cortex (Figures 11.1C, 11.2C). This elevation of baseline activity was followed by a further response increase evoked by the visual stimuli (Figure 11.1C).

Increases in baseline activity have also been found to depend on the expected task difficulty. Ress, Backus, and Heeger (2000) showed that increases in baseline activity in V1 were stronger when subjects expected a visual pattern that was difficult to discriminate compared to a pattern that was easy to discriminate. In areas that preferentially process a particular stimulus feature (e.g., color in V4 and TEO, or motion in MT/MST), increases in baseline activity were shown to be stronger during the expectation of a preferentially compared to a nonpreferentially processed stimulus feature (Chawla, Rees, & Friston, 1999; Shulman et al., 1999). The baseline increases found in human visual cortex may be subserved by increases in spontaneous firing rate similar to those found in the single-cell recording studies (Luck et al., 1997) but summed over large populations of neurons. The increases evoked by directing attention to a target location in anticipation of a behaviorally relevant stimulus at that attended location are thus likely to reflect a top-down feedback bias in favor of a preferred stimulus at an attended location. This bias signal has been demonstrated at each level of visual processing, including the LGN, striate, and extrastriate areas.

Comparison of Attention Effects across the Visual System

With fMRI, neural responses can be investigated at the population level and across a wide range of different processing stages, allowing for quantitative comparisons of a given modulatory effect across the visual system. For example, each attention effect can be quantified for each visual area by normalizing the mean fMRI signals and by computing index values, which are measures of the magnitude of the attentional effect. Such an approach was taken in one study, in which the attention effects of response enhancement, response suppression, and baseline increases, described previously, were investigated in the same subjects (O'Connor et al., 2002). A quantitative analysis of attention effects on the visual system is shown in Figure 11.2; larger index values indicate larger effects of attention. It should be noted that index values cannot be easily compared across attention effects due to differences in index definitions and attention tasks. In accordance with previous findings (Cook & Maunsell, 2002; Kastner, De Weerd, Desimone, & Ungerleider, 1998; Martinez et al., 1999; Mehta, Ulbert, & Schroeder, 2000), the magnitude of all attention effects increased from early to more advanced processing levels along both the ventral and dorsal pathways of visual cortex (Figure 11.2A–11.2C). This is consistent with the idea that attention operates through top-down signals that are transmitted via corticocortical feedback connections in a hierarchical fashion. Thereby, areas at advanced levels of visual cortical processing are more strongly controlled by attentional mechanisms than are early processing levels. This idea is supported by single-cell recording studies, which have shown that attentional effects in area TE of inferior temporal cortex have a latency of approximately 150 msec (Chelazzi, Duncan, Miller, & Desimone, 1998), whereas attentional effects in V1 have a longer latency, approximately 230 msec (Roelfsema, Lamme, & Spekreijse, 1998). According to this account, one would predict smaller attention effects in the LGN than in striate cortex. Surprisingly, it was found that all attention effects tended to be larger in the LGN than in striate cortex (Figure 11.2A–11.2C). This finding raises the possibility that attentional modulation in the LGN may be attributable not exclusively to corticothalamic feedback from striate cortex but may also reflect additional modulatory influences from other sources. Furthermore, it is possible that differences in strength of attentional effects at different processing levels may reflect the degree of parallel processing rather than a feedback mechanism that reverses the processing hierarchy.

In summary, selective attention affects information processing in the visual system in multiple ways. Single-cell physiology and neuroimaging studies provide convergent evidence that neural activity is enhanced when subjects attend to a stimulus, and it is suppressed when they ignore it. Further, directed attention to a spatial location in anticipation of the stimulus onset has been shown to lead to an increase of baseline activity.

MULTIPLE FUNCTIONS OF SELECTIVE ATTENTION IN THE VISUAL SYSTEM AND BEYOND

Multiple effects of attention—response enhancement and suppression and increases in baseline activity—have been demonstrated at various levels of visual processing. It is well known that each of the visual processing stages contributes differently to our visual perception. Therefore, it is possible that attentional modulation in the visual system serves different functions at different processing levels that are determined by the processing capabilities of each level. In this section, I discuss some of the evidence in support of such hypothesis. I argue that, at the thalamic level, attention may serve to control neural response gain. At early cortical processing stages, attention may affect contextual modulation of neural responses, which may serve important functions in basic mechanisms of scene segmentation and grouping (Ito & Gilbert, 1999). At intermediate cortical processing stages, attention may mediate the spatial filtering of unwanted information. These multilevel modulatory processes appear to be controlled by a higher-order frontoparietal network of brain areas (see also Shulman, Astafiev, & Corbetta, Chapter 9, this volume).

The LGN: An Early "Gatekeeper"?

In monkey physiology studies, attentional modulation of neural responses has been consistently found in cortical areas but not in the LGN (e.g., Mehta et al., 2000). These negative findings have led to the notion that selective attention is confined to cortical processing. This view has been recently challenged by demonstrating multiple effects of attention in the human LGN using fMRI, as reviewed in the last section (Figure 11.1; O'Connor et al., 2002). fMRI measures neural activity at a population level that may reveal even small modulatory effects that cannot be reliably found at the single-unit level when they are summed across large populations of neurons. Moreover, attention effects were found to be stronger in the LGN than in striate cortex (Figure 11.2A–11.2C). Due to its afferent input, the LGN may be in an ideal strategic position to serve as an early "gatekeeper" in attentional gain control. In addition to corticothalamic feedback projections from V1, the LGN receives inputs from the superior colliculus, which is part of a distributed network of areas controlling eye movements, and the thalamic reticular nucleus (TRN). For several reasons, the TRN has long been implicated in theoretical accounts of selective attention (Crick, 1984). First, all feedforward projections from the thalamus to the cortex as well as their reverse projections pass through the TRN. Second, the TRN receives inputs not only from the LGN and V1 but also from several extrastriate areas and the pulvinar. Thereby, it may serve as a node where several cortical areas and thalamic nuclei of the visual system can interact to modulate thalamocortical transmission through inhibitory connections to LGN neurons (Sherman & Guillery, 2001). And third, the TRN contains topographically organized representations of the visual field and can thereby modulate thalamocortical or corticothalamic transmission in spatially specific ways. Importantly, mechanisms of both response enhancement of attended stimuli and response suppression of unattended stimuli were found at the level of the LGN. This finding raises the possibility that neural response gain is controlled in the LGN by means of top-down influences on complex thalamocortical circuitry. Such a mechanism may determine at the earliest possible stage in the visual processing stream the degree to which information is represented at cortical stages. However, much remains to be learned about the role of thalamocortical circuits in attentional gain control and the precise nature of such a mechanism.

Spatial Filtering of Distracters in Areas V4 and TEO

At the thalamic level, attention may serve to control response gain, thereby increasing neural signals evoked by behaviorally relevant stimuli relative to background noise. At the cortical level, one important function of attention is to filter out another type of noise that is induced by the vast majority of visual information: the unwanted information from distracters (Reynolds & Desimone, 1999). Evidence from single-cell physiology and lesion studies in monkeys and fMRI studies in humans suggests that areas V4 and TEO are important sites where relevant information is selected and irrelevant information is filtered out (De Weerd, Peralta, Desimone, & Ungerleider, 1999; Kastner et al., 1998; Reynolds et al., 1999). In single-cell physiology studies, it has been demonstrated that (1) multiple stimuli present at the same time within a neuron's RF compete for neural representation, and (2) directed attention can influence this competition in favor of one of the stimuli. Competitive interactions among multiple stimuli were indicated by the finding that neural responses to a visual stimulus are reduced when the stimulus is presented together with a second stimulus in the same RF compared to when the stimulus is presented alone. These suppressive interactions have been found in several areas, including V2, V4, MT, MST, and IT (Miller, Gochin, & Gross, 1993; Recanzone, Wurtz, & Schwarz, 1997; Reynolds et al., 1999). When a monkey directed attention to one of two competing stimuli within a RF, the responses in extrastriate areas V2, V4, and MT were as large as those to that stimulus presented alone, thereby eliminating the suppressive influence of the competing stimulus (Moran & Desimone, 1985; Recanzone & Wurtz, 2000; Reynolds et al., 1999). These findings suggest that attention may resolve the competition among multiple stimuli by counteracting the suppressive influences of nearby stimuli, thereby enhancing information processing at the attended location. This may be an important mechanism by which attention filters out information from nearby distracters (Desimone & Duncan, 1995; Duncan, 1996). Importantly, this filter mechanism occurs most strongly at the level of the RF and will therefore operate optimally in extrastriate areas at intermediate processing stages, which have sufficiently large RFs to encompass multiple stimuli.

fMRI studies have demonstrated that similar mechanisms appear to operate in human extrastriate cortex (Kastner et al., 1998, 2001). Competitive interactions among multiple stimuli were probed in a paradigm in which four stimuli were presented to the periphery of the visual field under two presentation conditions, sequential and simultaneous. In the sequential presentation condition, a single stimulus appeared in one location, then another appeared in a different location, and so on, until each of the stimuli had been presented in the different locations. In the simultaneous presentation condition, the same stimuli appeared in the same locations, but they were presented together. Integrated over time, the physical stimulation parameters were identical in each of the stimulus locations in the two presentation conditions, but suppressive (competitive) interactions among stimuli could take place only in the simultaneous presentation condition. Based on the results from monkey physiology, we predicted that the fMRI signals would be smaller during the simultaneous than during the sequential presentation condition due to the presumed mutual suppression induced by the competitively interacting stimuli. The predicted differences in responses evoked by sequentially and simultaneously presented stimuli were found in areas V1, V2, V4, and TEO (Figure 11.3). The response differences were smallest in V1 and increased in magnitude toward extrastriate cortex, suggesting that the competitive interactions were scaled to the increasing RF sizes along the ventral visual pathway.

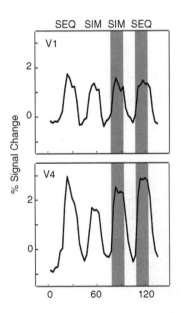

FIGURE 11.3. Competitive interactions and attentional modulation in visual cortex. fMRI time course signals obtained in V1 and V4, averaged across subjects ($n = 5$). Simultaneously presented stimuli (SIM) evoked less activity than sequentially presented stimuli (SEQ) in V4 and in V1, when the subjects' attention was directed away from the stimulus display (unshaded time series). The magnitude of the response differences were smallest in V1 and increased toward extrastriate areas, suggesting that suppressive (competitive) interactions were scaled to the RF size of neurons in visual cortex. Spatially directed attention (shaded time series) increased responses to simultaneously presented stimuli to a larger degree than to sequentially presented ones in V4. From Kastner, De Weerd, Desimone, and Ungerleider (1998).

The effects of spatially directed attention on multiple competing visual stimuli were probed by adding two additional conditions to the experimental design, described earlier, attended and unattended. During the unattended condition, attention was directed away from the peripheral visual display by having subjects count letters at fixation. In the attended condition, subjects were instructed to attend covertly to one of the stimulus locations in the display and to count the occurrences of one of the four stimuli. Based on the results from monkey physiology, we predicted that attention should reduce suppressive interactions among stimuli. Thus, responses evoked by the competing, simultaneously presented stimuli should be enhanced more strongly than responses evoked by the noncompeting sequentially presented stimuli. Such effects of directed attention on competitive interactions were found in areas V2, V4, and TEO (Figure 11.3). Importantly, the magnitude of the attentional effect scaled with the magnitude of the suppressive interactions among stimuli, with the strongest reduction of suppression occurring in areas V4 and TEO, suggesting that the effects scaled with RF size. These findings suggest that in both monkeys and humans, areas at intermediate levels of visual processing such as V4 and TEO appear to be important sites for the filtering of unwanted information by counteracting competitive interactions among stimuli at the level of the RF. This notion has also been supported by studies in a patient with an isolated V4 lesion and in monkeys with lesions of areas V4 and TEO (De Weerd et al., 1999; Gallant, Shoup, & Mazer, 2000). In these studies, subjects performed an orientation discrimination of a grating stimulus in the absence and in the presence of surrounding distracter stimuli. Significant performance deficits were observed in the distracter-present, but not in the distracter-absent condition, suggesting a deficit in the efficacy of the filtering of distracter information.

Frontal and Parietal Cortex: Sorting Out Sources and Sites

There is evidence from studies in patients suffering from attentional deficits due to brain damage and from functional brain imaging studies in healthy subjects performing attention tasks that attention-related modulatory signals are not generated within the visual system but, rather, derive from higher-order areas in parietal and frontal cortex and are transmitted via feedback projections to the visual system (Corbetta & Shulman, 2002; Kanwisher & Wojciulik, 2000; Kastner & Ungerleider, 2000; Nobre, 2001). A network consisting of areas in the superior parietal lobule (SPL), frontal eye fields (FEF), and supplementary eye field (SEF) has been shown to be consistently activated across subjects in a variety of visuospatial tasks (for meta-analyses, see Kastner & Ungerleider, 2000; Pessoa, Kastner, & Ungerleider, 2003), as illustrated for a single subject in Figure 11.4A. However, from these studies it is not clear whether the activity found in areas of frontal and parietal cortex reflects complex processing of visual information or whether this activity reflects the attentional operations themselves. To sort out "sources" that generate attentional feedback signals from "sites" that receive top-down modulatory signals, we analyzed the time courses of fMRI signals in the previously described experiment that probed attention-related baseline increases in the human visual system in the absence of visual stimulation (Kastner et al., 1999; O'Connor et al., 2002). Subjects were cued by a briefly presented marker close to fixation to direct attention to a peripheral target location and to expect the onset of visual stimuli; this expectation period was followed by attended presentations of visual stimuli. Thereby, the effects of directed attention in the presence and in the absence of visual stimuli could be dissociated. As described earlier and illustrated for area V4 in Figure 11.4C, in the visual system, the fMRI signals increased during the expectation period (textured epochs),

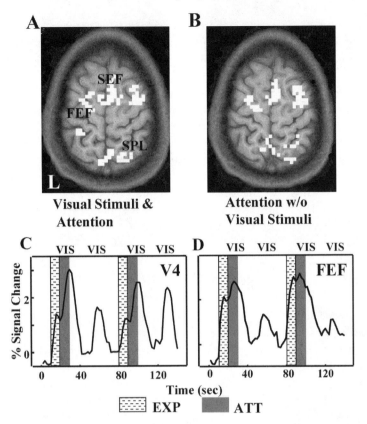

FIGURE 11.4. A frontoparietal network for spatial attention. Axial slice through frontal and parietal cortex from a single subject, obtained in the same scanning session. (A) When the subject directed attention to a peripheral target location and performed a discrimination task, a distributed frontoparietal network was activated including the SEF, the FEF, and the SPL. (B) The same network of frontal and parietal areas was activated when the subject directed attention to the peripheral target location in expectation of the stimulus onset, which is in the absence of any visual input. L indicates left hemisphere. (C) Time series of fMRI signals in V4. Directing attention to a peripheral target location in the absence of visual stimulation led to an increase of baseline activity (textured blocks), which was followed by a further increase after the onset of the stimuli (gray-shaded blocks). (D) Time series of fMRI signals in FEF. Directing attention to the peripheral target location in the absence of visual stimulation led to a stronger increase in baseline activity than in visual cortex; the further increase of activity after the onset of the stimuli was not significant. VIS, visual presentation block; EXP, expectation period; ATT, attended presentation block.

before any stimuli were present on the screen. This increase of baseline activity was followed by a further increase of activity evoked by the onset of the stimulus presentations (gray-shaded epochs).

In parietal and frontal cortex, the same distributed network for spatial attention was activated during directed attention in the absence of visual stimulation as during directed attention in the presence of visual stimulation, consisting of the FEF, the SEF, and the SPL (Figures 11.4A and 11.4B). The time course analysis of the fMRI signals revealed that, as in visual cortical areas, there was an increase in activity in these frontal and parietal areas due to directed attention in the absence of visual input. However, (1) this increase in activity was stronger in SPL, FEF, and SEF than the increase in activity seen in visual cortex (as exemplified for FEF in Figure 11.4D), and (2) there was no further increase in activity evoked by the attended stimulus presentations in these parietal and frontal areas. Rather, there was sustained activity throughout the expectation period and the attended presentations (Figure 11.4D). These results from parietal and frontal areas suggest that the activity reflected the attentional operations of the task and not visual processing. These findings therefore provide the first evidence that these parietal and frontal areas may be the sources of feedback that generated the top-down modulatory signals seen in visual cortex. The anatomical connections of SPL, FEF, and SEF put them in a position to serve as sources of top-down feedback signals that modulate neural processing in the visual system. In the monkey, FEF and SEF are reciprocally connected with ventral stream areas (Ungerleider, Gaffan, & Pelak, 1989; Webster, Bachevalier, & Ungerleider, 1994) and posterior parietal cortex (Cavada & Goldman-Rakic, 1989). The posterior parietal cortex is connected with ventral stream areas via the lateral intraparietal area (area LIP) (Webster et al., 1994).

CONCLUSIONS

Evidence from single-cell physiology and functional brain imaging reveals that attention operates at various processing levels within the visual system and beyond. First, the LGN appears to be the first stage in the processing of visual information that is modulated by attention, consistent with the idea that it may play an important role as an early gatekeeper in controlling neural gain. Second, areas at intermediate cortical processing levels such as V4 and TEO appear to be important sites at which attention filters out unwanted information by means of receptive field mechanisms. Third, the attention mechanisms that operate in the visual system appear to be controlled by a distributed network of higher-order areas in frontal and parietal cortex, which generate top-down signals that are transmitted via feedback connections to the visual system. The overall view that emerges is that neural mechanisms of selective attention operate at multiple levels in the visual system and beyond and are determined by the visual processing capabilities of each level. In this respect, attention can be considered a "multilevel selection" process (Braun, Koch, Lee, & Itti, 2001).

ACKNOWLEDGMENTS

I thank Hilda M. Fehd for help with preparing the manuscript. This work was supported by the National Institute of Mental Health and the Whitehall Foundation.

REFERENCES

Braun, J., Koch, C., Lee, K. D., & Itti, L. (2001). Perceptual consequences of multilevel selection. In J. Braun, C. Koch, & J. L. (Eds.), *Visual attention and cortical circuits* (pp. 215–241). Cambridge, MA: MIT Press.

Cameron, E. L., Tai, J. C., & Carrasco, M. (2002). Covert attention affects the psychometric function of contrast sensitivity. *Vision Research, 42,* 949–967.

Cavada, C., & Goldman-Rakic, P. S. (1989). Posterior parietal cortex in rhesus monkey: II. Evidence for segregated corticocortical networks linking sensory and limbic areas with the frontal lobe. *Journal of Comparative Neurology, 287,* 422–445.

Chawla, D., Rees, G., & Friston, K. J. (1999). The physiological basis of attentional modulation in extrastriate visual areas. *Nature Neuroscience, 2,* 671–676.

Chelazzi, L., Duncan, J., Miller, E. K., & Desimone, R. (1998). Responses of neurons in inferior temporal cortex during memory-guided visual search. *Journal of Neurophysiology, 80,* 2918–2940.

Connor, C. E., Gallant, J. L., Preddie, D. C., & Van Essen, D. C. (1996). Responses in area V4 depend on the spatial relationship between stimulus and attention. *Journal of Neurophysiology, 75,* 1306–1308.

Connor, C. E., Preddie, D. C., Gallant, J. L., & Van Essen, D. C. (1997). Spatial attention effects in macaque area V4. *Journal of Neuroscience, 17,* 3201–3214.

Cook, E., & Maunsell, J. (2002). Attentional modulation of behavioral performance and neuronal responses in middle temporal and ventral intraparietal areas of macaque monkey. *Journal of Neuroscience, 22,* 1994–2004.

Corbetta, M., & Shulman, G. L. (2002). Control of goal-directed and stimulus-driven attention in the brain. *Nature Neuroscience Reviews, 3,* 201–215.

Crick, F. (1984). Function of the thalamic reticular complex: The searchlight hypothesis. *Proceedings of the National Academy of Sciences USA, 81,* 4586–4590.

Desimone, R., & Duncan, J. (1995). Neural mechanisms of selective visual attention. *Annual Review of Neuroscience, 18,* 193–222.

De Weerd, P., Peralta, M. R., Desimone, R., & Ungerleider, L. G. (1999). Loss of attentional stimulus selection after extrastriate cortical lesions in macaques. *Nature Neuroscience, 2,* 753–758.

Duncan, J. (1996). Cooperating brain systems in selective perception and action. In T. Inui & J. L. McClelland (Eds.), *Attention and performance* (Vol. 16, pp. 549–578). Cambridge, MA: MIT Press.

Gallant, J. L., Shoup, R. E., & Mazer, J. A. (2000). A human extrastriate area functionally homologous to macaque V4. *Neuron, 27,* 227–235.

Haenny, P. E., Maunsell, J. H., & Schiller, P. H. (1988). State dependent activity in monkey visual cortex. II. Retinal and extraretinal factors in V4. *Experimental Brain Research, 69,* 245–259.

Ito, M., & Gilbert, C. D. (1999). Attentional modulates contextual influences in the primary visual cortex of alert monkeys. *Neuron, 22,* 593–604.

Kanwisher, N., & Wojciulik, E. (2000). Visual attention: Insights from brain imaging. *Nature Neuroscience Reviews, 1,* 91–100.

Kastner, S., De Weerd, P., Desimone, R., & Ungerleider, L. G. (1998). Mechanisms of directed attention in the human extrastriate cortex as revealed by functional MRI. *Science, 282,* 108–111.

Kastner, S., De Weerd, P., Pinsk, M. A., Elizondo, M. I., Desimone, R., & Ungerleider, L. G. (2001). Modulation of sensory suppression: Implications for receptive field sizes in the human visual cortex. *Journal of Neurophysiology, 86,* 1398–1411.

Kastner, S., Pinsk, M. A., De Weerd, P., Desimone, R., & Ungerleider, L. G. (1999). Increased activity in human visual cortex during directed attention in the absence of visual stimulation. *Neuron, 22,* 751–761.

Kastner, S., & Ungerleider, L. G. (2000). Mechanisms of visual attention in the human cortex. *Annual Review of Neuroscience, 23,* 315–341.

Lavie, N. (1995). Perceptual load as a necessary condition for selective attention. *Journal of Experimental Psychology: Human Perception and Performance, 21,* 451–468.

Lavie, N., & Tsal, Y. (1994). Perceptual load as a major determinant of the locus of selection in visual attention. *Perception and Psychophysics, 56,* 183–197.

Lu, Z. L., & Dosher, B. A. (1998). External noise distinguishes attention mechanisms. *Vision Research, 38,* 1183–1198.

Luck, S. J., Chelazzi, L., Hillyard, S. A., & Desimone, R. (1997). Neural mechanisms of spatial selective attention in areas V1, V2, and V4 of macaque visual cortex. *Journal of Neurophysiology, 77,* 24–42.

Martinez, A., Anllo-Vento, L., Sereno, M. I., Frank, L. R., Buxton, R. B., Dubowitz, D. J., et al. (1999). Involvement of striate and extrastriate visual cortical areas in spatial attention. *Nature Neuroscience, 2,* 364–369.

McAdams, C. J., & Maunsell, J. H. (1999). Effects of attention on orientation-tuning functions of single neurons in macaque cortical area V4. *Journal of Neuroscience, 19*, 431–441.

Mehta, A. D., Ulbert, I., & Schroeder, C. E. (2000). Intermodal selective attention in monkeys. I: Distribution and timing of effects across visual areas. *Cerebral Cortex, 10*, 343–358.

Miller, E. K., Gochin, P. M., & Gross, C. G. (1993). Suppression of visual responses of neurons in inferior temporal cortex of the awake macaque by addition of a second stimulus. *Brain Research, 616*, 25–29.

Moran, J., & Desimone, R. (1985). Selective attention gates visual processing in the extrastriate cortex. *Science, 229*, 782–784.

Motter, B. C. (1993). Focal attention produces spatially selective processing in visual cortical areas V1, V2, and V4 in the presence of competing stimuli. *Journal of Neurophysiology, 70*, 909–919.

Nobre, A. C. (2001). The attentive homunculus: Now you see it, now you don't. *Neuroscience and Biobehavioral Reviews, 25*, 477–496.

O'Connor, D. H., Fukui, M. M., Pinsk, M. A., & Kastner, S. (2002). Attention modulates responses in the human lateral geniculate nucleus. *Nature Neuroscience, 5*, 1203–1209.

Pessoa, L., Kastner, S., & Ungerleider, L. G. (2003). Neuroimaging studies of attention: From modulation of sensory processing to top-down control. *Journal of Neuroscience, 23*, 3990–3998.

Posner, M. I. (1980). Orienting of attention. *Quarterly Journal of Experimental Psychology, 32*, 3–25.

Recanzone, G. H., Wurtz, R. H., & Schwarz, U. (1997). Responses of MT and MST neurons to one and two moving objects in the receptive field. *Journal of Neurophysiology, 78*, 2904–2915.

Recanzone, G. H., & Wurtz, R. H. (2000). Effects of attention on MT and MST neuronal activity during pursuit initiation. *Journal of Neurophysiology, 83*, 777–790.

Rees, G., Frith, C. D., & Lavie, N. (1997). Modulating irrelevant motion perception by varying attentional load in an unrelated task. *Science, 278*, 1616–1619.

Ress, D., Backus, B. T., & Heeger, D. J. (2000). Activity in primary visual cortex predicts performance in a visual detection task. *Nature Neuroscience, 3*, 940–945.

Reynolds, J. H., Chelazzi, L., & Desimone, R. (1999). Competitive mechanisms subserve attention in macaque areas V2 and V4. *Journal of Neuroscience, 19*, 1736–1753.

Reynolds, J. H., & Desimone, R. (1999). The role of neural mechanisms of attention in solving the binding problem. *Neuron, 24*, 111–125.

Roelfsema, P. R., Lamme, V. A., & Spekreijse, H. (1998). Object-based attention in the primary visual cortex of the macaque monkey. *Nature, 395*, 376–381.

Sherman, S. M., & Guillery, R. W. (2001). *Exploring the thalamus*. San Diego, CA: Academic Press.

Shiu, L. P., & Pashler, H. (1995). Spatial attention and vernier acuity. *Vision Research, 35*, 337–343.

Shulman, G. L., Ollinger, J. M., Akbudak, E., Conturo, T. E., Snyder, A. Z., Petersen, S. E., et al. (1999). Areas involved in encoding and applying directional expectation to moving objects. *Journal of Neuroscience, 19*, 9480–9496.

Spitzer, H., Desimone, R., & Moran, J. (1988). Increased attention enhances both behavioral and neuronal performance. *Science, 240*, 338–340.

Spitzer, H., & Richmond, B. J. (1991). Task difficulty: Ignoring, attending to, and discriminating a visual stimulus yield progressively more activity in inferior temporal neurons. *Experimental Brain Research, 83*, 340–348.

Treue, S., & Martinez Trujillo, J. C. (1999). Feature-based attention influences motion processing gain in macaque visual cortex. *Nature, 399*, 575–579.

Treue, S., & Maunsell, J. H. (1996). Attentional modulation of visual motion processing in cortical areas MT and MST. *Nature, 382*, 539–541.

Ungerleider, L. G., Gaffan, D., & Pelak, V. S. (1989). Projections from inferior temporal cortex to prefrontal cortex via the uncinate fascicle in rhesus monkeys. *Experimental Brain Research, 76*, 473–484.

Webster, M. J., Bachevalier, J., & Ungerleider, L. G. (1994). Connections of inferior temporal areas TEO and TE with parietal and frontal cortex in macaque monkeys. *Cerebral Cortex, 5*, 470–483.

Yeshurun, Y., & Carrasco, M. (1998). Attention improves or impairs visual performance by enhancing spatial resolution. *Nature, 396*, 72–75.

12

Probing the Flexibility
of Attentional Orienting in the Human Brain

Anna Christina Nobre

Attentional orienting can be defined as the set of processes by which neural resources are deployed selectively toward specific attributes of events on the basis of changing motivation, expectation, or volition in order to optimize perception and action. Operationally, orienting can be measured through the behavioral consequences of changes in stimulus salience, predictability, or relevance. To date, the vast majority of research has investigated the nature of the neural systems and mechanisms involved in orienting attention to spatial locations and objects. The emerging view is that of a large-scale neural network built around a critical parietofrontal axis, which modulates information processing from early stages of perceptual analysis through top-down influences. One of the main objectives of research in my laboratory over the last 5 years has been to test the ubiquity of this attentional orienting system in the human brain. My colleagues and I have probed the ability to orient attention selectively to the contents of mental representations and the ability to orient attention to nonspatial attributes of perceptual events. We have used hemodynamic and electrophysiological measures of brain activity to reveal the neural systems and mechanisms involved. The central question is whether one general-purpose attentional orienting system is involved in all cases, modulating similar stages of information processing, or whether the brain areas and mechanisms involved in attentional orienting are determined by the domain in which orienting operates or the type of expectancies that can be formed. Our results suggest a flexible view, in which brain areas with relevant functional specializations participate in the networks involved and multiple alternative mechanisms exist for the optimization of perception and action.

VISUAL SPATIAL ORIENTING

Orienting Attention to Locations of Perceptual Events

Research on brain-lesioned patients with cognitive impairments related to visual spatial attention has implicated the posterior parietal cortex as well as frontal and subcortical structures in control systems of spatial attention (Husain & Rorden, 2003; Mesulam, 1999; Mort et al., 2003). Brain-imaging studies in normal participants over the last decade have

157

sharpened our anatomical resolution of the large-scale neural network for spatial orienting and have started to dissect the functional contributions of the various brain areas involved (Corbetta & Shulman, 2002; Giesbrecht & Mangun, in press; Kastner & Ungerleider, 2000; Mesulam, Small, Vandenberghe, Gitelman, & Nobre, in press; Nobre, 2001a). The task developed by Posner (1978, 1980) has provided a simple and effective tool with which to investigate visual spatial orienting. Using variants of the Posner task, our group and others have revealed the functional anatomy of visual spatial orienting to include a core set of regions in the posterior parietal cortex around the intraparietal sulcus and in the frontal eye fields (Beauchamp, Petit, Ellmore, Ingeholm, & Haxby, 2001; Corbetta, Miezin, Shulman, & Petersen, 1993; Gitelman et al., 1999; Hopfinger, Buonocore, & Mangun, 2000; Kim et al., 1999; Nobre et al., 1997; Vandenberghe et al., 2000; Wojciulik & Kanwisher, 1999; Yantis et al., 2002). These parietal and frontal areas overlap with areas participating in eye-movement control (Corbetta et al., 1998; Nobre, Gitelman, Dias, & Mesulam, 2000; Perry & Zeki, 2000; Rosen et al., 1999). The tight coupling between visual spatial orienting and oculomotor functions is also supported by the behavioral literature (Hoffman, 1998; Rizzolatti, Riggio, Dascola, & Umilta, 1987; Sheliga, Riggio, Craighero, & Rizzolatti, 1995) and suggests that the purely mental function of covert attentional orienting may be ancillary to this overt sensorimotor function, which shares many of its functional characteristics. Like attentional orienting, eye-movement control also requires the accurate and rapid online mapping, predicting, and updating of events within spatial frameworks (see Nobre, 2001a). Recordings of single-unit activity in nonhuman primates support the involvement of posterior parietal areas (most research has focused on the lateral intraparietal sulcus and inferior parietal lobule), and of the frontal eye fields in spatial orienting (Colby & Goldberg, 1999; Constantinidis & Steinmetz, 2001; Schall & Bichot, 1998) and highlight the sensitivity of neurons in these regions to both covert attention and oculomotor functions (Colby, Duhamel, & Goldberg, 1996; Moore & Armstrong, 2003; Moore & Fallah, 2001; Snyder, Batista, & Andersen, 1997, 1998).

The parietofrontal network for visual spatial orienting modulates, through top-down biasing signals, multiple levels of analysis of incoming events, starting from early perceptual stages. Hemodynamic studies show enhanced activations in regions coding attended locations within multiple visual areas, including primary visual cortex (Kastner, De Weerd, Desimone, & Ungerleider, 1998; Kastner, Pinsk, De Weerd, Desimone, & Ungerleider, 1999; Martinez et al., 1999, 2001; Tootell et al., 1998). Event-related potential (ERP) results recorded from human participants show relative enhancement of visual components generated in extrastriate cortex for items in attended locations (Clark & Hillyard, 1996; Eimer, 1998; Heinze et al., 1994; Hillyard & Mangun, 1987; Mangun, 1995; Van Voorhis & Hillyard, 1977). The early C1 component generated in primary visual cortex is not affected, suggesting that the modulation of activity in primary visual cortex observed in functional magnetic resonance imaging (fMRI) studies may reflect modulation of later, reentrant activity (Di Russo, Martinez, & Hillyard, 2003; Martinez et al., 1999, 2001). Single-unit recordings from nonhuman primates have shown that spatial attention optimizes perceptual analysis in extrastriate areas by increasing the tonic firing rate of neurons coding stimuli in relevant locations (Luck, Chelazzi, Hillyard, & Desimone, 1997), changing the effective size of receptive fields to filter out signals from stimuli in irrelevant locations (Moran & Desimone, 1985; Reynolds & Desimone, 1999), and increasing synchronization of high-frequency oscillatory activity (Fries, Reynolds, Rorie, & Desimone, 2001).

Studies of attentional orienting to objects or perceptual features have led to a very similar view of the neural systems and mechanisms. Posterior parietal and frontal areas are activated when attention is oriented toward visual objects or their constituent features (Giesbrecht, Woldorff, Song, & Mangun, 2003; Shulman, d'Avossa, Tansy, & Corbetta, 2002; Wojciulik & Kanwisher, 1999). As with spatial attention, the consequences of attentional modulation start from early stages of perceptual analysis. ERP results indicate modulation beginning in extrastriate cortex (Anllo-Vento & Hillyard, 1996; Anllo-Vento, Luck, & Hillyard, 1998; Hillyard & Munte, 1984; Valdes Sosa, Bobes, Rodriguez, & Pinilla, 1998), and hemodynamic studies show increased activations in brain areas specialized for the attended object features (Chawla, Rees, & Friston, 1999; Corbetta, Miezin, Dobmeyer, Shulman, & Petersen, 1990; O'Craven, Downing, & Kanwisher, 1999). Single-unit results suggest an equivalent set of cellular mechanisms for attentional selection based on features or objects compared to selection based on location. So far, feature and object attention studies have revealed tonic changes in firing rate of neurons encoding relevant objects or features and changes in receptive-field properties that filter out signals from irrelevant objects or features (Chelazzi, Miller, Duncan, & Desimone, 1993; Haenny & Schiller, 1988; Motter, 1994; Treue & Martinez Trujillo, 1999). However, as I have argued previously (Nobre, 2001a), several studies investigating attention to objects or features do not eliminate confounded spatial factors, making it difficult to draw firm conclusions about the generality of mechanisms for spatial versus object or feature attention (cf. Sabes, Breznen, & Andersen, 2002).

Orienting Attention to Locations in Mental Representations

To investigate the specificity of the neural systems of attentional orienting for mediating our interaction with the perceptual domain, my colleagues and I have begun to investigate the ability to orient attention to the contents of mental representations. As humans, much of our world is internal. We constantly build and manipulate mental representations based on experiences and expectancies. Intuition suggests that orienting attention to selective attributes of these internalized representations is a common aspect of our daily activity. One example may be our ability to reach toward the glass of beer without breaking gaze from pivotal action in the soccer game on the television.

Behavioral tasks designed to test the ability to orient attention to locations in mental representations held within working memory used spatial cues presented seconds after a stimulus array had disappeared (Griffin & Nobre, 2003). Tasks required participants to decide whether a probe stimulus presented at the end of a trial was present in the previous array (see Figure 12.1). Informative cues pointed to the relevant location in the preceding stimulus array with a high probability of accuracy. The impact of orienting attention to locations in mental representations was identified by comparing behavioral performance in trials with spatially informative *retro*cues with performance in trials with neutral cues, which provided no information about relevant locations in the array. Trials with spatially informative precues were also included in order to compare and contrast the effects of spatial orienting operating within working memory versus perceptual representations.[1]

Results have consistently confirmed the ability to orient selective spatial attention to internal representations (Figure 12.1) (Griffin & Nobre, 2003), at least when the number of objects and features in the array falls within the capacity of working memory (Luck & Vogel, 1997; Wheeler & Treisman, 2002). Orienting attention retrospectively to locations in previous arrays or prospectively to locations in future arrays yielded equivalent patterns of behavioral modulation. Similar attentional benefits and costs were observed for informative retrocues and precues over multiple experiments. In the case of retrocues, attentional effects

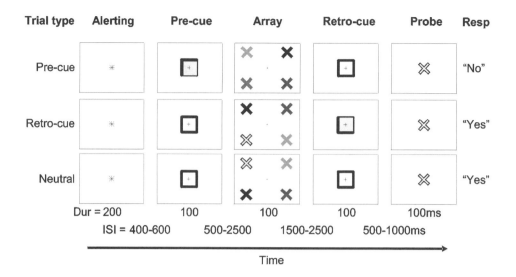

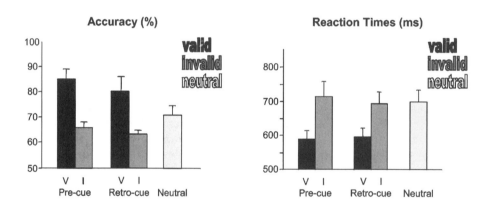

FIGURE 12.1. Example of experimental task investigating behavioral effects of orienting to locations within working-memory representations (Griffin & Nobre, 2003, Experiment 1). All trials contained a precue (100 msec), an array of four different-colored crosses (100 msec) (represented here in shades of gray), a retrocue (100 msec), and a probe stimulus (100 msec). In precue trials the spatially informative orienting cue (80% validity) was presented before the stimulus array. In retrocue trials the spatially informative orienting cue (80% validity) was presented after the stimulus array. In neutral trials there was no spatially informative orienting cue. Subjects (n = 10) responded according to whether the central probe stimulus had been present in the array (50% probability). The bottom panels show the behavioral results for "yes" trials, in which the probe was present in the array. On the left are mean reaction times (RTs) and standard errors for probe stimuli in precue, retrocue, and neutral trials, separated according to the factor of cue validity. Comparison between RTs in valid and invalid trials showed a main effect of cue validity, $F(1,9)$ = 13.8, p < 05, but no effect of or interaction with cue type (precue vs. retrocue). Comparison between RTs in valid and neutral trials showed significant cue benefits, $F(2,18)$ = 8.4, p < .05. Post-hoc tests showed that both valid precues and retrocues differed from neutral cues, but did not differ from one another. Comparisons between RTs in invalid and neutral trials did not reveal any significant cue costs. On the right are mean accuracies and standard errors for probe stimuli in precue, retrocue, and neutral trials, separated according to cue validity. Comparison between accuracies in valid and invalid trials showed a main effect of cue validity, $F(1,9)$ = 12.4, p < .05, but no effect of or interaction with cue type. Comparison between accuracies in valid and neutral trials revealed significant cue benefits, $F(2,18)$ = 6.2, p < .05, which post-hoc tests showed to occur only for precue versus neutral trials. Comparisons between accuracies in invalid and neutral trials revealed significant cue costs for "yes" trials, reflected in an interaction between response (yes, no) and cue type, $F(2,18)$= 4.191, p = .034. Subsidiary comparisons showed that "yes" trials in both invalid precues and retrocues differed from neutral cues, but did not differ from one another.

may have reflected spatially specific enhancement of representations in working memory. Changes in response criteria were ruled out as the only explanation for the effects (Griffin & Nobre, 2003).

To compare and contrast the neural systems that control attentional orienting to upcoming perceptual events and to previous events stored as mental representations, we used event-related fMRI (Nobre et al., 2004). The task required spatial orienting to a specific location in a forthcoming (precue trials) or previous (retrocue trials) stimulus array in order to decide whether a probe stimulus at the end of the trial matched the color of the item at the cued location (Figure 12.2a). We measured neural activity elicited by spatial versus neutral precues and retrocues. To isolate activations specific to cue stimuli, long and variable delays (2–15 seconds) were used between events within trials. Orienting attention to locations in perceptual and working-memory representations activated a largely overlapping network of occipital, parietal, and frontal areas (Figure 12.2b), consistent with that observed in other visuospatial orienting studies (Nobre, 2001a). Some degree of selectivity was also observed. A region in the right inferior parietal cortex was specifically activated by spatial precues whereas prefrontal regions were engaged specifically by spatial retrocues.

The extensive overlap of activations clearly supports the participation of a common set of brain areas in spatial orienting, whether the orienting act occurs within the perceptual or working-memory domain. The selective activations, however, leave open the question whether the networks for spatial orienting in the perceptual and working-memory domains are completely coextensive. Spatial precues and retrocues both triggered a shift toward or a zooming in on a relevant spatial location. However, in addition to the variable of interest, namely, the workspace of attentional orienting, spatial orienting by precues and retrocues differed in other ways. The selective activations could reflect differences in brain areas that participate in shifting or zooming attention in the perceptual versus working-memory domains. For example, some prefrontal regions could provide top-down biasing signals during the shifting or zooming of the focus of spatial attention (Desimone & Duncan, 1995) when this occurs within a working-memory context. Alternatively, selective brain activations could reflect different functions, complementary to shifting or zooming the attentional focus, afforded by precues and retrocues during spatial orienting. In our task, spatial orienting toward an upcoming perceptual array triggered by precues involved prolonged periods of directionally specific expectancy, where a spatial focus was maintained. Inferior parietal areas have previously been linked to maintaining a spatial focus (Awh & Jonides, 2001; Vandenberghe, Gitelman, Parrish, & Mesulam, 2001). Spatial orienting toward an array held in working memory did not require a sustained spatial focus. Instead, spatial retrocues afforded the selection of object information from the relevant array location and inhibition of object information from irrelevant locations, and required the maintenance of online target identity or color. Prefrontal regions could have been involved in selecting targets from among distractors (Thompson Schill, D'Esposito, Aguirre, & Farah, 1997) or maintaining object or feature information.

To track the temporal dynamics of brain activity involved in spatial orienting to events in the perceptual or working-memory domains, we recorded ERPs (Griffin & Nobre, 2003). The task was the same as that used in the fMRI study, except that it included many more trials and the intervals between trial events were shorter (Figure 12.2a). Waveforms elicited by spatially informative relative to neutral precues and retrocues both contained lateralized early posterior and later frontal potentials (Figure 12.2c). The pattern was consistent with previous ERP studies of visuospatial orienting (Harter, Anllo-Vento, & Wood, 1989; Hopf & Mangun, 2000; Nobre, Sebestyen, & Miniussi, 2000; Yamaguchi, Tsuchiya, &

FIGURE 12.2. Examples of experimental tasks used for hemodynamic and ERP studies comparing orienting to locations within perceptual versus working-memory representations.

(A) The structure of the task was the same for experiments using event-related fMRI (Nobre et al., 2004) and event-related potentials (Griffin & Nobre, 2003) except for the number of trials and the duration of intervals between trial events. All trials contained a stimulus that indicated the onset of a trial (200 msec), a precue (100 msec), an array of four different-colored crosses (100 msec) (represented here in shades of gray), a retrocue (100 msec), and a probe stimulus (100 msec). The interstimulus interval (ISI) between events is shown below the task diagram for the two types of methods. In the event-related fMRI experiment the intervals were of sufficient variability and duration (2–15 seconds) to measure individual hemodynamic responses elicited by individual events within the trial. In precue trials, the spatially informative cue appeared before the stimulus array. In retrocue trials, the spatially informative cue appeared after the array. In all trials participants responded according to whether the probe stimulus had been present at the cued location (50% probability). Behavioral results for both hemodynamic (n = 10 subjects) and ERP experiments (n = 12 subjects) showed no significant difference in reaction times or accuracies between precue and retrocue trials, and consistently faster responses in "yes" trials, in which the probe item matched the location indicated.

(B) fMRI activations. Significant activations are overlaid on different views of a standardized brain volume (Collins, Neelin, Peters, & Evans, 1994; Talairach & Tournoux, 1988). From left to right, activations are shown on the left and right lateral surface. The top row shows brain areas that were significantly more activated by precues than retrocues ([spatial minus neutral precues] – [spatial – neutral retrocues], masked inclusively [p < .001 uncorrected] by spatial precue activations). The arrow points to the only significant activation (the threshold was set to p < .001 corrected for false-discovery rates [Genovese et al., 2002]) that was specific for precues, in the right posterior angular gyrus (Talairach coordinate: 33 –87 15). The middle row shows brain areas that were significantly activated by both spatial precues and retrocues ([spatial precue – neutral precue], masked by [spatial precue] and [spatial retrocue – neutral retrocue], masked by [spatial retrocue]). An extensive network of parietal, frontal, and visual areas was activated. The bottom row shows brain areas that were preferentially activated by retrocues ([spatial minus neutral retrocues] minus [spatial minus neutral precues], masked by spatial retrocue activations). Activations in some parietal areas within the common network were enhanced, and specific activations were obtained in medial (Talairach coordinate: –03 24 39) and lateral prefrontal regions (Talairach coordinates: 36 24 –12, 51 39 21, 48 45 21, –54 21 33) (see arrows).

(C) ERP waveforms. Results are illustrated by grand-averaged waveforms (positive polarity is plotted upward) from lateral posterior (PO7/PO8) and lateral frontal (F3/F4) electrodes; and by scalp topographies isolating effects of interest. The horizontal electrooculogram (HEOG) waveform is also shown for the principle comparisons to demonstrate the lack of systematic eye movements during task performance. The electrode montage is shown at the top of the figure. (1) The top panel compares orienting attention to the left (thick line) and right (thin line) by precues. To isolate effects of spatial orienting, both attend-left and attend-right waveforms have had the waveform from the neutral cue stimulus that occurred at the same time point subtracted from them. Arrows indicate the presence of statistically significant effects. The scalp topographies plot the difference in grand-averaged ERPs elicited by precues when subjects attended the right versus left, and are shown from a bird's-eye perspective. The gray scale uses black isocontour lines for positive polarity and white isocontour lines for negative polarity, and shows the range of possible voltage values in the topographies (bar on the right). The anterior scalp is shown at the top and the right scalp is shown at the right side in this and subsequent figures. (2) The middle panel compares orienting attention to the left (thick line) and right (thin line) by retrocues. To isolate effects of spatial orienting, both attend-left and attend-right waveforms have had the waveform from the neutral cue stimulus that occurred at the same time point subtracted from them. The scalp topographies plot the difference in grand-averaged ERPs elicited by retro-cues when subjects attended the right versus left. (3) The bottom panel compares grand-averaged waveforms elicited by precue stimuli (thin line) and retrocue stimuli (thick line). The waveforms are averaged over the direction of attention. To isolate effects of spatial orienting, both precue and retrocue waveforms have had the waveform from the neutral cue stimulus that occurred at the same time point subtracted from them. Scalp topographies show significant differences in grand-averaged ERPs elicited by retrocues versus precues.

A. Behavioral tasks for fMRI and ERP experiments

Trial type	Alerting	Precue	Array	Retrocue	Probe	Resp
Precue						"Yes"
Retrocue						"No"

| | Dur = 200 | 100 | 100 | 100 | 100ms | |

| fMRI task ISI = | 2-16 | 2-16 | 2-16 | 2-16sec | |
| ERP task ISI = | 400-600 | 500-2500 | 1500-2500 | 500-1000ms | |

Time

B. fMRI activations

Precue

Common

Retrocue

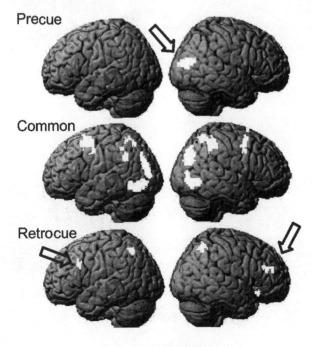

FIGURE 12.2A–B.

C. ERP waveforms

1. Precue

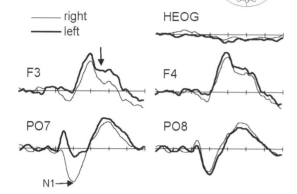
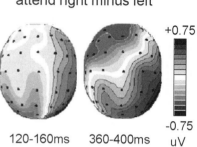

2. Retrocues

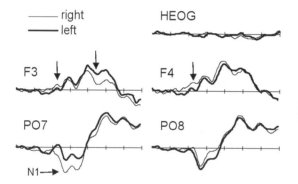
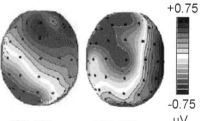

3. Retrocues x Precues

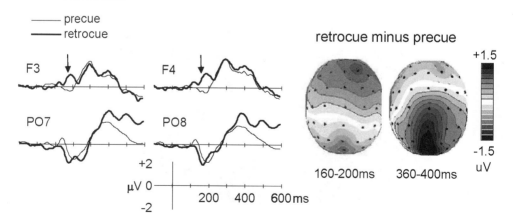

FIGURE 12.2C.

Kobayashi, 1994) and is likely to reflect activity in the parietofrontal network activated for both types of cues. In addition to the common ERP modulations, retrocues elicited an early potential over the frontal scalp that was modulated by the direction of spatial orienting. To the extent that this ERP component reflects activity in some of the prefrontal regions activated selectively by retrocues in the fMRI study (Nobre et al., 2004), it suggests an early involvement of at least some of the prefrontal areas in spatial orienting when working-memory representations are involved. For example, shifting or zooming attention within a mnemonic context could involve a frontal top-down biasing signal (Desimone & Duncan, 1995) to guide the retrieval, maintenance, selection, or filtering of information within working memory. The exact functional significance of this effect, however, remains to be resolved.

So far, studies comparing the effect of the perceptual versus mnemonic workspace of attentional orienting have emphasized common behavioral consequences and neural systems. The behavioral consequences of orienting attention to spatial locations of internal representations were equivalent to those when spatial attention is deployed toward upcoming perceptual representations. The neural systems showed extensive anatomical overlap and similar time course of neural modulation. However, it is likely that some prefrontal regions selectively participate in orienting attention within a working-memory context. The selective activation of prefrontal regions by spatial retrocues, coupled with the early ERP component over frontal scalp that was sensitive to attentional orienting, suggests that prefrontal areas may play an early role in the orienting act in this case, for example, by providing a top-down biasing signal. Further experiments will continue to investigate the limits and properties of our ability to orient attention within mental representations and the neural systems and mechanisms involved. To decipher the nature of prefrontal contributions, experiments will manipulate working-memory load, target selection, and other critical variables during retrocueing tasks.

ORIENTING ATTENTION TO TEMPORAL MOMENTS

A complementary approach to investigate the generality of attentional orienting is to examine the behavioral consequences of building different types of expectancies about the unfolding world. To date, most research on attentional orienting has focused on expectancies about perceptual parameters such as locations or object features. One critical dimension left out of attentional orienting research has been that of time.[2] In a dynamic world, objects appear, move, and change over time. Common sense suggests the ability to use temporal information to build expectancies and optimize behavior.

The warning-signal literature has long shown that behavioral performance can be improved when target stimuli occur at a constant and predictable time after a cue (Niemi & Naeaetaenen, 1981). Information about the temporal relationship between a cue and a target enables participants to reach and maintain a state of alertness (Posner & Boies, 1971). Alerting builds up after the cue in a state of minivigilance until preparatory and expectation processes peak in anticipation of the target (Posner & Petersen, 1990). Effects of alerting can be separated from effects of visual spatial attention in orienting tasks by using nonspatial warning cues (Beane & Marrocco, Chapter 23, this volume). Alerting induces reliable performance benefits, which probably contribute significantly to the overall effects measured in selective attention tasks. However, this literature has not indicated whether these preparatory processes can come under flexible cognitive control—that is, whether we can use information about different predicted time intervals to orient attention flexibly to any point in time at which a stimulus is expected, in order to optimize behavior by specific temporal expectancies.

To explore the consequences of temporal *orienting* on performance, we developed temporal-cueing variants of the Posner task. In these tasks, a cue stimulus predicts with high probability the specific temporal interval at which a target stimulus will appear (see Figure 12.3). Behavioral results have consistently shown performance benefits for detecting or discriminating events that occur at expected relative to unexpected intervals (Griffin, Miniussi, & Nobre, 2001; Griffin & Nobre, in press; Nobre, 2001b). We have recently also developed a more naturalistic task for testing temporal orienting and for comparing it with spatial orienting (see Figure 12.3). In this task, an object moves across a screen and disappears behind an occluding strip. The object moves with predictable or random spatial or temporal trajectory. Participants use spatial or temporal expectancies formed online to make detection or discrimination judgments upon the reappearance of the object. Performance in this task is equally facilitated by temporal or spatial expectancies (Doherty, Griffin, Rao, & Nobre, 2003).

A comparison of the neural systems involved in spatial and temporal orienting using hemodynamic measures shows a large degree of overlap in the networks involved, as well as some degree of specialization (Figure 12.4a) (Coull & Nobre, 1998). Participants detected the brief appearance of target stimuli that occurred at one of two peripheral locations (left, right) and at one of two time intervals (300, 1,500 msec). Across different conditions, predictive cues indicated (80% validity) the likely spatial location, time interval, or both the location and the interval of the subsequent target. In one additional condition, neutral cues provided no predictive information. All task conditions contained equivalent stimulus parameters and response requirements. Only the type of expectancy varied. When compared to a visual-fixation baseline task, both spatial and temporal orienting conditions activated a largely overlapping network of occipital, parietal, and frontal areas, consistent with that observed in other visuospatial orienting studies (Nobre, 2001a). Analysis of the main effects of temporal versus spatial orienting revealed differential contributions from some parietal and frontal areas. Spatial orienting preferentially activated the right inferior parietal lobule, whereas temporal orienting preferentially activated left inferior parietal and left inferior lateral premotor/prefrontal cortex (Coull & Nobre, 1998). Though alerting may contribute to spatial and temporal orienting effects generally, direct comparisons between alerting and orienting conditions showed that these effects are dissociable in terms of participating brain areas and pharmacological manipulations (Coull, Nobre, & Frith, 2001).

The extensive overlap of activations in temporal and spatial orienting suggests that a common set of brain areas participate in orienting attention based on very different types of expectancies. Activation of this parietofrontal network by temporal orienting occurs even when the task uses only foveal stimuli (Coull, Frith, Buchel, & Nobre, 2000). The selective activations, however, suggest that the attentional orienting is not achieved by a rigid network. Instead, brain areas with useful specializations may participate depending on the type of expectancy. It is difficult to pinpoint the exact contribution of the areas specifically involved in the spatial or temporal orienting conditions. The right inferior parietal area could contribute to the maintenance of a spatial focus, as was argued for the results in spatial precue versus retrocue conditions. The left inferior parietal and left inferior premotor areas activated preferentially during temporal orienting are very similar to areas involved in motor-preparation and motor-attention tasks, which are thought to reflect sensorimotor circuits for the control of hand movements (Rushworth, Johansen-Berg, Goebel, & Devlin, 2003). Temporal orienting cues in our task may have optimised performance in large part through the timely selection and execution of manual responses by these sensorimotor circuits (Nobre, 2001a, 2001b).

Despite the largely overlapping networks involved in temporal and spatial orienting, ERP studies have shown that temporal and spatial orienting can have very different consequences on the analysis of incoming stimuli. In direct comparisons of temporal and spatial orienting tasks using equivalent stimulus presentation parameters and response requirements, we found clearly distinct patterns of modulation of the perceptual and motor components of the ERPs (Figure 12.4b) (Griffin, Miniussi, & Nobre, 2002). Consistently with the vast previous literature, spatial orienting enhanced early contralateral visual components that reflect extrastriate processing (P1 and N1). Temporal orienting did not affect these visual components in a retinotopically specific way, though in some cases a diffuse modulation of the ERPs was observed within an early period still usually associated with perceptual processing. Instead, pronounced effects were observed upon later potentials linked to decisions and responses, which were not observed in the spatial orienting conditions (Miniussi, Wilding, Coull, & Nobre, 1999). For example, the latency of the P300 component was diminished for targets appearing at the predicted temporal interval. We have recently obtained a similar pattern of findings using the more naturalistic temporal and spatial orienting task involving the movement of an object behind an occluding strip (Doherty et al., 2003).

Results from ERP studies thus highlight the impressive flexibility of attentional orienting systems in how they optimize perception and action. Instead of operating always at the same level of stimulus analysis, as would be expected if there were fixed bottleneck points at which resource capacities were limited, such as in the classic Broadbent model (Broadbent, 1958), top-down signals can act on multiple levels to bias perceptual analysis or facilitate the selection or execution of relevant responses. The levels of information processing affected will depend on the nature of the expectancies and their affordances.

In our tasks, temporal orienting has had more pronounced effects on motor-related processing, whereas spatial orienting has exerted greater perceptual modulation. However, our tasks have required speeded motor responses and have involved relatively low perceptual demands. In tasks emphasizing perceptual factors over motor factors, temporal orienting may influence perceptual analysis. For example, Correa, Lupiáñez, and Tudela (2003) have recently shown improvements in the sensitivity measures (d') of the accuracy to detect targets briefly presented within rapid–serial–visual–presentation streams in delayed-response tasks. Future research should reveal the array of possible consequences of temporal orienting on information processing.

Little is known about the cellular mechanisms of temporal orienting. Only a few single-unit studies have been completed to date. Recent research has revealed that changes in receptive-field properties in V4 neurons are highly temporally correlated with the probability that the relevant stimulus change will occur at that given time (Ghose & Maunsell, 2002). Changes in oscillatory activity in V4 reflecting local synchronization of neuronal activity may be similarly correlated with temporal expectancies (Liang, Bressler, Desimone, & Fries, 2003). Recordings from the lateral bank of the intraparietal sulcus (LIP) have also recently revealed the ability to anticipate the timing of behaviorally relevant events. In this area, thought to participate in control of visuospatial orienting and oculomotor control, increases in cellular activity are correlated with the conditional probability that a relevant event will occur at a given moment in time (Janssen & Shadlen, 2003). In these experiments, spatial

FIGURE 12.3. Behavioral tasks and reaction-time results in representative temporal orienting experiments. In all diagrams time flows from top to bottom. In cued temporal orienting tasks (a–b), stimulus and interval durations are indicated in the corresponding frames.

(A) Task for comparison between spatial and temporal orienting using hemodynamic measures (Coull & Nobre, 1998; see Figure 12.4). A central symbolic cue indicated (80% validity) the likely spatial location (S) (brightening of one of the diamond sides indicated left of right), temporal interval (T) (brightening of one of the circles indicated 300 or 1,500 msec), both location and interval (ST) (combined brightening of one diamond side and circle), or provided no information regarding location or interval (N) (brightening of entire cue stimulus). Mean reaction times and standard errors are shown for the targets following informative (S, T, ST) and neutral (N) cues are shown. Behavioral comparisons ($n = 12$) showed that participants were significantly faster for trials with informative cues relative to neutral cues, $F(3,33) = 5.3$, $p < .05$.

(B) Task using foveal stimuli and manipulating temporal orienting only (Griffin et al., 2001, Experiment 2). The cue predicted the likely appearance of the target at either a short (300 msec) or long (700 msec) interval (cue-to-target stimulus-onset asynchrony [SOA]). There were nine possible SOAs (shown along the x axis of the behavioral graph). The cue predicted the correct interval on 80% of the trials. On remaining, invalid, trials, the target could appear at any one of the eight remaining SOAs. The graph shows mean reaction times and standard errors ($n = 9$ subjects) for targets appearing at a given interval separated according to when subjects were cued to expect the target. Circles represent trials in which subjects were cued that targets would occur at the short (300 msec) interval, whereas squares represent trials in which subjects were cued that targets would occur at the long (700 msec) interval. Reaction times for valid trials are plotted with filled symbols. The results showed an interaction between cue validity and SOA, $F(8,64) = 8.5$, $p < .05$, indicating that temporal orienting cues optimized performance more in trials with relatively short SOAs. There was also a main effect of SOA, showing that subjects respond faster in trials with relatively long SOAs, $F(8,64) = 15.7$, $p < .05$.

(C) Task in which spatial or temporal expectancies are developed online from the movement of a ball across the screen (Doherty et al., 2003). A ball moved across the screen from left to right in a straight or random spatial trajectory, in either constant (550 msec/step) or random (200–900 msec/step) temporal steps, and passed under an occluding strip. Predictable linear spatial trajectory afforded online buildup of spatial expectancy (S) about the reappearance of the ball. Regular temporal steps afforded the buildup of temporal expectancy about the reappearance of the ball. Random spatial and temporal trajectories afforded no specific spatial or temporal expectancy (N). The graph plots averaged median reaction times ($n = 17$) for discriminating a change in the target stimulus upon its reappearance in the different expectancy conditions. The results showed a main effect of the type of expectancy afforded by the movement of the ball, $F(2,32) = 8.0$, $p < .05$. Planned post-hoc comparisons showed that both spatial (S) and temporal (T) expectancies improved reaction times relative to no-expectancy (N) trials, and that the advantages conferred by spatial and temporal expectancies did not differ from one another.

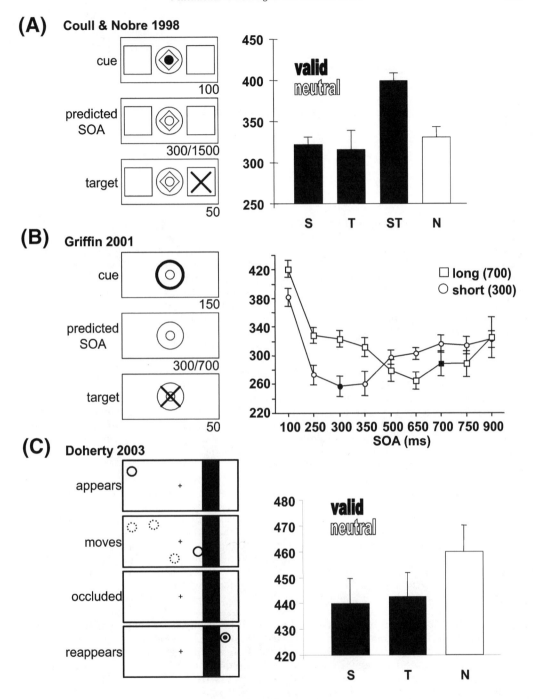

FIGURE 12.3.

FIGURE 12.4. Hemodynamic and ERP studies comparing spatial and temporal orienting.

(A) Hemodynamic results for experimental task shown in Figure 12.3a (Coull & Nobre, 1998). In active task conditions, cues predicted either the spatial location of the target (S), its temporal interval (T), both its location and interval (ST), or made no specific prediction (N). A low-level visual-fixation baseline condition (B) was also included. Significant activations obtained using positron emission tomography (PET) are overlaid on lateral surface views of a standardized brain volume (Collins et al., 1994; Talairach & Tournoux, 1988). The top row shows brain areas that were significantly activated in task conditions including spatial cueing relative to conditions without spatial cueing (main effect of spatial cueing: [(S–B) and (ST–T)] $p < .001$ uncorrected; masked by the simple effect of spatial cueing [S – B] at $p < .001$ uncorrected). Spatial cueing preferentially activated the right inferior parietal lobule (Talairach coordinates: 62 –46 32 and 58 –44 42) as well as left occipitotemporal cortex and a region in the left cerebellum. The middle row shows brain areas that were significantly activated by both spatial and temporal cues [(S – B) and (T – B)] $p < .001$. An extensive network including parietal, frontal, and visual cortical areas was commonly activated by both types of cues. The bottom row shows brain areas that were significantly activated in task conditions including temporal cueing (main effect of temporal cueing: [(T–B) and (ST–S)] $p < .001$ uncorrected; masked by the simple effect of temporal cueing [T–B] at $p < .001$ uncorrected). Temporal cueing preferentially activated left inferior premotor/prefrontal cortex and left parietal cortex (Talairach coordinates: –42 –48 48, –44 –44 38, and –44 4 20), as well as a different region in the left cerebellum.

(B) ERP results (Griffin et al., 2002, Experiment 2). The task was similar to that used for the hemodynamic experiment. A brief cue (100 msec) preceded a unilateral peripheral stimulus (100 msec). Across conditions the cue oriented attention to the spatial locations or temporal instants of the peripheral stimulus. In the spatial condition, the cue consisted of the brightening of one side of a central diamond stimulus, which formed an arrow indicating the relevant stimulus location. In the temporal condition, the cue consisted of the brightening of an inner or outer circle, indicating the relevant time at which the peripheral stimulus would occur (600 msec or 1,200 msec). The subjects ($n = 12$) were required to respond when they viewed a prespecified target stimulus appearing at the cued location or interval. Targets occurred on 19% of trials, and differed from the standard foil stimuli in subtle visual characteristics. To compare and contrast the effects of spatial versus temporal orienting upon the analysis of visual stimuli, ERP waveforms were compared to the standard foil stimuli, which occurred with equal probability at the two stimulus locations (left, right) and time intervals (short-, long-SOA). ERP results are illustrated by grand-averaged waveforms elicited by standard peripheral stimuli at the short SOA (positive polarity is plotted upward) from midline parietal (PZ) and lateral posterior (PO7/PO8) electrodes. Stimuli appearing in the left and right visual field have been averaged together, but preserving their positions relative to contralateral and ipsilateral electrodes. The electrode montage is shown at the top of the figure. (1) The top panel compares waveforms elicited by standard stimuli occurring at the valid (thick line) and invalid (thin line) spatial location. The visual P1 component was not conspicuous in the waveforms. The visual N1 component was significantly larger for attended relative to unattended stimuli, especially over the contralateral scalp. Invalid stimuli elicited a significantly larger late P300 potential. (2) The bottom panel compares waveforms elicited by standard stimuli at the short SOA when the interval predicted was valid (short-SOA, thick line) or invalid (long-SOA, thin line). Temporal orienting did not affect the amplitude of the visual P1 or N1 components, or the amplitude of the later P300 component. Instead, temporal orienting exerted a significant effect on the latency of the P300 component, which was earlier for stimuli at attended (338 msec) relative to unattended (358 msec) intervals.

A.   PET activations: comparison of neural systems

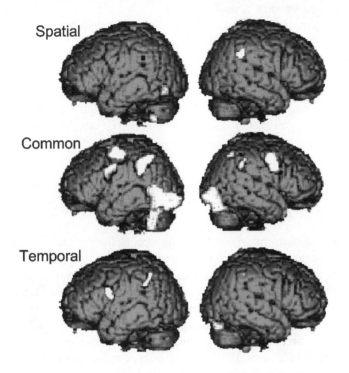

B.   ERP waveforms: different mechanisms of modulation

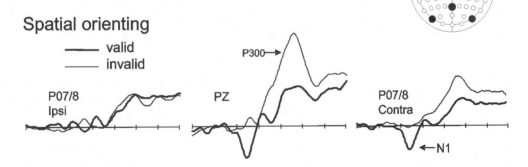

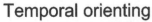

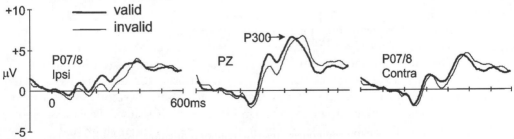

FIGURE 12.4.

factors were also at play in stimulus selection. Future studies that reduce spatial factors and record from other brain areas should be very revealing.

In addition to any lesson that research on temporal orienting may yield regarding the nature and flexibility of attentional orienting, its robust behavioral and neural effects warrant a much greater regard for temporal factors in cognitive research in general, and attention-related research in particular. Effects of temporal expectancies may be insidious in many types of experiments. For example, the use of a fixed or a narrow range of intervals between stimuli is very common and may inadvertently engender temporal expectancies that could determine or interact with the experimental factors of interest (Griffin & Nobre, in press).

GENERAL PRINCIPLES OF ATTENTIONAL ORIENTING

Working Hypotheses

Our experiments manipulating the domain in which orienting occurs (perceptual or mnemonic) or the types of expectancies that guide attentional orienting (spatial or temporal) reveal a flexible but not anarchic view of attentional orienting. In all cases, the posterior parietal and dorsal premotor/prefrontal areas are engaged by the orienting cues. The findings suggest that spatial coordinates may provide a useful scaffold on which to construct and manipulate perceptual as well as mnemonic representations to guide action, providing a means to link the various constituent attributes and modalities of the relevant events (Treisman & Gelade, 1980). Parietofrontal sensorimotor circuits that transform perception into action within spatial frameworks appear to provide a core axis for attentional orienting. The oculomotor circuit, with the ability to map, predict, and update events in retinotopic coordinates with great speed, may be particularly useful (Andersen & Buneo, 2002; Cohen & Andersen, 2002). Undoubtedly there is much complexity to be revealed within parietofrontal networks guiding spatially directed attention. Space is represented over multiple coordinate frames (egocentric, object centered, allocentric), and according to the different action systems (gazing, grasping, reaching) (Andersen & Buneo, 2002; Colby & Duhamel, 1996; Snyder, Batista, & Andersen, 2000). Indeed, in tasks in which attention is oriented toward specific manual responses (motor-attention tasks), the specific parietal and frontal areas involved differ from those involved in visuospatial orienting tasks, and oculomotor areas need not be recruited (Rushworth, Ellison, & Walsh, 2001; Rushworth, Johansen-Berg, Goebel, & Devlin, 2003). The roles of the different spatial coordinate frames and effector systems engaged by different tasks are beginning to be explored (Astafiev et al., 2003; Connolly, Goodale, Desouza, Menon, & Vilis, 2000; Scherberger, Goodale, & Andersen, 2003; Weissman, Giesbrecht, Song, Mangun, & Woldorff, 2003).

Brain areas with relevant functional specializations join core parietofrontal networks depending on the context of attentional orienting and the types of expectancies involved. Here, I have reviewed our findings that lateral prefrontal areas participate when spatial orienting occurs within a mental representation, and that sensorimotor areas involved in hand responses participate when orienting to moments in time. We have recently also started to investigate the ability to orient attention to semantic categories (Cristescu, Devlin, & Nobre, 2003a, 2003b; see also Neely, 1977). Our brain-imaging results so far show that cues predicting semantic categories selectively recruit activity in multimodal areas involved in semantic analysis before any word stimuli are presented. Other examples of participation of additional brain areas depending on the context of attentional orienting come from studies that have manipulated motivational factors. Lateral orbitofrontal cortex[3] is selectively activated when expectancies are breached (Nobre, Coull, Frith, & Mesulam, 1999), and other limbic areas also come online when attentional orienting occurs within a strong reward context (Small, Gitelman, Bloise, Parrish, & Mesulam, 2002). Other examples involving different types of expectancies come from experiments manipulating attention to object features, such as color or motion (Giesbrecht et al., 2003; Shulman et al., 1999, 2002). For example, Giesbrecht and colleagues (2003) have recently reported selective activation of posterior inferior occipitotemporal cortex by cues that oriented attention to the color of objects versus cues that orient attention to spatial locations. In this case, visual areas specialized for color processing may have participated in the control of feature-based orienting of attention (though this is not the authors' favored explanation).

These attentional orienting networks, assembled flexibly around the core sensorimotor parietofrontal axis, can influence ongoing information processing at multiple stages and in different ways. The level at which attentional orienting modulates stimulus analysis probably depends on the affordances of the different types of expectancies. For example, whereas spatial expectancies can be easily translated into receptive-field properties of neurons, temporal expectancies alone cannot lead easily to selective early perceptual modulation. Instead, they can prepare response-related areas for timely action. The cellular mechanisms mediating attentional modulations continue to be unveiled, and these may differ in different types of brain areas and according to different types of expectancies.

Directions for Future Research

One important caveat hangs over current research on the neural bases of attentional orienting. Most neuroscientific studies of attentional orienting, including those in my laboratory, have used motor responses as the main behavioral dependent variable, and most tasks have emphasized speeded action. It is possible that the parietofrontal networks, which translate perception into action, are critical because action is *in control* in these tasks. Motor action is the main behavioral goal. It is possible, in principle, for attentional orienting to optimize other aspects of our interaction with the world. For example, attention could be deployed to selective stimulus attributes in order to enhance perception, memory, or emotional impact, independently of the need for imminent action. It will be very important to develop tasks in which attentional benefits can be measured in these other aspects of behavior. Such experiments will provide a strong test of the generality of the principles regarding the neural organization of attention that have emerged from action-based experiments.

ACKNOWLEDGMENTS

Research on attentional orienting in my laboratory has been supported by project grants awarded by The Wellcome Trust and by a 21st Century Research Award in Bridging Brain, Mind and Behavior from the James S McDonnell Foundation. As ever, I am indebted to my friends and collaborators, Marsel Mesulam, Jenny Coull, Matthew Rushworth, Joe Devlin; and the members of the Brain & Cognition laboratory, especially Ivan Griffin, Carlo Miniussi, Anling Rao, Tamara Cristescu, and Joanna Doherty for helping shape the work and the ideas presented here.

NOTES

1. The experimental design borrows from the classic partial-report experiments by Sperling (1960), in which spatial cues prompted retrieval of items from immediately preceding arrays held in very short-term iconic memory. Cues presented after stimulus arrays are within working memory have also been used before in attentional experiments, but not as attention-orienting cues. Instead, postcues have been typically used to signal the location at which a decision was required (Downing, 1988; Hawkins et al., 1990; Luck & Hillyard, 1994) or to facilitate decisions about predefined targets (Kinchla, Chen, & Evert, 1995).
2. Note that previous research has considered temporal factors in terms of temporal constraints of attention to locations (inhibition of return) and objects (psychological refractory period, attentional dwell time, attentional blink, repetition blindness).
3. Inferior parietal areas are also activated during invalid trials (Corbetta, Kincade, Ollinger, McAvoy, & Shulman, 2000; Nobre, Coull, Frith, & Mesulam, 1999). Its involvement is thought to reflect reorienting functions.

REFERENCES

Andersen, R. A., & Buneo, C. A. (2002). Intentional maps in posterior parietal cortex. *Annual Review of Neuroscience, 25*, 189–220.

Anllo-Vento, L., & Hillyard, S. A. (1996). Selective attention to the color and direction of moving stimuli: Electrophysiological correlates of hierarchical feature selection. *Perception and Psychophysics, 58*(2), 191–206.

Anllo-Vento, L., Luck, S. J., & Hillyard, S. A. (1998). Spatio-temporal dynamics of attention to color: Evidence from human electrophysiology. *Human Brain Mapping, 6*(4), 216–238.

Astafiev, S. V., Shulman, G. L., Stanley, C. M., Snyder, A. Z., Van Essen, D. C., & Corbetta, M. (2003). Functional organization of human intraparietal and frontal cortex for attending, looking, and pointing. *Journal of Neuroscience, 23*, 4689–4699.

Awh, E., & Jonides, J. (2001). Overlapping mechanisms of attention and spatial working memory. *Trends in Cognitive Sciences, 5*(3), 119–126.

Beauchamp, M. S., Petit, L., Ellmore, T. M., Ingeholm, J., & Haxby, J. V. (2001). A parametric fMRI study of overt and covert shifts of visuospatial attention. *NeuroImage, 14*(2), 310–321.

Broadbent, D. E. (1958). *Perception and communication.* New York: Pergamon Press.

Chawla, D., Rees, G., & Friston, K. J. (1999). The physiological basis of attentional modulation in extrastriate visual areas. *Nature Neuroscience, 2*(7), 671–676.

Chelazzi, L., Miller, E. K., Duncan, J., & Desimone, R. (1993). A neural basis for visual search in inferior temporal cortex. *Nature, 363*, 345–347.

Clark, V. P., & Hillyard, S. A. (1996). Spatial selective attention affects early extrastriate but not striate components of the visual evoked potential. *Journal of Cognitive Neuroscience, 8*(5), 387–402.

Cohen, Y. E., & Andersen, R. A. (2002). A common reference frame for movement plans in the posterior parietal cortex. *Nature Review of Neuroscience, 3*, 553–562.

Colby, C. L., & Duhamel, J. R. (1996). Spatial representations for action in parietal cortex. *Brain Research: Cognitive Brain Research, 5*(1–2), 105–115.

Colby, C. L., Duhamel, J. R., & Goldberg, M. E. (1996). Visual, presaccadic, and cognitive activation of single neurons in monkey lateral intraparietal area. *Journal of Neurophysiology, 76*(5), 2841–2852.

Colby, C. L., & Goldberg, M. E. (1999). Space and attention in parietal cortex. *Annual Review of Neuroscience, 22*, 319–349.

Collins, D. L., Neelin, P., Peters, T. M., & Evans, A. C. (1994). Automatic 3D intersubject registration of MR volumetric data in standardized Talairach space. *Journal of Computer Assisted Tomography, 18*(2), 192–205.

Connolly, J. D., Goodale, M. A., Desouza, J. F., Menon, R. S., & Vilis, T. (2000). A comparison of frontoparietal fMRI activation during anti-saccades and anti-pointing. *Journal of Neurophysiology, 84*(3), 1645–1655.

Constantinidis, C., & Steinmetz, M. A. (2001). Neuronal responses in area 7a to multiple-stimulus displays: I. neurons encode the location of the salient stimulus. *Cerebral Cortex, 11*(7), 581–591.

Corbetta, M., Akbudak, E., Conturo, T. E., Snyder, A. Z., Ollinger, J. M., Drury, H. A., et al. (1998). A common network of functional areas for attention and eye movements. *Neuron, 21*(4), 761–773.

Corbetta, M., Kincade, J. M., Ollinger, J. M., McAvoy, M. P., & Shulman, G. L. (2000). Voluntary orienting is dissociated from target detection in human posterior parietal cortex. *Nature Neuroscience, 3*(3), 292–297.

Corbetta, M., Miezin, F. M., Dobmeyer, S., Shulman, G. L., & Petersen, S. E. (1990). Attentional modulation of neural processing of shape, color, and velocity in humans. *Science, 248*, 1556–1559.

Corbetta, M., Miezin, F. M., Shulman, G. L., & Petersen, S. E. (1993). A PET study of visuospatial attention. *Journal of Neuroscience, 13*(3), 1202–1226.

Corbetta, M., & Shulman, G. L. (2002). Control of goal-directed and stimulus-driven attention in the brain. *Nature Review of Neuroscience, 3*(3), 201–215.

Correa, A., Lupiáñez, J., & Tudela, P. (2003, September). *Attentional preparation based on temporal expectancy modulates processing at perceptual-level.* Paper presented at the XIII Conference of the European Society of Cognitive Psychology, Granada.

Coull, J. T., Frith, C. D., Buchel, C., & Nobre, A. C. (2000). Orienting attention in time: Behavioural and neuroanatomical distinction between exogenous and endogenous shifts. *Neuropsychologia, 38*(6), 808–819.

Coull, J. T., & Nobre, A. C. (1998). Where and when to pay attention: the neural systems for directing attention to spatial locations and to time intervals as revealed by both PET and fMRI. *Journal of Neuroscience, 18*, 7426–7435.

Coull, J. T., Nobre, A. C., & Frith, C. D. (2001). The noradrenergic alpha2 agonist clonidine modulates behavioural and neuroanatomical correlates of human attentional orienting and alerting. *Cerebral Cortex, 11*(1), 73–84.

Cristescu, T., Devlin, J. T., & Nobre, A. C. (2003a). *Brain areas involved in orienting attention to semantic categories* (Program No. 873.10.2003). Washington, DC: Society for Neuroscience.

Cristescu, T., Devlin, J. T., & Nobre, A. C. (2003b, June). *Orienting attention to semantic categories.* Paper presented at the 9th International Conference on Functional Mapping of the Human Brain, New York.

Desimone, R., & Duncan, J. (1995). Neural mechanisms of selective visual attention. *Annual Review of Neuroscience, 18*, 193–222.

Di Russo, F., Martinez, A., & Hillyard, S. A. (2003). Source analysis of event-related cortical activity during visuo-spatial attention. *Cerebral Cortex, 13*(5), 486–499.

Doherty, J., Griffin, I. C., Rao, A., & Nobre, A. C. (2003). Spatial versus temporal expectancies derived from object movement differentially modulate stimulus processing (Program No. 228.10.2003). Washington, DC: Society for Neuroscience.

Downing, C. J. (1988). Expectancy and visual-spatial attention: Effects on perceptual quality. *Journal of Experimental Psychology: Human Perception and Performance, 14*(2), 188–202.

Eimer, M. (1998). Mechanisms of visuospatial attention: Evidence from event-related potentials. *Visual Cognition, 5*(1–2), 257–286.

Fries, P., Reynolds, J. H., Rorie, A. E., & Desimone, R. (2001). Modulation of oscillatory neuronal synchronization by selective visual attention. *Science, 291*, 1560–1563.

Ghose, G. M., & Maunsell, J. H. (2002). Attentional modulation in visual cortex depends on task timing. *Nature, 419*, 616–620.

Giesbrecht, B., & Mangun, G. R. (in press). Identifying the neural systems of top-down attentional control: A meta-analytic approach. *NeuroImage.*

Giesbrecht, B., Woldorff, M. G., Song, A. W., & Mangun, G. R. (2003). Neural mechanisms of top-down control during spatial and feature attention. *NeuroImage, 19*(3), 496–512.

Gitelman, D. R., Nobre, A. C., Parrish, T. B., LaBar, K. S., Kim, Y. H., Meyer, J. R., et al. (1999). A large-scale distributed network for covert spatial attention: Further anatomical delineation based on stringent behavioural and cognitive controls. *Brain*, *122*(Pt. 6), 1093–1106.

Griffin, I. C., Miniussi, C., & Nobre, A. C. (2001). Orienting attention in time. *Frontiers in Bioscience*, *6*, D660–D671.

Griffin, I. C., Miniussi, C., & Nobre, A. C. (2002). Multiple mechanisms of selective attention: Differential modulation of stimulus processing by attention to space or time. *Neuropsychologia*, *40*(13), 2325–2340.

Griffin, I. C., & Nobre, A. C. (2003). Orienting attention to locations in internal representations. *Journal of Cognitive Neuroscience*, *15*(8), 1176–1194.

Griffin, I. C., & Nobre, A. C. (in press). Temporal orienting of attention. In L. Itti, G. Rees, & J. Tsotsos (Eds.), *Neurobiology of attention*. New York: Academic Press/Elsevier Science.

Haenny, P. E., & Schiller, P. H. (1988). State dependent activity in monkey visual cortex. I. Single cell activity in V1 and V4 on visual tasks. *Experimental Brain Research*, *69*(2), 225–244.

Harter, M. R., Anllo-Vento, L., & Wood, F. B. (1989). Event-related potentials, spatial orienting, and reading disabilities. *Psychophysiology*, *26*(4), 404–421.

Hawkins, H. L., Hillyard, S. A., Luck, S. J., Mouloua, M., Downing, C. J., & Woodward, D. P. (1990). Visual attention modulates signal detectability. *Journal of Experimental Psychology: Human Perception and Performance*, *16*(4), 802–811.

Heinze, H. J., Mangun, G. R., Burchert, W., Hinrichs, H., Scholz, M., Munte, T. F., et al. (1994). Combined spatial and temporal imaging of brain activity during visual selective attention in humans. *Nature*, *372*, 543–546.

Hillyard, S. A., & Mangun, G. R. (1987). Sensory gating as a physiological mechanism for visual selective attention. *Electroencephalography and Clinical Neurophysiology*, *40*(Suppl.), 61–67.

Hillyard, S. A., & Munte, T. F. (1984). Selective attention to color and location: An analysis with event-related brain potentials. *Perception and Psychophysics*, *36*(2), 185–198.

Hoffman, J. E. (1998). Visual attention and eye movements. In H. Pashler (Ed.), *Attention* (pp. 119–154). Hove, UK: Psychology Press.

Hopf, J. M., & Mangun, G. R. (2000). Shifting visual attention in space: an electrophysiological analysis using high spatial resolution mapping. *Clinical Neurophysiology*, *111*(7), 1241–1257.

Hopfinger, J. B., Buonocore, M. H., & Mangun, G. R. (2000). The neural mechanisms of top-down attentional control. *Nature Neuroscience*, *3*(3), 284–291.

Husain, M., & Rorden, C. (2003). Non-spatially lateralized mechanisms in hemispatial neglect. *Nature Review of Neuroscience*, *4*(1), 26–36.

Janssen, P., & Shadlen, M. N. (2003). *Representation of the hazard function of elapsed time by neurons in macaque area LIP* (Program No. 767.1.2003). Washington, DC: Society for Neuroscience.

Kastner, S., De Weerd, P., Desimone, R., & Ungerleider, L. G. (1998). Mechanisms of directed attention in the human extrastriate cortex as revealed by functional MRI. *Science*, *282*, 108–111.

Kastner, S., Pinsk, M. A., De Weerd, P., Desimone, R., & Ungerleider, L. G. (1999). Increased activity in human visual cortex during directed attention in the absence of visual stimulation. *Neuron*, *22*(4), 751–761.

Kastner, S., & Ungerleider, L. G. (2000). Mechanisms of visual attention in the human cortex. *Annual Review of Neuroscience*, *23*, 315–341.

Kim, Y. H., Gitelman, D. R., Nobre, A. C., Parrish, T. B., LaBar, K. S., & Mesulam, M. M. (1999). The large-scale neural network for spatial attention displays multifunctional overlap but differential asymmetry. *NeuroImage*, *9*(3), 269–277.

Kinchla, R. A., Chen, Z., & Evert, D. (1995). Precue effects in visual search: Data or resource limited? *Perception and Psychophysics*, *57*(4), 441–450.

Liang, H., Bressler, S. L., Desimone, R., & Fries, P. (2003). Attention-modulated gamma frequency activity in macaque V4 reflects task timing and performance (Program No. 385.13.2003). Washington, DC: Society for Neuroscience.

Luck, S. J., Chelazzi, L., Hillyard, S. A., & Desimone, R. (1997). Neural mechanisms of spatial selective attention in areas V1, V2, and V4 of macaque visual cortex. *Journal of Neurophysiology*, *77*(1), 24–42.

Luck, S. J., & Hillyard, S. A. (1994). Spatial filtering during visual search: evidence from human electrophysiology. *Journal of Experimental Psychology: Human Perception and Performance*, 20(5), 1000–1014.

Luck, S. J., & Vogel, E. K. (1997). The capacity of visual working memory for features and conjunctions. *Nature*, 390, 279–281.

Mangun, G. R. (1995). Neural mechanisms of visual selective attention. *Psychophysiology*, 32(1), 4–18.

Martinez, A., Anllo-Vento, L., Sereno, M. I., Frank, L. R., Buxton, R. B., Dubowitz, D. J., et al. (1999). Involvement of striate and extrastriate visual cortical areas in spatial attention. *Nature Neuroscience*, 2(4), 364–369.

Martinez, A., DiRusso, F., Anllo-Vento, L., Sereno, M. I., Buxton, R. B., & Hillyard, S. A. (2001). Putting spatial attention on the map: Timing and localization of stimulus selection processes in striate and extrastriate visual areas. *Vision Research*, 41(10–11), 1437–1457.

Mesulam, M. M. (1999). Spatial attention and neglect: Parietal, frontal and cingulate contributions to the mental representation and attentional targeting of salient extrapersonal events. *Philosophical Transactions of the Royal Society of London B (Biological Sciences)*, 354, 1325–1346.

Mesulam, M. M., Small, D., Vandenberghe, R., Gitelman, D. R., & Nobre, A. C. (in press). A heteromodal large-scale network for spatial attention. In L. Itti, G. Rees, & J. Tsotsos (Eds.), *Neurobiology of attention*. New York: Academic Press/Elsevier Science.

Miniussi, C., Wilding, E. L., Coull, J. T., & Nobre, A. C. (1999). Orienting attention in time. Modulation of brain potentials. *Brain*, 122(Pt. 8), 1507–1518.

Moore, T., & Armstrong, K. M. (2003). Selective gating of visual signals by microstimulation of frontal cortex. *Nature*, 421, 370–373.

Moore, T., & Fallah, M. (2001). Control of eye movements and spatial attention. *Proceedings of the National Academy of Sciences USA*, 98(3), 1273–1276.

Moran, J., & Desimone, R. (1985). Selective attention gates visual processing in the extrastriate cortex. *Science*, 229, 782–784.

Mort, D. J., Malhotra, P., Mannan, S. K., Rorden, C., Pambakian, A., Kennard, C., et al. (2003). The anatomy of visual neglect. *Brain*, 126(Pt. 9), 1986–1997.

Motter, B. C. (1994). Neural correlates of attentive selection for color or luminance in extrastriate area V4. *Journal of Neuroscience*, 14(4), 2178–2189.

Neely, J. H. (1977). The effects of visual and verbal satiation on a lexical decision task. *American Journal of Psychology*, 90(3), 447–459.

Niemi, P., & Naeaetaenen, R. (1981). Foreperiod and simple reaction time. *Psychological Bulletin*, 89(1), 133–162.

Nobre, A. C. (2001a). The attentive homunculus: Now you see it, now you don't. *Neuroscience and Biobehavioral Reviews*, 25(6), 477–496.

Nobre, A. C. (2001b). Orienting attention to instants in time. *Neuropsychologia*, 39(12), 1317–1328.

Nobre, A. C., Coull, J. T., Frith, C. D., & Mesulam, M. M. (1999). Orbitofrontal cortex is activated during breaches of expectation in tasks of visual attention. *Nature Neuroscience*, 2(1), 11–12.

Nobre, A. C., Coull, J. Vandeberghe, R., Maquet, P., Frith, C. D., & Mesulam, M. M. (2004). Directing attention to locations in perceptual versus mental representations. *Journal of Cognitive Neuroscience*, 16(3).

Nobre, A. C., Gitelman, D. R., Dias, E. C., & Mesulam, M. M. (2000). Covert visual spatial orienting and saccades: overlapping neural systems. *NeuroImage*, 11(3), 210–216.

Nobre, A. C., Sebestyen, G. N., Gitelman, D. R., Mesulam, M. M., Frackowiak, R. S., & Frith, C. D. (1997). Functional localization of the system for visuospatial attention using positron emission tomography. *Brain*, 120(Pt. 3), 515–533.

Nobre, A. C., Sebestyen, G. N., & Miniussi, C. (2000). The dynamics of shifting visuospatial attention revealed by event-related potentials. *Neuropsychologia*, 38(7), 964–974.

O'Craven, K. M., Downing, P. E., & Kanwisher, N. (1999). fMRI evidence for objects as the units of attentional selection. *Nature*, 401, 584–587.

Perry, R. J., & Zeki, S. (2000). The neurology of saccades and covert shifts in spatial attention: An event-related fMRI study. *Brain*, 123(Pt. 11), 2273–2288.

Posner, M. I. (1978). *Chronometric explorations of mind.* Hillsdale, NJ: Erlbaum.

Posner, M. I. (1980). Orienting of attention. *Quarterly Journal of Experimental Psychology, 32*(1), 3–25.

Posner, M. I., & Boies, S. J. (1971). Components of attention. *Psychological Review, 78,* 391–408.

Posner, M. I., & Petersen, S. E. (1990). The attention systems of the human brain. *Annual Review of Neuroscience, 13,* 25–42.

Reynolds, J. H., & Desimone, R. (1999). The role of neural mechanisms of attention in solving the binding problem. *Neuron, 24*(1), 19–29, 111–125.

Rizzolatti, G., Riggio, L., Dascola, I., & Umilta, C. (1987). Reorienting attention across the horizontal and vertical meridians: evidence in favor of a premotor theory of attention. *Neuropsychologia, 25*(1a), 31–40.

Rosen, A. C., Rao, S. M., Caffarra, P., Scaglioni, A., Bobholz, J. A., Woodley, S. J., et al. (1999). Neural basis of endogenous and exogenous spatial orienting. A functional MRI study. *Journal of Cognitive Neuroscience, 11*(2), 135–152.

Rushworth, M. F., Ellison, A., & Walsh, V. (2001). Complementary localization and lateralization of orienting and motor attention. *Nature Neuroscience, 4*(6), 656–661.

Rushworth, M. F., Johansen-Berg, H., Goebel, S. M., & Devlin, J. T. (2003). The left parietal and premotor cortices: motor attention and selection. *NeuroImage, 20*(Suppl. 1), S89–S100.

Sabes, P. N., Breznen, B., & Andersen, R. A. (2002). Parietal representation of object-based saccades. *Journal of Neurophysiology, 88*(4), 1815–1829.

Schall, J. D., & Bichot, N. P. (1998). Neural correlates of visual and motor decision processes. *Current Opinion in Neurobiology, 8*(2), 211–217.

Scherberger, H., Goodale, M. A., & Andersen, R. A. (2003). Target selection for reaching and saccades share a similar behavioral reference frame in the macaque. *Journal of Neurophysiology, 89*(3), 1456–1466.

Sheliga, B. M., Riggio, L., Craighero, L., & Rizzolatti, G. (1995). Spatial attention-determined modifications in saccade trajectories. *Neuroreport, 6*(3), 585–588.

Shulman, G. L., d'Avossa, G., Tansy, A. P., & Corbetta, M. (2002). Two attentional processes in the parietal lobe. *Cerebral Cortex, 12,* 1124–1131.

Shulman, G. L., Ollinger, J. M., Akbudak, E., Conturo, T. E., Snyder, A. Z., Petersen, S. E., et al. (1999). Areas involved in encoding and applying directional expectations to moving objects. *Journal of Neuroscience, 19,* 9480–9496.

Small, D. M., Gitelman, D. R., Bloise, S., Parrish, T. B., & Mesulam, M. M. (2002, June). *Influence of reward and punishment upon spatial attention: Interaction between the limbic system and the spatial attention network.* Paper presented at the 8th International Conference Functional Mapping of the Human Brain, Sendai, Japan.

Snyder, L. H., Batista, A. P., & Andersen, R. A. (1997). Coding of intention in the posterior parietal cortex. *Nature, 386,* 167–170.

Snyder, L. H., Batista, A. P., & Andersen, R. A. (1998). Change in motor plan, without a change in the spatial locus of attention, modulates activity in posterior parietal cortex. *Journal of Neurophysiology, 79*(5), 2814–2819.

Snyder, L. H., Batista, A. P., & Andersen, R. A. (2000). Intention-related activity in the posterior parietal cortex: A review. *Vision Research, 40*(10–12), 1433–1441.

Sperling, G. (1960). The information available in brief visual presentation. *Psychological Monographs, 74*(11, Whole No. 498), 29.

Talairach, J., & Tournoux, P. (1988). *A co-planar stereotaxic atlas of the human brain.* Stuttgart, Germany: Thieme.

Thompson Schill, S. L., D'Esposito, M., Aguirre, G. K., & Farah, M. J. (1997). Role of left inferior prefrontal cortex in retrieval of semantic knowledge: A reevaluation. *Proceedings of the National Academy of Sciences USA, 94,* 14792–14797.

Tootell, R. B., Hadjikhani, N., Hall, E. K., Marrett, S., Vanduffel, W., Vaughan, J. T., et al. (1998). The retinotopy of visual spatial attention. *Neuron, 21*(6), 1409–1422.

Treisman, A. M., & Gelade, G. (1980). A feature-integration theory of attention. *Cognitive Psychology, 12*(1), 97–136.

Treue, S., & Martinez Trujillo, J. C. (1999). Feature-based attention influences motion processing gain in macaque visual cortex. *Nature, 399,* 575–579.

Valdes Sosa, M., Bobes, M. A., Rodriguez, V., & Pinilla, T. (1998). Switching attention without shifting the spotlight object-based attentional modulation of brain potentials. *Journal of Cognitive Neuroscience, 10*(1), 137–151.

Vandenberghe, R., Duncan, J., Arnell, K. M., Bishop, S. J., Herrod, N. J., Owen, A. M., et al. (2000). Maintaining and shifting attention within left or right hemifield. *Cerebral Cortex, 10*(7), 706–713.

Vandenberghe, R., Gitelman, D. R., Parrish, T. B., & Mesulam, M. M. (2001). Functional specificity of superior parietal mediation of spatial shifting. *NeuroImage, 14*(3), 661–673.

Van Voorhis, S., & Hillyard, S. A. (1977). Visual evoked potentials and selective attention to points in space. *Perception and Psychophysics, 22*(1), 54–62.

Weissman, D. H., Giesbrecht, B., Song, A. W., Mangun, G. R., & Woldorff, M. G. (2003). Conflict monitoring in the human anterior cingulate cortex during selective attention to global and local object features. *NeuroImage, 19*(4), 1361–1368.

Wheeler, M. E., & Treisman, A. M. (2002). Binding in short-term visual memory. *Journal of Experimental Psychology: General, 131*(1), 48–64.

Wojciulik, E., & Kanwisher, N. (1999). The generality of parietal involvement in visual attention. *Neuron, 23*(4), 747–764.

Yamaguchi, S., Tsuchiya, H., & Kobayashi, S. (1994). Electroencephalographic activity associated with shifts of visuospatial attention. *Brain, 117*(Pt. 3), 553–562.

Yantis, S., Schwarzbach, J., Serences, J. T., Carlson, R. L., Steinmetz, M. A., Pekar, J. J., et al. (2002). Transient neural activity in human parietal cortex during spatial attention shifts. *Nature Neuroscience, 5,* 995–1002.

13

Cortical Mechanisms of Visual Attention

Electrophysiological and Neuroimaging Studies

Lourdes Anllo-Vento, Mircea A. Schoenfeld, and Steven A. Hillyard

The cognitive system for visual attention includes a top-down control network of interconnected cortical and subcortical structures that initiate and maintain the selectivity of perception. Studies using neuroimaging and neuropsychological techniques have identified specific regions of the frontal, posterior parietal, and superior temporal lobes and the cingulate gyrus as major components of this network (reviewed in Hopfinger, Woldroff, Fletcher, & Mangun, 2001; see Nobre, Chapter 12, and Shulman, Astafiev, & Corbetta, Chapter 9, this volume). It is hypothesized that the control network influences perceptual processing via anatomical projections to appropriate levels of the visual pathways that exert facilitatory and/ or inhibitory influences on cell populations that encode incoming sensory information (Desimone & Duncan, 1995; see Reynolds, Chapter 10, this volume). This attentional system has enormous flexibility and may select visual stimuli for preferential processing based on their locations, feature properties, or object category.

The operating principles of the attention system can be investigated in humans by obtaining noninvasive measures of brain activity from persons engaged in tasks requiring stimulus selection. To discover how sensory inputs are modulated by the top-down network, it is essential to obtain information about both the anatomical sites where the modulations occur and their exact timing. This can be achieved by using neuroimaging techniques that offer anatomical precision such as functional magnetic resonance imaging (fMRI) together with recordings of electrical or magnetic field changes that accurately reflect the time course of activity patterns within the participating neuronal populations. This chapter reviews recent studies that have combined these methods to analyze the neural substrates of visual attention to location, to different types of nonspatial features, and to multifeature objects.

ATTENTION TO LOCATION

Voluntarily directing attention to a particular location in visual space results in faster and more accurate detections of stimuli presented there. Some cognitive theorists have proposed that improved processing of attended-location stimuli results from an early facilitation of sensory inputs (Posner & Dehaene 1994) while others attributed these effects to the biasing of later decision processes (Sperling, 1984). Evidence from noninvasive scalp recordings of event-related brain potentials (ERPs) and event-related magnetic fields (ERFs) from early levels of the visuocortical pathways has helped to resolve this traditional controversy of early versus late selection mechanisms.

As shown in Figure 13.1A, a briefly flashed stimulus triggers an ERP over the scalp that consists of a characteristic sequence of voltage deflections or components that reflect the time course of sensory processing in the visuocortical areas with a resolution of millisec-

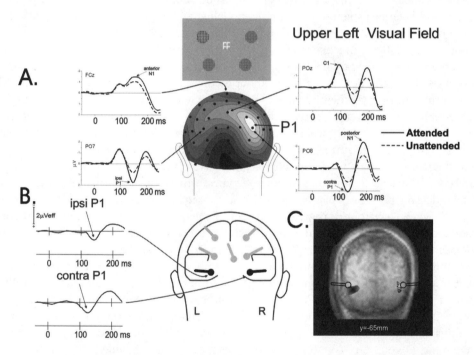

FIGURE 13.1. (A) Effect of spatial attention on the visual ERP. Grand average ERPs (over 23 subjects) recorded from four scalp sites in response to stimuli in the upper left visual field in a spatial attention experiment by Di Russo et al. (2003). Stimuli were small circular checkerboards flashed in random order to the upper left and right visual fields at intervals varying between 250 and 550 msec, while subjects attended to one field at a time. Superimposed ERP waveforms compare conditions when the upper left stimuli were attended (solid lines) versus when stimuli in the opposite field were attended (dashed lines). Voltage negativity is plotted upward. Note that the P1 (80–130 msec) and N1 (140–200 msec) components were enhanced in amplitude by spatial attention. Head with voltage map shows the contralateral occipital scalp distribution of the late phase of the P1 (100–130 msec) that is enhanced by attention. (B) Dipole modeling of the neural generators of the enhanced P1 component in the grand average waveforms using the BESA algorithm indicates dipolar sources in ventral occipital cortex. At the left are the calculated source waveforms giving the time course of activity in the contralateral and ipsilateral dipoles. (C) Co-registration of dipolar sources of the enhanced P1 with group-average fMRI activations (shaded spots) in the ventral fusiform gyrus obtained from the same subjects performing the same experiment in a different session.

onds. The earliest component is a voltage-negative "C1" wave (onset latency of 50–60 msec) that is distributed over the midline occipital scalp, which is followed by positive P1 (onset at 70–90 msec) and negative N1 (onset at 130–150 msec) components that are largest over lateral occipital areas. A separate frontal N1 component (onset at 100–120 msec) is largest over the anterior scalp. Typically, stimuli flashed to attended locations elicit enlarged P1 and/or N1 components, while leaving the earlier C1 unaffected (reviewed in Di Russo, Martinez, & Hillyard, 2003; Hillyard & Anllo-Vento, 1998). These attention effects usually take the form of amplitude modulations of the P1 and N1 components with little change in their timing or scalp distribution (Figure 13.1A), suggesting that spatial attention acts as a gain control or amplification mechanism that produces a multiplicative increase in the stimulus-evoked neural response according to the amount of attention allocated to the stimulus location (Hillyard, Vogel, & Luck, 1998). This amplification presumably enhances the signal-to-noise ratio of attended-location inputs and may do so by increasing their effective contrast as proposed by Reynolds (Chapter 10, this volume).

The localization of the P1 and N1 amplitude modulations within the visuocortical pathways has been investigated with dipole modeling techniques in conjunction with neuroimaging of the active brain regions using fMRI (Di Russo et al., 2003; Mangun et al., 2001; Martinez et al., 2001a). In these studies ERPs were recorded in one session, and the dipolar sources that best fit the scalp fields of the attention effects were calculated (Figure 13.1B). In a second session the same task was carried out by the same subjects while undergoing fMRI, and co-localization of the hemodynamic activations with the estimated dipolar sources allowed inferences to be made about both the timing and localization of the attention effects (Figure 13.1C). Using this approach, the early phase of the P1 amplification with attention (at 70–100 msec) was localized to lateral extrastriate cortex in or near visual areas V3 and V3a and adjacent regions of the middle occipital gyrus (Figure 13.2). The later phase of the P1 at 100–130 msec was found to originate from ventral occipital cortex in or near area V4 and the adjacent posterior fusiform gyrus. The subsequent attention-related enhancements of the N1 wave were found to arise from multiple generators in extrastriate visual cortex, including a posterior parietal source at 140–160 msec and a ventral occipital source at 160–200 msec (see also Hopf, Vogel, Woodman, Heinze, & Luck, 2002).

Amplitude modulations of the P1 and N1 components have been observed in a variety of spatial attention tasks including sustained attention to a location, voluntary and reflexive spatial cueing, and visual search (reviewed in Hopfinger, Luck, & Hillyard, in press; Luck & Hillyard, 2000). While the P1 and N1 are often modulated in concert, they may be dissociated under certain conditions and thus appear to reflect different aspects of spatial selection. For example, in voluntary (symbolic) spatial cueing tasks that included a "neutral" (distributed attention) condition, it was found that P1 but not N1 was suppressed to stimuli at noncued locations relative to neutral cueing, whereas N1 but not P1 was enhanced in amplitude for cued relative to neutral conditions. Furthermore, in tasks that involved reflexive spatial cueing, the capture of attention by a nonpredictive peripheral cue resulted in larger P1 amplitudes at precued locations without any N1 modulation. Based on these and other dissociations, Luck and associates have proposed that the P1 modulations reflect an early gain control mechanism that suppresses irrelevant-location inputs, while the N1 reflects the limited-capacity discriminative processing of stimuli at attended locations (Hopf et al., 2002; Luck & Hillyard, 2000).

These results from ERP and fMRI studies provide strong support for an early selection mechanism in visual spatial attention. The finding that spatial selection is first manifested by the early P1 component that originates from extrastriate visuocortical areas (V3, V3a, V4)

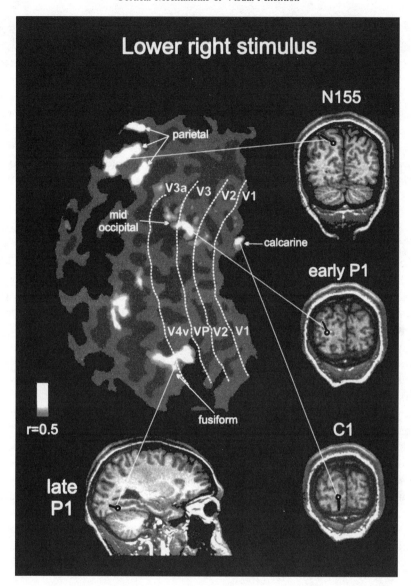

FIGURE 13.2. Visuocortical areas giving rise to different ERP components, including the attention-sensitive P1 and N1 waves. Coronal and sagittal sections show the calculated positions of dipoles accounting for different components of the visual ERP (based on grand average waveforms) to be co-localized with fMRI activations produced by the same stimuli (circular checkerboards flashed to the lower right visual field) in a single subject. These fMRI activations are projected onto a flattened cortical representation of the left hemisphere, where the dashed white lines represent the boundaries between the different visual areas determined by visual field sign mapping. From Di Russo, Martinez, Sereno, Pitzalis, and Hillyard (2001). Copyright 2001 by Wiley-Liss. Reprinted by permission.

in which only elementary stimulus features are represented argues against a late selection mechanism in which attention only acts after stimuli are fully analyzed. Neurophysiological studies in monkeys have also demonstrated that stimulus-evoked activity in these early cortical areas can be enhanced by spatial attention (see Reynolds, Chapter 10, this volume). Moreover, ERP studies of attention to multifeature stimuli have found that selection of nonspatial features such as color or motion can be contingent upon the earlier selection for location, which is also inconsistent with late selection theory (Hillyard & Anllo-Vento, 1998). Finally, irrelevant "probe" stimuli presented to an attended location similiarly elicit enlarged P1 components, consistent with an early selection mechanism that is based solely on location and does not take into account higher-order features of the stimuli (Luck & Hillyard, 2000).

The Role of Primary Visual Cortex

Several lines of evidence indicate that the earlier C1 component, which is not modulated by attention (Figure 13.1A), represents the initial wave of evoked activity in primary visual cortex (V1). Dipole modeling of the C1's voltage and magnetic field distributions points to a source in calcarine cortex, and the polarity inversion of the calcarine dipole for upper versus lower field stimuli accords with the retinotopic organization of area V1 (Di Russo et al., 2003; Noesselt et al., 2002). The insensitivity of the C1 to manipulations of attention seems at first glance to be at odds with reports that neural activity in area V1 as indexed by fMRI is increased in a retinotopic fashion when attention is directed to stimuli in the contralateral visual field (reviewed in Martinez et al., 2001). This apparent discrepancy may be resolved, however, by ERP and ERF data showing that attentional modulation of V1 activity may occur at a longer latency (140–200 msec), well beyond the initial response in V1 that is manifested in the C1 (Di Russo et al., 2003; Noesselt et al., 2002). This attention-related V1 activity has been interpreted as reflecting delayed feedback from the higher extrastriate areas where attention initially enhances the neural response to the stimulus. In support of such a mechanism, intracranial recordings in monkeys have shown that attention can affect visual processing in extrastriate areas V2 and V4 at a shorter latency than in area V1 (Schroeder, Mehta, & Foxe, 2001). This delayed feedback to area V1 may improve figure/ground segregation and heighten the salience of stimuli at attended locations (Lamme & Spekreijse, 2000).

ATTENTION TO NONSPATIAL FEATURES

When stimuli are selected according to whether they contain a particular value of a nonspatial feature such as color or shape, the associated ERP components differ from the P1/N1 modulation characteristic of spatial attention. Stimuli having the attended value (e.g., attended red flashes intermixed with irrelevant blue flashes) typically elicit initial ERP modulations that reflect processing of the specific feature that is being attended (reviewed in Hillyard & Anllo-Vento, 1998). For example, paying attention to stimulus color is associated with an early positivity (PD130) having an onset latency of 100 msec and an occipitoparietal scalp distribution (Anllo-Vento, Luck, & Hillyard, 1998). When the attended feature is spatial frequency, the earliest ERP modulations are also observed at approximately 100 msec poststimulus, but they differ in polarity and hemispheric predominance depending on whether the attended spatial frequency is high or low (Kenemans, Lijffijt,

Comfferman, & Verbaten, 2002; Martinez, Di Russo, Anllo-Vento, & Hillyard, 2001). These short-latency attention effects presumably reflect increased neural activity in the extrastriate visual areas where the features are initially selected for further processing.

These early ERP modulations are followed by a prominent negative wave that reflects the selective processing of any type of attended nonspatial feature in the visual modality, be it color, spatial frequency, orientation, or shape. This component, the selection negativity (SN), typically onsets at around 140–180 msec, has its maximal amplitude over occipital areas of the scalp and may extend for several hundreds of msec (Anllo-Vento et al., 1998; Martinez et al., 2001). The SN is best observed in difference potentials in which the ERP elicited by stimuli having an unattended feature (e.g., blue stimuli when red is attended) is subtracted from the ERP elicited by the same stimuli when they are attended (e.g., blue stimuli when blue is attended). The onset of the SN can provide a high-resolution measure of the time at which a particular feature is discriminated and selectively processed according to its task relevance. Moreover, localizing the neural generators of the SN can help to identify the specific brain areas that are engaged in the attentional selection of different stimulus features.

While stimuli may be selected on the basis of a single relevant feature, attention may also select objects consisting of multiple features or conjunctions of features. According to proposals by Desimone and Duncan (1995), distinct objects compete for processing resources within hierarchically organized areas of the ventral visual stream, such as V4 and IT. Different features or properties of the same object, however, are accessible together and in parallel. The cortical events associated with these two stages in the selection of multifeature objects can be studied by analyzing the timing and brain sources of (1) the SNs associated with selection of the individual features, and (2) the SN accompanying selection of the conjunction of features that correspond to a given object (e.g., Previc & Harter, 1982; Smid, Jakob, & Heinze, 1999). In an experiment of this type (Anllo-Vento & Hillyard, 1996), we presented subjects with sequences of bar gratings that were oriented either vertically or horizontally and were colored either red or orange (see Figure 13.3A). On a given run, subjects attended to only one of these four feature conjunctions (e.g., red vertical bars) with the task of responding to occasional targets defined as having one shortened bar in the attended array.

On different runs, subjects attended to each of the four color-orientation conjunctions in turn. Therefore, each stimulus could share one feature, two features, or none with the attended combination. ERPs were then averaged across all runs to stimuli having the relevant feature combination (C+O+), stimuli sharing its color but not orientation (C+O-), stimuli sharing its orientation but not color (C-O+), and stimuli that did not share either of the features of the relevant conjunction (C-O-). The SN associated specifically with color selection was obtained by subtracting the ERP to stimuli having the unattended color and orientation (C-O-) from the ERP to stimuli having the attended color and unattended orientation (C+O-) (difference wave 2–4 in Figure 13.3B); this SN had an onset latency of 180 msec. Similarly, orientation selection was accompanied by a SN with an onset of 140 msec, which was obtained by subtracting the (C-O-) ERP from the ERP to stimuli with the relevant orientation but the irrelevant color (C-O+) (difference wave 3–4). The SN corresponding to the selection of the conjunction was obtained by subtracting the (C-O-) ERP from the ERP to the relevant combination of the two features (C+O+) (difference wave 1–4). This latter SN also had an onset latency of about 140 msec.

If selective processing of the two features defining the attended conjunction proceeded independently or in parallel, the SN wave associated with selection of the attended conjunction would equal the sum of the SNs accompanying color selection and orientation selec-

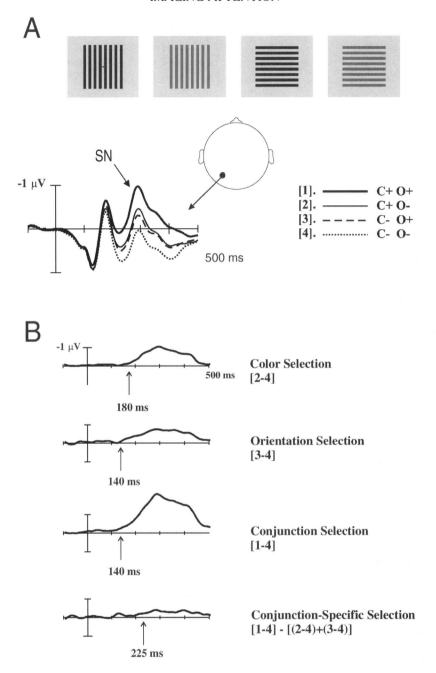

FIGURE 13.3. (A) Diagram of the four standard stimuli, which were presented one at a time in random order. Bars in the display could be horizontal or vertical, and red (dark bars) or orange (light bars). Subjects attended to a particular combination of bar color and orientation. At the left are ERPs averaged across 15 subjects and recorded over left ventral occipital scalp. Superimposed waveforms were elicited by (1) stimuli that shared both relevant features (C+O+); (2) stimuli having the relevant color and the irrelevant orientation (C+O+); (3) stimuli having the relevant orientation and the irrelevant color (C-O+); and (4) stimuli having neither of the relevant features (C-O-). (B) Selection negativities in difference waveforms corresponding to selection of the relevant color, the relevant orientation, the relevant conjunction of color and orientation, and the difference between the conjunction SN and the sum of the color and orientation difference waves.

tion. Any deviation from such additivity would indicate additional neural activity associated with the selective processing of the conjunction itself (Hansen & Hillyard, 1983; Woods, Alho, & Algazi, 1994). Such conjunction-specific processing is thus represented in the difference ERP formed by subtracting the sum of the SNs associated with the separate feature selections from the SN associated with selection of the conjunction (Figure 13.4B, bottom waveform). This difference ERP shows that conjunction-specific processing is reflected in a SN that begins at around 225 msec. These data thus indicate that a stage of independent, parallel feature selection takes place over the time interval 140–225 msec, and that selective processing of the conjunction itself starts at around 225 msec and continues for several hundred msec (along with continued parallel processing of the color and orientation features).

To estimate the locations of the cortical areas in which feature and conjunction-selective processing take place, topographical voltage maps were constructed for the respective SNs (Figure 13.4A). The SNs for color and orientation selection showed very similar narrowly focused distributions over the occipital scalp, whereas the conjunction-specific SN had a broader and more lateral scalp distribution. Dipole modeling showed that the SN distributions for the independent color and orientation selections could be fit accurately in both cases by a pair of dipoles located in ventral occipitotemporal cortex. In contrast, the

A. Voltage Topography of SN

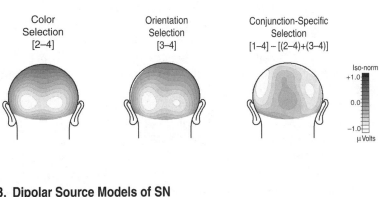

B. Dipolar Source Models of SN

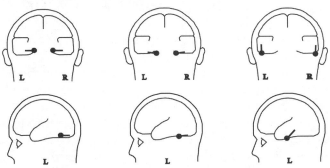

FIGURE 13.4. (A) Voltage topographies of the SNs shown in Figure 13.3B. Voltage isocontours are normalized to ±1.0 µV. (B) Coronal and sagittal views of the dipole models of the neural generators of the grand-average SNs shown in (A), obtained using the brain electric source analysis (BESA) algorithm. Dipole pairs in the left and right hemispheres were constrained to have mirror-image locations and orientations. Note that the conjunction-specific SN dipoles were situated more anteriorly in ventral temporal cortex.

conjunction-specific SN was best fit by a dipole pair situated more anteriorly, in ventral temporal areas. These data indicate that paying attention to a multifeature object involves distinct sequential but overlapping stages of processing carried out in different cortical areas. Starting at around 140 msec there was an initial parallel selection of the relevant features that was localized to ventral extrastriate areas known to encode simple features such as color and elementary shapes. Conjunction-specific processing began some 70–80 msec later in more anterior temporal areas in which higher-order feature combinations and objects are encoded. These ERP data thus reinforce current conceptions of the hierarchical organization of the ventral visual pathways for feature and object encoding (Tanaka, 1997). They also demarcate the timing of two separate stages in the selective processing of multifeature objects: an initial stage of parallel feature selection and a subsequent phase in which the task-relevant conjunction is selected. Both of these stages take place well before the ultimate motor response for target detection, which occurred with reaction times averaging 580 msec in this task.

OBJECT-SELECTIVE ATTENTION AND FEATURE BINDING

The experiments described earlier show that specific processing of an attended feature conjunction follows independent selection of the individual features. It is not clear from such results, however, whether the attention mechanism actually selects the integrated object or simply registers when the two task-relevant features are present. Behavioral studies have provided evidence that visual attention does select out whole objects as integrated feature ensembles by showing, for example, that paying attention to one part of an object improves processing of its other parts as well (Scholl, 2001). An important fMRI study (O'Craven, Downing, & Kanwisher, 1999) reinforced the view that integrated objects may serve as the units of attention by showing that directing attention to one feature of an object produces activation of the neural representations of all its features, including those not relevant to the current task. Given the poor time resolution of fMRI, however, it was not possible to determine whether the activation of irrelevant features occurs rapidly enough to participate in the feature-binding process that leads to the perception of a unitary object.

The question of the timing of irrelevant feature activation and binding was investigated in a recent study that combined recordings of ERPs and ERFs with fMRI (in separate sessions) as subjects attended to multifeature objects formed by moving dot arrays (Schoenfeld et al., 2003). Subjects viewed a video display in which 100 stationary white dots were present continuously on the screen during the intertrial intervals (Figure 13.5A). On each trial a random half of the dots moved to the left while the other half moved to the right for 300 msec, thereby producing the perception of two transparent surfaces moving in opposite directions. On each block of trials the subject was cued to attend to the surface moving in one direction and judge its velocity while ignoring the surface moving in the opposite direction. On a random basis the color of the left- or right-moving dot array could either remain white or change to red during the period of movement. This resulted in six equiprobable types of trials (3 color combinations × 2 attention conditions) as schematized in Figure 13.5B. The color of the moving dot arrays was always irrelevant to the task of directional velocity judgment.

The main questions here were (1) whether the irrelevant color feature would show increased activation in its specialized cortical module when it belonged to the attended surface and (2) how rapidly this activation would occur. This was assessed by comparing the ERP/

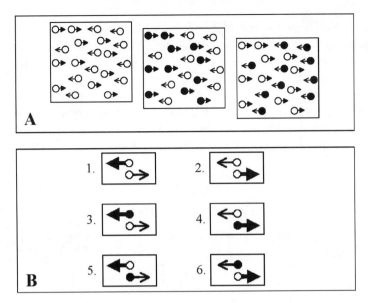

FIGURE 13.5. (A). Schematic diagram of the three possible stimulus arrays in the study of Schoenfeld et al. (2003). The right-moving or left-moving dot arrays could be either red (filled dots) or white (open dots) on a random basis. Bold arrows indicate the attended direction (right-moving in this case), which was cued prior to each block of trials. The subject's task was to detect and respond to occasional faster-moving arrays (targets) in the attended direction. (B). Schematic depiction of the six experimental conditions defined by the colors of the moving arrays and the direction of attention. From Schoenfeld et al. (2003). Copyright 2003 by The National Academy of Sciences of the USA. Reprinted by permission.

ERF waveforms on trials where the attended versus the unattended surface changed color (Figure 13.6A). Increased ERP/ERF amplitudes were found beginning at 200–240 msec when the attended-direction surface changed color (Figure 13.6B), and the source of this effect was localized through dipole modeling to the fusiform gyrus of the ventral occipital cortex (Figure 13.6C, 13.6D). This localization was confirmed in separate sessions with event-related fMRI, where the same comparisons (attended vs. unattended surface changing color) showed bilateral activations in the fusiform gyrus (Figure 13.6D). This enhanced fusiform activity associated with the attended surface being colored was more specifically localized to retinotopically mapped visual area V4v (Figure 13.7).

These converging fMRI and ERP/ERF data indicated that processing of the irrelevant color feature was facilitated rapidly in ventral occipital cortex (area V4v) when the color belonged to the attended surface. This V4v area has been identified previously as harboring a specialized module for the processing of color information (e.g. McKeefry & Zeki, 1997). The timing of the irrelevant color activation in this cortical area (200–240 msec) is comparable to the timing of the selection of task-relevant feature conjunctions involving color (180–260 msec) as reported in previous studies (e.g., Cortese, Bernstein, & Alain, 1999; Karayanidis & Michie, 1996; Smid et al., 1999; see also Figure 13.3B). Because the irrelevant feature activation observed here occurs in the same time frame as when relevant features are conjoined and selected, we conclude that enhanced processing of the irrelevant feature of the attended object in its specialized module can occur rapidly enough to participate in the feature-binding process that underlies the perceptual unity of the attended object.

These data reinforce previous evidence that multifeature objects can serve as the units of visual attention and provide strong support for the "integrated competition" model of object-selective attention (Duncan, Humphreys, & Ward, 1997). According to this model, the neural basis for perceptual integration of an attended object consists of the competitive activation of a network of specialized modules that encode its individual features. Directing attention to one of an object's features will produce a competitive advantage for the object in the module encoding that feature, which is then transmitted to the modules that encode the object's other features, including those that are irrelevant to the task at hand. The conse-

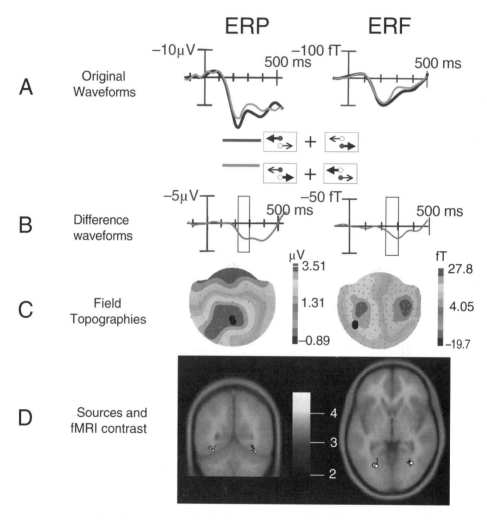

FIGURE 13.6. The effect of attention on irrelevant color processing in the study of Schoenfeld et al. (2003). (A). Concurrently recorded ERP and ERF waveforms (averaged over attend-left and attend-right conditions) on trials where the dot array moving in the attended (black lines) or unattended (gray lines) direction changed color from white to red. (B). Difference waveforms formed by subtracting the gray from the black waveforms shown in A. (C). Surface field topographies of the difference ERP and ERF waveforms shown in B over the time interval 220–300 msec. (D). Projections of the calculated source dipoles accounting for the surface topographies of the difference waveforms shown in C and the corresponding fMRI activations for the attention effect on irrelevant color processing (same contrast as in A). All data shown are across-subject averages. From Schoenfeld et al. (2003). Copyright 2003 by The National Academy of Sciences of the USA. Reprinted by permission.

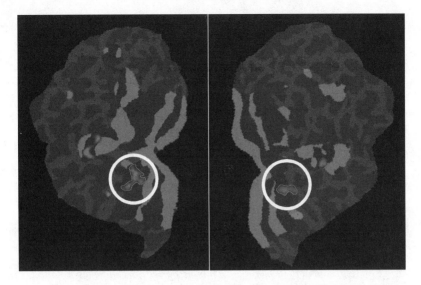

Left Hemisphere   Right Hemisphere

FIGURE 13.7. Projection of single-subject fMRI activations derived from the contrast illustrated in Figure 13.6 onto flat-maps of that subject's retinotopic visuocortical areas. These activations representing the effect of attention on processing of the irrelevant color feature were localized to visual area V4v.

quent activation of the entire network of specialized modules through mutually supportive interconnections is proposed to underlie the binding of features into a unified perceptual object.

CONCLUSION

The studies reviewed in this chapter make it clear that measures of the timing of neural activity patterns like those provided by ERP/ERF recordings are essential for unraveling the dynamic mechanisms of visual attention in humans. Hemodynamic neuroimaging experiments have been highly successful in identifying the multiplicity of brain areas that participate in attentional control and selection, but the intricate interplay among those areas will remain obscure in the absence of timing information. For example, the critical question of whether selective modulation of neural activity at a particular level of the visual pathways (such as V1) results from an early selection during the feedforward sweep of input or a late selection at a higher level that is relayed via feedback connections may be difficult to answer if the precise timing of the modulation is unknown. Indeed, there is increasing evidence that feedforward and feedback (recurrent) processes play distinctive roles in visual perception. As reviewed by Lamme and Roelfsema (2000), recurrent neural activity has been implicated in the identification of fine details in visual patterns, the enhancement of figure–ground relationships, the attentional selection of objects, and even in visual awareness itself. Further study of visual perception and attention in humans will require the adroit combination of time-sensitive and location-sensitive methodologies (e.g., Marinkovic et al., 2003).

REFERENCES

Anllo-Vento, L., & Hillyard, S. A. (1996). Following the time course of feature extraction with event-related brain potentials. *NeuroImage, 3,* 173.

Anllo-Vento, L., Luck, S. J., & Hillyard, S. A. (1998). Spatio-temporal dynamics of attention to color: evidence from human electrophysiology. *Human Brain Mapping, 6,* 216–238.

Cortese, F. Bernstein, I. J., & Alain, C. (1999). Binding visual features during high-rate serial presentation. *Neuroreport, 10,* 1565–1570.

Desimone, R., & Duncan, J. (1995). Neural mechanisms of selective visual attention. *Annual Review of Neuroscience, 18,* 193–222.

Di Russo, F., Martinez, A., & Hillyard, S. A. (2003). Source analysis of event-related cortical activity during visio-spatial attention. *Cerebral Cortex, 13,* 486–499.

Di Russo, F., Martinez, A., Sereno, M. I., Pitzalis, S., & Hillyard, S. A. (2001). Cortical sources of the early components of the visual evoked potential. *Human Brain Mapping, 15,* 95–111.

Duncan, J., Humphreys, G., & Ward, R. (1997). Competitive brain activity in visual attention. *Current Opinion in Neurobiology, 7,* 255–261.

Hansen, J. C., & Hillyard, S. A. (1983). Selective attention to multidimensional auditory stimuli in man. *Journal of Experimental Psychology: Human Perception and Performance, 9,* 1–19.

Hillyard, S. A., & Anllo-Vento, L. (1998). Event-related brain potentials in the study of visual selective attention. *Proceedings of the National Academy of Sciences USA, 95,* 781–787.

Hillyard, S. A., Vogel, E. K., & Luck, S. J. (1998). Sensory gain control (amplification as a mechanism of selective attention: electrophysiological and neuroimaging evidence. *Philosophical Transactions of the Royal Society of London B (Biological Sciences), 353,* 1257–1270.

Hopf, J.-M., Vogel, E., Woodman, G., Heinze, H.-J., & Luck, S. J. (2002). Localizing visual discrimination processes in space and time. *Journal of Neurophysiology, 88,* 2088–2095.

Hopfinger, J. B., Luck, S. J., & Hillyard, S. A. (in press). Selective attention: Electrophysiological and neuromagnetic studies. In M. S. Gazzaniga (Ed.), *The newest cognitive neurosciences* (3rd ed.). Cambridge, MA: MIT Press.

Hopfinger, J. B., Woldroff, M. G., Fletcher, E. M., & Mangun, G. R. (2001). Dissociating top-down attentional control from selective perception and action. *Neuropsychologia, 39,* 1277–1291.

Karayanidis, F., & Michie, P. T. (1996). Frontal processing negativity in a visual selective attention task. *Electroencephalography and Clinical Neurophysiology, 99,* 38–56.

Kenemans, J. L., Lijffijt, M., Camfferman, G., & Verbaten, M. N. (2002). Split-second sequential selective activation in human secondary visual cortex. *Journal of Cognitive Neuroscience, 14,* 48–61.

Lamme, V. A. F., & Roelfsema, P. R. (2000). The distinct modes of vision offered by feedforward and recurrent processing. *Trends in Neuroscience, 23,* 571–579.

Lamme, V. A. F., & Spekreijse, H. (2000). Contextual modulation in primary visual cortex and scene perception. In M. S. Gazzaniga (Ed.), *The new cognitive neurosciences* (2nd ed., pp. 279–290). Cambridge, MA: MIT Press.

Luck, S. J., & Hillyard, S. A. (2000). The operation of selective attention at multiple stages of processing: Evidence from human and monkey electrophysiology. In M. S. Gazzaniga (Ed.), *The new cognitive neurosciences* (2nd ed., pp. 687–700). Cambridge, MA: MIT Press.

Mangun, G. R., Hinrichs, H., Scholz, M., Mueller-Gaertner, H. W., Herzog, H., Krause, B. J., et al. (2001). Integrating electrophysiology and neuroimaging of spatial selective attention to simple isolated visual stimuli. *Vision Research, 41,* 1423–1435.

Marinkovic, K., Dhond, R. P., Dale, A. M., Glessner, M., Carr, V., & Halgren, E. (2003). Spatiotemporal dynamics of modality-specific and supramodal word processing. *Neuron, 38,* 487–497.

Martinez, A., Di Russo, F., Anllo-Vento, L., & Hillyard, S. A. (2001). Electrophysiological analysis of cortical mechanisms of selective attention to high and low spatial frequencies. *Clinical Neurophysiology, 112,* 1980–1998.

Martinez, A., Di Russo, F., Anllo-Vento, L., Sereno, M. I., Buxton, R. B., & Hillyard, S. A. (2001).

Putting spatial attention on the map: Timing and localization of stimulus selection processes in striate and extrastriate visual areas. *Vision Research, 41,* 1437–1457.

McKeefry, D., & Zeki, S. (1997). The position and topography of the human color center as revealed by functional magnetic resonance imaging. *Brain, 120,* 2229–2242.

Noesselt, T., Hillyard, S. A., Woldorff, M. G., Hagner, T., Jaencke, H., Tempelmann, C., et al. (2002). Delayed striate cortical activation during spatial attention. *Neuron, 35,* 575–587.

O'Craven, K. M., Downing, P. E., & Kanwisher, N. (1999). fMRI evidence for objects as the units of attentional selection. *Nature, 401,* 584–587.

Posner, M. I., & Dehaene, S. (1994). Attentional networks. *Trends in Neuroscience, 17,* 75–79.

Previc, F. H., & Harter, M. R. (1982). Electrophysiological and behavioral indicants of selective attention to multifeature gratings. *Perception and Psychophysics, 32,* 465–472.

Schoenfeld, M. A., Tempelmann, C., Martinez, A., Hopf, J.-M., Sattler, C., Heinze, H.-J., et al. (2003). *Proceedings of the National Academy of Sciences USA, 100,* 11806–11811.

Scholl, B. J. (2001). Objects and attention: The state of the art. *Cognition, 80,* 1–46.

Schroeder, C. E., Mehta, A. D., & Foxe, J. J. (2001). Determinants and mechanisms of attentional modulation of neural processing. *Frontiers in Bioscience, 6,* 672–684.

Smid, H. G., Jakob, A., & Heinze, H. J. (1999). An event-related brain potential study of visual selective attention to conjunctions of color and shape. *Psychophysiology, 36,* 264–279.

Sperling, G. (1984). A unified theory of attention and signal detection. In R. Parasuraman & D. R. Davies (Eds.), *Varieties of attention* (pp. 103–181). Orlando, FL: Academic Press.

Tanaka, K. (1997). Mechanisms of visual object recognition: monkey and human studies. *Current Opinion in Neurobiology, 7,* 523–529.

Woods, D. L., Alho, K., & Algazi A. (1994). Stages of auditory feature conjunction: an event-related brain potential study. *Journal of Experimental Psychology: Human Perception and Performance, 20,* 81–94.

14

Mechanisms of Attention in Audition as Revealed by the Event-Related Potentials of the Brain

Risto Näätänen and Kimmo Alho

In this chapter, we examine event-related potential (ERP) work on auditory attention, starting with studies aimed at determining the extent and quality of the processing that occurs in the absence of attention to provide a baseline against which the effects of attention can be evaluated.

AUDITORY PROCESSING IN THE ABSENCE OF ATTENTION

There is one component in the auditory ERP—the *mismatch negativity* (MMN)—that is really informative with regard to the actual processing of the unattended input. This is of great importance as on the basis of mere behavioral data, it is very hard and risky, sometimes even impossible (e.g., infants and several patient groups), to make inferences with regard to the extent and quality of automatic processing in audition. Studies using the MMN, isolated from the "N2" wave or the "N2-P3a" wave complex by Näätänen, Gaillard, and Mäntysalo (1978), suggest, as reviewed later, that the physical sound features of even unattended stimuli are fully processed at least under most attention conditions. Furthermore, the MMN can be recorded even in newborns and infants, providing objective information on the development of their central auditory-processing abilities, and also in different patient groups that cannot produce reliable behavioral data.

In fact, the MMN, elicited when some regularity in auditory stimulation is violated by a change (deviant stimulus), can be best observed when the subject's attention is directed away from this stimulus sequence. Otherwise, deviant stimuli elicit, besides the MMN, also the N2b (Fitzgerald & Picton, 1983; Näätänen, Simpson, & Loveless, 1982), a negative component overlapping the later part of the MMN, and a subsequent P3a positivity (Squires, Squires, & Hillyard, 1975), an index of involuntary attention switch (Escera, Alho,

Winkler, & Näätänen, 1998; Schröger, 1996) also often elicited in ignore conditions. The MMN is usually evaluated from the difference wave obtained by subtracting the ERP to the standard (repetitive) stimulus from that elicited by the deviant stimulus.

An MMN in response to a minor change in tonal frequency is illustrated in Figure 14.1 (Sams, Paavilainen, Alho, & Näätänen, 1985). Each stimulus block was composed of standard stimuli (80%) of 1,000 Hz and deviant stimuli (20%) differing in frequency from the standards, delivered in random order and at a constant interstimulus interval (ISI) of 1 second. The frequency of the deviant stimulus was, in separate blocks, either 1,004, 1,008, 1,016, or 1,032 Hz. The subject was instructed to ignore the auditory stimuli and to concentrate on reading a book.

The N1 wave in response to the different deviant stimuli was similar to the one evoked by the standard stimulus and did not vary in amplitude or latency with the degree of deviance. As shown by the difference waveforms in Figure 14.1, a clear MMN was elicited by deviant stimuli with frequencies higher than 1,008 Hz. Even the 1,008-Hz stimuli, which were found in a separate condition to be near the discrimination threshold, elicited an MMN, although a very small one. Further, the MMN peaked earlier for larger deviations in pitch. When the magnitude of deviation was further increased, the decreased MMN latency resulted in an increasing overlap between the MMN and N1 components, which must be taken into account in assessing the strength of the MMN-generator process. In Figure 14.1, a small P3a is seen to follow the MMN. Such data suggest that even minor stimulus changes are detected in the absence of attention, implicating that the physical stimulus features are thoroughly processed even in the absence of attention.

The MMN can also be elicited by other types of auditory changes, being, in fact, elicited by any discriminable change in acoustic input. Furthermore, numerous studies (for a re-

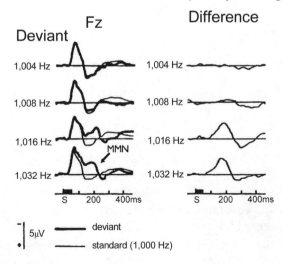

FIGURE 14.1. *Left:* Frontal (Fz) ERPs (averaged across subjects) to 1,000-Hz standard (thin line) and to deviant (thick line) stimuli of different frequencies, as indicated on the left side. *Right:* The difference waves obtained by subtracting the standard-stimulus ERP from the corresponding deviant-stimulus ERP. From Näätänen and Picton (1987). Copyright 1987 by Blackwell. Reprinted by permission.

view, see Näätänen, 2001) established that the MMN provides an index of perceptual discrimination accuracy such that if an MMN is elicited when one stimulus is used as the
standard and the other as the deviant, then the two stimuli can be behaviorally discriminated (Kraus et al., 1996). Consequently, the MMN can serve as an objective measure of perceptual discrimination and thus of sound-processing accuracy.

Several studies have tested the assumed independence of attention of the MMN. For example, Alho, Woods, Algazi, and Näätänen (1992) found that the MMN to slightly higher-
pitched deviant tones in an auditory stimulus sequence was of very similar amplitude during
easy and difficult visual discrimination tasks demanding very different amounts of attention.
However, this MMN appeared to be larger in amplitude when subjects attended to auditory
stimuli than when they attended to visual stimuli, suggesting some attentional enhancement
of the MMN amplitude. In a similar vein, Trejo, Ryan-Jones, and Kramer (1995) found that
the MMN amplitude for a frequency change in a binaural repetitive tone was larger when
subjects attended to this tone sequence than when they attended to a concurrent narrative.
In contrast, several selective-listening studies with an instruction to attend to stimuli in a
designated ear and to ignore a concurrent stimulus sequence in the opposite ear obtained
MMNs of very similar amplitudes to occasional frequency changes in both the attended and
unattended ears (Alho, Sams, Paavilainen, Reinikainen, & Näätänen, 1989; Näätänen,
Paavilainen, Tiitinen, Jiang, & Alho, 1993; Paavilainen, Tiitinen, Alho, & Näätänen, 1993).

In contrast, Woldorff, Hackley, and Hillyard (1991) and Näätänen and colleagues
(1993) found that the MMN elicited by occasional decrements in tone intensity in the unattended ear was attenuated in amplitude (but was not totally abolished) relative to that for
the attended ear tones. In addition, Woldorff, Hillyard, Gallen, Hampson, and Bloom
(1998) demonstrated that the MMNm (the magnetic equivalent of the MMN) amplitude for
intensity decrements of identical magnitude was larger in the attended than in the unattended ear.

Nevertheless, no data exist that cast doubt on MMN elicitation even by a slight sound
change in the absence of attention. Furthermore, the automaticity of the MMN is strongly
supported by results demonstrating that an MMN can be elicited even in comatose patients
by changes in tone frequency (Kane, Curry, Butler, & Cummins, 1993; Kane et al., 1996) or
duration (Fischer et al., 1999; Morlet, Bouchet, & Fischer, 2000) (when these patients were
going to return into consciousness within the next few days).

Woldorff and colleagues (1991, 1998), however, interpreted the attenuation of the
MMNm amplitude in the unattended channel as suggesting attenuated sensory processing in
the absence of attention. Näätänen (1991), however, proposed that attention might affect
the MMN amplitude but not necessarily the threshold of the MMN-generator activation. If
this threshold is not affected (as is the case if the MMN is not abolished by the withdrawal
of attention), then an attenuated MMN amplitude cannot be taken, according to him, as
suggesting that sensory processing is deteriorated in the unattended channel, for even a very
weak MMN-generator process implicates differential antecedent processing (and encoding
to sensory memory) of standard and deviant stimuli (i.e., apparently, the full sensory processing in the unattended channel). (Of course, these very weak MMN-generator activations
might fail to trigger further processes, those leading to attention switch to, and conscious
perception of, sound change; see Näätänen, 1992, pp. 204–206.)

As for the intracranial generators of the MMN, the largest amplitudes are recorded
over the frontocentral scalp areas. The source modeling of the ERP (e.g., Giard et al., 1995;
Scherg, Vajsar, & Picton, 1989) and of the MMNm (Alho et al., 1998; Jemel, Achenbach,
Müller, Röpke, & Oades, 2002; Levänen, Ahonen, Hari, McEvoy, & Sams, 1996) suggests

bilateral generators in the auditory cortices, explaining, at least in part, the large MMN amplitudes over the frontocentral scalp (for corroborating intracranial recordings, see Halgren et al., 1995; Kropotov et al., 1995, 2000; Liasis, Towell, & Boyd, 1999, 2000).

In addition, scalp-current density maps (Giard, Perrin, Pernier, & Bouchet, 1990; Rinne, Alho, Ilmoniemi, Virtanen, & Näätänen, 2000) suggest a further MMN generator in the prefrontal cortex. Corroborating lesion data were obtained by Alho, Woods, Algazi, Knight, and Näätänen (1994) and Alain, Woods, and Knight (1998); functional magnetic resonance imaging (fMRI) data by Schall, Johnston, Todd, Ward, and Michie (2003), Celsis and colleagues (1999), and Opitz, Rinne, Mecklinger, von Cramon, and Schröger (2002); and positron emission tomography (PET) data by Dittmann-Balcar, Jüptner, Jentzen, and Schall (2001) and Müller, Jüptner, Jentzen, and Müller (2002). fMRI (e.g., Schall et al., 2003) and PET (e.g., Müller et al., 2002) studies have also verified the auditory-cortex source of the MMN.

As to the functional significance of these two principal generator processes of the MMN, it appears that the preperceptual auditory-cortex process comparing the present input with that represented by the sensory-memory trace developed by preceding stimuli generates the auditory-cortex subcomponent of the MMN. The frontal subcomponent of the MMN, triggered by the initiation of the MMN process in the auditory cortex in response to sound change (Giard et al., 1990; Näätänen, 1992; Rinne et al., 2000), might, in turn, be generated by a frontal processs belonging to the chain of cerebral events leading to attention switch to, and conscious perception of, sound change (Giard et al., 1990; Näätänen, 1990). This conscious change detection is associated with the activation of the autonomous nervous system (Lyytinen, Blomberg, & Näätänen, 1992), accompanied by a distracting effect on the subject's task performance in the primary task (Escera et al., 1998), and by the P3a ERP component which has a scalp distribution anterior to that of the P3b (Alho et al., 1998; Escera et al., 1998; Sams et al., 1985; Squires et al., 1975).

When subjects attend to auditory stimuli in order to detect occasional deviant sounds in a sequence of standard sounds, then the MMN to these target sounds is followed, and often partly overlapped, by another negative component, the one called the N2b (Sams et al., 1985; for reviews, see Näätänen, 1992; Näätänen & Gaillard, 1983), which is, in turn, succeeded by the P3a and P3b components (Donchin & Coles, 1988; Picton, 1992; Squires et al., 1975). Thus, the N2b, P3a, and P3b appear to be associated with conscious change detection. Moreover, the speed of detecting deviant target sounds seems to be governed by the preattentive change-detection process generating the MMN, as the MMN peak latency which decreases with an increasing stimulus change strongly correlates with the reaction time (RT) and the N2b latency for deviant target sounds (Novak, Ritter, Vaughan, & Wiznitzer, 1990; Tiitinen, May, Reinikainen, & Näätänen, 1994).

SELECTIVE ATTENTION

In their pioneering ERP study on selective attention, Hillyard, Hink, Schwent, and Picton (1973) presented tones with varying short intervals (100–800 msec) in a random order to the left and right ears. Subjects were instructed to attend either to the left- or right-ear tones and to discriminate slightly higher, deviant tones among the standard-pitch tones delivered to the attended ear. The standard tones in the attended ear elicited a larger N1 deflection than did similar tones when attention was directed to the opposite ear. The authors proposed that this attention effect was caused by selective tonic facilitation of the processing of the attended input and, further, that this facilitation might underlie the stimulus-set mode of selective attention of Broadbent (1958, 1970).

This view was soon challenged, however, by Näätänen and his colleagues (Näätänen, Gaillard, & Mäntysalo, 1978; Näätänen & Michie, 1979), who suggested that the effect of selective attention on auditory ERPs was caused by a separate attentional selection mechanism rather than by simple amplification of processing attended inputs. More specifically, they proposed that the N1 attention effect reported by Hillyard and colleagues (1973) was not caused by the modulation of the N1 response but rather by an endogenous attention-related negative ERP component, with its early portion overlapping with the exogenous component(s) of the N1. Näätänen and colleagues (1978) used a similar paradigm to that of Hillyard and colleagues except that the tones were now delivered at constant, 800-msec intervals. Under these conditions, the attention effect appeared as a slow, endogenous negative ERP component, which Näätänen and colleagues termed the processing negativity (PN). This PN commenced at the N1 latency and continued for several hundreds of milliseconds. Further studies suggested that the negative difference (Nd; Hansen & Hillyard, 1980) between ERPs to attended and unattended sounds consists of at least two components: an early one at the N1 latency and a more frontally distributed one typically peaking at 300–400 msec from sound onset (e.g., Alho, Woods, & Algazi, 1994; Giard, Perrin, Pernier, & Peronnet, 1988; Hansen & Hillyard, 1980; Woods & Clayworth, 1987). As reviewed later, it appears that both types of effects have been confirmed by subsequent studies, suggesting the presence of two different types of selective-attention mechanisms in audition. The attentional enhancement of the exogenous N1 might be associated with coarse selection of sounds (e.g., sounds at the left vs. sounds at the right) in conditions with high stimulus rates (e.g., 4 Hz) and strongly focused attention (cf. Woldorff & Hillyard, 1991), whereas the selective-attention mechanism generating the PN would be capable of selecting attended sounds that are delivered at lower rates and differ less from unattenuated sounds (cf. Alho, 1992; Alho, Donauer, et al., 1987; Alho, Töttölä, Reinikainen, Sams, & Näätänen, 1987; Alho, Lavikainen, Reinikainen, Sams, & Näätänen, 1990).

Näätänen (1982, 1990, 1992) proposed that the earlier PN component, explaining the attention effect at the N1 latency, is generated by the selection of attended stimuli for further analysis in a gradual matching process, in which each sound is compared with what he called the attentional trace. According to this theory, the attentional trace is an actively maintained cortical representation of the physical feature(s) of to-be-attended sounds (e.g., their pitch, location, or both), separating them from the unattended sounds (see also Alho et al., 1989). He further proposed that the attended sounds perfectly match with this trace and therefore elicit a large and long-duration PN, whereas other (i.e., unattended) sounds mismatch with the trace and are rejected from further processing. Furthermore, the speed of this rejection depends on how much the unattended sounds differ from the attended sounds on the critical dimension(s), with more different sounds being rejected earlier and thus generating shorter-duration PNs than sounds that are less easily discriminable from the attended sounds. These suggestions, illustrated schematically in Figure 14.2, were supported by the results of several studies (Alho, Donauer, et al., 1987; Alho, Paavilainen, Reinikainen, & Näätänen, 1986; Alho, Töttölä, et al., 1987; Hari et al., 1989; Michie, Solowij, Crawford, & Glue, 1993).

According to Näätänen (1982, 1990, 1992), the attentional trace is formed in the auditory cortex by rehearsal of the sensory-memory representation of the attended stimulus and therefore depends on the sensory reinforcement provided by the attended sounds. This is supported by results indicating no differences between ERPs to attended and unattended

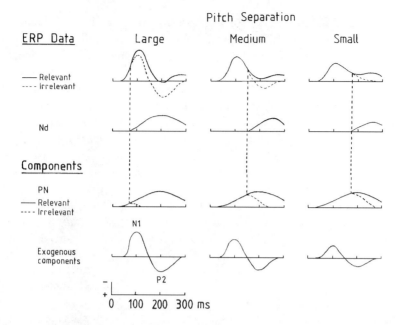

FIGURE 14.2. First row: A schematic illustration of ERPs to relevant (to-be-attended) and irrelevant (to-be-ignored) sounds for "large," "medium," and "small" pitch separations between the relevant and irrelevant sounds. (The model is also valid for "large," "medium," and "small" location separations.) Second row: The respective negative difference (Nd waves) obtained by subtracting the ERPs to irrelevant sounds from those to relevant sounds. Third row: The processing negativities (PNs) to the relevant and irrelevant sounds (only the earlier component of the PN is illustrated). The PNs summate to the exogenous evoked potential (EP) components (shown on the fourth row). The attenuation of the Nd amplitude and the increase of the Nd onset latency with a decreasing pitch separation (illustrated on the third row) result from the coinciding increase and prolongation of the PN to irrelevant sounds, whereas pitch separation has no effect on the PN elicited by the relevant sounds. Fourth row: The attenuation of the N1 and P2 components (identical for relevant and irrelevant sounds) explains the effects of pitch separation on relevant-sound ERPs and a part of the effects of pitch separation on irrelevant-sound ERPs (for simplicity, the different subcomponents of the exogenous N1 and P2 are not illustrated). From Alho, Töttölä, Reinikainen, Sams, and Näätänen (1987). Copyright 1987 by Elsevier. Reprinted by permission.

sounds for the first two or three stimuli in the beginning of the selective-listening task (Hansen & Hillyard, 1988) or for sounds that are delivered with very long intervals (Alho et al., 1990). These findings are in line with behavioral results showing that several presentations of to-be-attended sounds are necessary before they can be effectively attended and other sounds rejected and ignored (Treisman, Squire, & Green, 1974).

As already mentioned, the early Nd at the N1 latency is followed by a late Nd with a frontally dominant scalp distribution (Alho, Teder, Lavikainen, & Näätänen, 1994; Alho, Woods, & Algazi, 1994; Giard et al., 1988; Hansen & Hillyard, 1980; Näätänen & Michie, 1979; Näätänen, Teder, Alho, & Lavikainen, 1992; Teder, Alho, Reinikainen, & Näätänen, 1993; Woods & Clayworth, 1987). This late Nd, caused by the later component of the PN, might be generated by the active rehearsal of the attentional trace after each occurrence of an attended sound (Näätänen, 1982, 1990, 1992), and presumably originates from the frontal lobes (Alcaini, Giard, & Perrin, 1995; Giard et al., 1988). The important role of the frontal lobes in maintaining selective auditory attention indicated by the PN is also suggested by the results of Knight, Hillyard, Woods, and Neville (1981) who observed that patients with unilateral lesions of the dorsolateral prefrontal cortex have attenuated PNs in relation to those of healthy controls. Moreover, the parietal cortical areas, too, are involved in auditory selective attention, as PN amplitudes at latencies longer than 150 msec from sound onset are attenuated in patients with unilateral parietal or temporoparietal lesions (Woods, Knight, & Scabini, 1993). Interestingly, these lesions did not affect the ERP attention effect at shorter latencies (i.e., at the N1 latency range), although attenuated exogenous N1 responses were observed in patients with temporoparietal lesions. These patient studies are in line with PET results also suggesting the involvement of the prefrontal and parietal cortices in auditory attention. In one of these studies, Alho and colleagues (1999) delivered tones to the left and right ears at a very fast rate (6 Hz for each ear), supposed to lead to strongly focused attention (cf. Woldorff & Hillayrd, 1991). Subjects selectively attended either to the left- or right-ear tones. In a control condition, they were instructed to ignore all tones and to attend to visual stimuli (presented also in the auditory attention conditions). Selective listening increased activity bilaterally in auditory and prefrontal cortices and unilaterally in the right parietal cortex (Figure 14.3; see also O'Leary et al., 1996; Tzourio et al., 1997; Zatorre, Mondor, & Evans, 1999).

However, there are also results that are not in keeping with the attentional-trace theory. According to Woldorff and Hillyard (1991), the similar time courses of the N1 and the early attention effect elicited at the N1 latency with fast stimulation rates support Hillyard and colleagues' (1973) original proposal that the early Nd is caused by an enhancement of the exogenous N1. This "gain theory" of selective attention (see Näätänen, 1986) is further supported by the magnetoencephalographic (MEG) studies on selective auditory attention using fast stimulus rates and finding no significant differences between the auditory-cortex generators of the magnetic counterparts of the exogenous N1 (the N1m) and the attention effect at

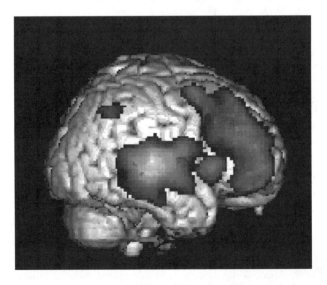

FIGURE 14.3. PET data indicating activations (shaded area) in the prefrontal, parietal, and auditory cortices of the right hemisphere when subjects selectively attended to tones delivered to the left ear and ignored right-ear tones and visual stimuli, relative to a condition in which attention was directed away from the left- and right-ear tones to visual stimuli. Similar results were obtained in the condition in which subjects selectively attended to the right-ear tones. Prefrontal and auditory-cortex activations were also observed in the right hemisphere for both selective-listening conditions. Unpublished data from Alho et al. (1999).

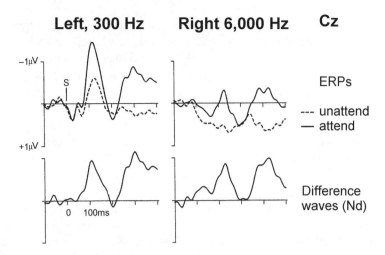

FIGURE 14.4. Top row: ERPs to the 300-Hz left-ear tones and 6,000-Hz right-ear tones delivered at a very fast rate when they were attended and when they were ignored during attention to the other tones. Note the negative N1 deflection peaking at 120 msec from the onset of the 300-Hz, left-ear tones but not elicited (or elicited with a minimal amplitude) by the 6,000-Hz right-ear tones. Bottom row: The corresponding attended–unattended ERP difference waves indicating that an early negative difference (Nd) peaking at about 120 msec and a later Nd peaking around 300 ms were elicited with similar amplitudes by the 300-Hz left-ear and 6,000-Hz right-ear tones. These data support the proposal that the Nds are caused by endogenous PNs rather than by an attentional modulation of the exogenous ERP components such as the N1 components. From Näätänen, Teder, Alho, and Lavikainen (1992). Copyright 1992 by Lippincott, Williams & Wilkins. Reprinted by permission.

the N1m latency (Kaufman & Williamson, 1987; Rif, Hari, Hämäläinen, & Sams, 1991; Woldorff et al., 1993). However, it should be noted that several studies found different scalp distributions for the exogenous N1 and the coinciding attention effect observed in fast-rate conditions (Alho, Teder, et al., 1994; Näätänen et al., 1992; Woods & Clayworth, 1987). For example, the exogenous N1 is typically larger over the hemisphere contralateral to the stimulated ear than over the ipsilateral hemisphere, whereas the early Nd shows less or no such contralaterality. Moreover, Näätänen and colleagues (1992) observed a much larger N1 for unattended 300-Hz left-ear tones than for unattended 6,000-Hz right-ear tones, whereas the Nd effects at the N1 latency had similar amplitudes for both tones (Figure 14.4). This finding, too, suggests that the early attention effect is caused by a PN component separable from the exogenous N1, as do also the aforementioned results of Woods and colleagues (1993) that temporoparietal lesions lead to attenuated N1 responses but do not affect the attention effect at the N1 latency. All these results suggest that the attention effect at the N1 latency is caused, at least partly, by an endogenous PN overlapping with the exogenous N1. However, these findings cannot rule out the possibility that attention also enhances some exogenous component of the N1. Moreover, it must be noted that the attentional-trace theory cannot explain the more positive ERPs to attended than unattended sounds at 20–50 msec from sound onset (Woldorff & Hillyard, 1991; Woldorff et al., 1993), suggesting enhanced processing of attended sounds at a very early processing stage. Therefore, it must be concluded that there might be two attentional selection mechanisms, (1) a gain mechanism underlying these early positive-polarity attention effects and possibly some enhancement of the exogenous N1, and (2) the one generating the PN (see also Hansen & Hillyard, 1980). However, as noted by Alho (1992), the gain mechanism may be operational only in conditions with very fast stimulus rates and large differences between the attended and unattended stimuli, whereas the selection based on the attentional trace generating the PN occurs even for sounds delivered at slower rates and for small pitch and location differences between the attended and unattended sounds (Alho et al., 1986; Alho, Donauer, et al., 1987; Alho, Töttölä, et al., 1987), encountered in everyday listening situations.

Furthermore, the attentional-trace theory has also been challenged by findings from multidimensional selective-listening situations first studied with ERPs by Hansen and Hillyard (1983). For example, when subjects selectively attend to sounds with a certain combination of pitch and location, the to-be-ignored sounds sharing the location of the attended sounds but clearly differing from them in pitch, or vice versa, may elicit long-duration (small-amplitude) PNs (Alho et al., 1989; Woods, Alho, & Algazi, 1994; Woods & Alain, 2001). These PNs appear to be associated with the exhaustive processing of the unattended sounds on the dimension on which they match with the attentional trace. As Woods and Alain (2001) pointed out, this finding is difficult to explain with the attentional-trace theory because one might assume that once an unattended stimulus is found not to match with the attentional trace on one dimension (e.g., location) the processing (i.e., comparison with the attentional trace) of its other features (e.g., pitch) should also terminate. Thus it appears that the attentional selection of sounds on the basis of their location and that on the basis of their pitch are carried out by separate mechanisms, or in terms of the attentional-trace theory, by separate attentional traces. This proposal is further supported by different scalp distributions (indicating different generators) observed for such location-specific and pitch-specific PNs (Woods et al., 1994; Woods & Alain, 2001).

REFERENCES

Alain, C., Woods, D. L., & Knight, R. T. (1998). A distributed cortical network for auditory sensory memory in humans. *Brain Research, 812,* 23–37.

Alcaini, M., Giard, M. H., & Perrin, F. (1995). Selective auditory attention modulates effects in tonotopically organized cortical areas: A topographic ERP study. *Human Brain Mapping, 2,* 159–169.

Alho, K. (1992). Selective attention in auditory processing as reflected by event-related brain potentials. *Psychophysiology, 29,* 247–263.

Alho, K., Donauer, N., Paavilainen, P., Reinikainen, K., Sams, M., & Näätänen, R. (1987). Stimulus selection during auditory spatial attention as expressed by event-related potentials. *Biological Psychology, 24,* 153–162.

Alho, K., Lavikainen, J., Reinikainen, K., Sams, M., & Näätänen, R. (1990). Event-related brain potentials in selective listening to frequent and rare stimuli. *Psychophysiology, 27,* 73–86.

Alho, K., Medvedev, S. V., Pakhomov, S. V., Roudas, M. S., Zeffiro, T., Tervaniemi, M., et al. (1999). Selective tuning of the left and right auditory cortices during spatially directed attention. *Cognitive Brain Research, 7,* 335–342.

Alho, K., Paavilainen, P., Reinikainen, K., & Näätänen, R. (1986). Small pitch separation and the selective-attention effect on the ERP. *Psychophysiology, 23,* 189–197.

Alho, K., Sams, M., Paavilainen, P., Reinikainen, K., & Näätänen, R. (1989). Event-related brain potentials reflecting processing of relevant and irrelevant stimuli during selective listening. *Psychophysiology, 26,* 514–528.

Alho, K., Teder, W., Lavikainen, J., & Näätänen, R. (1994). Strongly focused attention and auditory event-related potentials. *Biological Psychology, 38,* 73–90.

Alho, K., Töttölä, K., Reinikainen, K., Sams, M., & Näätänen, R. (1987). Brain mechanisms of selective listening reflected by event-related potentials. *Electroencephalography and Clinical Neurophysiology, 68,* 458–470.

Alho, K., Winkler, I., Escera, C., Huotilainen, M., Virtanen, J., Jääskeläinen, I. P., et al. (1998). Processing of novel sounds and frequency changes in the human auditory cortex: Magnetoencephalographic recordings. *Psychophysiology, 35,* 211–224.

Alho, K., Woods, D.L., & Algazi, A. (1994). Processing of auditory stimuli during auditory and visual attention as revealed by event-related potentials. *Psychophysiology, 31,* 469–479.

Alho, K., Woods, D. L., Algazi, A., Knight, R. T., & Näätänen, R. (1994). Lesions of frontal cortex diminish the auditory mismatch negativity. *Electroencephalography and Clinical Neurophysiology, 91,* 353–362.

Alho, K., Woods, D. L., Algazi, A., & Näätänen, R. (1992). Intermodal selective attention II: Effects of attentional load on processing auditory and visual stimuli in central space. *Electroencephalography and Clinical Neurophysiology, 82,* 356–368.

Broadbent, D. E. (1958). *Perception and communication.* New York: Pergamon Press.

Broadbent, D. E. (1970). Stimulus set and response set: Two kinds of selective attention. In D. I. Mostofsky (Ed.), *Attention: Contemporary theory and analysis* (pp. 51–60). New York: Appleton-Century-Crofts.

Celsis, P., Boulanouar, K., Doyon, B., Ranjeva, J. P., Berry, I., Nespoulous, J. L., et al. (1999). Differential fMRI responses in the left posterior superior temporal gyrus and left supramarginal gyrus to habituation and change detection in syllables and tones. *NeuroImage, 9,* 135–144.

Dittmann-Balcar, A., Jüptner, M., Jentzen, W., & Schall, U. (2001). Dorsolateral prefrontal cortex activation during automatic auditory duration-mismatch processing in humans: A positron emission tomography study. *Neuroscience Letters, 308,* 119–122.

Donchin, E., & Coles, M. G. H. (1998). Is the P300 component a manifestation of context updating? *The Behavioral and Brain Sciences, 11,* 357–374.

Escera, C., Alho, K., Winkler, I., & Näätänen R. (1998). Neural mechanisms of involuntary attention switching to novelty and change in the acoustic environment. *Journal of Cognitive Neuroscience, 10,* 590–604.

Fischer, C., Morlet, D., Bouchet, P., Luaute, J., Jourdan, C., & Salord, F. (1999). Mismatch negativity and late auditory evoked potentials in comatose patients. *Clinical Neurophysiology, 110,* 1601–1610.

Fitzgerald, P. G., & Picton, T. W. (1983). Event-related potentials recorded during the discrimination of improbable stimuli. *Biological Psychology, 17,* 241–276.

Giard, M.-H., Perrin, F., Pernier, J., & Peronnet, F. (1988). Several attention-related waveforms in auditory areas: a topographic study. *Electroencephalography and Clinical Neurophysiology, 69,* 371–384.

Giard, M.-H., Perrin, F., Pernier, J., & Bouchet, P. (1990). Brain generators implicated in processing of auditory stimulus deviance: A topographic event-related potential study. *Psychophysiology, 27,* 627–640.

Giard, M.-H., Lavikainen, J., Reinikainen, K., Bertrand, O., Pernier, J., & Näätänen, R. (1995). Separate representation of stimulus frequency, intensity, and duration in auditory sensory memory: An event-related potential and dipole-model analysis. *Journal of Cognitive Neuroscience, 7,* 133–143.

Halgren, E., Baudena, P., Clarke, J. M., Heit, G., Liegois, C., Chauvel, P., et al. (1995). Intracerebral potentials to rare target and distractor auditory and visual stimuli. I. Superior temporal plane and parietal lobe. *Electroencephalography and Clinical Neurophysiology, 94,* 191–220.

Hansen, J. C., & Hillyard, S. A. (1980). Endogenous brain potentials associated with selective auditory attention. *Electroencephalography and Clinical Neurophysiology, 49,* 277–290.

Hansen, J. C., & Hillyard, S. A. (1983). Selective attention to multidimensional auditory stimuli. *Journal of Experimental Psychology: Human Perception and Performance, 9,* 1–19.

Hansen, J. C., & Hillyard, S. A. (1988). Temporal dynamics of human auditory selective attention. *Psychophysiology, 25,* 316–329.

Hari, R., Hämäläinen, M., Kaukoranta, E., Mäkelä, J., Joutsiniemi, S.-L., & Tiihonen, J. (1989). Selective listening modifies activity of the human auditory cortex. *Experimental Brain Research, 74,* 463–470.

Hillyard, S. A., Hink, R. F., Schwent, V. L., & Picton, T. W. (1973). Electrical signs of selective attention in the human brain. *Science*, 182, 177–180.

Jemel, B., Achenbach, C., Müller, B. W., Röpke, B., & Oades, R. D. (2002). Mismatch negativity results from bilateral asymmetric dipole sources in the frontal and temporal lobes. *Brain Topography*, 15, 13–27.

Kane, N. M., Curry, S. H., Butler, S. R., & Cummins, B. H. (1993). Electrophysiological indicator of awakening from coma. *Lancet*, 341, 688.

Kane, N. M., Curry, S. H., Rowlands, C. A., Manara, A. R., Lewis, T., Moss, T., et al. (1996). Event-related potentials—Neurophysiological tools for predicting emergence and early outcome from traumatic coma. *Intensive Care Medicine*, 22, 39–46.

Kaufman, L., & Williamson, S. J. (1987). Recent developments in neuromagnetism. In C. Barber & T. Blum (Eds.), *Evoked potentials* (Vol. 3, pp. 100–113). Boston: Butterworths.

Knight, R. T., Hillyard, S. A., Woods, D. L., & Neville, H. J (1981). The effects of frontal cortex lesions on event-related potentials during auditory selective attention. *Electroencephalography and Clinical Neurophysiology*, 52, 571–582.

Kraus, N., McGee, T. J., Carrell, T. D., Zecker, S. G., Nicol, T. G., & Koch, D. B. (1996). Auditory neurophysiologic responses and discrimination deficits in children with learning problems. *Science*, 273, 971–973.

Kropotov, J. D., Alho, K., Näätänen, R., Ponomarev, V. A., Kropotova, O. V., Anichkov, A. D., et al. (2000). Human auditory-cortex mechanisms of preattentive sound discrimination. *Neuroscience Letters*, 280, 87–90.

Kropotov, J. D., Näätänen, R., Sevostianov, A. V., Alho, K., Reinikainen, K., & Kropotova, O. V. (1995). Mismatch negativity to auditory stimulus change recorded directly from the human temporal cortex. *Psychophysiology*, 32, 418–422.

Levänen, S., Ahonen, A., Hari, R., McEvoy, L., & Sams, M. (1996). Deviant auditory stimuli activate human left and right auditory cortex differently. *Cerebral Cortex*, 6, 288–296.

Liasis, A., Towell, A., & Boyd, S. (1999). Intracranial auditory detection and discrimination potentials as substrates of echoic memory in children. *Cognitive Brain Research*, 7, 503–506.

Liasis, A., Towell, A., & Boyd, S. (2000). Intracranial evidence for differential encoding of frequency and duration discrimination responses. *Ear and Hearing*, 21, 252–256.

Lyytinen, H., Blomberg, A. P., & Näätänen R. (1992). Event-related potentials and autonomic responses to a change in unattended auditory stimuli. *Psychophysiology*, 29, 523–534.

Michie, P. T., Solowij, N., Crawford, J. M., & Glue L. C. (1993). The effects of between-source discriminability on attended and unattended auditory ERPs. *Psychophysiology*, 30, 205–220.

Morlet, D., Bouchet, P., & Fischer, C. (2000). Mismatch negativity and N100 monitoring: Potential clinical value and methodological advances. *Audiology and Neuro-Otology*, 5, 198–206.

Müller, B. W., Jüptner, M., Jentzen, W., & Müller, S. P. (2002). Cortical activation to auditory mismatch elicited by frequency deviant and complex novel sounds: A PET study. *NeuroImage*, 17, 231–239.

Näätänen, R. (1982). Processing negativity: An evoked-potential reflection of selective attention. *Psychological Bulletin*, 92, 605–640.

Näätänen, R. (1986). The neural-specificity theory of visual selective attention evaluated: A commentary on Harter and Aine. *Biological Psychology*, 23, 281–295.

Näätänen, R. (1990). The role of attention in auditory information processing as revealed by event-related potentials and other brain measures of cognitive function. *Behavioral and Brain Sciences*, 13, 201–288.

Näätänen, R. (1991). Mismatch negativity (MMN) outside strong attentional focus: A commentary on Woldorff et al. *Psychophysiology*, 28, 478–484.

Näätänen, R. (1992). *Attention and brain function*. Hillsdale, NJ: Erlbaum.

Näätänen, R. (2001). The perception of speech sounds by the human brain as reflected by the mismatch negativity (MMN) and its magnetic equivalent MMNm. *Psychophysiology*, 38, 1–21.

Näätänen, R., & Gaillard, A. W. K. (1983) The orienting reflex and the N2 deflection of the event-related potential (ERP). In A. W. K. Gaillard & W. Ritter (Eds.), *Tutorials in event related potential research: Endogenous components* (pp. 119–141). Amsterdam: North Holland.

Näätänen, R., Gaillard, A. W. K., & Mäntysalo, S. (1978). Early selective-attention effect on evoked potential reinterpreted. *Acta Psychologica*, 42, 313–329.

Näätänen, R., & Michie, P. T. (1979). Early selective attention effects on the evoked potential. A critical review and reinterpretation. *Biological Psychology*, 8, 81–136.

Näätänen, R., Paavilainen, P., Tiitinen, H., Jiang, D., & Alho, K. (1993). Attention and mismatch negativity. *Psychophysiology*, 30, 436–450.

Näätänen, R., & Picton, T. W. (1987). The N1 wave of the human electric and magnetic response to sound: A review and an analysis of component structure. *Psychophysiology*, 24, 375–425.

Näätänen, R., Simpson, M., & Loveless, N. E. (1982). Stimulus deviance and evoked potentials. *Biological Psychology*, 14, 53–98.

Näätänen, R., Teder, W., Alho, K., & Lavikainen, J. (1992). Auditory attention and selective input modulation: A topographical ERP study.: *NeuroReport*, 3, 493–496.

Novak, G., Ritter, W., Vaughan, H. G., Jr., & Wiznitzer, M. L. (1990). Differentiation of negative event-related potentials in an auditory discrimination task. *Electroencephalography and Clinical Neurophysiology*, 75, 255–275.

O'Leary, D. D., Andreasen, N. C., Hurtig, R. R., Hichwa, R. D., Watkins, L., Ponto, L. L. B., et al. (1996). A positron emission tomography study of binaurally and dichotically presented stimuli: Effects of level of language and directed attention. *Brain and Language*, 53, 20–39.

Opitz, B., Rinne, T., Mecklinger, A., von Cramon, D. Y., & Schröger, E. (2002). Differential contribution of frontal and temporal cortices to auditory change detection: fMRI and ERP results. *NeuroImage*, 15, 167–174.

Paavilainen, P., Tiitinen, H., Alho, K., & Näätänen, R. (1993). Mismatch negativity to slight pitch changes outside strong attentional focus. *Biological Psychology*, 37, 23–41.

Picton, T. W. (1992). The P300 wave of the human event-related potential. *Journal of Clinical Neurophysiology*, 9, 456–479.

Rif, J., Hari, R., Hämäläinen, M. S., & Sams, M. (1991). Auditory attention affects two different areas in the human supratemporal cortex. *Electroencephalography and Clinical Neurophysiology*, 79, 464–472.

Rinne, T., Alho, K., Ilmoniemi, R. J., Virtanen, J., & Näätänen, R. (2000). Separate time behaviors of the temporal and frontal mismatch negativity sources. *NeuroImage*, 12, 14–19.

Sams, M., Paavilainen, P., Alho, K., & Näätänen, R. (1985). Auditory frequency discrimination and event-related potentials. *Electroencephalography and Clinical Neurophysiology*, 62, 437–448.

Schall, U., Johnston, P., Todd, J., Ward, P. B., & Michie, P. T. (2003). Functional neuroanatomy of auditory mismatch processing: An event-related fMRI study of duration-deviant oddballs. *NeuroImage*, 20, 729–736.

Scherg, M., Vajsar, J., & Picton, T. W. (1989). A source analysis of the late human auditory evoked potentials. *Journal of Cognitive Neuroscience*, 1, 336–355.

Schröger, E. (1996). A neural mechanism for involuntary attention shifts to changes in auditory stimulation. *Journal of Cognitive Neuroscience*, 8, 527–539.

Squires, N. K., Squires, K. C., & Hillyard, S. A. (1975). Two varieties of long-latency positive waves evoked by unpredictable auditory stimuli in man. *Electroencephalography and Clinical Neurophysiology*, 38, 387–401.

Teder, W., Alho, K., Reinikainen, K., & Näätänen, R. (1993). Interstimulus interval and the selective attention effect on auditory ERPs: "N1 enhancement" vs. processing negativity. *Psychophysiology*, 30, 71–81.

Tiitinen, H., May, P., Reinikainen, K., & Näätänen, R. (1994). Attentive novelty detection in humans is governed by pre-attentive sensory memory. *Nature*, 372, 90–92.

Treisman, A. M., Squire, R., & Green, J. (1974). Semantic processing in dichotic listening? A replication. *Memory and Cognition*, 2, 641–646.

Trejo, L. J., Ryan-Jones, D. L., & Kramer, A. F. (1995). Attentional modulation of the mismatch negativity elicited by frequency differences between binaurally presented tone bursts. *Psychophysiology*, 32, 319–328.

Tzourio, N., El Massioui, F., Crivello, F., Joliot, M., Renault, B., & Mazoyer, B. (1997). Functional anatomy of auditory attention studied with PET. *NeuroImage, 5,* 63–77.

Woldorff, M. G., Gallen, C. G., Hampson, S. A., Hillyard, S. A., Pantev, C., Sobel, D., et al. (1993). Modulation of early sensory processing in human auditory cortex during auditory selective attention. *Proceedings of the National Academy of Sciences USA, 90,* 8722–8726.

Woldorff, M. G., Hackley, S. A., & Hillyard, S. A. (1991). The effects of channel-selective attention on the mismatch negativity wave elicited by deviant tones. *Psychophysiology, 28,* 30–42.

Woldorff, M. G., & Hillyard, S. A. (1991). Modulation of early auditory processing during selective listening to rapidly presented tones. *Electroencehalography and Clinical Neurophysiology, 79,* 170–191.

Woldorff, M. G., Hillyard, S. A., Gallen, C. C., Hampson, S. R., & Bloom, F. E. (1998). Magnetoencephalographic recordings demonstrate attentional modulation of mismatch-related neural activity in human auditory cortex. *Psychophysiology, 35,* 283–292.

Woods, D. L., & Alain, C. (2001). Conjoining three auditory features: An event-related brain potential study. *Journal of Cognitive Neuroscience, 13,* 492–509.

Woods, D. L., Alho, K., & Algazi, A. (1994). Stages of auditory feature conjunction: An event-related brain potential study. *Journal of Experimental Psychology: Human Perception and Performance, 20,* 81–94.

Woods, D. L., & Clayworth, C. C. (1987). Scalp topographies dissociate N1 and Nd components during auditory selective attention. In R. Johnson Jr., J. W. Rohrbaugh, & R. Parasuraman (Eds.), *Current trends in event-related brain potential research* (pp. 155–160). Amsterdam: Elsevier.

Woods, D. L., Knight, R. T., & Scabini, D. (1993). Anatomical substrates of auditory selective attention: Behavioral and electrophysiological effects of posterior association cortex lesions. *Cognitive Brain Research, 1,* 227–240.

Zatorre, R. J., Mondor, T. A., & Evans, A. C. (1999). Auditory attention to space and frequency activates similar cerebral systems. *NeuroImage, 10,* 544–554.

15

Multimodal Studies of Cingulate Cortex

George Bush

The principles that guide my laboratory's work are simple. To truly understand neuropsychiatric diseases, we must first develop a solid knowledge base about normal brain physiology and mechanisms—only then can we adequately develop and test neurobiological models for defined illness. In turn, elucidating the neural bases for neuropsychiatric disorders can inform our understanding of normal brain function in ways that studying solely healthy volunteers cannot.

More specifically, my research seeks to achieve two main goals: (1) to determine how cingulate cortex subdivisions contribute to normal cognitive, motor, and emotional processes, and (2) to determine if, and how, cingulate dysfunction plays a role in the pathophysiology of neuropsychiatric disorders—especially attention-deficit/hyperactivity disorder (ADHD). Toward these ends, we employ a combination of techniques—including functional magnetic resonance imaging (fMRI) and intracranial recordings (ICRs), in conjunction with novel cognitive, motor, and emotional activation paradigms—in our efforts to understand how the different cingulate subdivisions work and how their malfunction may lead to symptoms. In the following sections, I (1) provide background information on cingulate subdivisions, (2) outline our current thinking on how dorsal anterior cingulate cortex (the "cognitive division") contributes to attention, (3) detail why we focus on integrating fMRI in humans and single-unit electrophysiology studies in monkeys, (4) introduce our recent efforts to combine fMRI and intracranial recordings in humans, and (5) briefly summarize our approach to studying ADHD.

CINGULATE SUBDIVISIONS

Determining the nature of ACC function, with special attention to the different roles of its subterritories, is particularly vital to understanding the neurobiology of many neuropsychiatric disorders. Straddling the fence between cognition and emotion, ACC has been suggested to be involved in the pathophysiology of ADHD (Bush et al., 1999), posttraumatic stress disorder (Shin et al., 2001), depression (Davidson et al., 2002; Drevets, 2001; Mayberg et al., 1999), obsessive–compulsive disorder (Jenike et al., 1991), schizophrenia, bipolar disorder, akinetic mutism, panic disorder, Tourette's syndrome (Benes, 1993), and Alzheimer's disease (Vogt, Vogt, Nimchinsky, & Hof, 1997). It is not surprising that ACC has been associated with such a wide variety of disorders, as it encompasses a large territory and its subregions are vital to many cognitive, motor, and emotional processes (Vogt, Finch, & Olson, 1992). Many studies have reported ACC activation as if it were a single homogeneous region, but to truly understand how it may be involved in neuropsychiatric disorders, the functions of different ACC subregions in normal humans must be determined.

ACC encompasses at least two major subdivisions that subserve distinct functions, including (1) dorsal ACC (dACC; areas 32' and/or 24c'), which has been shown to be involved in cognition (Bush, Luu, & Posner, 2000; Devinsky, Morrell, & Vogt, 1995; Vogt et al., 1992) and reward-based decision making (Bush et al., 2002), and (2) perigenual ACC (pACC; rostral/subgenual areas 24, 25, 32, and 33), which is involved in processing affective/emotional information, including assigning emotional valence to internal and external stimuli, conditioned emotional learning, regulation of autonomic and endocrine functions, vocalizations expressing internal states, assessing motivation, and maternal–infant interactions (Devinsky et al., 1995; Vogt et al., 1992; Vogt, Berger, & Derbyshire, 2003; Vogt, Derbyshire, & Jones, 1996; Whalen et al., 1998). These subterritories are distinguishable based on cytoarchitectural (Vogt, 1993) and connectivity patterns (Vogt & Pandya, 1987) as well as convergent evidence from studies using a variety of experimental techniques, including lesion studies, electrophysiology, and functional neuroimaging (see Bushet al., 2000). Cognitive tasks tend to activate dACC. Conversely, pACC has been activated by affectively related tasks, including studies of obsessive–compulsive disorder symptom provocation, simple phobia, posttraumatic stress disorder, and depression (see Bush et al., 2000; Whalen et al., 1998; and Figure 15.1). (For more complete reviews of other cingulate subdivisions, including the caudal cingulate motor area and posterior cingulate cortex, see Picard and Strick [2001]; Vogt [1993]; Vogt et al. [2003].)

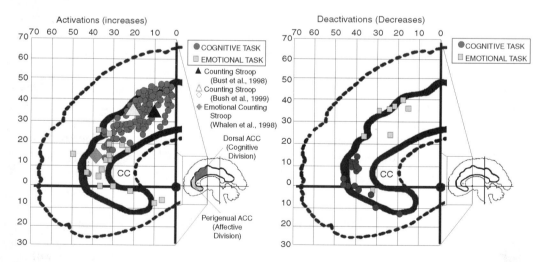

FIGURE 15.1. Meta-analysis of activations and deactivations in response to cognitive and emotional tasks. Cognitive tasks (e.g., Stroop and Stroop-like tasks, divided-attention tasks, and response-selection tasks—coded with dark circles) tend to activate dACC and deactivate pACC. Conversely, emotion tasks (light squares) tend to activate pACC and deactivate dACC. From Bush, Luu, and Posner (2000). Copyright 2000 by Elsevier. Adapted by permission.

Notably, to assess the dichotomy of dACC/pACC subdivisions more directly, two Stroop-like interference tasks with differing causes of interference (i.e., one cognitive [Bush et al., 1998] and one affective [Whalen et al., 1998]) were validated in fMRI studies run with the *same* subjects during the *same* scanning session. In an interesting double dissociation (depicted in Figure 15.1, left), the cognitively interfering Counting Stroop produced dACC activation but not pACC activation, whereas the affectively interfering Emotional Counting Stroop produced pACC activation but not dACC activation.

Figure 15.1 (right) also raises the basis of our laboratory's interest in task-induced deactivations (TIDs). Namely, as we, and others, have noted (Binder et al., 1999; Bush et al., 2000; Drevets & Raichle, 1998; Mayberg et al., 1999; Raichle et al., 2001), cognitive tasks not only tend to activate dACC, but "deactivate" the affective subdivision (pACC). Conversely, while emotional tasks tend to activate pACC, they deactivate the cognitive subdivision (dACC). The nature of these deactivations is a matter of intense debate, and we hope that our combined fMRI and intracranial recordings methodology (described later) will soon be able to contribute to this discussion.

DORSAL ANTERIOR CINGULATE CORTEX: THE "COGNITIVE DIVISION"?

Knowing that different divisions of anterior cingulate are important for processing different types of information is intrinsically interesting, and having such information can assist one in developing testable models of psychiatric disorder. However, even a meta-analysis of all tasks activating ACC still would not provide an answer to how the subterritories actually function mechanistically—a point that is crucial to elucidating their potential role in disease. Specifically, developing models for how the different ACC subdivisions support the various cognitive, motor, and emotional functions is vital to determining how they might contribute to the pathophysiology of different neuropsychiatric disorders.

Here we will take dACC as an example. dACC has long been associated with the motor system, based on nonhuman primate studies of cingulate projections/connections (Bates & Goldman-Rakic, 1993; Biber, Kneisley, & LaVail, 1978; Dum & Strick, 1991, 1993; Morecraft & Van Hoesen, 1992; Pandya, Van Hoesen, & Mesulam, 1981; Vogt, Pandya, & Rosene, 1987), electrical stimulation (Luppino, Matelli, Camarda, Gallese, & Rizzolatti, 1991), and electrophysiology studies (Shima et al., 1991). As seen in Figure 15.1, dACC has also been activated during performance of cognitive-interference tasks, divided-attention tasks, and response-selection/inhibition tasks in normal subjects—supporting the conclusion that dACC plays a critical role in attention (Colby, 1991; Goldman-Rakic, 1987, 1988; Posner & Dehaene, 1994; Posner & Driver, 1992; Posner & Petersen, 1990; Raichle et al., 1994). Notably, in a study of divided and selective attention (Corbetta, Miezen, Dobmeyer, Shulman, & Petersen, 1991), dACC was active in the divided-attention condition but *not* active in any of the selective attention conditions. Furthermore, dACC was not activated in positron emission tomography (PET) studies of simple sustained-attention tasks (Pardo, Fox, & Raichle, 1991) or during the cognitively demanding reading and semantic processing tasks examined by Petersen, Fox, Snyder, and Raichle (1990). These facts combine to show that dACC is not merely recruited any time focused/selective attention is needed but, rather, that dACC plays specific roles in difficult cognitive and attentional tasks. But how . . . ?

INTEGRATING HUMAN AND MONKEY STUDIES:
THE HETEROGENEITY "MODEL"

Based primarily on work in humans, different functions have been ascribed to dACC, including attention-for-action/target selection, motivational valence assignment, motor response selection, error detection/performance monitoring, competition monitoring, anticipation, working memory, novelty detection, and reward assessment—but no single unifying model has been able to explain the diverse results from neuroimaging and electrophysiological studies (Bush et al., 2000, 2002). Here we turned to the monkey electrophysiologists for guidance.

Single-unit recording studies of the putative monkey homologue of dACC (rostral cingulate motor area) have repeatedly shown it is populated by a heterogeneous group of cells. Niki and Watanabe (1979) identified timing (stimulus anticipation) units and others sensitive to targets, motor responses, rewards, or errors. Nishijo and colleagues (1997) found ACC cells that were anticipatory, stimulus-related, response-related, and reward-related—adding that subsets responded to novel objects whereas others could discriminate rewarding, aversive, and neutral objects. Procyk, Tanaka, and Joseph (2000) recorded from dACC cells that reacted to targets, rewards, or error cues and others involved in routine and nonroutine motor-sequencing behaviors in macaques.

Though it has been established in monkeys that dACC consists of many different cell types, the problem of how to link this literature to humans remains. Fortunately, a single-unit recording study provided a key piece of information. Shima and Tanji (1998) recorded from dACC (CMAr) cells in *Macaca fuscata* during a reward-based decision-making task. As in the other studies, the authors noted that different populations of cells responded to target detection, motor response, constant rewards, and reduced rewards. Critically, Shima and Tanji also reported that *the proportions of each cell type were not equal in dACC*—five times as many cells responded specifically to movement selection based on reduced reward (37%) as opposed to constant reward (7%). We believed that such a large difference in the proportions of cells could be exploited in fMRI studies (i.e., that this would produce measurable, differential fMRI activation).

Based on these monkey single-unit recordings, we hypothesized that human dACC consists of mixed cells that variously anticipate and detect targets, indicate novelty, influence motor responses, encode reward values, and signal errors. As an initial test of this conceptualization, we conducted an fMRI study using a reward-based decision-making task (modeled after Shima and Tanji's task) to isolate responses from a subpopulation of dACC cells sensitive to reward reduction. On each trial of this task, subjects were asked to press one of two buttons depending on the feedback they received on the previous trial. If, as on 80% of trials, they had received the full "constant reward" (15¢), they were to press the same button as on the previous trial. If instead, they had received either a "reduced reward" (9¢), or had seen a "SWITCH" command, they were trained to press the other button.

As predicted, seven of eight subjects showed significant ($p < 10^{-4}$) dACC activation when contrasting reduced reward (REDrew) trials to fixation (FIX). Confirmatory group analyses then corroborated the predicted ordinal relationships of fMRI activation expected during each trial type (REDrew > SWITCH > constant reward (CONrew) $\geq$ FIX (see Figure 15.2). The data supported a role for dACC in reward-based decision making, and by linking the human and monkey literatures, provided initial support for the existence of heterogeneity within dACC.

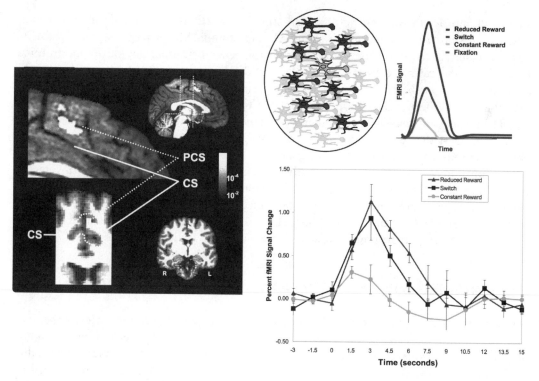

FIGURE 15.2. Dorsal anterior cingulate cortex fMRI responses during reward-based decision making. We used the "local heterogeneity concept" to predict dACC responses to a reward-based decision-making task (Bush et al., 2002). Assuming that each voxel within human dACC is comprised of different cell types in roughly the same proportions seen in the monkey (per Shima & Tanji, 1998—schematized in the upper-right corner) allowed us to successfully predict the fMRI responses in dACC, pACC, and cCMA. Here, the observed dACC responses (lower right) show the predicted responses.

The "local heterogeneity concept" is by no means a new one (in fact, electrophysiologists see it as patently obvious that not all cells in a region will respond the same way). However, the point that may be overlooked (and is essential for understanding fMRI results) is that the patterns of local heterogeneity (i.e., the proportions and interconnections of cell types) vary widely among different brain regions)—and a more refined understanding of these interregional differences can be used to better predict the fMRI responses of the different brain regions. For example, not only could the relative proportions of cell types in monkey dACC be used to predict its response in our human fMRI study, but data from Shima and Tanji's (1998) study showing that the caudal cingulate motor area (CMA) did not contain significant numbers of REDrew cells allowed us to successfully predict that we would *not* observe caudal CMA activation (Bush et al., 2002).

Confirmation of the existence of such a local intracortical network of heterogeneous cell types within dACC would be important, as it would allow us to advance beyond current hypotheses of the pathophysiology of psychiatric disorders by providing a framework for how the brain normally processes cognitive information. The mechanism of how such a local dACC network might operate and contribute to cognition is straightforward and consistent with observed behavior. Signaling from anticipatory/timing cells would have predictive value and improve the processing of salient stimuli. Novelty detection and target detection cells would similarly enhance attention to relevant stimuli. Motor response cells in dACC have been shown to contribute to complex motor behaviors, especially during nonroutine tasks. Of course, reward cells and error cells would provide invaluable feedback that would guide future actions based on experience. Thus, support exists for such a dynamic interaction among heterogeneous cell types within dACC.

The reward angle may be particularly germane to psychiatric illnesses. Taken together, the data suggest that dACC may play a role in reward circuitry—particularly in reward-based decision making, learning, and especially the performance novel (nonautomatic) tasks—functions known to be substantially influenced by dopamine. Moreover, this line of inquiry may have clinical relevance, given the implication of dopaminergic pathways in the pathophysiology of attention-deficit disorder (Biederman & Spencer, 1999) and observed dysfunction of dACC in this illness (Bush et al., 1999). Similar arguments could be made and tested with respect to schizophrenia, depression, and anxiety disorders.

COMBINED fMRI AND INTRACRANIAL RECORDINGS IN HUMANS

Although the data supporting the "local heterogeneity conceptualization" are compelling, they do call for one to rely on the assumption of a close homology between monkey and human brains—a reasonable but unproven assumption. Thus, our recent efforts to explore this issue further involve the use of combined fMRI and intracranial recordings performed in some fairly unique populations of awake behaving humans: patients having cingulotomies for intractable obsessive–compulsive disorder or depression and patients having depth electrode assessments prior to neurosurgical treatment of intractable seizures. To date, intra-operative recordings have been performed in two patients using the reward-based decision-making task that was described previously and used in our recent fMRI study of dACC (Bush et al., 2002). Figure 15.3 shows some preliminary data identifying a cell in dACC that responds preferentially to reward reduction trials—showing the feasibility of this approach. By combining and correlating fMRI and intracranial recordings, we hope to shed light on a number of unresolved issues of the mechanisms of cingulate subdivisions as well as the nature of the neuron–fMRI relationship. Specifically, we hope to determine whether the fMRI activation in dACC confirms the predictions of the local heterogeneity conceptualization and to quantitatively compare the proportions of cell types within human dACC to those observed in monkeys. Also, as indicated in Figure 15.3, it should be possible, within single subjects, to directly relate cognition-induced fMRI deactivations of pACC to decreases in pACC neuronal activity.

ANTERIOR CINGULATE CORTEX:
RELEVANCE TO PSYCHIATRIC DISORDERS

While the issues of how cingulate cortex subdivisions contribute to normal cognition, motor control, and emotion are of intrinsic interest to cognitive and emotional neuroscientists, it is important to relate this basic science information to the study of neuropsychiatric disorders. Specifically, we seek to apply this information to (1) understand pathophysiology, (2) explain and improve drug effects, and (3) develop neuroimaging-based clinical tests for neuro-

Dorsal ACC Activation

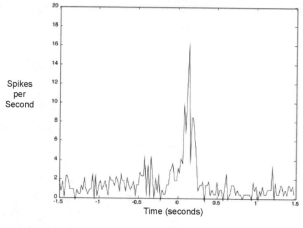

Perigenual ACC Deactivation

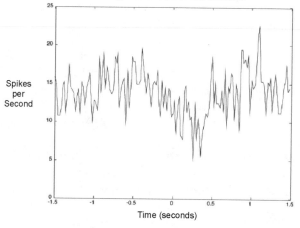

FIGURE 15.3. Intracranial recording of human dACC and pACC neuronal responses. During cingulotomy, single unit recordings were made as subjects performed a reward-based decision-making task (see Bush et al., 2002). Here (above) a single dACC neuron (aligned to reduced reward feedback at *t* = 0) was observed to respond preferentially to reduced reward trials. Other dACC neurons (data not shown) responded to anticipation of cues, cue presentation and motor response—supporting the "local heterogeneity concept." Below, a pACC neuron with a high tonic firing rate was conversely seen to decrease firing during the task—consistent with fMRI and PET findings of cognitive task-induced deactivations of pACC, as described in the text.

psychiatric disorders. As an example of our approach, I briefly overview our recent work on ADHD.

ADHD and dACC

Determining the underlying neurobiology of ADHD is of great importance. It has been estimated to affect 3–5% in school-age children and to persist, to a lesser degree, into adulthood (Biederman & Spencer, 1999). As such, it is a source of great morbidity and makes a huge impact on society with regard to its influence on affected children and their families, its attendant financial cost, disruption of schools, and its potential to lead to criminality and substance abuse.

If one had to guess which of the ACC subdivisions might be abnormal in ADHD, dACC would, of course, be the obvious choice, even without specifically knowing how dACC works mechanistically. dACC dysfunction could play primary roles in producing the inattention and hyperactivity of ADHD by disrupting normal processes of target selection, distracter filtering, response selection, reward/error assessment, and/or motivation evaluation.

We initially tested our hypothesis of dACC dysfunction in ADHD by scanning adults with ADHD and closely matched healthy controls using fMRI and the Counting Stroop (Bush et al., 1999). The Counting Stroop (Bush et al., 1998) is a Stroop variant cognitive interference task that pits two competing information-processing operations against one another. Specifically, reading and counting processes compete, as subjects are instructed to report via button-press the number of words (1–4) on the screen, regardless of word meaning. Neutral trials contain common animals (e.g., *dog* written three times; answer: "three"), while interference trials contain number words that are incongruent with the correct response (e.g., *two* written three times; answer: "three").

As predicted (Figure 15.4), the expected fMRI activation was observed in the dACC of the normal controls, but *no* dACC activation was found in the group with ADHD. Furthermore, normal bilateral activation *was* seen in dorsolateral prefrontal and parietal cortex (Brodmann areas 46/9 and 7, respectively) in the ADHD subjects—indicating that the ADHD subjects were able to produce significant activation in *other* brain regions that have been shown to support performance of the Counting Stroop, and suggesting that ADHD may involve a specific deficit of dACC.

While such group-averaged studies are very important, as they can shed light on pathophysiology, such tasks are not clinically useful as they do not have the capacity to distinguish patients from healthy subjects at the individual level. Seeking to develop a clinically useful task, our recent work has also included the development and use of the Multi-Source Interference Task (MSIT; Bush et al., 2003)—a cognitive-interference task that robustly and

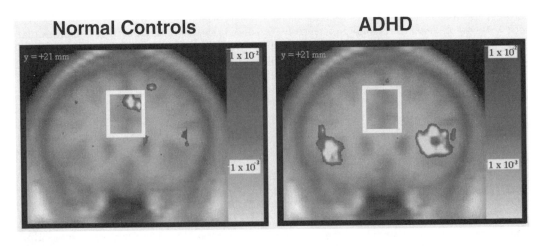

FIGURE 15.4. Dorsal ACC (cognitive division) activates in healthy controls, but not in subjects with ADHD, during the Counting Stroop. From Bush et al. (1999). Copyright 1999 by the Society of Biological Psychiatry. Reprinted with permission.

reliably activates dACC, dorsolateral prefrontal cortex, and parietal cortex in individual subjects during fMRI.

During the MSIT, subjects are given a button-press with buttons representing 1, 2, and 3 from left to right. They are instructed that sets of three numbers (1, 2, 3, and/or 0) will appear together, and that one number will be different from the other two (matching distractor) numbers. Subjects report, via button-press, the identity of the number that is different from the other two numbers. In control trials (e.g., see 100, correct answer = press button 1) the target number matches its position on the button press (e.g., the number 1 would appear in the first [leftmost] position, and the distractors are always zeroes [in the case of the original Bush et al., 2003, paper, distractors were the letter x]). In contrast, during interference trials (e.g., see 232, correct answer = press button 3) the target never matches its position on the button-press and the distractors are other potential target numbers. The difficult interference trials reliably and robustly activate dACC within single subjects.

Ongoing work in our lab, done in close collaboration with ADHD clinical researchers, including Drs. Joseph Biederman, Thomas Spencer, and Larry Seidman, has involved the use of the MSIT to study ADHD pathophysiology as well as to characterize the effects of drugs such as methylphenidate and galantamine. In addition, collaborative efforts are aimed at using the MSIT to study cognition and attention processing in schizophrenia, mood disorders, obsessive–compulsive disorder, posttraumatic stress disorder, Alzheimer's dementia, Tourette's syndrome, sleep disorders, dyslexia, and HIV-related cognitive deficits. In turn, it is hoped that by improving our understanding of these disorders, in particular the specificity of the patterns of brain dysfunction associated with each disorder, we can better characterize the normal mechanisms of attention.

SUMMARY

By no means do we fully comprehend how this marvelous little collection of functional subdivisions collectively known as ACC operates or interacts, but the combined efforts of anatomists, electrophysiologists, neurochemists, clinicians, and neuroimagers are drawing an ever clearer picture of how the various ACC subdivisions work in normal cognitive and emotional processing, as well as how they might fail and thus contribute to psychopathology. We have seen regional specificity of function in normal humans, and observed how this information can help us develop and test refined disorder-specific hypotheses. We have also seen how animal work and human studies can inform one another to reveal new understanding of the mysterious mechanisms underlying normal human cognition and reward processing. The challenges ahead are to continue extending our knowledge on all these fronts and to continually seek to leverage the emerging knowledge in the service of developing clinically meaningful neuroimaging-based diagnostic tests and therapy-monitoring procedures that can be used to help our patients.

ACKNOWLEDGMENTS

I would like to thank Brent Vogt, Mike Posner, Scott Rauch, Mike Jenike, and Bruce Rosen for their invaluable mentoring; Paul Whalen, Lisa Shin, Jennifer Holmes, Joe Biederman, Jean Frazier, Craig Surman, Eve Valera, Tom Spencer, and Larry Seidman for help with cingulate and ADHD studies; and

Ziv Williams, Emad Eskandar, and Rees Cosgrove for assistance with cingulotomy studies. In addition, I thank the National Institute of Mental Health, the National Science Foundation, the National Alliance for Research on Schizophrenia and Depression, and the MIND Institute for financial support.

REFERENCES

Bates, J. F., & Goldman-Rakic, P. S. (1993). Prefrontal connections of medial motor areas in the rhesus monkey. *Journal of Comparative Neurology, 336*, 211–228.

Benes, F. M. (1993). Relationship of cingulate cortex to schizophrenia and other psychiatric disorders. In B. A. Vogt & M. Gabriel (Eds.), *Neurobiology of cingulate cortex and limbic thalamus: A comprehensive handbook* (pp. 581–605). Boston: Birkhäuser.

Biber, M. P., Kneisley, L. W., & LaVail, J. H. (1978). Cortical neurons projecting to the cervical and lumbar enlargements of the spinal cord in young and adult rhesus monkeys. *Experimental Neurology, 59*, 492–508.

Biederman, J., & Spencer, T. (1999). Attention-deficit/hyperactivity disorder (ADHD) as a noradrenergic disorder. *Biological Psychiatry, 46*, 1234–1242.

Binder, J. R., Frost, J. A., Hammeke, T. A., Bellgowan, P. S., Rao, S. M., & Cox, R. W. (1999). Conceptual processing during the conscious resting state. A functional MRI study. *Journal of Cognitive Neuroscience, 11*(1), 80–95.

Bush, G., Frazier, J. A., Rauch, S. L., Seidman, L. J., Whalen, P. J., Jenike, M. A., et al. (1999). Anterior cingulate cortex dysfunction in attention-deficit/hyperactivity disorder revealed by fMRI and the Counting Stroop. *Biological Psychiatry, 45*, 1542–1552.

Bush, G., Luu, P., & Posner, M. I. (2000). Cognitive and emotional influences in anterior cingulate cortex. (2000) *Trends in Cognitive Sciences, 4*, 215–222.

Bush, G., Shin, L. M., Holmes, J., Rosen, B. R., & Vogt, B. A. (2003). The Multi-Source Interference Task: Validation study with fMRI in individual subjects. *Molecular Psychiatry, 8*, 60–70.

Bush, G., Vogt, B. A., Holmes, J., Dale, A., Greve, D., Jenike, M. A., et al. (2002). Dorsal anterior cingulate cortex: A role in reward-based decision-making. *Proceedings of the National Academy of Sciences USA, 99*, 523–528.

Bush, G., Whalen, P. J., Rosen, B. R., Jenike, M. A., McInerney, S. C., & Rauch, S. L. (1998). The Counting Stroop: An interference task specialized for functional neuroimaging—validation study with functional MRI. *Human Brain Mapping, 6*, 270–282

Colby, C. L. (1991). The neuroanatomy and neurophysiology of attention. *Journal of Child Neurology, 6*(Suppl.), S88–S116.

Corbetta, M., Miezen, F. M., Dobmeyer, S., Shulman, G. L., & Petersen, S. E. (1991). Selective and divided attention during visual discriminations of shape, color, and speed: Functional anatomy by positron emission tomography. *Journal of Neuroscience, 11*, 2383–2402.

Davidson, R. J., Lewis, D. A., Alloy, L. B., Amaral, D. G., Bush, G., Cohen, J. D., et al. (2002). Neural and behavioral substrates of mood and mood regulation. *Biological Psychiatry, 52*(6), 478–502.

Devinsky, O., Morrell, M. J., & Vogt, B. A. (1995). Contributions of anterior cingulate cortex to behavior. *Brain, 118*, 279–306.

Drevets, W. C. (2001). Neuroimaging and neuropathological studies of depression: Implications for the cognitive-emotional features of mood disorders. *Current Opinion in Neurobiology, 11*(2), 240–249.

Drevets, W. C., & Raichle, M. E. (1998). Reciprocal suppression of regional cerebral blood flow during emotional versus higher cognitive processes: Implications for interactions between emotion and cognition. *Cognition and Emotion, 12*, 353–385.

Dum, R. P., & Strick, P. L. (1991). The origin of corticospinal projections from the premotor areas in the frontal lobe. *Journal of Neuroscience, 11*, 667–689.

Dum, R. P., & Strick, P. L. (1993). Cingulate motor areas. In B. A. Vogt & M. Gabriel (Eds.), *Neurobiology of cingulate cortex and limbic thalamus: A comprehensive handbook* (pp. 415–441). Boston: Birkhäuser.

Goldman-Rakic, P. S. (1987). Circuitry of primate prefrontal cortex and regulation of behavior by representational knowledge. In F. Plum & V. Mountcastle (Eds.), *The handbook of physiology. Sec. 1, The nervous system, Vol. V, Higher functions of the brain, Pt. 1* (pp. 373–416). Bethesda, MD: American Physiological Society.

Goldman-Rakic, P. S. (1988). Topography of cognition: Parallel distributed networks in primate association cortex. *Annual Review of Neuroscience, 11*, 137–156.

Jenike, M. A., Baer, L., Ballantine, H. T., Martuza, R. L., Tynes, S., Girunas, I., et al. (1991). Cingulotomy for refractory obsessive-compulsive disorder: A long-term follow-up of 33 patients. *Archives of General Psychiatry, 48*, 548–555.

Luppino, F., Matelli, M., Camarda, R. M., Gallese, V., & Rizzolatti, F. (1991). Multiple representations of body movements in mesial area 6 and the adjacent cingulate cortex: An intracortical microstimulation study in the macaque monkey. *Journal of Comparative Neurology, 311*, 463–482.

Mayberg, H. S., Liotti, M., Brannan, S. K., McGinnis, S., Mahurin, R. K., Jerabek, P. A., et al. (1999). Reciprocal limbic–cortical function and negative mood: Converging PET findings in depression and normal sadness. *American Journal of Psychiatry, 156*, 675–682.

Morecraft, R. J., & Van Hoesen, G. W. (1992). Cingulate input to the primary and supplementary motor cortices in the rhesus monkey: Evidence for somatotopy in Areas 24c and 23c. *Journal of Comparative Neurology, 322*, 471–489.

Niki, H., & Watanabe, M. (1979). Prefrontal and cingulate unit activity during timing behavior in the monkey. *Brain Research, 171*, 213–224.

Nishijo, H., Yamamoto, Y., Ono, T., Uwano, T., Yamashita, J., & Yamashima, T. (1997). *Neuroscience Letters, 227*, 79–82.

Pandya, D. N., Van Hoesen, G. W., & Mesulam, M. M. (1981). Efferent connections of the cingulate gyrus in the rhesus monkey. *Experimental Brain Research, 42*, 319–330.

Pardo, J. V., Fox, P. T., & Raichle, M. E. (1991). Localization of a human system for sustained attention by positron emission tomography. *Nature, 349*, 61–64.

Petersen, S. E., Fox, P. T., Snyder, A. Z., & Raichle, M. E. (1990). Activation of extrastriate and frontal cortical areas by visual words and word-like stimuli. *Science, 249*, 1041–4.

Picard, N., & Strick, P. L. (2001). Imaging the premotor areas. *Current Opinions in Neurobiology, 11*, 663–72.

Posner, M. I., & Dehaene, S. (1994). Attentional networks. *Trends in Neuroscience, 17*, 75–79.

Posner, M. I., & Driver, J. (1992). The neurobiology of selective attention. *Current Opinions in Neurobiology, 2*, 165–169.

Posner, M. I., & Petersen, S. E. (1990). The attention system of the human brain. *Annual Review of Neuroscience, 13*, 25–42.

Procyk, E., Tanaka, Y. L., & Joseph, J. P. (2000). Anterior cingulate activity during routine and nonroutine sequential behaviors in macaques. *Nature Neuroscience, 3*, 502–508.

Raichle, M. E., Fiez, J. A., Videen, T. O., MacLeod, A. K., Pardo, J. V., Fox, P. T., et al. (1994). Practice-related changes in human brain functional anatomy during nonmotor learning. *Cerebral Cortex, 4*, 8–26.

Raichle, M. E., MacLeod, A. M., Snyder, A. Z., Powers, W. J., Gusnard, D. A., & Shulman, G. L. (2001). A default mode of brain function. *Proceedings of the National Academy of Sciences USA, 98*(2), 676–82.

Shima, K., Aya, K., Mushiake, H., Inase, M., Aizawa, H., & Tanji, J. (1991). Two movement-related foci in the primate cingulated cortex observed in signal-triggered and self-paced forelimb movements. *Journal of Neurophysiology, 65*, 188–202.

Shima, K., & Tanji, J. (1998). Role for cingulate motor area cells in voluntary movement selection based on reward. *Science, 282*, 1335–1338.

Shin, L. M., Whalen, P. J., Pitman, R. K., Bush, G., Macklin, M. L., Lasko, N. B., et al. (2001). An fMRI study of anterior cingulate function in posttraumatic stress disorder. *Biological Psychiatry, 50*, 932–42.

Vogt, B. A. (1993). Structural organization of cingulate cortex: Areas, neurons, and somatodendritic transmitter receptors. In B. A. Vogt & M. Gabriel (Eds.), *Neurobiology of cingulate cortex and limbic thalamus: A comprehensive handbook* (pp. 19–70). Boston: Birkhäuser.

Vogt, B. A., Berger, G. R., & Derbyshire, S. W. G. (2003). Structural and functional dichotomy of human midcingulate cortex. *European Journal of Neuroscience, 18,* 3134–3144.

Vogt, B. A., Derbyshire, S., & Jones, A. K. P. (1996). Pain processing in four regions of human cingulate cortex localized with co-registered PET and MR imaging. *European Journal of Neuroscience, 8,* 1461–1473.

Vogt, B. A., Finch, D. M., & Olson, C. R. (1992). Functional heterogeneity in cingulate cortex: The anterior executive and posterior evaluative regions. *Cerebral Cortex, 2,* 435–443.

Vogt, B. A., Nimchinsky, E. A., Vogt, L. J., & Hof, P. R. (1995). Human cingulate cortex: Surface features, flat maps, and cytoarchitecture. *Journal of Comparative Neurology, 359,* 490–506.

Vogt, B. A., & Pandya, D. N. (1987). Cingulate cortex of the rhesus monkey: II. Cortical afferents. *Journal of Comparative Neurology, 262,* 271–289.

Vogt, B. A., Pandya, D. N., & Rosene, D. L. (1987). Cingulate cortex of the rhesus monkey: I. Cytoarchitecture and thalamic afferents. *Journal of Comparative Neurology, 262,* 256–270.

Vogt, B. A., Vogt, L. J., Nimchinsky, E. A., & Hof, P. R. (1997). Primate cingulate cortex chemoarchitecture and its disruption in Alzheimer's disease. In F. E. Bloom, A. Björklund, & T. Hökfelt (Eds.), *Handbook of chemical neuroanatomy. Vol. 13: The primate nervous system* (pp. 455–527). Amsterdam: Elsevier Science.

Whalen, P. J., Bush, G., McNally, R. J., Wilhelm, S., McInerney, S. C., Jenike, M. A., et al. (1998). The emotional counting Stroop paradigm: An fMRI probe of the anterior cingulate affective division. *Biological Psychiatry, 44,* 1219–1228.

Zametkin, A. J., Nordahl, T. E., Gross, M., King, A. C., Semple, W. E., Rumsey, J., et al. (1990). Cerebral glucose metabolism in adults with hyperactivity of childhood onset. *New England Journal of Medicine, 323,* 1361–1366.

16

Anterior Cingulate Cortex, Selection for Action, and Error Processing

Clay B. Holroyd, Sander Nieuwenhuis, Rogier B. Mars, and Michael G. H. Coles

The concepts of "attention to action" (Norman & Shallice, 1986) and "selection for action" (Allport, 1987) refer to how particular cognitive intentions and sensory inputs are selected and coupled with the effector system for the control of action production. A central role in this process has been attributed to the anterior cingulate cortex (ACC) (Posner, Petersen, Fox, & Raichle, 1988; see also Mesulam, 1981; Posner & Dehaene, 1994; Posner & DiGirolamo, 1998; Posner & Petersen, 1990). According to this view, the ACC contributes to executive or strategic aspects of motor control by allowing only particular sources of information access to the output system. More specifically, the ACC appears to be involved in selecting actions or action plans that are consistent with task goals, that is, to transform intentions into actions. This proposition has been supported by converging evidence from a broad array of empirical techniques, including functional neuroimaging, neuroanatomical, neurophysiological, intracranial stimulation, and lesion studies in humans and animals (Bush, Luu, & Posner, 2000; Devinsky, Morrell, & Vogt, 1995; Dum & Strick, 1993; Goldberg, 1992; Paus, 2001; Picard & Strick, 1996). This research has indicated that a caudal/dorsal area of the ACC appears to be involved in the cognitive control of motor behavior.

Consistent with this role, the ACC is also thought to be involved in error processing (Holroyd & Coles, 2002; cf. Botvinick, Braver, Barch, Carter, & Cohen, 2001). This position holds that the ACC is sensitive to incorrect or inappropriate behaviors and suggests that one aspect of the ACC control function involves bringing erroneous behaviors in line with desired goals. The motivation for this proposal is due primarily to observations of the error-related negativity (ERN), a component of the event-related brain potential (ERP) associated with error commission, which appears to be generated in the ACC. In this chapter, we review these ERN studies and discuss what insights they have provided into ACC function. We begin by describing the initial investigations that demonstrated that ERN is produced by an error-processing system. Then, we review studies that suggested that the ERN is generated in the ACC and, thus, that the ACC is involved in error processing. We next present a recent theory that holds that the ERN is produced by the impact of reinforcement learning signals conveyed by the mesencephalic dopamine system on the ACC, and that the ACC uses that information to improve performance on the task at hand. Finally, we provide empirical support for this theory.

THE ERN AND ERROR PROCESSING

The ERN is a negative deflection in the ERP that peaks about 80 msec after subjects make an incorrect response in speeded response-time tasks (Figure 16.1a). Although a similar component can be seen in the reports of several studies appearing in the 1980s (e.g., McCarthy, 1984; Renault, Ragot, & Lesevre, 1980), a paper by Falkenstein and his colleagues in Dortmund (Falkenstein, Hohnsbein, Hoormann, & Blanke, 1990) seems to have acted as a stimulus for a recent surge of interest in brain potentials associated with errors. The report from Dortmund was followed by observations from laboratories at Illinois (Gehring, Goss, Coles, Meyer, & Donchin, 1993) and Oregon (Dehaene, Posner, & Tucker, 1994). One thing that intrigued these early investigators was that the onset of this negative potential preceded the overt erroneous response, suggesting that the cognitive system "knew" about the error as it was being made.

These early reports were followed by studies of the influence of various factors on the amplitude and latency of the component, and of the relationship between the component and remedial actions that appeared to be consequences of erroneous behavior (see Falkenstein, Hohnsbein, & Hoormann, 1995; Gehring, Coles, Meyer, & Donchin, 1995).

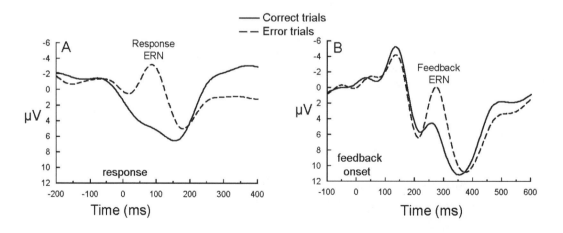

FIGURE 16.1. The error-related negativity (ERN). (A) The response ERN. (B) The feedback ERN. Negative is plotted up by convention. From Nieuwenhuis et al. (2002). Copyright 2002 by Psychonomic Society, Inc. Adapted by permission.

The amplitude of the ERN increases with the importance of errors (Falkenstein et al., 1995; Gehring et al., 1993) defined by speed versus accuracy instructions, and with the degree of error, defined by the number of movement parameters that differ between incorrect and correct responses (Bernstein, Scheffers, & Coles, 1995; Falkenstein et al., 1995). The ERN is present when errors cannot be corrected by a second motor response, as in a go/no-go task (Scheffers, Coles, Bernstein, Gehring, & Donchin, 1996), and it decreases as the quality of performance declines with fatigue (Scheffers, Humphrey, Stanny, Kramer, & Coles, 1999) or with degraded stimuli (Scheffers & Coles, 2000). Finally, the amplitude of the ERN appears to be related to remedial actions that compensate for the fact that an error is or has been made. These remedial actions include error correction, error force, and an increase in reaction time on trials following an error (Gehring et al., 1993).

A second line of research was stimulated by the observation that a similar brain response occurs when subjects receive feedback indicating that they have just made an erroneous response. Miltner, Braun, and Coles (1997) observed ERN-like activity in a time-estimation task when subjects received feedback that their previous time estimate was incorrect (see also Badgaiyan & Posner, 1998). This phenomenon has been called the "feedback ERN" to distinguish it from its counterpart, the "response ERN" (Figure 16.1b). Importantly, the discovery of the feedback ERN seemed to indicate that ERN production does not depend directly on motor processes associated with error commission (such as remedial actions that follow the error) but, rather, on processes that can occur subsequent to the error, such as the detection of the error or learning from the error. Also important was the observation that the feedback ERN was produced independently of whether the feedback was delivered in the auditory, somatosensory, or visual modalities (Miltner et al., 1997). In like fashion, subsequent research demonstrated that the response ERN was produced by errors committed not only with the hands but also with the feet (Holroyd, Dien, & Coles, 1998), the eyes (Nieuwenhuis, Ridderinkhof, Blom, Band, & Kok, 2001; Van't Ent & Apkarian, 1999), and the voice (Masaki, Tanaka, Takasawa, & Yamazaki, 2001), as well as by slow (but correct) responses in tasks in which speed is of the essence (Johnson, Otten, Boeck, & Coles, 1997; Luu, Flaisch, & Tucker, 2000). These findings indicate that the system that produces the ERN is involved in a "generic" form of error processing that is sensitive to error information regardless of its type or source.

Taken together, these results motivated the theory that the ERN is elicited either by a process of error detection or by a process that is engaged following the detection of the error (Falkenstein, Hohnsbein, & Hoormann, & Blanke, 1991; Gehring et al., 1993). As articulated by Coles, Scheffers, and Holroyd (2001), the theory proposes that error detection involves a comparison between two response representations: (1) a representation of the response that is being executed, derived from efference copy; and (2) a representation of the response that should be executed, derived from further stimulus processing and application of the appropriate stimulus–response mapping rule. (In most cases, the ERN has been investigated in situations in which errors occur as the result of impulsive action, such that further processing of the stimulus can lead to a representation of the correct response.) When the comparison process detects a mismatch between these two representations, or when error feedback is provided, an error signal is generated. The signal provides an input to the remedial action system whose function is to deal with the fact that an error is being made, or has been made.

THE ERN AND THE ACC

Coincident with the effort to understand the function of the system that produces the ERN was a search to identify where in the brain the ERN is produced. Early studies suggested that the ERN was generated in the ACC. This inference was based on the component's frontocentral scalp distribution, which suggested that the ERN was generated by "a system involving the anterior cingulate cortex and supplementary motor areas" (Gehring et al., 1993, p. 389), but also on the results of primate studies that reported that neurons in the ACC were activated by errors (e.g., Gemba, Sasaki, & Brooks, 1986) and by the absence of expected rewards (Niki & Watanabe, 1979). A recent study has further indicated that some ACC neurons are sensitive to both error responses and error feedback (Ito, Stuphorn, Brown, & Schall, 2003). Source localization studies of the ERN were also consistent with this hypothesis, with dipole modeling of the difference in activity between correct and incorrect responses yielding a single source located in the inferior ACC (Dehaene et al., 1994). Follow-up studies showed ACC sources irrespective of whether the errors were made with hands or feet (Holroyd et al., 1998), and magnetoencephalographic studies yielded similar results (e.g. Miltner et al., 2003). Analyses of the feedback ERN also showed an ACC source, irrespective of whether the feedback was presented in the visual, the auditory, or the somatosensory modality (Miltner et al., 1997; see also Gehring & Willoughby, 2002).

Imaging studies using rapid event-related functional magnetic resonance imaging (fMRI) confirmed the dipole models, reporting activation in the ACC (BA 24/32) in response to errors (Carter et al., 1998). A number of studies have indicated that the rostral–caudal extent of the ACC is activated more to errors than to correct responses (e.g., Kiehl, Liddle, & Hopfinger, 2000; Menon, Adleman, White, Glover, & Reiss, 2001; Ullsperger & Von Cramon, 2001). Initial investigations aimed at identifying the locus of feedback-related error activity were less successful (e.g., Van Veen, Holroyd, Cohen, Stenger, & Carter, 2002), but recent imaging studies have found that a dorsal region of the ACC is activated by error feedback (Ullsperger & Von Cramon, 2003) and by unexpected decreases in rewards (e.g., Bush et al., 2002). Furthermore, a recent study showed that a single area in caudal and dorsal ACC is activated by both error responses and by error feedback (Holroyd et al., in press). These results indicate that this region of the ACC comprises part of a generic error-processing system that is sensitive to both internal and external sources of error information and are consistent with the hypothesis that this brain region produces both the response ERN and the feedback ERN.

The suggestion that the ACC produces the ERN was corroborated by findings in patients with focal brain lesions. Stemmer, Segalowitz, Witzke, and Schoenle (2004) studied patients with a ruptured aneurysm of the anterior communicating artery, resulting in damage to the ACC and adjacent regions. They reported that these patients, although showing error rates comparable to normal control subjects, did not produce ERNs following error responses. A similar result was obtained by Swick and Turken (2002), who studied a patient with a rostral-to-middorsal ACC lesion. Gehring and Knight (2000) showed that patients with lateral prefrontal damage produced an ERN following incorrect trials but also following correct trials. In contrast, Ullsperger and colleagues found a reduced ERN in people with lateral prefrontal lesions (Ullsperger, Von Cramon, & Müller, 2002). Although these two results are in disagreement, they both suggest an interaction between the ACC and the prefrontal cortex in error processing.

Finally, involvement of the ACC in ERN production has been suggested by studies of clinical populations. Key among these populations are people with obsessive–compulsive disorder and people with Gilles de la Tourette syndrome, who have been shown to produce abnormally large ERNs (Gehring, Himle, & Nisenson, 2000; Hajcak & Simons, 2002; Johannes, Wieringa, Müller-Vahl, Dengler, & Münte, 2002). These disorders disrupt high-level error processing and motor control functions and are believed to affect a neural network involving the ACC and the basal ganglia (Devinsky et al., 1995; Wise & Rapoport, 1991).

REINFORCEMENT LEARNING THEORY OF THE ERN

Although these studies established a role for the ACC in error processing and in the production of the ERN, they were less specific about the details of that role. In contrast, a recent theory has formalized these ideas in a computational model that makes explicit the functional significance and neural implementation of the error-processing system that gives rise to the ERN (Holroyd & Coles, 2002; for a contrasting view, see Botvinick et al., 2001; Yeung, Botvinick, & Cohen, 2003). The theory is based on previous research that indicates that the basal ganglia monitor ongoing events and continuously predict whether the outcomes of those events will end favorably or unfavorably (Barto, 1995; Houk, Adams, & Barto, 1995; Montague, Dayan, & Sejnowski, 1996). According to this position, when the basal ganglia revise their predictions for the worse (indicating that ongoing events are "worse than expected"), they produce a negative error signal. Conversely, when the basal ganglia revise their predictions for the better (indicating that ongoing events are "better than expected"), they produce a positive error signal. These negative and positive error signals are conveyed from the basal ganglia as phasic decreases and increases, respectively, of the tonic activity of the mesencephalic dopamine system. In turn, the dopamine system conveys the signals back to the basal ganglia, where they are used to improve the predictions, and to frontal cortex (for reviews of this phasic activity, see Schultz, 1998, 2002).

The ERN theory builds on this theoretical framework by proposing that the ACC uses these dopamine signals to improve performance on the task at hand according to principles of reinforcement learning (Holroyd & Coles, 2002; see also Sutton & Barto, 1998). According to the theory (Figure 16.2), the ACC receives motor command information from multiple neural sources (called "controllers"), including dorsolateral prefrontal cortex, orbitofrontal cortex, the amygdala, and other areas. Because the commands from the different systems can sometimes conflict, the function of the ACC is to give control over the motor system to the controller that is best suited to carry out the task. Thus, consistent with its putative role in selection for action, the ACC acts as a "control filter" that decides which high-level executive commands gain control over the motor system. The theory also holds that the dopamine signals modulate and reinforce ACC activity such that the filtering function is optimized, a position that is consistent with the established role played by dopamine in reinforcement learning (for reviews, see Schultz, 1998, 2002) and with dopaminergic modulation of ACC activity (e.g., Crino, Morrison, & Hof, 1993; Porrino, 1993; Richardson & Gratton, 1998; Vogt, Vogt, Nimchinsky, & Hof, 1997; Wilkinson et al., 1998). According to the theory, furthermore, the impact of the dopamine signals on the apical dendrites of motor neurons in the ACC modulates the amplitude of the ERN, such that phasic decreases in dopamine activity (indicating that ongoing events are worse than expected) are associated with large ERNs, and phasic increases in dopamine (indicating that ongoing events are better than expected) are associated with small ERNs. Thus, response ERNs and feedback ERNs are elicited, respectively, by unpredicted error responses and error feedback.

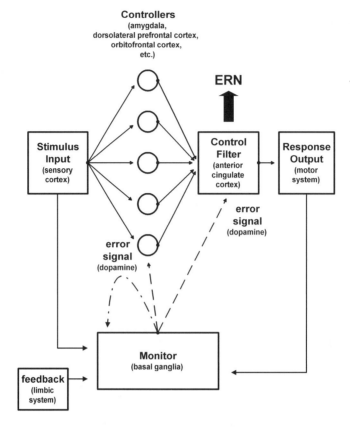

FIGURE 16.2. Reinforcement learning theory of the ERN. Multiple controllers in the brain process sensory input and produce motor commands. These commands are filtered by a control area in the anterior cingulate cortex, such that a subset of appropriate, nonconflicting commands are passed to the motor system. Simultaneously, a monitor located in the basal ganglia processes sensory information from the external environment, feedback information (such as rewards and punishments), and efference copies of the response in progress. The monitor produces error signals that are conveyed by the mesencephalic dopamine system to other parts of the brain, including anterior cingulate cortex, where they reinforce processes that contribute to optimal task performance. The amplitude of the ERN is determined by the impact of the error signals on the control area in the anterior cingulate cortex.

This "reinforcement learning theory of the ERN" (RL-ERN theory) has inspired several empirical studies of the feedback ERN (reviewed by Nieuwenhuis, Holroyd, Mol, & Coles, 2003). All these studies have employed a pseudo trial-and-error learning paradigm in which, on each trial, subjects select one of several response options and are then told the outcome of their choice by means of a feedback stimulus. The first of these studies tested a fundamental prediction of the theory, which is that the ERN should occur following the first indication that ongoing events are worse than expected. Thus, if a negative feedback stimulus is not predicted by prior events, then presentation of the feedback stimulus should elicit the ERN. On the other hand, if the subject has learned a set of stimulus–response mappings and the feedback merely confirms the application of an inappropriate mapping, then the ERN should occur at the time of the error response and not at the time of feedback presentation. According to the theory, on trials when the system detects the error at the time of the response, there is a negative prediction error and a large ERN. Therefore, when the feedback is presented the system has already detected the error, and there is no change in prediction and no ERN associated with the feedback. These predictions were confirmed in two recent experiments involving a probabilistic learning task: The response ERN was elicited on trials in which the feedback was fixed and the stimulus–response mappings could be learned, and the feedback ERN was elicited on trials in which the feedback was random and the stimulus–response mappings could not be learned (Holroyd & Coles, 2002; Nieuwenhuis et al., 2002). Furthermore, in an event-related fMRI study that adopted a similar task design, a caudal and dorsal area of the ACC was activated following error responses on trials with fixed mappings and following error feedback on trials with random mappings, consistent with the ERN results (Holroyd et al., in press).

These studies also demonstrated that the changes in the predictions are not all-or-none: The relative size of the response ERN and feedback ERN is highly sensitive to the degree to which a response is predictive of the value of the feedback (Nieuwenhuis et al., 2002), and even when the feedback is delivered at random, the amplitude of the feedback ERN tracks the size of the prediction error on a trial-by-trial basis (Holroyd & Coles, 2002). Furthermore, in a study in which the global probability of rewards and punishments was varied by condition, it was found that the amplitude of the feedback ERN was largest when the unfavorable outcomes were infrequent (and therefore less likely to be predicted) compared to when the unfavorable outcomes were frequent (and therefore more likely to be predicted) (Holroyd, Nieuwenhuis, Yeung, & Cohen, 2003).

Other recent studies have investigated how the monitoring system determines whether an outcome is good or bad. In one such study, feedback stimuli conveyed information along two different dimensions: a "gain/loss" dimension, indicating whether the subject's choice led to a gain or loss of money, and a "correct/error" dimension, indicating whether the subject's choice was better or worse than the alternative choice that the subject could have made (Nieuwenhuis, Yeung, Holroyd, Schurger, & Cohen, in press). The results demonstrated that the feedback ERN was sensitive to both the gain/loss information and the correct/error information conveyed by the feedback, depending on which dimension of the feedback was made most salient to the subjects. Results from another study are consistent with this view (Gehring & Willougby, 2002). These findings support the notion that the ERN is sensitive to any performance-related feedback information indicating favorable or unfavorable outcomes.

In these studies, the feedback indicated explicitly whether an outcome was favorable or unfavorable (such as a red square of color indicating monetary loss and a green square of color indicating monetary gain). However, the question arises as to how the monitoring system determines the favorableness of an outcome when that information is not made explicit by the feedback. To address this question, Holroyd, Larsen, and Cohen (in press) varied the range of possible outcomes by condition. On each trial of a "win" condition, subjects either won nothing, won a small reward, or won a large reward, and on each trial of a "lose" condition, subjects either lost nothing, lost a small reward, or lost a large reward. It was found that winning nothing in the win condition elicited a large ERN whereas losing nothing in the lose condition did not elicit an ERN, even though these two outcomes were identical (no change in total reward), and that small losses in the lose condition and small wins in the win condition elicited ERNs of comparable amplitude, even though these outcomes were different (wins vs. losses). These results indicate that the monitoring system determines whether an outcome is good or bad relative to the range of outcomes possible: For example, a $500 reward is good when the alternative is nothing, but a $500 is bad when the alternative is $1,000 (but see also Mars, de Bruijn, Hulstijn, Miltner, & Coles, in press). The results also dovetail with those of Yeung and Sanfey (2003), who showed that ERN amplitudes elicited by large losses in the context of large gains and losses are about the same size as ERN amplitudes elicited by small losses in the context of small gains and losses.

In all these studies, the feedback stimuli indicated only the outcome of each trial (e.g., win vs. loss) but not what should be done to improve performance at the task (e.g., press the left button). According to the RL-ERN theory, the error information carried by the mesencephalic dopamine system describes only whether an event was favorable or unfavorable but not how that information should be used.[1] By default, then, the theory holds that a different neural system processes error information that indicates what a subject should do to improve performance. To investigate this issue, Mars and colleagues (in press) conducted a reinforcement learning experiment that included two conditions, one in which the feedback indicated only the outcome, and a second in which the feedback also indicated how performance should be improved. They found that the feedback ERN was smaller in the second condition, consistent with the position that the associated error information was processed by a different neural system.

Other studies have investigated the neural basis of the theory—in particular, whether the mesencephalic dopamine system contributes to ERN production. Although the results of these studies must be viewed as only suggestive, many of the findings are consistent with the theory and provide some preliminary support for it. For example, ERN amplitude is increased by administration of d-amphetamine, which releases dopamine and inhibits its reuptake, suggesting that dopamine affects the mechanism that produces the ERN (de Bruijn, Hulstijn, Verkes, Ruigt, & Sabbe, 2003). Conversely, alcohol consumption reduces ERN amplitude (Ridderinkhof et al., 2002), possibly because dopamine receptors may contribute to the reinforcing aspects of alcohol addiction (Holroyd & Yeung, 2003). Although Parkinson's disease disrupts the mesencephalic dopamine system, evidence of abnormal ERNs in people with mild to moderate Parkinson's disease has been mixed (Falkenstein et al., 2001; Holroyd, Praamstra, Plat, & Coles, 2002). On the other hand, ERN amplitude is smaller in older adults, perhaps because of age-related changes of the dopamine system (Nieuwenhuis et al., 2002). Moreover, dopamine dysfunction is thought to be an important factor underlying schizophrenia (e.g., Dolan et al., 1995; for review, see Davis, Kahn, Ko, & Davidson, 1991; Harrison, 2000), and people with schizophrenia evidence abnormal ERNs (Bates, Kiehl, Laurens, & Liddle, 2002; Kopp & Rist, 1999; Mathalon et al., 2002). Also suggestive is the finding of abnormally large ERNs in people with Gilles de la Tourette syndrome (Johannes et al., 2002), because hyperactivity of the midbrain dopamine system has been proposed to be the main neurochemical abnormality underlying this disorder (Devinsky, 1983; Singer, Butler, Tune, Seifert, & Coyle, 1982).

CONCLUSION

In a recent review of the ACC, Paus (2001) concluded that

> the ACC is a prime example of a brain structure in which a regulatory network, composed of cells from the modulatory brainstem nuclei, interacts with an executive network, composed of local-circuit neurons. . . . By virtue of their action on ACC neurons, neuromodulators such as dopamine . . . are in a powerful position to regulate the interaction between cognition and motor control in relation to changes in emotional and motivational states. (p. 423)

In this view, the selection for action process mediated by the ACC is fine-tuned by the reward-related functions associated with midbrain dopamine. Research into the ERN has provided insight into how such a process might occur. In particular, the RL-ERN theory has specified how the ERN may provide a window into this control mechanism. The principles underlying the theory are computationally robust and, in other domains, have been used to teach autonomous systems how to operate in uncertain and variable environments (Sutton & Barto, 1998), including how and where to deploy attention (Ballard, 1991; Whitehead & Lin, 1995). These successes afford the hope that the same principles can be used to understand the contribution of the ACC to attention and action selection.

ACKNOWLEDGMENTS

This research was supported in part by postdoctoral fellowship No. MH63550 from the National Institute of Mental Health (to Clay B. Holroyd) and by the Netherlands Organization for Scientific Research (to Sander Nieuwenhuis).

NOTE

1. The midbrain dopamine system is sometimes said to convey a "scalar" signal (one piece of information: good vs. bad), as opposed to a "vector" signal (many pieces of information: good vs. bad and how the behavior should be modified).

REFERENCES

Allport, A. (1987). Selection for action: Some behavioral and neurophysiological considerations of attention and action. In H. Heuer & A. F. Sanders (Eds.), *Perspectives on perception and action* (pp. 395–419). Hillsdale, NJ: Erlbaum.

Badgaiyan, R. D., & Posner, M. I. (1998). Mapping the cingulate cortex in response selection and monitoring. *NeuroImage, 7,* 255–260.

Ballard, D. H. (1991). Animate vision. *Artificial Intelligence, 48,* 57–86.

Barto, A. G. (1995). Adaptive critics and the basal ganglia. In J. Houk, J. Davis, & D. Beiser (Eds.), *Models of information processing in the basal ganglia* (pp. 215–232). Cambridge, MA: MIT Press.

Bates, A. T., Kiehl, K. A., Laurens, K. R., & Liddle, P. F. (2002). Error-related negativity and correct response negativity in schizophrenia. *Clinical Neurophysiology, 113,* 1454–1463.

Bernstein, P. S., Scheffers, M. K., & Coles, M. G. H. (1995). "Where did I go wrong?" A psychophysiological analysis of error detection. *Journal of Experimental Psychology: Human Perception and Performance, 21,* 1312–1322.

Botvinick, M., Braver, T. S., Barch, D. M., Carter, C. S., & Cohen, J. D. (2001). Conflict monitoring and cognitive control. *Psychological Review, 108,* 624–652.

Bush, G., Luu, P., & Posner, M. I. (2000). Cognitive and emotional influences in anterior cingulate cortex. *Trends in Cognitive Sciences, 4,* 215–222.

Bush, G., Vogt, B. A., Homes, J., Dale, A. M., Greve, D., Jenike, M. A., et al. (2002). Dorsal anterior cingulate cortex: A role in reward-based decision making. *Proceedings of the National Academy of Sciences USA, 99,* 523–528.

Carter, C. S., Braver, T. S., Barch, D. M., Botvinick, M. M., Noll, D., & Cohen, J.D. (1998). Anterior cingulate cortex, error detection, and the online monitoring of performance. *Science, 280,* 747–749.

Coles, M. G. H., Scheffers, M. K., & Holroyd, C. B. (2001). Why is there an ERN/Ne on correct trials? Response representations, stimulus-related components, and the theory of error-processing. *Biological Psychology, 56,* 191–206.

Crino, P. B., Morrison, J. H., & Hof, P. R. (1993). Monoaminergic innervation of cingulate cortex. In B. A. Vogt & M. Gabriel (Eds.), *Neurobiology of cingulate cortex and limbic thalamus: A comprehensive handbook* (pp. 285–310). Boston: Birkhauser.

Davis, K. L., Kahn, R. S., Ko, G., & Davidson, M. (1991). Dopamine in schizophrenia: A review and reconceptualization. *American Journal of Psychiatry, 148,* 1474–1486.

de Bruijn, E. R. A., Hulstijn, W., Verkes, R. J., Ruigt, G. S. F., & Sabbe, B. G. C. (2003). *Drug-induced stimulation and suppression of action monitoring.* Manuscript submitted for publication.

Dehaene, S., Posner, M. I., & Tucker, D. M. (1994). Localization of a neural system for error detection and compensation. *Psychological Science, 5,* 303–305.

Devinsky, O. (1983). Neuroanatomy of Gilles de la Tourette's syndrome. *Annals of Neurology, 40,* 508–514.

Devinsky, O., Morrell, M. J., & Vogt, B. A. (1995). Contributions of anterior cingulate cortex to behaviour. *Brain, 118,* 279–306.

Dolan, R. J., Fletcher, P., Frith, C. D., Friston, K. J., Frackowiak, R. S. J., & Grasby, P. M. (1995). Dopaminergic modulation of impaired cognitive activation in the anterior cingulate cortex in schizophrenia. *Nature, 378,* 180–182.

Dum, R. P., & Strick, P. L. (1993). Cingulate motor areas. In B. A. Vogt & M. Gabriel (Eds.), *Neurobiology of cingulate cortex and limbic thalamus: A comprehensive handbook* (pp. 415–441). Boston: Birkhauser.

Falkenstein, M., Hielscher, H., Dziobek, I., Schwarzenau, P., Hoormann, J., Sundermann, B., et al. (2001). Action monitoring, error detection, and the basal ganglia: An ERP study. *Neuroreport, 12,* 157–161.

Falkenstein, M., Hohnsbein, J., & Hoormann, J. (1995). Event-related potential correlates of errors in reaction tasks. In G. Karmos, M. Molnar, V. Csepe, I. Czigler, & J. E. Desmedt (Eds.), *Perspectives of event-related potentials research (EEG Suppl. 44)* (pp. 287–296). Amsterdam: Elsevier Science.

Falkenstein, M., Hohnsbein, J., Hoormann, J., & Blanke, L. (1990). Effects of errors in choice reaction tasks on the ERP under focused and divided attention. In C. Brunia, A. Gaillard, & A. Kok (Eds.), *Psychophysiological brain research* (pp 192–195). Tilburg, The Netherlands: Tilburg University Press.

Falkenstein, M., Hohnsbein, J., Hoormann, J., & Blanke, L. (1991). Effects of crossmodal divided attention on late ERP components: II. Error processing in choice reaction tasks. *Electroencephalography and Clinical Neurophysiology, 78,* 447–455.

Gehring, W. J., Coles, M. G. H., Meyer, D. E., & Donchin, E. (1995). A brain potential manifestation of error-related processing. In G. Karmos, M. Molnar, V. Csepe, I. Czigler, & J. E. Desmedt (Eds.), *Perspectives of event-related potentials research (EEG Suppl. 44)* (pp. 261–272). Amsterdam: Elsevier Science.

Gehring, W. J., Goss, B., Coles, M. G. H., Meyer, D. E., & Donchin, E. (1993). A neural system for error detection and compensation. *Psychological Science, 4,* 385–390.

Gehring, W. J., Himle, J., & Nisenson, L.G. (2000). Action-monitoring dysfunction in obsessive–compulsive disorder. *Psychological Science, 11,* 1–6.

Gehring, W. J., & Knight, R. T. (2000). Prefrontal-cingulate interactions in action monitoring. *Nature Neuroscience, 3,* 516–520.

Gehring, W. J., & Willoughby, A. R. (2002). The medial frontal cortex and the rapid processing of monetary gains and losses. *Science, 295,* 2279–2282.

Gemba, H., Sasaki, K., & Brooks, V. B. (1986). "Error" potentials in limbic cortex (anterior cingulate area 24) of monkeys during motor learning. *Neuroscience Letters, 70,* 223–227.

Goldberg, G. (1992). Premotor systems, attention to action, and behavioral choice. In J. Kien, C. R. McCrohan, & W. Winslow (Eds.), *Neurobiology of motor programme selection: New approaches to the study of behavioural choice* (pp. 225–249). Oxford, UK: Pergamon Press.

Hajcak, G., & Simons, R. F. (2002). Error-related brain activity in obsessive-compulsive undergraduates. *Psychiatry Research, 110,* 63–72.

Harrison, P. J. (2000). Dopamine and schizophrenia—proof at last? *The Lancet, 356,* 958–959.

Holroyd, C. B., & Coles, M. G. H. (2002). The neural basis of human error processing: Reinforcement learning, dopamine, and the error-related negativity. *Psychological Review, 109,* 679–709.

Holroyd, C. B., Dien, J., & Coles, M. G. H. (1998). Error-related scalp potentials elicited by hand and foot movements: Evidence for an output-independent error-processing system in humans. *Neuroscience Letters, 242,* 65–68.

Holroyd, C. B., Larsen, J. T., & Cohen, J. D. (in press). Context dependence of the event-related brain potential associated with reward and punishment. *Psychophysiology.*

Holroyd, C., B., Nieuwenhuis, S., Yeung, N., & Cohen, J. D. (2003). Reward prediction errors are reflected in the event-related brain potential. *Neuroreport, 14,* 2481–2484.

Holroyd, C. B., Nieuwenhuis, S., Yeung, N., Nystrom, L. E., Mars, R. B., Coles, M. G. H., & Cohen, J. D. (in press). Dorsal anterior cingulate cortex shows fMRI response to internal and external error signals. *Nature Neuroscience.*

Holroyd, C. B., Praamstra, P., Plat, E., & Coles, M. G. H. (2002). Spared error-related potentials in mild to moderate Parkinson's disease. *Neuropsychologia, 1419,* 1–9.

Holroyd, C. B., & Yeung, N. (2003). Alcohol and error processing. *Trends in Neurosciences, 26,* 402–404.

Houk, J. C., Adams, J. L., & Barto, A. G. (1995). A model of how the basal ganglia generate and use neural signals that predict reinforcement. In J. Houk, J. Davis, & D. Beiser (Eds.), *Models of information processing in the basal ganglia* (pp. 249–270). Cambridge, MA: MIT Press.

Ito, S., Stuphorn, V., Brown, J. W., & Schall, J. D. (2003). Performance monitoring by anterior cingulate cortex during saccade countermanding. *Science, 302,* 120–122.

Johannes, S., Wieringa, B. M., Müller-Vahl, K. R., Dengler, R., & Münte, T. F. (2002). Excessive action monitoring in Tourette syndrom. *Journal of Neurology, 249,* 961–966.

Johnson, T., M., Otten, L. J., Boeck, K., & Coles, M. G. H. (1997). Am I too late? The neural consequences of missing a deadline. *Psychophysiology, 34,* S48.

Kiehl, K. A., Liddle, P. F., & Hopfinger, J. B. (2000). Error processing and the rostral anterior cingulate: An event-related fMRI study. *Psychophysiology, 37,* 216–223.

Kopp, B., & Rist, F. (1999). An event-related brain potential substrate of disturbed response monitoring in paranoid schizophrenic patients. *Journal of Abnormal Psychology, 108,* 337–346.

Luu, P., Flaisch, T., & Tucker, D. M. (2000). Medial frontal cortex in action monitoring. *Journal of Neuroscience, 20,* 464–469.

Mars, R. B., de Bruijn, E. R. A., Hulstijn, W., Miltner, W. H. R., & Coles, M. G. H. (in press). What if I told you: "You were wrong"? Brain potentials and behavioral adjustments elicited by feedback in a time-estimation task. In M. Ullsperger & M. Falkenstein (Eds.), *Errors, conflicts and the brain: Current opinions on performance monitoring.* Leipzig: MPI of Cognitive Neuroscience.

Masaki, H., Tanaka, H., Takasawa, N., & Yamazaki, K. (2001). Error-related brain potentials elicited by vocal errors. *Neuroreport, 12,* 1851–1855.

Mathalon, D. H., Fedor, M., Faustman, W. O., Gray, M., Askari, N., & Ford, J. M. (2002). Response-monitoring dysfunction in schizophrenia: An event-related brain potential study. *Journal of Abnormal Psychology, 111,* 22–41.

McCarthy, G. (1984). Stimulus evaluation time and P300 latency. In E. Donchin (Ed.), *Cognitive psychophysiology: Event-related potentials and the study of cognition* (pp. 254–287). Hillsdale, NJ: Erlbaum.

Menon, V., Adleman, N. E., White, C. D., Glover, G. H., & Reiss, A. L. (2001). Error-related brain activation during a go/nogo response inhibition task. *Human Brain Mapping, 12,* 131–143.

Mesulam, M.-M. (1981). A cortical network for directed attention and unilateral neglect. *Annals of Neurology, 10,* 309–325.

Miltner, W. H. R., Braun, C. H., & Coles, M. G. H. (1997). Event-related brain potentials following incorrect feedback in a time-estimation task: Evidence for a "generic" neural system for error detection. *Journal of Cognitive Neuroscience, 9,* 788–798.

Miltner, W. H. R., Lemke, U., Weiss, T., Holroyd, C. B., Scheffers, M. K., & Coles, M. G. H. (2003). Implementation of error-processing in the human anterior cingulate cortex: A source analysis of the magnetic equivalent of the error-related negativity. *Biological Psychology, 64,* 157–166.

Montague, P. R., Dayan, P., & Sejnowski, T. J. (1996). A framework for mesencephalic dopamine systems based on predictive Hebbian learning. *Journal of Neuroscience, 16,* 1936–1947.

Nieuwenhuis, S., Holroyd, C. B., Mol, N., & Coles, M. G. H. (2003). *Reward-related brain potentials from medial frontal cortex: A review.* Manuscript in preparation.

Nieuwenhuis, S., Ridderinkhof, K. R., Blom, J., Band, G. P. H., & Kok, A. (2001). Error-related potentials are differentially related to awareness of response errors: Evidence from an antisaccade task. *Psychophysiology, 38,* 752–760.

Nieuwenhuis, S., Ridderinkhof, K. R., Talsma, D., Coles, M. G. H., Holroyd, C. B., Kok, A., et al. (2002). A computational account of altered error processing in older age: Dopamine and the error-related negativity. *Cognitive, Affective, and Behavioral Neuroscience, 2,* 19–36.

Nieuwenhuis, S., Yeung, N., Holroyd, C. B., Schurger, A., & Cohen, J. D. (in press). Sensitivity of electrophysiological activity from medial frontal cortex to utilitarian and performance feedback. *Cerebral Cortex.*

Niki, H., & Watanabe, M. (1979). Prefrontal and cingulate unit activity during timing behavior in the monkey. *Brain Research, 171,* 213–224.

Norman, D. A., & Shallice, T. (1986). Attention to action: Willed and automatic control of behavior. In R. J. Davidson, G. E. Schwartz, & D. Shapiro (Eds.), *Consciousness and self-regulation* (Vol. 4, pp. 1–19). New York: Plenum Press.

Paus, T. (2001). Primate anterior cingulate cortex: Where motor control, drive and cognition interface. *Nature Reviews Neuroscience, 2,* 417–424.

Picard, N., & Strick, P. L. (1996). Motor areas of the medial wall: A review of their location and functional activation. *Cerebral Cortex, 6,* 342–353.

Porrino, L. J. (1993). Cortical mechanisms of reinforcement. In B. A. Vogt & M. Gabriel (Eds.), *Neurobiology of cingulate cortex and limbic thalamus: A comprehensive handbook* (pp. 445–460). Boston: Birkhauser.

Posner, M. I., & Dehaene, S. (1994). Attentional networks. *Trends in Neurosciences, 17,* 75–79.

Posner, M. I., & DiGirolamo, G. J. (1998). Executive attention: Conflict, target detection, and cognitive control. In R. Parasuraman (Ed.), *The attentive brain* (pp. 401–423). Cambridge, MA: MIT Press.

Posner, M. I., & Petersen, S. E. (1990). The attention system of the human brain. *Annual Review of Neuroscience, 13,* 25–42.

Posner, M. I., Petersen, S. E., Fox, P. T., & Raichle, M. E. (1988). Localization of cognitive operations in the human brain. *Science, 240,* 1627–1631.

Renault, B., Ragot, R., & Lesevre, N. (1980). Correct and incorrect responses in a choice reaction time task and the endogenous components of the evoked potential. *Progress in Brain Research, 54,* 647–654.

Richardson, N. R., & Gratton, A. (1998). Changes in medial prefrontal cortical dopamine levels associated with response-contingent food reward: An electrochemical study in rat. *Journal of Neuroscience, 18,* 9130–9138.

Ridderinkhof, K. R., de Vlugt, Y., Bramlage, A., Spaan, M., Elton, M., Snel, J., et al. (2002). Alcohol consumption impairs detection of performance errors in mediofrontal cortex. *Science, 298,* 2209–2211.

Scheffers, M. K., & Coles, M. G. H. (2000). Performance monitoring in a confusing world: Error-related brain activity, judgments of response accuracy, and types of errors. *Journal of Experimental Psychology: Human Perception and Performance, 26,* 141–151.

Scheffers, M. K., Coles, M. G. H., Bernstein, P., Gehring, W. J., & Donchin, E. (1996). Event-related brain potentials and error-related processing: An analysis of incorrect responses to go and no-go stimuli. *Psychophysiology, 33,* 42–53.

Scheffers, M. K., Humphrey, D. G., Stanny, R. R., Kramer, A. F., & Coles, M. G. H. (1999). Error-related processing during a period of extended wakefulness. *Psychophysiology, 36,* 149–157.

Schultz, W. (1998). Predictive reward signal of dopamine neurons. *Journal of Neurophysiology, 80,* 1–27.

Schultz, W. (2002). Getting formal with dopamine and reward. *Neuron, 36,* 241–263.

Singer, H. S., Butler, I. J., Tune, L. E., Seifert, W. E., & Coyle, J. T. (1982). Dopaminergic dysfunction in Tourette syndrome. *Annals of Neurology, 12,* 361–366.

Stemmer, B., Segalowitz, S. J., Witzke, W., & Schoenle, P. W. (2004). Error detection in patients with lesions to the medial prefrontal cortex: An ERP study. *Neuropsychologia, 42,* 118–130.

Sutton, R. S., & Barto, A. G. (1998). *Reinforcement learning: An introduction.* Cambridge, MA: MIT Press.

Swick, D., & Turken, A. U. (2002). Dissociation between conflict detection and error monitoring in the human anterior cingulate cortex. *Proceedings of the National Academy of Sciences USA, 99,* 16354–16359.

Ullsperger, M., & Von Cramon, D. Y. (2001). Subprocesses of performance monitoring: A dissociation of error processing and response competition revealed by event-related fMRI and ERPs. *NeuroImage, 14,* 1387–1401.

Ullsperger, M., & Von Cramon, D. Y. (2003). Error processing using external feedback: Specific roles of the habenular complex, the reward system, and the cingulate motor area revealed by fMRI. *Journal of Neuroscience, 23,* 4308–4314.

Ullsperger, M., Von Cramon, D. Y., & Muller, N. G. (2002). Interactions of focal cortical lesions with error processing: Evidence from event-related brain potentials. *Neuropsychology, 16,* 548–561.

Van Veen, V., Holroyd, C. B., Cohen, J. D., Stenger, A. W., & Carter, C. S. (2002). *Errors without conflict don't activate the anterior cingulate cortex: Implications for performance monitoring theories (Program No. 16.1. 2002)* [Online]. Washington, DC: Society for Neuroscience. Available: http://sfn.scholarone.com/itin2002/

Van't Ent, D., & Apkarian, P. (1999). Motoric response inhibition in finger movement and saccadic eye movement: A comparative study. *Clinical Neurophysiology, 110,* 1058–1072.

Vogt, B. A., Vogt, L. J., Nimchinsky, E. A., & Hof, P. R. (1997). Primate cingulate cortex chemoarchitecture and its disruption in Alzheimer's disease. In F. E. Bloom, A. Bjorklund, & T. Hokfelt (Eds.), *Handbook of chemical neuroanatomy: Vol. 13. The primate nervous system, part I* (pp. 455–528). Amsterdam: Elsevier.

Whitehead, S. D., & Lin, L.-J. (1995). Reinforcement learning of non-Markov decision processes. *Artificial Intelligence, 73,* 271–306.

Wilkinson, L. S., Humby, T., Killcross, A. S., Torres, E. M., Everitt, B. J., & Robbins, T. W. (1998). Dissociations in dopamine release in medial prefrontal cortex and ventral striatum during the acquisition and extinction of classical aversive conditioning in rat. *European Journal of Neuroscience, 10,* 1019–1026.

Wise, S. P., & Rapoport, J. L. (1991). Obsessive–compulsive disorder: Is it basal ganglia dysfunction? In J. L. Rapoport (Ed.), *Obsessive–compulsive disorder in children and adolescents* (pp. 327–344). Washington, DC: American Psychiatric Press.

Yeung, N., Botvinick, M. M., & Cohen, J. D. (in press). The neural basis of error detection: Conflict monitoring and the error-related negativity. *Psychological Review.*

Yeung, N., & Sanfey, A. (2003). *Discrete coding of magnitude and valence in the human brain.* Manuscript submitted for publication.

17

The Anterior Cingulate Cortex

Regulating Actions in Context

Phan Luu and Stacey M. Pederson

Prior to the advent of noninvasive neuroimaging technologies, knowledge about human cognitive functions and how they mapped onto neuroanatomy had to be gleaned primarily from animal studies and studies of patients with known cerebral lesions. In the 1980s and 1990s availability of noninvasive neuroimaging technologies, such as positron emission tomography (PET) and functional magnetic resonance imaging (fMRI), allowed precise localization of cognitive functions in the intact human brain (see (Posner & DiGirolamo, 1998; Posner, Petersen, Fox, & Raichle, 1988). Of particular interest to this volume is a series of PET studies examining regions involved in word reading, which suggested that the anterior cingulate cortex (ACC) is involved in a form of attention referred to as *attention for action* (Posner & Dehaene, 1994; Posner et al., 1988).

Attention for action describes cognitive operations that allow for voluntary (i.e., controlled) processes to override or exert influence over automatic processes (Posner, 1978). This attention system is not sensory or cognitive operation specific. Attention for action has been described as executive attention (Vogt, Finch, & Olson, 1993). Consistent with the idea of attention for action, executive attention is thought to be engaged when routine functions are insufficient or ongoing behavior must be adjusted to meet environmental demands (Posner & DiGirolamo, 1998).

In this chapter we describe our current understanding of ACC function and attention for action based on research using dense-array electroencephalography (EEG) technology. Dense-array EEG technology is relatively new, being in common use only within the past decade. Traditionally, event-related potential (ERP) technology was valued for its direct reflection of neuronal function, unlike fMRI and PET methodologies, which rely on indirect measures of neuronal activity. However, unlike these hemodynamic-based technologies that provide precise spatial localization of cognitive functions, traditional ERP methods have poor spatial resolution. With dense-array ERP technology, localization is improved and has been shown to be both accurate and capable of discriminating nearby sources (see Cuffin,

Schomer, Ives, & Blume, 2001; Laarne, Tenhunen-Eskelinen, Hyttinen, & Eskola, 2000; Lantz, Grave de Peralta, Spinelli, Seeck, & Michel, 2003; Luu, Tucker, Derryberry, Reed, & Poulsen, 2003).

Using ERP methodologies, we study a particular component of executive attention of the ACC: action monitoring. In action monitoring, the appropriateness of an action must be monitored within a given context. Inappropriateness of the response, defined as errors, is evaluated relative to the context of the action. Violations of action relative to action context are essentially expectancy violations, and the detection of these violations is understood as a core component of attention for action.

THE ERROR-RELATED NEGATIVITY:
AN INDEX OF ACTION MONITORING

The error-related negativity (ERN) or the error negativity (Ne), was first reported in the early 1990s by Falkenstein, Hohnsbein, Hoormann, and Blanke (1991) and Gehring, Goss, Coles, Meyer, and Donchin (1993). The ERN is recorded as a negative deflection in the ongoing EEG with a peak negativity approximately 50–150 msec after an erroneous response (see Figure 17.1). The ERN has a mediofrontal distribution, and using dense-array EEG recordings Dehaene, Posner, and Tucker (1994) localized the source generator of the scalp re-

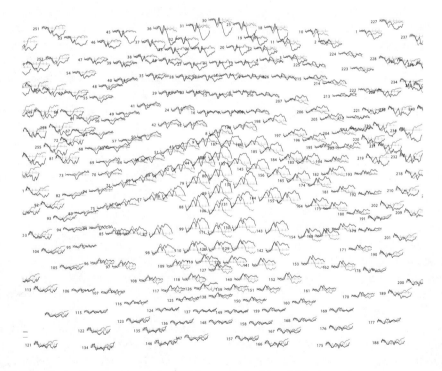

FIGURE 17.1. Scalp distribution of the ERN recorded with a 256–channel sensor array. View is top looking down with nose at the front. The ERN is observed at the top of the head (center of figure starting at channel 8 and extending caudally) as a negative deflection approximately 100 ms after erroneous button press. Also prominent in this figure is the Pe, the large positive deflection immediately after the ERN. The Pe spans an interval approximately between 300 and 500 msec after an erroneous button press.

corded ERN to the ACC. This important localization finding was later confirmed both in other dense-array EEG (Luu, Collins, & Tucker, 2000; Miltner, Braun, & Coles, 1997) and fMRI studies (Kiehl, Liddle, & Hopfinger, 2000; Menon, Adleman, White, Glover, & Reiss, 2001; Ullsperger & von Cramon, 2001).

Functional significance of the ERN remains controversial, and at least three competing functional theories exist. The first theory claims that the ERN reflects the output of an error detection system (Holroyd & Coles, 2002). Rather than reflecting error detection per se, the conflict-monitoring theory claims that the ACC's detection of conflict produces the ERN, and that errors are merely associated with increased conflict (Carter, Botvinick, & Cohen, 1999; Carter et al., 1998). Incorporating the vast human and animal literatures, we propose that the ERN is not merely a reflection of the evaluation of an error or of conflict but instead reflects the affective consequence of expectancy violations (Luu & Tucker, 2004; Luu et al., 2003). We do not perceive our proposal to be inconsistent with the error or conflict-monitoring theories. Rather, in our theory the limbic functions of the ACC are emphasized; error or conflict within a particular task induces affective evaluations of expectancy violations.

ACTION IN CONTEXT: EXPECTANCY VIOLATIONS

There is a large body of literature on brain responses to context violations (see Pritchard, Shappell, & Brandt, 1991). These studies have examined effects of context violation at different levels (stimulus feature discrepancies, semantic violations, etc.). In this chapter we limit our brief review of context violations to situations in which violations are immediately relevant to action control; that is, context is established to direct appropriate behaviors.

Initially, it was believed that the elicitation of the ERN required explicit recognition that an error has been committed (Dehaene et al., 1994). If an error response is not recognized as such, an error feedback is required, which is adequate for the elicitation of a mediofrontal, stimulus-locked negativity thought to be equivalent to the ERN (Kopp, Rist, & Mattler, 1996; Miltner et al., 1997; Ruchsow, Grothe, Spitzer, & Kiefer, 2002). The feedback provides information regarding violation of the task context and thus elicits a negativity with a peak latency between 250 and 400 msec poststimulus that we refer to as the medial frontal negativity (MFN; see Gehring & Willoughby, 2002; Tucker, Luu, Frishkoff, Quiring, & Poulsen, 2003).

Interestingly, this finding of error feedback inducing a mediofrontal response was anticipated by the findings of Gevins and colleagues (1989), who reported a mediofrontal theta response, at about the same time as the MFN, after presentation of an error feedback. It is likely that the MFN is part of the N2 complex known to index both automatic and controlled detection of context violation (Pritchard et al., 1991), but this relation remains to be clarified.

Other studies have shown the MFN to be similar to the ERN in several ways. Kopp and Wolff (2000) studied contingency learning in humans and found that when established contingencies are violated, a negative component over mediofrontal recording sites is observed. In sequence learning paradigms as subjects learn the sequence, violations of a position within the sequence elicit an N2 with a mediofrontal distribution, and this N2 response is larger as subjects learn the sequence (Eimer, Goschke, Schlaghecken, & Stürmer, 1996; Schlaghecken, Stürmer, & Eimer, 2000). These findings suggest that as subjects learn the context of appropriate action, violations of that context elicit larger ACC responses.

Using an old/new memory paradigm, Nessler and Mecklinger (2003) found that an MFN-like component indexes correct recognition of new but semantically similar items (i.e., lures) in this recognition test of previously learned items. The authors found that the correctly rejected lures elicited a larger MFN-like response than did items that were correctly recognized as old (i.e., previously studied) or lures that were incorrectly classified as old (i.e., falsely recognized).

Based on the view that all learning occurs in a context defined by the specific features of the task at hand (Balsam, 1985), one interpretation of this finding is that the larger MFN in the presence of lures reflects the ACC's detection of a context violation. Explicitly stated in the context of this recognition paradigm, the lures violate the background context of previously encountered items. To the extent that this context violation is detected—as indexed by a larger MFN—the more likely the lures will be correctly recognized as newly presented items. The failure of this detection—as evidenced by a lack of or smaller MFN—results in the erroneous identification of the lures as old.

Schnider, Valenza, Morand, and Michel (2002) used a memory paradigm to investigate brain responses to suppression of irrelevant stimuli—as defined by the current context of the study—that had been previously encountered. Examining the responses to nontarget items revealed that as subjects were exposed to a second run of nontarget items, the ERP to these items were differentiated from the target items by a lack of an MFN. Similar to Nessler and Mecklinger's (2003) findings, targets appear to be defined electrophysiologically, and perhaps cognitively, by how they "stand out" from the context of the task.

PROTECTION AGAINST NEGATIVE OUTCOMES AS A CONTEXT FOR ACTION

In monkeys and humans, the cingulate motor area (CMA) is activated when a change of behaviors is required due to reductions of an expected reward (Bush et al., 2002; Shima & Tanji, 1998). Shima and Tanji observed that cells in the rostral CMA (CMAr) are activated only when reduction of reward is associated with a corresponding "corrective" response. Bush and colleagues (2002) extended these results to humans, adding that a non–reward-related behavioral switch signal was not sufficient to activate the CMA. These studies confirm the role of the ACC in compensatory behaviors when expectations are violated.

Further evidence of MFN reactivity to motivational consequences of context violation comes from studies investigating MFN responses to affective feedback. Gehring and Willoughby (2002) found that rather than responding to the correctness of a response, the MFN was sensitive to loss, with MFNs larger on trials following loss trials than those following gain trials. We used a delayed feedback paradigm to investigate brain responses to evaluative feedback (Luu et al., 2003). Each trial began with a feedback stimulus (a letter grade), based on performance from five trials previous, which indicated both speed of response and the correctness of the response. Similar to Gehring and Willoughby's findings, the MFN was sensitive to feedback type and of larger amplitude for feedback indicating negative feedback, which was not necessary indicative of errors. Extending this finding, the larger MFN to negative feedback was also not necessarily indicative of a loss of points. In other studies, we have found MFNs that differentiated between good and bad target locations, which signaled whether points could be earned or lost, respectively (Tucker, Hartry-Speiser, McDougal, Luu, & deGrandpre, 1999), and good and bad self-descriptive trait words (Tucker et al., 2003). These findings are consistent with the concept of attention for action, suggesting that there is a bias in context–action representations and that this bias is for prevention of loss or negative evaluation. Core to this bias is evaluation of expectancy violations along a negative affect dimension.

There is increasing evidence that ERN amplitude varies with negative affect (Gehring, Himle, & Nisenson, 2000; Johannes, Wieringa, Nager, Dengler, & Münte, 2001; Luu et al., 2000; Pailing & Segalowitz, in press). It is possible that the violation of context representation (i.e., expectancy) is inherently aversive and that mechanisms originally developed for evaluating the unpleasantness of physical and psychological pain are also used for the evaluation of context violations (Luu et al., 2000; Luu & Tucker, 2002, 2004), which is consistent with the role of the ACC in pain evaluation (Rainville, Duncan, Price, Carrier, & Bushnell, 1997).

ACTION REGULATION: EVALUATING ACTION AGAINST CONTEXT

When an MFN in response to error feedback was first recorded, it was assumed to be equivalent to the response-locked ERN. We recently investigated this possibility using the delayed-feedback paradigm described earlier (Luu et al., 2003). This paradigm removes response control properties associated with immediate feedback presentation while preserving affective responses that can influence subsequent performance, thus providing access to both ERN and MFN measures in the same subject.

Based on extensive cytoarchitectural, lesion, electrophysiology, and imaging evidence that the ACC can be functionally differentiated by cognitive (dorsal) and affective (rostroventral) subdivisions (for a review, see Bush, Luu, & Posner, 2000), we first estimated the ERN sources using one dipole in the region of the dorsal ACC and a second dipole in the rostral extent of the ACC using BESA (2000) software (see Figure 17.2). We then applied the same source model to the MFN. Surprisingly, when the ERN model was applied to the MFN, only the dorsal ACC source was active. van Veen and Carter (2002) have also reported a dorsal ACC source for both ERN and N2 (i.e., MFN) components. Therefore, it appears that when an actual error is committed, the rostral ACC is additionally engaged.

Because the rostral ACC source appears to be active only after error commission and is best seen in response-locked data, we speculated that the rostral ACC is involved in response monitoring. In contrast, because the MFN is locked to the stimulus and is active when either an error is committed or a feedback is presented, we proposed that the dorsal ACC may be involved in monitoring the action context (Luu et al., 2003). Consistent with the cognitive–affective division, the dorsal ACC tracks parameters of the task (such as feedback and conflicting task demands), and the rostroventral ACC tracks the affective evaluation of response outcomes. Similar results have been obtained using fMRI methodologies. For example, Elliot and Dolan (1998) found dorsal ACC activity when subjects had to formulate a hypothesis about what would constitute a correct response given a set of stimuli. In contrast, the rostral ACC was active only when subjects made a choice.

We (Makeig, Luu, & Tucker, 2002) further investigated this response monitoring/action context duality using independent components analysis (ICA). ICA decomposes the multichannel EEG data by "blind" separation of the single-trial data into independent components that contribute separate information to the data. Makeig and colleagues (2002) found that the ERN is the sum of several components, with one component varying with the actual response and the second varying with the parameters of the task, (i.e., being responsive to target onset, response deadline, and feedback presentation). Although the number of com-

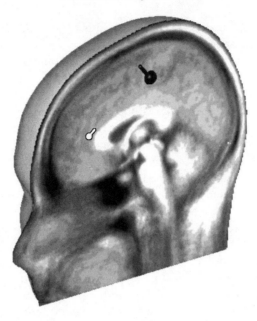

FIGURE 17.2. The generators of the ERN as estimated by equivalent dipoles. The first dipole is located in the rostral ACC and the second dipole is located in the dorsal ACC/supplementary motor area.

ponents contributing to the ERN varies between subjects, they generally can be separated along this response tracking versus context division.

Thus, it appears that the ACC is involved in associating an appropriate response within a given context, monitoring the outcome of the action, and switching behaviors when outcomes are not as expected. We refer to these functions as action regulation. As such, the ERN is expected to index basic learning processes. Current direct evidence for the role of the ERN in learning is limited, but the indirect evidence is compelling. We have reviewed this possibility extensively elsewhere (see Luu & Tucker, 2002, 2004) and provide a brief summary below.

ACTION REGULATION AND LEARNING

Electrophysiological evidence for the involvement of the EEG theta rhythm (4–7 Hz for humans) in learning comes from animal studies. Adey (1967) found that in early stages of learning, when animals were trying to learn the association between a conditioned stimulus and reward, an EEG theta rhythm was prominent and phased-locked to the auditory cue. As the animals' performance marked proficiency on the task, theta amplitude decreased, and this was due to either a loss of phase-locked activity or a modulation of the frequency. However, when the cue was reversed, EEG theta activity reappeared and was again phase-locked to the stimulus.

Buzsáki, Grastyán, Tveritskaya, and Czopf (1979) observed similar effects. When an animal has to remember whether the current stimulus is the same or different from a previous stimulus in order to determine which response to make, Givens (1996) found that EEG theta rhythm recorded in the dentate gyrus became phase-locked to the stimulus. However, when performing a much simpler, well-learned task of stimulus–response mapping, EEG theta activity was not phase-locked to the stimulus.

How to integrate these animal findings with the ERN literature has been difficult until we discovered that the ERN reflects that part of the EEG theta rhythm phase-locked to the response (Luu & Tucker, 2001). We reported that when the ERN data are filtered with a 4–7 Hz bandpass, it is clear that the ERN is but one part of an ongoing midline oscillation, and that when errors are committed this midline oscillation alternates with potentials recorded over the motor cortex, which are also oscillatory in nature. Examining single-trial data, the theta origin of the ERN becomes quite clear: The ERN reflects the phase-locked component of the midline theta rhythm (Luu, Tucker, & Makeig, in press). When phase-locked data are subtracted from total theta activity, leaving nonphase locked activity, differences between error and correct trials are still observed.

When a EEG theta source model, based on the two midline sources identified as necessary to account for a frontal midline theta process (Asada, Fukuda, Tsunoda, Yamaguchi, & Tonoike, 1999), was fitted to the ERN data, the source distribution and phase relation between the sources were almost identical to those obtained for midline theta rhythm (Luu et al., 2003). Neurophysiologically, it has been proposed that the EEG theta rhythm is the mechanism by which distant cortical structures exchange information of local networks (Miller, 1991). If the ERN is integrally related to ongoing EEG theta rhythms, the ERN may index basic learning mechanisms of limbic networks. That is, rather than reflecting the functions of a single ACC region, the ERN may reflect theta coordination of the broader action–regulation functions of the limbic system.

ACTION REGULATION AND AWARENESS

The role of executive attention in awareness was previously discussed by Posner (1994). Here we briefly discuss the electrophysiological evidence regarding the role of awareness in error commission and expectancy violation. Awareness in this context is defined by subjects' report of being aware of either making an error or of the presence of an action–context violation. As noted previously, it was thought that a subject must be aware of making an error at the time of error commission in order to elicit an ERN (Dehaene et al., 1994), and later studies showed that if a subject is not aware of making an error, presentation of an error feedback generated an ERN-like response (Miltner et al., 1997).

Addressing this issue directly, Scheffers and Coles (2000) asked subjects to rate the degree to which they believed a response was correct or in error. These authors found that when subjects rated a correct response as being erroneous, the ERN associated with this response was much larger than ones associated with responses rated as correct. Similarly, those incorrect responses rated as correct elicited smaller ERNs than those error responses rated as incorrect. We attempted to address this issue by examining late responses—that is, responses that are executed correctly but are too late according to an imposed reaction-time (RT) deadline (Luu, Flaisch, & Tucker, 2000). We divided the responses into three levels of lateness, with the logic being that as subjects become increasing late they also become aware of the status of the late response. For example, those responses that barely exceed the RT deadline will not be easily perceived as erroneous compared to those responses that are very late. We found that as subjects became increasingly late in their response, the ERN increased in amplitude. However, the latest responses still elicited a smaller ERN than an ERN associated with an error of commission. This later finding is consistent with subjective experience because in speeded response tasks subjects are immediately aware of committing the wrong response.

Using an antisaccade task and asking subjects to rate whether they were aware of making a saccadic error, Nieuwenhuis, Ridderinkhof, Blom, Band, and Kok (2001) showed that unperceived errors elicited an ERN, a finding that is at odds with the previous two studies. However, it is possible that awareness is not the binary phenomenon Nieuwenhuis and colleagues conceived. It is also possible that awareness of an error is not necessary for eliciting the ERN but that awareness modulates the mediofrontal response to violations of expectancies.

Eimer and colleagues' studies of implicit and explicit serial learning (Eimer et al., 1996; Schlaghecken et al., 2000) help to shed light on this issue. In this task, subjects were required to make rapid responses to letter stimuli that were each mapped to a unique finger response. Participants were not informed of the appearance of a regular series of stimuli but were later sorted into those who reported the existence of a regular sequence of stimuli and those who did not. Periodically, a position in the series was replaced with a deviant stimulus. Behaviorally, RTs on deviant trials and trials following deviant trials were longer than standard trials. The RT slowdown after a deviant trial is similar to the posterror slowing often observed in speeded-response tasks. Subjects who did not report explicit knowledge of the stimulus sequence exhibited less of a slowdown after deviant trials, suggesting that they were less aware that a violation of the context had occurred. Comparing the electrophysiological response, these authors found that deviant stimuli elicited a larger N2 (i.e., MFN) than standard stimuli and that this response was larger in those subjects who were aware of a regular sequence. Thus, it appears that awareness of an error or context violation may not be necessary to elicit the ERN or MFN, but awareness does appear to modulate their amplitudes.

CONCLUSION

There are many theories of ACC function. Common to most theories is the belief that the ACC is engaged when rapid changes in behaviors are required. That is, contributions from the ACC are required when ongoing actions are inadequate or do not match up with current demands. The concept of attention for action is used to describe the cognitive processes that are engaged under situations that require control, although cognitive control may not be implemented by the ACC (see Garavan, Ross, Murphy, Roche, & Stein, 2002; MacDonald, Cohen, Stenger, & Carter, 2000). The results from ERP studies of action monitoring reviewed in this chapter reveal that this concept is still appropriate for describing ACC functions, particularly because it emphasizes the role of action in cognition. It is likely that the ACC has evolved to regulate behaviors such that they are adaptive to sudden changes in the environment and should be important to early stages of learning. Indeed, in animal models of associative learning, the ACC is a critical component of a network responsible for rapid association between a stimulus and a required response (Gabriel, Burhans, Talk, & Scalf, 2002).

We use the construct of action regulation to describe ACC function because it emphasizes the role of the ACC in adapting behaviors to a given context. Recent evidence implicates the ACC in at least three processes involved in action regulation: (1) monitoring context violation (i.e., expectancy violation), (2) monitoring response relative to the context, and (3) evaluating the motivational or affective consequence of the expectancy violations.

These basic functions support adaptive regulation of behaviors and are manifested as learning. The ACC is one structure within this circuit, with the amygdala, mediodorsal nucleus of the thalamus, and the basal ganglia making up the other key structures (Gabriel et al., 2002). The coordinating mechanism of activity between structures within this circuit remains to be elucidated, and we offer the EEG theta rhythm as a strong candidate.

REFERENCES

Adey, W. R. (1967). Intrinisic organization of cerebral tissue in alterting, orienting, and discriminative reponses. In G. C. Quarton, T. Melnechuck, & F. O. Schmitt (Eds.), *The neurosciences* (pp. 615–633). New York: Rockefeller Univerisity Press.

Asada, H., Fukuda, Y., Tsunoda, S., Yamaguchi, M., & Tonoike, M. (1999). Frontal midline theta rhythms reflect alternative activation of prefrontal cortex and anterior cingulate cortex in humans. *Neuroscience Letters, 274,* 29–32.

Balsam, P. D. (1985). The functions of context in learning and performance. In P. D. Balsam & A. Tomie (Eds.), *Context and learning* (pp. 1–22). Hillsdale: Erlbaum.

Bush, G., Luu, P., & Posner, M. I. (2000). Cognitive and emotional influences in anterior cingulate cortex. *Trends in Cognitive Sciences, 4,* 215–222.

Bush, G., Vogt, B. A., Holmes, J., Dale, A. M., Greve, D., Jenike, M. A., et al. (2002). Dorsal anterior cingulate cortex: a role in reward-based decision making. *Proceedings of the National Academy of Sciences USA, 99,* 523–528.

Buzsáki, G., Grastyán, E., Tveritskaya, I. N., & Czopf, J. (1979). Hippocampal evoked potentials and EEG changes during classical conditioning in the rat. *Electroencephalography and Clinical Neurophysiology, 47,* 64–74.

Carter, C. S., Botvinick, M. M., & Cohen, J. D. (1999). The contribution of the anterior cingulate cortex to executive processes in cognition. *Reviews in Neuroscience, 10,* 49–57.

Carter, C. S., Braver, T. S., Barch, D. M., Botvinick, M. M., Noll, D., & Cohen, J. D. (1998). Anterior cingulate cortex, error detection, and the online monitoring of performance. *Science, 280,* 747–749.

Cuffin, B. N., Schomer, D. L., Ives, J. R., & Blume, H. (2001). Experimental tests of EEG source localization accuracy in spherical head models. *Clinical Neurophysiology, 112,* 46–51.

Dehaene, S., Posner, M. I., & Tucker, D. M. (1994). Localization of a neural system for error detection and compensation. *Psychological Science, 5,* 303–305.

Eimer, M., Goschke, T., Schlaghecken, F., & Stürmer, B. (1996). Explicit and implicit learning of event sequences: Evidence from event-related brain potentials. *Journal of Experimental Psychology: Learning, Memory, and Cognition, 22,* 970–987.

Elliot, R., & Dolan, R. J. (1998). Activation of different anterior cingulate foci in association with hypothesis testing and response selection. *NeuroImage, 8,* 17–29.

Falkenstein, M., Hohnsbein, J., Hoormann, J., & Blanke, L. (1991). Effects of crossmodal divided attention on late ERP components. II. Error processing in choice reaction tasks. *Electroencephalography and Clinical Neurophysiology, 78,* 447–455.

Gabriel, M., Burhans, L., Talk, A., & Scalf, P. (2002). Cingulate cortex. In V. S. Ramachandran (Ed.), *Encyclopedia of the human brain* (pp. 775–791): Amsterdam: Elsevier Science.

Garavan, H., Ross, T. J., Murphy, K., Roche, R. A. P., & Stein, E. A. (2002). Dissociable executive functions in the dynamic control of behavior: Inhibition, error detection, and correction. *NeuroImage, 17,* 1820–1829.

Gehring, W. J., Goss, B., Coles, M. G. H., Meyer, D. E., & Donchin, E. (1993). A neural system for error detection and compensation. *Psychological Science, 4,* 385–390.

Gehring, W. J., Himle, J., & Nisenson, L. G. (2000). Action monitoring dysfunction in obsessive-compulsive disorder. *Psychological Science, 11,* 1–6.

Gehring, W. J., & Willoughby, A. R. (2002). The medial frontal cortex and the rapid processing of monetary gains and losses. *Science, 295,* 2279–2282.

Gevins, A. S., Cutillo, B. A., Bressler, S. L., Morgan, N. H., White, R. M., Illes, J., et al. (1989). Event-related covariances during a bimanual visuomotor task. II. Preparation and feedback. *Electroencephalography and Clinical Neurophysiology, 74,* 147–160.

Givens, B. (1996). Stimulus-evoked resetting of the dentate theta rhythm: Relation to working memory. *Neuroreport, 8,* 159–163.

Holroyd, C. B., & Coles, M. G. H. (2002). The basis of human error processing: Reinforcement learning, dopamine, and the error-related negativity. *Psychological Review, 109,* 679–709.

Johannes, S., Wieringa, B. M., Nager, W., Dengler, R., & Münte, T. F. (2001). Oxazepam alters action monitoring. *Psychopharmacology, 155,* 100–106.

Kiehl, K. A., Liddle, P. F., & Hopfinger, J. B. (2000). Error processing and the rostral anterior cingulate: An event-related fMRI study. *Psychophysiology, 37,* 216–223.

Kopp, B., Rist, F., & Mattler, U. (1996). N200 in the flanker task as a neurobehavioral tool for investigating executive control. *Psychophysiology, 33,* 282–294.

Kopp, B., & Wolff, M. (2000). Brain mechanisms of selective learning: event-related potentials provide evidence for error-driven learning in humans. *Biological Psychology, 51,* 223–246.

Laarne, P. H., Tenhunen-Eskelinen, M. L., Hyttinen, J. K., & Eskola, H. J. (2000). Effect of EEG electrode density on dipole localization accuracy using two realistically shaped skull resistivity models. *Brain Topography, 12,* 249–254.

Lantz, G., Grave de Peralta, R., Spinelli, L., Seeck, M., & Michel, C. M. (2003). Epileptic source localization with high density EEG: how many electrodes are needed? *Clinical Neurophysiology, 114,* 63–69.

Luu, P., Collins, P., & Tucker, D. M. (2000). Mood, personality, and self-monitoring: negative affect and emotionality in relation to frontal lobe mechanisms of error monitoring. *Journal of Experimental Psychology: General, 129,* 43–60.

Luu, P., Flaisch, T., & Tucker, D. M. (2000). Medial frontal cortex in action monitoring. *Journal of Neuroscience, 20,* 464–469.

Luu, P., & Tucker, D. M. (2001). Regulating action: Alternating activation of human prefrontal and motor cortical networks. *Clinical Neurophysiology, 112,* 1295–1306.

Luu, P., & Tucker, D. M. (2002). Self-regulation and the executive functions: electrophysiological clues. In A. M. Preverbio (Ed.), *The cognitive electrophysiology of mind and brain* (pp. 199–223). San Diego, CA: Academic Press.

Luu, P., & Tucker, D. M. (2004). Self-regulation by the medial frontal cortex: limbic representation of motive set-points. In M. Beauregard (Ed.), *Consciousness, emotional self-regulation and the brain* (pp. 123–161). Amsterdam: John Benjamin.

Luu, P., Tucker, D. M., Derryberry, D., Reed, M., & Poulsen, C. (2003). Activity in human medial frontal cortex in emotional evaluation and error monitoring. *Psychological Science, 14,* 47–53.

Luu, P., Tucker, D. M., & Makeig, S. (in press). Limbic theta and the error-related negativity: Neurophysiological mechanisms of action regulation. *Clinical Neuropsychology.*

MacDonald, A. W., Cohen, J. D., Stenger, V. A., & Carter, C. S. (2000). Dissociating the role of the dorsolateral prefrontal and anterior cingulate cortex in cognitive control. *Science, 288,* 1835–1838.

Makeig, S., Luu, P., & Tucker, D. M. (2002). *Do "brainstorms" help turn intentions into attentions?* Paper presented at the Human Brain Mapping conference, Sendai, Japan.

Menon, V., Adleman, N. E., White, C. D., Glover, G. H., & Reiss, A. L. (2001). Error-related brain activation during a go/nogo response inhibition task. *Human Brain Mapping, 12,* 131–143.

Miller, R. (1991). *Cortico-hippocampal interplay and the representation of contexts in the brain.* New York: Springer-Verlag.

Miltner, W. H. R., Braun, C. H., & Coles, M. G. H. (1997). Event-related brain potentials following incorrect feedback in a time-estimation task: Evidence for a "generic" neural system for error detection. *Journal of Cognitive Neuroscience, 9,* 787–797.

Nessler, D., & Mecklinger, A. (2003). ERP correlates of true and false recognition after different retention delays: stimulus- and response-related processes. *Psychophysiology, 40,* 146–159.

Nieuwenhuis, S., Ridderinkhof, K. R., Blom, J., Band, G. P., & Kok, A. (2001). Error-related brain potentials are differentially related to awareness of response errors: Evidence from an antisaccade task. *Psychophysiology, 38,* 752–760.

Pailing, P. E., & Segalowitz, S. J. (in press). The error-related negativity (ERN/Ne) as a state and trait measure: Motivation, personality, and ERPs in response to errors. *Psychophysiology.*

Posner, M. I. (1978). *Chronometric explorations of mind.* Hillsdale, NJ: Erlbaum.

Posner, M. I. (1994). Attention: The mechanisms of consciousness. *Proceedings of the National Academy of Sciences USA, 91,* 7398–7403.

Posner, M. I., & Dehaene, S. (1994). Attentional networks. *Trends in Neuroscience, 17,* 75–79.

Posner, M. I., & DiGirolamo, G. (1998). Executive attention: Conflict, target detection and cognitive control. In R. Parasuraman (Ed.), *The attentive brain* (pp. 401–423). Cambridge, MA: MIT Press.

Posner, M. I., Petersen, S. E., Fox, P. T., & Raichle, M. E. (1988). Localization of cognitive operations in the human brain. *Science, 240,* 1627–1631.

Pritchard, W. S., Shappell, S. A., & Brandt, M. E. (1991). Psychophysiology of N200/N400: A review and classification scheme. In P. K. Ackles & M. G. Coles (Eds.), *Advances in psychophysiology* (pp. 43–106). London: Jessica Kingsley.

Rainville, P., Duncan, G. H., Price, D. D., Carrier, B., & Bushnell, C. M. (1997). Pain affect encoded in human anterior cingulate but not somatosensory cortex. *Science, 277,* 968–971.

Ruchsow, M., Grothe, J., Spitzer, M., & Kiefer, M. (2002). Human anterior cingulate cortex is activated by negative feedback: Evidence from event-related potentials in a guessing task. *Neuroscience Letters, 325,* 203–206.

Scheffers, M. K., & Coles, M. G. H. (2000). Performance monitoring in a confusing world: Error-related brain activity, judgments of response accuraccy, and types of errors. *Journal of Experimental Psychology: Human Perception and Performance, 26,* 141–151.

Schlaghecken, F., Stürmer, B., & Eimer, M. (2000). Chunking processes in the learning of event sequences: Electrophysiological indicators. *Memory and Cognition, 28,* 821–831.

Schnider, A., Valenza, N., Morand, S., & Michel, C. M. (2002). Early cortical distinction between memories that pertain to onging reality and memories that don't. *Cerebral Cortex, 12,* 54–61.

Shima, K., & Tanji, J. (1998). Role for cingulate motor area cells in voluntary movement selection based on reward. *Science, 282,* 1335–1338.

Tucker, D. M., Hartry-Speiser, A., McDougal, L., Luu, P., & deGrandpre, D. (1999). Mood and spatial memory: Emotion and the right hemisphere contribution to spatial cognition. *Biological Psychology, 50,* 103–125.

Tucker, D. M., Luu, P., Desmond, R. E., Hartry-Speiser, A. L., Davey, C., & Flaisch, T. (2003). Corticolimbic Mechanisms in Emotional Decisions. *Emotion, 3,* 127–149.

Tucker, D. M., Luu, P., Frishkoff, G., Quiring, J., & Poulsen, C. (2003). Frontolimbic response to negative feedback in clinical depression. *Journal of Abnormal Psychology, 112,* 667–678.

Ullsperger, M., & von Cramon, D. Y. (2001). Subprocesses of performance monitoring: A dissociation of error processing and response competition revealed by event-related fMRI and ERPs. *NeuroImage, 14,* 1387–1401.

van Veen, V., & Carter, C. S. (2002). The timing of action monitoring processes in anterior cingulate cortex. *Journal of Cognitive Neuroscience, 14,* 593–602.

Vogt, B. A., Finch, D. M., & Olson, C. R. (1993). Functional heterogeniety in the cingulate cortex: The anterior executive and posterior evaluative regions. *Cerebral Cortex, 2,* 435–443.

IV

SYNAPTIC AND GENETIC STUDIES

18

Molecular Genetics of Visuospatial Attention and Working Memory

Raja Parasuraman and Pamela Greenwood

A long-held goal of psychology is to understand how genetic variation contributes to individual differences in behavior, through interaction with development, learning, and other environmental factors. A century ago, Spearman (1904) observed that individuals who do well on one test of intellectual functioning (e.g., verbal ability) tend to do well on others (e.g., memory and general reasoning). He argued that this was evidence of a general cognitive ability or g, which has since been shown in numerous studies to be highly heritable (Plomin, DeFries, McClearn, & McGuffin, 2001). Despite this, little is known of the particular genes underlying the heritability not only of g but also the equally heritable cognitive functions that contribute to g. However, with the recent specification of the human genome (Ventner et al., 2001), the individual genes contributing to specific cognitive functions have become the object of intensive investigation.

In this chapter we discuss the molecular genetics of two aspects of cognition: visuospatial attention and working memory. We also consider the effects of genetic variation in these cognitive domains in relation to adult aging. Attention provides a useful model system to examine for a number of reasons. First, the neural basis of attention—in terms of the associated brain networks and their neurochemical innervation—has become increasingly well specified in recent years (Everitt & Robbins, 1997; Parasuraman, 1998; Posner & Petersen, 1990), thereby allowing close ties to be forged to emerging findings from molecular genetics. In addition, some components of attention have been shown to be heritable in twin studies (Fan, Wu, Fossella, & Posner, 2001; Swan & Carmelli, 2002). These components of attention are also markedly affected, although in different ways, by normal aging as well as by Alzheimer's disease (AD) and related dementias (Greenwood & Parasuraman, 1997; Parasuraman & Greenwood, 1998).

THE ALLELIC ASSOCIATION APPROACH
TO THE GENETICS OF COGNITION

Much of what we know about the genetics of cognition has come from twin studies in which identical and fraternal twins are compared to assess the heritability of a trait. The twin paradigm, which has been the methodological workhorse of behavioral genetics for the past century, is powerful for showing the *existence and degree* of genetic influence for a particular trait. However, this approach cannot identify the *particular genes* involved in that trait. Recent advances in molecular genetics now allow a different, complementary approach to behavioral genetics, that of *allelic association*. Most commonly used to associate the likelihood of disease with candidate genes, the allelic association method can also be used to relate specific genes to behavioral performance measures in healthy persons (Plomin & Crabbe, 2000). This method has been recently applied to the study of individual differences in cognition in healthy individuals, revealing evidence of modulation of cognitive task performance by specific genes (Fan et al., 2001; Fossella, Posner, Fan, Swanson, & Pfaff, 2001; Fossella et al., 2002; Greenwood, Sunderland, Friz, & Parasuraman, 2000).

Our approach combines the allelic association method of behavioral genetics with the methods of modern cognitive neuroscience. Figure 18.1 shows a general schema of the approach. Such an approach allows for theory-based, empirical analysis of the role of particular polymorphic genes in cognition. Allelic association requires identification of candidate genes—genes deemed likely to influence a given cognitive ability or trait due to the func-

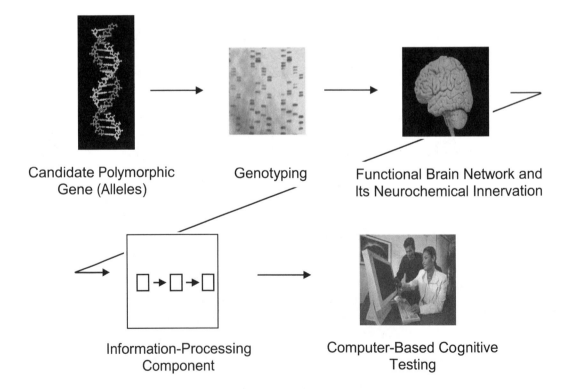

Candidate Polymorphic Gene (Alleles)

Genotyping

Functional Brain Network and Its Neurochemical Innervation

Information-Processing Component

Computer-Based Cognitive Testing

FIGURE 18.1. Molecular genetics of cognition: The allelic association approach.

tional role of each gene's protein product in the brain. The completion of the Human Genome Project (Ventner et al., 2001) and the attendant burgeoning literature on the function of individual genes and single nucleotide polymorphisms (SNPs) permits investigation into the genetics of cognition at the level of individual genes. We illustrate this approach by considering its application to the role of specific genes in individual differences in visuospatial attention and working memory.

More than 99% of individual DNA sequences in the human genome do not differ between individuals and hence are of limited interest in investigating individual differences in normal cognition. However, a few DNA base pairs (bp) occur in different forms or alleles. Allelic variation is due to slight differences in the chain of nucleic acids making up the gene—commonly the result of a substitution of one nucleotide for another—a SNP. Consequently, the protein whose production is directed by that gene is correspondingly altered. SNPs occur at a rate of about 1 in every 1,000 bp in unrelated individuals. There are thought to be about 1.8 million SNPs, but only about 5–10% of these are likely to be associated with disease (Plomin et al., 2001).

Polymorphisms can influence brain function through effects with a range of specificities. At one extreme, the effects may be limited to one receptor type involving a particular neurotransmitter. Such effects are likely to be more specific than those involving whole-brain effects, such as genes that have broad-based effects on neuron health.

The goal of determining the role of a particular gene in a given cognitive phenotype poses a challenge. Even given that SNPs with functional significance for behavior represent only a small part of the human genome, there are still so many of them that forging valid links to cognition may prove difficult. However, the general problem of establishing a reliable association between genotype and phenotype may be mitigated by using the allelic association approach within a theoretical framework in which the "intermediate steps" between genotype and phenotype (see Figure 18.2) are specified (to a degree). Such a framework can capitalize on the breakthroughs in understanding the neural bases of cognition that have been made possible by modern cognitive neuroscience. Although no such broad framework for all of cognition currently exists, enough is known to begin to undertake such an approach for particular cognitive domains. For example, Posner has proposed an influential "attentional network" theory in which three separate attentional functions—orienting, alerting, and executive function—are linked to the activation of separate but overlapping cortical and subcortical networks (Posner & Petersen, 1990). Posner and colleagues have also argued that performance on psychological tests of these attentional functions can serve as phenotypes against which candidate genes can be tested (Fan et al., 2001; Fan, Fossella, Sommer, Wu, & Posner, 2003; Fossella et al., 2002). We have also argued that specific information-processing tests aimed at particular attentional functions can serve as behavioral assays of the integrity of mediating cortical networks, thereby allowing for assessment of the effects of the underlying genes (Greenwood et al., 2000; Parasuraman, Greenwood, & Sunderland, 2002) as well of the effects of neurodegeneration on these networks (Parasuraman & Greenwood, 1998).

The neurochemical innervation of brain networks subserving particular cognitive functions are being increasingly well specified (Everitt & Robbins, 1997; Goldman-Rakic, 1998). For example, with respect to attentional function, a growing body of evidence from lesion and electrophysiological studies in animals and neuroimaging and pharmacological studies in humans points to the role of cholinergically mediated posterior brain networks in spatial attention and dopaminergically rich frontal networks in executive attention. It therefore follows that if progress is also made in delineating the genes and their protein

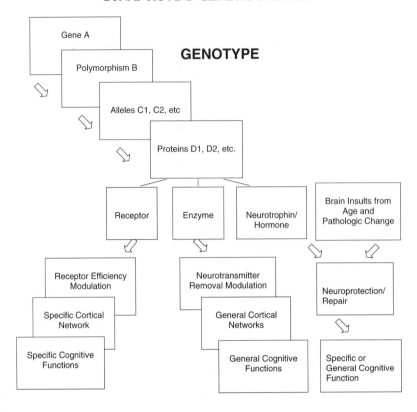

PHENOTYPE

FIGURE 18.2. Schematic of the relation between a hypothetical gene with a behaviorally relevant polymorphism and specific or general effects on cognition. The possible "intermediate steps" between genotype and phenotype are indicated.

products that influence these neurochemical pathways, links can be established between genes and different aspects of cognitive function. Figure 18.2 provides an illustration of these links.

As Figure 18.2 indicates, the protein products of particular genes can affect cognition through a number of pathways, including receptor modulation, neurotransmitter modulation, or neuroprotection. Genes with a role in neuroprotection and neuronal repair may be particularly important in aging and following brain injury. Chemical neurotransmitters, such as dopamine and acetylcholine, bind to specialized receptors on postsynaptic sites. This binding causes the ion channel in the receptor to open with the ensuing ion flow through the receptor channel producing the neuronal signal. Variations in receptor structure as a consequence of minor variations in the corresponding gene have been shown to affect the efficiency of receptor transmission (e.g., Steinlein et al., 1997). Even after a neurotransmitter is released into the synapse, its physiological fate can be influenced by genes. There is a need for efficient removal of a neurotransmitter from the synaptic cleft because continued exposure of receptors to transmitter can desensitize the receptors. Neurotransmitters can be removed from the cleft by diffusion, by enzyme degradation, and by reuptake. The latter two mechanisms are controlled by genes.

The polymorphisms known to exist in brain dopaminergic and cholinergic systems generally involve receptor and transporter molecules. A polymorphism in a gene controlling part of a specific receptor type would at least initially only affect neurotransmission through that receptor type. In contrast, a polymorphism in a gene controlling an enzyme which degrades a family of neurotransmitters could have broader effects. A third category of genes plays a role in neuroprotection and thus can have either specific or broad effects.

In summary, our approach involves several methods.

Genotyping for Candidate Polymorphic Genes (Alleles)

Once a candidate polymorphism has been identified, individuals are genotyped for the polymorphism from DNA extracted from buccal (cheek) tissue samples for polymerase chain reaction–based assays. This method is safe and reliable and provides a convenient, low-cost alternative to blood samples for obtaining genomic DNA (Richards et al., 1993). In our lab we use the MasterAMP Buccal Swab DNA Extraction Kit (Epicentre Technologies, Madison, WI). It is no longer necessary to have an in-house genotyping facility because recent advances in the field of nucleic acid measurement technology have lowered the cost and increased the ease and speed for the reliable assay of specific genetic polymorphisms. Commercial genotyping services obtain reliable genotypes from buccal swabs using mass spectroscopy for approximately $2.50/genotype with extremely high throughput.

Identification of a Functional Brain Network and Its Neurochemical Innervation

This is a fundamental assumption of the approach. It is assumed that normal genetic variation in neurotransmitter genes can lead to individual differences in cognitive functions that are measurable behaviorally. Allelic variation results in differences between individuals in the level, rate of transport or clearance, or regulation of neurotransmitters and enzymes. Such differences are important for the efficient activation of a functional brain network and can lead to differences in the cognitive function mediated by that network.

Identification of Information-Processing Components of Cognition

The cognitive neuroscience literature is used to link particular components of cognition to the functional brain network and its neurochemical innervation (e.g., executive attention and working memory to the dopaminergic prefrontal cortex). It is assumed that individual differences in the efficiency of these processing components—reflected in performance measures—are the result of variations in the activation of the underlying functional brain network.

Computer-Based Cognitive Testing

Finally, participants who have been previously genotyped (as in step 1) for a specific polymorphism are tested on well-validated, theoretically derived, information-processing tests developed on the basis of prior research as in step 3.

There are some limitations in the combined allelic association/cognitive neuroscience approach outlined here. No component of cognition is likely to be modified by only one gene and the interpretation of individual differences in a particular cognitive function will ultimately involve specification of the role of many genes as well as environmental factors (Plomin & Crabbe, 2000). It is also important that SNPs or other candidate genes are chosen in a theory-based manner for their functional significance for cognition, to minimize the probability of type I error in finding gene–cognition links. Nevertheless, as discussed herein, certain genes appear to contribute in relatively specific ways to individual differences in aspects of cognition. By using this approach, the knowledge of cognitive neuroscience can be brought to bear on molecular genetics in order to begin to specify the links between genotypes and their expression in phenotypes, as shown in Figure 18.2.

We illustrate our approach by considering the role of neurotransmitter genes, dopaminergic and cholinergic, in modulating individual differences in attention and working memory. We also examine the role of a gene that has more broad-based effects on neuronal health, the apolipoprotein E (APOE) gene, and also consider its role in cognitive aging (for a more detailed review, see Greenwood and Parasuraman, 2003).

NEUROTRANSMITTER RECEPTOR GENES

Dopaminergic Genes

Dopaminergic receptor genes are likely candidates for genetic effects on attention due to the importance of dopaminergic innervation for working memory and executive functions. Dopamine agents have been shown to modulate working memory in monkeys (Sawaguchi & Goldman-Rakic, 1991) and humans (Muller, von Cramon, & Pollmann, 1998), and dopaminergic receptor genes have been linked to aspects of attention (Faraone, Doyle, Mick, & Biederman, 2001). Executive attention involves a complex of functions, including conflict resolution, difficult processing, and multitasking (Posner & DiGirolamo, 1998), as well as the process by which contents of memory storage are used in planning and execution of tasks (Smith & Jonides, 1999). This aspect of attention appears to depend on prefrontal cortex (PFC). Dopamine plays an important role not only in PFC-mediated processes of working memory but also in hippocampal inputs to that region (Gurden, Jakita, & Jay, 2000). In humans, the binding potential of DRD1 but not D2 dopamine receptors modulates working-memory performance (Abi-Dargham et al., 2002). Drug-induced blockade of D2 receptors down-regulates DRD1 receptors in PFC and impairs working memory—both reversible by administration of a D1 agonist (Castner, Williams, & Goldman-Rakic, 2000). Thus, genes with a role in the dopaminergic system are good candidates for modulation of working memory.

Several studies have found components of executive control to be highly heritable (Fan et al., 2001; Swan & Carmelli, 2002). Dopaminergic innervation of the mediators of executive control and working memory in PFC suggests that a contributor to that heritability could be genes that control the dopaminergic degradation pathway, such as the COMT (Egan et al., 2001) and DRD4 genes (Fossella et al., 2002). Another candidate is the DBH gene, which is involved in converting dopamine to norepinephrine in adrenergic vesicles (Kohnke et al., 2002). A polymorphism in the DBH gene, a G to A substitution at 444, exon 2 (G444A) on chromosome 9, has been associated with familial cases of attention deficit hyperactivity disorder (Daly, Hawi, Fitzgerald, & Gill, 1999). We therefore examined its role in attention and working memory (Greenwood, Fossella, & Parasuraman, 2003).

We genotyped a group of healthy adults ages 18–68 years for the G444A polymorphism of the DBH gene and tested them on tasks of working memory and visuospatial attention (described later). This is a functional polymorphism, as the A allele is associated with

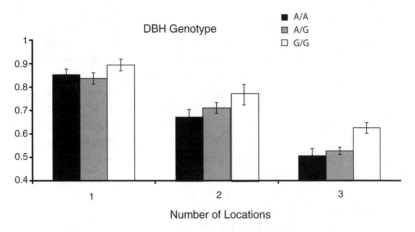

FIGURE 18.3. Effects of allelic variation in the DBH gene on match accuracy as a function of number of spatial locations to be maintained in working memory. From Greenwood, Fossella, and Parasuraman (2003). Reprinted by permission of the authors.

lower plasma and cerebrospinal fluid (CSF) DBH levels, and the G allele with higher DBH levels (Cubells et al., 2000). The working-memory task involved maintaining a representation of up to three spatial locations over a period of 3 seconds. After a fixation cross, participants were shown target circles at one to three locations. Following a 3-second delay during which the circles disappeared, participants had to decide whether a test circle presented at a location was one of the original target locations (match) or not (mismatch). Matching accuracy decreased as the number of locations to be maintained in working memory increased. More important, accuracy was lower for individuals with one A allele compared to those with none, and lower still for those with two A alleles (Figure 18.3). This "gene dose" effect of the A allele was particularly marked at the highest memory load (three locations). At the same time, individual differences in performance of a visuospatial attention task (described later) were not significantly related to allelic variation in the DBH gene. Thus, this pattern of results (single dissociation) is suggestive of a specific link between the DBH gene, plasma DBH levels, and working memory.

Cholinergic Genes

Cholinergic genes are also good candidates for examining genetic contributions to attention. Cholinergic receptors are known to modulate neuronal function in hippocampus and parietal cortex (Xiang, Huguenard, & Prince, 1998). Although a majority of cholinergic receptors are muscarinic, nicotinic receptors are important in regulating fast synaptic transmission (Alkondon, Pereira, Eisenberg, & Albuquerque, 2000). This may underlie the important functional role that nicotinic receptors play in attention (Levin & Simon, 1998). Nicotinic acetylcholine receptors are composed of subunits that assemble together to form the receptor itself. There are seven alpha-like subunits (alpha-2 to 7 and alpha-9) and three beta-like subunits (beta-2, beta-3, and beta-4). The most widely distributed nicotinic receptor in the central nervous system is composed of alpha-4 and beta-2 subunits assembled together (Flores, DeCamp, Kilo, Rogers, & Hargreaves, 1996). Another major nicotine receptor consists of alpha-7 subunits assembled together.

Polymorphisms in cholinergic receptor subunit genes have functional consequences for behavior. A polymorphism in the gene controlling the alpha-4 subunit, CHRNA4, has been linked to cortical excitability in the P50 defect in schizophrenics (Freedman et al., 1997) as well as to performance on a sustained attention task (Cullum et al., 1993). The lack of an association of the CHRNA7 gene with attention-deficit/hyperactivity disorder (ADHD) (Kent et al., 2001) and the absence of the P50 defect in adults with ADHD (Olincy et al., 2000) suggests that the effects of this polymorphism are not general. However, the number of studies in this area is as yet small, and further work is needed to determine the specificity of the observed cognitive effects of both of these nicotinic receptor polymorphisms.

To examine the role of the CHRNA4 gene, we used a visuospatial attention task as well as the working-memory task described earlier (Greenwood, Fossella, & Parasuraman, 2003). This gene is expressed in parietal cortex, which is known to mediate visuospatial attention (Corbetta, 1998; Corbetta, Kincade, Ollinger, McAvoy, & Shulman, 2000; Nobre et al., 1997). The same sample of participants who were genotyped for the DBH gene were also typed for CHRNA4, specifically for a T to C exchange polymorphism (T1545C) (Steinlein et al., 1997). In the visuospatial attention task, an arrow cue indicated which of two locations to the left or right of fixation would contain a letter target. Following a cue-target delay of 200–2,000 msec, the target letter appeared. Participants were required to make a speeded decision as to whether the target was a consonant or vowel. Cue validity (valid, invalid, neutral) was varied so that both benefits (neutral cue RT–valid cue RT) and costs (invalid cue RT–neutral cue RT) of cueing could be obtained, following the procedure developed by Posner (1980). Both reaction time (RT) benefits of valid cues and RT costs of invalid cues on letter discrimination varied in a systematic manner with CHRNA4 genotype (Figure 18.4) but not with DBH genotype. With an increased "gene dose" of the C allele (from 0 to 1 to 2 C alleles), RT benefits increased progressively (Figure 18.4A) whereas RT costs decreased, also in a similarly progressive manner (Figure 18.4B). These systematic results provide the first evidence of a specific role for the CHRNA4 polymorphism in visuospatial attention.

When the results for the DBH and CHRNA4 genes are taken together, they provide converging evidence for the relative roles of different neurotransmitter genes. Working memory—measured in the ability to retain memory for a spatial location over a 3-second delay, was modulated by DBH genotype (Figure 18.3) but was unaffected by CHRNA4 genotype. Visuospatial attention—assessed using a cued letter-discrimination task, was affected by CHRNA4 (Figure 18.4) but not by DBH. Thus, a double dissociation was observed with visuospatial attention modulated by a cholinergic but not a dopaminergic gene and spatial working memory modulated by a dopaminergic but not a cholinergic gene.

THE APOE GENE

The genes discussed thus far are involved in controlling relatively specific aspects of neurotransmission. Those genes whose protein products are receptor subunits—such as the CHRNA4 and CHRNA7 subunits—exert effects on the particular cholinergic receptor of which their subunit is a part. Effects of variation in subunit genes can be predicted to be greatest on networks mediated by the particular neurotransmitter. More general effects may be exerted by genes controlling the enzymes that degrade neurotransmitters following release, such as DBH and COMT. A third category of genetic effects on cognition involves genes that exert their effects on neuron health and plasticity and thus may play a role in pro-

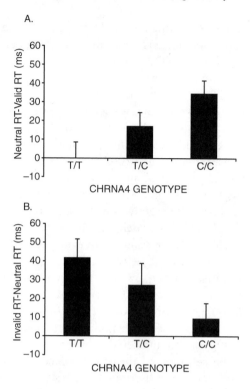

FIGURE 18.4. Effects of allelic variation in the CHRNA4 gene on visuospatial attention as a function of validity of cue location. (A) Benefits of valid cues (neutral RT – valid RT). (B) Costs of invalid cues (invalid RT – neutral RT). From Greenwood, Fossella, and Parasuraman (2003). Reprinted by permission of the authors.

cesses of neuroprotection following injury and aging. Such genes exert broad effects on cognition, consistent with their apparently widespread sites of action.

The best-known gene in this category is APOE, which is involved in cholesterol transport and strongly linked to AD risk (Corder et al., 1993). The APOE gene has also been linked to poorer prognosis in other neurodegenerative disorders, such as multiple sclerosis (Fazekas et al., 2001) and amyotrophic lateral sclerosis (Drory, Birnbaum, Korczyn, & Chapman, 2001), suggesting that it has broad effects on neuronal health and plasticity.

The polymorphic APOE gene on chromosome 19 occurs as one of three alleles (ϵ2, ϵ3, and ϵ4), with mean frequencies in the general population of about 8%, 78%, and 14%, respectively (Utermann, Langenbeck, Beisiegel, & Weber, 1980). The ϵ4 allele modifies risk of AD in a "gene dose" manner, increasing with the number of ϵ4 alleles inherited from both parents, from 0 (noncarriers), to 1 (heterozygotes), to 2 (homozygotes) (Corder et al., 1993). While 34–65% of individuals with AD carry the APOE ϵ4 allele, it is present in only approximately 24–31% of the nonaffected adult population (Saunders et al., 1993). It has been repeatedly confirmed that carriers of the ϵ4 allele are at increased risk of developing AD (Henderson et al., 1995; Katzman et al., 1997).

The product of the APOE gene is a plasma protein involved in the transport of cholesterol and other hydrophobic molecules. APOE is the principal apolipoprotein in the brain and its role as a lipid carrier may allow it to remove lipids from degenerating cells and supply lipid for growing neuronal processes (Rebeck et al., 1998). It has been postulated that glia recycle cholesterol from degenerating terminals, combine it with APOE, and supply it to neurons actively engaged in remodeling synapses and extending dendrites (Poirier, 1994). In support of this view, a complex of APOE and cholesterol has recently been identified as a strong promoter of synapse development (Ullian, Sapperstein, Christopherson, & Barres, 2001). Following injury to hippocampal neurons, an increase in ε4 allele expression was associated with decreased neuronal sprouting, while an increase in ε4 expression was associated with increased neuronal sprouting (Teter et al., 2002).

The APOE gene has been linked to cognitive changes in healthy adults in a growing number of studies (see Parasuraman et al., 2002, for a review). The ε4 allele is linked to faster decline in IQ from age 11 to age 80 in normal individuals (Deary et al., 2002). Furthermore, the ε4 allele has been associated with cortical hypometabolism (Reiman et al., 1996) and altered cerebral blood flow activation patterns related to task performance in healthy adults (Smith et al., 1999). This evidence suggests that the APOE gene begins to impact cognitive integrity in adulthood, consistent with evidence that APOE has a role in brain neuronal health and repair (Arendt et al., 1997).

To examine this hypothesis further, we examined changes in components of visuo-spatial attention and working memory in a sample of middle-age adults (mean age = 58 years) genotyped for the APOE gene (Greenwood et al., 2000). The same test of visuospatial attention (letter discrimination) described earlier, as well as a cued visual search task (Greenwood & Parasuraman, 1999) was administered. These tasks were chosen because we had previously found them to be sensitive to the effects of early-stage AD (Parasuraman & Greenwood, 1998). On the cued letter-discrimination task, carriers of the APOE-ε4 allele were particularly slow to respond when the location precue was invalid. On the cued visual search task, APOE-ε4 carriers showed reduced effects of precue precision compared to noncarriers. These results are particularly noteworthy because the pattern of attentional impairment in this healthy, nondemented sample of APOE-ε4 carriers was qualitatively (but not quantitatively) the same as those observed in older patients clinically diagnosed with AD (Greenwood, Parasuraman, & Alexander, 1997; Parasuraman, Greenwood, Haxby, & Grady, 1992).

In a follow-up study, we confirmed and extended these results (Greenwood, Lambert, Sunderland, & Parasuraman, in press). The tasks were the letter-discrimination task, the working-memory task described earlier in the DBH and CHRNA4 studies, and a task combining location cueing with spatial working memory. We observed that the ability to (1) redirect visuospatial attention, (2) retain memory for location, and (3) benefit from precue precision in retention of memory for location were each affected by gene dose (0, 1, or 2) of the APOE-e4 allele. Thus all three tasks were influenced by the APOE genotype, although there were some differences in the magnitude and pattern of effects across tasks. In general, APOE genotype affected component processes of several cognitive domains in a group of healthy, middle-age adults, only some of whom are likely to develop AD later in life (Henderson et al., 1995). This is consistent with the emergence in adulthood of a cognitive phenotype of the APOE-ε4 allele.

DISCUSSION AND CONCLUSIONS

We have outlined an approach to investigating the molecular genetics of cognition that combines the allelic association paradigm of behavioral genetics with the methods of cognitive neuroscience. The approach allows for theory-based, empirical analysis of the role of particular polymorphic genes in cognition. The overall approach, as illustrated in Figures 18.1 and 18.2, involves several steps, from the selection of candidate SNPs or other genetic polymorphisms to the identification of functional brain networks and their neurochemical innervation to the use of information-processing tasks as behavioral assays of the activation of these networks.

The utility of this approach was shown in analyses of individual differences in two areas of cognition—visuospatial attention and working memory. Specifically, application of the approach provided evidence for a double dissociation in gene–cognition links: Individual differences in visuospatial attention were related to allelic variation in CHRNA4 but not DBH gene, whereas working memory was modulated by CHRNA4 but not a DBH. The relatively specific effects of the CHRNA4 and DBH genes may be consistent with the role of these genes as neurotransmitter receptor modulators. In contrast, allelic variation in the APOE gene was shown to be related to changes in both visuospatial attention and working memory, and in studies in other labs, to other aspects of cognition (see Parasuraman et al., 2002, for a review). These broader effects are consistent with a putative role of APOE and other neuroprotective genes in processes of neuronal repair and health.

It has been known for some time that genetic variation at the level of single polymorphisms can affect cognition, but mainly in the context of devastating brain disorders such as Huntington's disease and AD. The question we addressed in this chapter was whether, in the absence of frank disorder, some polymorphisms modulate cognitive function within normal limits. The evidence suggests that they do. Hence, one main conclusion is that allelic variation in specific single genes can be reliably linked to individual differences in particular components of cognition in healthy adults. However, much remains to be learned about the specificity, generality, and replicability of the effects reported to date.

The single-gene approach can be criticized on the grounds that there could be increased likelihood of type I error. A basis for such criticism is that findings from studies of *disease* often do not replicate. In a recent large-scale meta-analysis of 36 genes in 370 genetic association studies, Ioannidis, Ntzani, Trikalinos, and Contopoulos-Ioannidis (2001) found that the strongest effects were usually seen by the first study reporting an association between a particular gene and a given disease. The authors suggested both publication bias and population diversity as factors. Therefore, evidence from initial association studies needs to be replicated so that type I errors can be avoided. Of course, the conclusions of Ionnidis and colleagues may apply primarily to association studies of disease, in which a gene is linked to the presence or absence of a diagnostic category. Whether single-gene studies of normal cognition, in which genes are linked to continuous variation in a cognitive phenotype, are subject to the same limitation is not presently known, because only a few such studies have been conducted. In addition, as discussed previously, a theory-driven approach to selection of candidate genotypes, as opposed to one based on an open search of the human genome, can serve to limit the probability of such false positives. Nevertheless, the possibility must be entertained, particularly if findings are not replicated.

In addition to consideration of type I error and effect size, cognitive phenotypes used in allelic association studies must also be chosen on the basis of high heritability and reliability. Unfortunately, in contrast to phenotypes developed by psychometricians, such as IQ, for which there is evidence of both high heritabilility and high reliability (Plomin et al., 2001), cognitive psychologists who have developed information-processing tests have not typically paid much attention to these issues. However, this is not to say that there is no such evidence. The spatial attention task developed by Posner (1980) has been shown in a twin study to have moderate heritability (Fan et al., 2001). Furthermore, in unpublished work we have found high test–retest reliabilities for the spatial attention tasks used in the genetic studies described in this chapter.

Another critical issue in the allelic association approach that needs to be addressed is the effect size associated with single-gene studies. If the APOE literature can be taken as an example, most studies of elderly APOE-ε4 carriers do consistently find cognitive deficits and studies of middle-age APOE-ε4 carriers similarly find reliable evidence either of cognitive deficits or brain change. Effect sizes typically range from 0.14–0.4 in the APOE studies. However, APOE may exert an unusually strong influence, and effect sizes for other genes may be smaller. The issue needs to be addressed empirically. Nevertheless, it is encouraging to note that other polymorphisms have been shown to have effects on cognition with medium to large effect sizes. For example, the effect sizes in the results for neurotransmitter receptor genes that we reported were .19 for the DBH gene and .3 for the CHRNA4 gene, and Egan and colleagues (2001) reported an effect size of .41 in their study of the COMT gene and executive function.

Individual differences in cognition have long been recognized. The small but emergent and growing literature using the allelic association approach indicates that such individual differences may owe something to what is viewed as normal genetic variation. Future work assessing genetic effects on cognitive processes would benefit from selecting genes based on links to known brain networks, as in the genetic studies of visuospatial attention and working memory reviewed in this chapter. Such links can provide a reliable foundation for relating particular genetic polymorphisms to cognition.

ACKNOWLEDGMENT

Preparation of this chapter was supported by Grant No. R01 AG19653 from the National Institute on Aging.

REFERENCES

Abi-Dargham, A., Mawlawi, O., Lombardo, I., Gil, R., Martinez, D., Huang, Y., et al. (2002). Prefrontal dopamine D1 receptors and working memory in schizophrenia. *Journal of Neuroscience, 22,* 3708–3719.

Alkondon, M., Pereira, E. F., Eisenberg, H. M., & Albuquerque, E. X. (2000). Nicotinic receptor activation in human cerebral cortical interneurons: A mechanism for inhibition and disinhibition of neuronal networks. *Journal of Neuroscience, 20,* 66–75.

Arendt, T., Schindler, C., Bruckner, M. K., Eschrich, K., Bigl, V., Zedlick, D., et al. (1997). Plastic neuronal remodeling is impaired in patients with Alzheimer's disease carrying apolipoprotein epsilon 4 allele. *Journal of Neuroscience, 17,* 516–529.

Castner, S. A., Williams, G. V., & Goldman-Rakic, P. S. (2000). Reversal of antipsychotic-induced working memory deficits by short-term dopamine D1 receptor stimulation. *Science, 287,* 2020–2022.

Corbetta, M. (1998). Frontoparietal cortical networks for directing attention and the eye to visual locations: Identical, independent, or overlapping neural systems? *Proceedings of the National Academy of Sciences USA, 95,* 831–838.

Corbetta, M., Kincade, J. M., Ollinger, J. M., McAvoy, M. P., & Shulman, G. L. (2000). Voluntary orienting is dissociated from target detection in human posterior parietal cortex. *Nature Neuroscience, 3*(3), 292–297.

Corder, E. H., Saunders, A. M., Strittmatter, W. J., Schmechel, D. E., Gaskell, P. C., Small, G. W., et al.

(1993). Gene dose of Apolipoprotein E type 4 allele and the risk of Alzheimer's disease in late onset families. *Science, 261,* 921–923.

Cubells, J. F., Kranzler, H. R., McCance-Katz, E., Anderson, G. M., Malison, R. T., Price, L. H., et al. (2000). A haplotype at the DBH locus, associated with low plasma dopamine beta-hydroxylase activity, also associates with cocaine-induced paranoia. *Molecular Psychiatry, 5*(1), 56–63.

Cullum, C. M., Harris, J. G., Waldo, M. C., Smernoff, E., Madison, A., Nagamoto, H. T., et al. (1993). Neurophysiological and neuropsychological evidence for attentional dysfunction in schizophrenia. *Schizophrenia Research, 10*(2), 131–141.

Daly, G., Hawi, Z., Fitzgerald, M., & Gill, M. (1999). Mapping susceptibility loci in attention deficit hyperactivity disorder: Preferential transmission of parental alleles at DAT1, DBH and DRD5 to affected children. *Molecular Psychiatry, 4*(2), 192–196.

Deary, I. J., Whiteman, M. C., Pattie, A., Starr, J. M., Hayward, C., Wright, A. F., et al. (2002). Ageing: Cognitive change and the APOE varepsilon 4 allele. *Nature, 418,* 932.

Drory, V. E., Birnbaum, M., Korczyn, A. D., & Chapman, J. (2001). Association of APOE epsilon4 allele with survival in amyotrophic lateral sclerosis. *Journal of Neurological Science, 190*(1–2), 17–20.

Egan, M. F., Goldberg, T. E., Kolachana, B. S., Callicott, J. H., Mazzanti, C. M., Straub, R. E., et al. (2001). Effect of COMT Val108/158 Met genotype on frontal lobe function and risk for schizophrenia. *Proceedings of the National Academy of Sciences USA, 98*(12), 6917–6922.

Everitt, B. J., & Robbins, T. W. (1997). Central cholinergic systems and cognition. *Annual Review of Psychology, 48,* 649–684.

Fan, J., Fossella, J. A., Sommer, T., Wu, Y., & Posner, M. I. (2003). Mapping the genetic variation of attention onto brain activity. *Proceedings of the National Academy of Sciences USA, 100,* 7406–7411.

Fan, J., Wu, Y., Fossella, J. A., & Posner, M. I. (2001). Assessing the heritability of attentional networks. *BMC Neuroscience, 2*(1), 14–18.

Faraone, S. V., Doyle, A. E., Mick, E., & Biederman, J. (2001). Meta-analysis of the association between the 7–repeat allele of the dopamine D(4) receptor gene and attention deficit hyperactivity disorder. *American Journal of Psychiatry, 158*(7), 1052–1057.

Fazekas, F., Strasser-Fuchs, S., Kollegger, H., Berger, T., Kristoferitsch, W., Schmidt, H., et al. (2001). Apolipoprotein E epsilon 4 is associated with rapid progression of multiple sclerosis. *Neurology, 57*(5), 853–857.

Flores, C. M., DeCamp, R. M., Kilo, S., Rogers, S. W., & Hargreaves, K. M. (1996). Neuronal nicotinic receptor expression in sensory neurons of the rat trigeminal ganglion: Demonstration of alpha3beta4, a novel subtype in the mammalian nervous system. *Journal of Neuroscience, 16,* 7892–7901.

Fossella, J., Posner, M. I., Fan, J., Swanson, J. M., & Pfaff, D. W. (2001). Attentional phenotypes for the analysis of higher mental function. *Scientific World, 2,* 217–223.

Fossella, J., Sommer, T., Fan, J., Wu, Y., Swanson, J. M., Pfaff, D. W., et al. (2002). Assessing the molecular genetics of attention networks. *BMC Neuroscience, 3*(1), 14.

Freedman, R., Coon, H., Myles-Worsley, M., Orr-Urtreger, A., Olincy, A., Davis, A., et al. (1997). Linkage of a neurophysiological deficit in schizophrenia to a chromosome 15 locus. *Proceedings of the National Academy of Sciences USA, 94*(2), 587–592.

Goldman-Rakic, P. S. (1998). The cortical dopamine system: Role in memory and cognition. *Advances in Pharmacology, 42,* 707–711.

Greenwood, P. M., Fossella, J. F., & Parasuraman, R. (2003, April). *Double dissociation of modulation of visuospatial attention and working memory by normal allelic variation in cholinergic and dopaminergic genes.* Paper presented at the annual meeting of the Cognitive Neuroscience Society, New York City.

Greenwood, P., Lambert, J. C., Sunderland, T., & Parasuraman, R. (2003). *Evidence for a "cognitive" phenotype of the apolipoprotein Ee4 allele in healthy middle-aged adults: Effects on spatial attention, working memory, and their interaction.* Manuscript submitted for publication.

Greenwood, P. M., & Parasuraman, R. (1997). Attention in aging and Alzheimer's disease: Behavior and neural systems. In J. A. Burack & J. T. Enns (Eds.), *Attention, development and psychopathology* (pp. 288–317). New York: Guilford Press.

Greenwood, P. M., & Parasuraman, R. (1999). Scale of attentional focus in visual search. *Perception and Psychophysics, 61,* 837–859

Greenwood, P., & Parasuraman, R. (2003). Normal genetic variation, cognition, and aging. *Behavioral and Cognitive Neuroscience Reviews, 2,* 1–29.

Greenwood, P. M., Parasuraman, R., & Alexander, G. E. (1997). Controlling the focus of spatial attention during visual search: Effects of advanced aging and Alzheimer disease. *Neuropsychology, 11*(1), 3–12.

Greenwood, P. M., Sunderland, T., Friz, J. L., & Parasuraman, R. (2000). Genetics and visual attention: Selective deficits in healthy adult carriers of the varepsilon 4 allele of the apolipoprotein E gene. *Proceedings of the National Academy of Sciences USA, 97,* 11661–11666.

Gurden, H., Takita, M., & Jay, T. M. (2000). Essential role of D1 but not D2 receptors in the NMDA receptor-dependent long-term potentiation at hippocampal–prefrontal cortex synapses *in vivo. Journal of Neuroscience, 20,* RC106.

Henderson, A. S., Easteal, S., Jorm, A. F., Mackinnon, A. J., Korten, A. E., Christensen, H., et al. (1995). Apolipoprotein E allele epsilon 4, dementia, and cognitive decline in a population sample. *Lancet, 346,* 1387–1390.

Ioannidis, J. P., Ntzani, E. E., Trikalinos, T. A., & Contopoulos-Ioannidis, D. G. (2001). Replication validity of genetic association studies. *Nature Genetics, 29*(3), 306–309.

Katzman, R., Zhang, M. Y., Chen, P. J., Gu, N., Jiang, S., Saitoh, T., et al. (1997). Effects of apolipoprotein E on dementia and aging in the Shanghai Survey of Dementia. *Neurology, 49*(3), 779–785.

Kent, L., Green, E., Holmes, J., Thapar, A., Gill, M., Hawi, Z., et al. (2001). No association between CHRNA7 microsatellite markers and attention-deficit hyperactity disorder. *American Journal of Medical Genetics, 105,* 686–689.

Kohnke, M. D., Zabetian, C. P., Anderson, G. M., Kolb, W., Gaertner, I., Buchkremer, G., et al. (2002). A genotype-controlled analysis of plasma dopamine beta-hydroxylase in healthy and alcoholic subjects: Evidence for alcohol-related differences in noradrenergic function. *Biological Psychiatry, 52,* 1151–1158.

Levin, E. D., & Simon, B. B. (1998). Nicotinic acetylcholine involvement in cognitive function in animals. *Psychopharmacology (Berlin), 138*(3–4), 217–230.

Muller, U., von Cramon, D. Y., & Pollmann, S. (1998). D1- versus D2-receptor modulation of visuospatial working memory in humans. *Journal of Neuroscience, 18*(7), 2720–2728.

Nobre, A. C., Sebestyen, G. N., Gitelman, D. R., Mesulam, M. M., Frackowiak, R. S., & Frith, C. D. (1997). Functional localization of the system for visuospatial attention using positron emission tomography. *Brain, 120,* 515-533.

Olincy, A., Ross, R. G., Harris, J. G., Young, D. A., McAndrews, M. A., Cawthra, E., et al. (2000). The P50 auditory event-evoked potential in adult attention-deficit disorder: Comparison with schizophrenia. *Biological Psychiatry, 47,* 969–977.

Parasuraman, R. (1998). *The attentive brain.* Cambridge, MA: MIT Press.

Parasuraman, R., & Greenwood, P. M. (1998). Selective attention in aging and dementia. In R. Parasuraman (Ed.), *The attentive brain* (pp. 461–488). Cambridge, MA: MIT Press.

Parasuraman, R., Greenwood, P. M., Haxby, J. V., & Grady, C. L. (1992). Visuospatial attention in dementia of the Alzheimer type. *Brain, 115,* 711–733.

Parasuraman, R., Greenwood, P. M., & Sunderland, T. (2002). The apolipoprotein E gene, attention, and brain function. *Neuropsychology, 16,* 254–274.

Plomin, R., & Crabbe, J. (2000). DNA. *Psychological Bulletin, 126*(6), 806–828.

Plomin, R., DeFries, J. C., McClearn, G. E., & McGuffin, P. (2001). *Behavioral genetics* (4th ed.). New York: Worth.

Poirier, J. (1994). Apolipoprotein E in animal models of CNS injury and in Alzheimer's disease. *Trends in Neuroscience, 17,* 525–530.

Posner, M. I. (1980). Orienting of attention. *Quarterly Journal of Experimental Psychology, 32,* 3–25.

Posner, M. I., & DiGirolamo, G. J. (1998). Executive attention: Conflict, target detection, and cognitive control. In R. Parasuraman (Ed.), *The attentive brain* (pp. 401–423). Cambridge, MA: MIT Press.

Posner, M. I., & Petersen, S. E. (1990). The attention system of the human brain. *Annual Review of Neuroscience, 13,* 25–42.

Rebeck, G. W., Alonzo, N. C., Berezovska, O., Harr, S. D., Knowles, R. B., Growdon, J. H., et al. (1998). Structure and functions of human cerebrospinal fluid lipoproteins from individuals of different APOE genotypes. *Experimental Neurology, 149*(1), 175–182.

Reiman, E. M., Caselli, R. J., Yun, L. S., Chen, K., Bandy, D., Minoshima, S., et al. (1996). Preclinical evidence of Alzheimer's disease in persons homozygous for the epsilon 4 allele for apolipoprotein E. *New England Journal of Medicine, 334,* 752–758.

Richards, B., Skoletsky, J., Shuber, A. P., Balfour, R., Stern, R. C., Dorkin, H. L., et al. (1993). Multiplex PCR amplification from the CFTR gene using DNA prepared from buccal brushes/swabs. *Human Molecular Genetics, 2*(2), 159–163.

Saunders, A. M., Strittmatter, W. J., Schmechel, D., St. George-Hyslop, P. H., Pericak-Vance, M. A., Joo, S. H., et al. (1993). Association of apolipoprotein E allele (4 with late-onset familial and spordic Alzheimer's disease. *Neurology, 43,* 1467–1472.

Sawaguchi, T., & Goldman-Rakic, P. S. (1991). D1 dopamine receptors in prefrontal cortex: Involvement in working memory. *Science, 251,* 947–950.

Smith, C. D., Andersen, A. H., Kryscio, R. J., Schmitt, F. A., Kindy, M. S., Blonder, L. X., et al. (1999). Altered brain activation in cognitively intact individuals at high risk for Alzheimer's disease. *Neurology, 53*(7), 1391–1396.

Smith, E. E., & Jonides, J. (1999). Storage and executive processes in the frontal lobes. *Science, 283,* 1657–1661.

Spearman, C. (1904). "General intelligence," objectively determined and measured. *American Journal of Psychology, 15,* 201–293.

Steinlein, O. K., Deckert, J., Nothen, M. M., Franke, P., Maier, W., Beckmann, H., et al. (1997). Neuronal nicotinic acetylcholine receptor alpha 4 subunit (CHRNA4) and panic disorder: An association study. *American Journal of Medical Genetics, 74*(2), 199–201.

Swan, G. E., & Carmelli, D. (2002). Evidence for genetic mediation of executive control: A study of aging male twins. *Journal of Gerontology. B: Psychological Science and Social Science, 57*(2), P133–P143.

Teter, B., Xu, P. T., Gilbert, J. R., Roses, A. D., Galasko, D., & Cole, G. M. (2002). Defective neuronal sprouting by human apolipoprotein E4 is a gain-of-negative function. *Journal of Neuroscience Research, 68*(3), 331–336.

Ullian, E. M., Sapperstein, S. K., Christopherson, K. S., & Barres, B. A. (2001). Control of synapse number by glia. *Science, 291,* 657–661.

Utermann, G., Langenbeck, U., Beisiegel, U., & Weber, W. (1980). Genetics of the apolipoprotein E system in man. *American Journal of Human Genetics, 32*(3), 339–347.

Ventner, J. C., Adams, M. D., Myers, E. W., Li, P. W., Mural, R. J., Sutton, G. G., et al. (2001). The sequence of the human genome. *Science, 291,* 1304–1351.

Xiang, Z., Huguenard, J. R., & Prince, D. A. (1998). Cholinergic switching within neocortical inhibitory networks. *Science, 281,* 985-988.

19

A Molecular Genetic Approach to the Neurobiology of Attention Utilizing Dopamine Receptor-Deficient Mice

David K. Grandy and Paul J. Kruzich

Early efforts to understand the neurobiological underpinnings of attention, in particular decision making and related executive functions involving human patients with psychiatric illnesses, provided many important insights. With the instrumentation and enhanced sophistication of imaging technology (recently acknowledged with a Nobel Prize for Medicine or Physiology in 2003), noninvasive visualization of specific regions in the functioning human brain during attentional tasks is now possible. Of the areas thus identified, the dorsal anterior cingulate cortex is particularly noteworthy (Bush, Lu, & Posner, 2000). Not only is this brain region robustly activated during executive functioning tasks, but it also receives considerable dopaminergic input from the ventral tegmental area (Bush et al., 2000). However, in spite of the elegant and important imaging work and the use of behavioral genetics with human subjects (see Parasuraman & Greenwood, Chapter 18, this volume), the feasibility of manipulating molecular targets (e.g., altering neurotransmission) in human subjects is rigorously and rightfully restricted. Therefore, animal models are necessary to complement human imaging studies and fully investigate molecular targets held to mediate attention, by such means as measuring gene expression or inducing targeted mutagenesis in genes of interest.

As more selective pharmacological tools became available and identification of their molecular targets became better understood through cloning, the neurochemical bases of several psychiatric disorders have become more clear (Civelli, Bunzow, & Grandy, 1993; Lachowicz & Sibley, 1997). Although some relatively selective pharmacological agents have been developed for dopamine receptor proteins *in vitro*, their selectivity *in vivo* is questionable. Consequently, the traditional pharmacological approach to describing a given behavior in terms of a particular dopamine receptor subtype has proven to be frustrating. As molecular biological approaches revealed the DNA blueprint of five dopamine receptor genes and even more subtypes, it quickly became apparent that new animal models would have to be developed if our understanding of the molecular events underlying dopamine's actions in the living brain was to improve. Therefore, in an effort to develop a model system wherein ligand selectivity is not an issue, we genetically modified mice so that their offspring possess one or no alleles of genes that accurately code for dopamine D_2 or dopamine D_4 receptors. Mice lacking these receptors have now been evaluated pharmacologically, electrophysiologically, neurochemically, anatomically, and behaviorally (prepulse inhibition and novelty seeking). Numerous studies involving both lines of dopamine receptor-deficient mice have provided evidence that individual dopamine receptor subtypes uniquely contribute to decision making and executive functioning.

MOLECULAR COMPLEXITY OF DOPAMINE SIGNALING IN THE BRAIN

Dopamine is recognized as an important modulator of several neuronal circuits involved in normal and pathological psychomotor behaviors (Graybiel, 1990; reviewed by Robbins, Millstein, & Dalley, Chapter 21, this volume). Originally, two functionally and anatomically distinct subtypes of G protein-coupled (adenylyl cyclase-linked) receptor were proposed based on their ability to stimulate (D_1-like) or inhibit (D_2-like) activation of adenylyl cyclase (Cools & van Rossum, 1976; Kebabian & Calne, 1979). These two subtypes were thought to mediate all of dopamine's biological effects. However, this simple concept eventually gave way to the realization that five distinct dopamine receptor genes exist in humans and rodents: two distinct D_1-like dopamine receptors (D_1 and D_5) and three D_2-like receptors (D_2, D_3 and D_4), and at least three of these subtypes yield alternatively spliced transcripts (subtypes within a subtype, such as the $D_{4.7}$ receptor documented by Deth, Kuznetsova, & Waly, Chapter 20, this volume) giving rise to several distinct receptor proteins (Civelli et al., 1993).

With the discovery that there are five dopamine receptor genes in rodents and primates, there was considerable interest in establishing whether each dopamine receptor subtype heterologously expressed in fibroblasts could be specifically distinguished from the others using commercially available D_1 and D_2 receptor-selective dopamine antagonists. These *in vitro* studies revealed that antagonists of the D_1-like receptors were not capable of specifically discriminating between the two D_1-like subtypes, D_1 and $D_{5/1b}$. Similarly, antagonists of the D_2-like receptors were unable to reliably discriminate between D_2, D_3, and D_4 receptors (Neve & Neve, 1997). Consequently, in light of the multiplicity of dopamine receptor subtypes and the lack of selective ligands, behavioral responses held to involve a specific dopamine receptor subtype became suspect.

In addition to greatly facilitating the pharmacological characterization of individual dopamine receptor subtypes as well as human allelic variants (Bunzow et al., 1988; Grandy et al., 1991; Van Tol et al., 1991; Zhou et al., 1990), the ability to heterologously express dopamine receptor-encoding sequences *in vitro* offered a means by which to investigate their ability to activate various second messenger signaling pathways. Although heterologous systems provide a well-established approach that has yielded interesting insights, it is important to recall an often overlooked limitation of these types of studies: The cells typically employed for heterologous expression of cloned G protein-coupled receptors are transformed fibroblasts that do not recapitulate the neuronal milieu in which these receptors normally exist. Consequently, the receptor-mediated second messenger coupling cascades studied *in vitro* are not necessarily of relevance *in vivo*. If the goal is to link an element of behavior to the activity of a specific dopamine receptor subtype, one must consider approaches that are more precise than traditional *in vivo* pharmacological manipulations, such as targeted mutagenesis of an animal's genome.

Another complicating aspect of dopamine receptor biology, yet one that is crucial if dopamine signaling *in vivo* is to be completely understood, concerns the localization of these proteins. Anatomically, the D_1 and $D_{5/1b}$ receptors are postsynaptic with respect to dopamine synthesis and release. Whereas the D_2 subtype is both pre- and postsynaptic with respect to dopamine (Pickel, Garzon, & Mengual, 2002), both D_4 and D_3 receptors appear to be postsynaptic (Bouthenet et al., 1991; Mrzljak et al., 1996). At the cellular level, dopamine receptor proteins are usually thought to reside in the plasma membrane of neurons where they encounter extracellular dopamine. However, these receptors are not static entities. Rather, they experience a life cycle that can last days to weeks and includes passing through the endoplasmic reticulum and golgi bodies on their way to the cell membrane. Following dopamine stimulation, dopamine receptors are either recycled or degraded in response to various cyclic AMP- (D_1 and D_5) or phosphoinositide (D_2)-mediated second-messenger signaling cascades. The trafficking of dopamine receptors occurs in cell bodies, dendrites, and synaptic terminal fields of dopamine-producing presynaptic neurons of the ventral tegmental area as well as in postsynaptic glutamtergic and GABA-ergic neurons of the dorsal cingulate cortex. Unfortunately, the paucity of high-affinity antisera specific for each of the dopamine receptor subtypes continues to hinder efforts to study dopamine receptor trafficking and cellular localization.

A MOLECULAR GENETIC APPROACH TO STUDYING THE NEUROBIOLOGY OF ATTENTION

Prior to the realization that a family of dopamine receptor subtypes exists, human diseases (e.g., schizophrenia and Parkinson's disease), pharmacological manipulations involving dopamine receptor antagonists, and neuroanatomical lesions were used to convincingly demonstrate the important contributions of dopamine signaling to attentional performance (Nieoullon, 2002; Robbins, 2002; Robbins et al., Chapter 21, this volume). However, once it was established that there are five dopamine receptor genes and that they code for numerous receptor subtypes, it was apparent that a molecular genetic approach might provide an unambiguous means of establishing each dopamine receptor subtype's role in complex behaviors—such as attention.

In spite of the fact that rats had been used extensively to study the neurobiological basis of various behaviors, we felt there were several compelling reasons to develop dopamine receptor-deficient mice. Not only do mice offer several practical advantages over rats in that they reproduce more quickly, tend to have larger litters, and thus are more efficient to maintain, pluripotent mouse embryonic stem cells were available (Capecchi, 1994; Smith, 2001), essential elements of any successful targeted mutagenesis effort. By engineering a targeting vector to genomic sequences of specific dopamine receptors that permitted homologous recombination and ultimately the inactivation of a particular dopamine receptor subtype of interest, it was possible to generate mice that possessed one functioning allele (heterozygous) or two nonfunctional mutant alleles (homozygous) of one or more dopamine receptor subtype without inadvertently interfering with the expression of other genes (transcriptomes), as can occur when expression cassettes become randomly integrated into genomic DNA.

Although elegant in both its selectivity and simulation of a genetically inherited trait or disorder (e.g., phenylketonuria), the inactivation of a mouse gene by homologous recombination dictates that the animal develop in the absence of the inactivated gene product—a situation fraught with potentially unexpected ramifications. Consequently, caution should be exercised when attempting to attribute a specific phenotype to the absence of a particular receptor subtype. The situation is further complicated by the fact that the initial establishment of a line of knockout mice not only implies that homologous recombination did occur, but also that behavioral differences may be the product of the mixing different background inbred strains and not the actual targeted mutation. Although strain differences in specific behaviors potentially confound the interpretation of experimental results obtained from mice that are the product of less than 5 generations of backcrossing to the inbred strain of one's choice, the issue can be addressed with repeated backcrossing of mice carrying the mutant allele to a single inbred strain of mice for at least 20 or more generations. Theoretically, most alleles should be homozygous with the exception of the mutant allele and the sequences surrounding it because they come from the original recombinant embryonic stem cell and are under positive selection.

Given that it is usually difficult, if not impossible, to actually achieve homozygosity at every gene locus with repeated backcrossing with gene knockout models, there has been much interest in employing recent technical advances, such as use of polymerase chain reaction-based primers selective for genomic markers of the original founder strains that permit the tracking of strain-specific regions of the mouse genome (Phillips et al., 2002). Being able to judiciously select the animal whose genome most closely matches the desired inbred strain offers the potential of significantly expediting inbreeding. Furthermore, by knowing at each generation the exact genetic material inherited from each parental strain, one could take advantage of the extant phenotypical differences that exist between inbred strains of mice and correlate the appearance or disappearance of phenotype with the presence or absence of particular strain-related haplotypes. In the meantime, conservative investigators adhere to the philosophy that it is only after repeated testing of many mice over several generations that one can begin to feel some confidence in assigning a particular phenotype to the absence of a particular dopamine receptor subtype.

THE NEUROBIOLOGY OF ATTENTION BENEFITS FROM STUDIES OF DOPAMINE RECEPTOR SUBTYPE-DEFICIENT MICE

So that we could begin to evaluate the contribution of each dopamine receptor subtype to a particular phenotype, lines of mice representing both parental genotypes (C57Bl/6J and two 129 substrains) each carrying a disrupted allele were established. Fortunately, the mutant allele of interest can be easily passed on to the genetic background of the investigator's choosing in order to exploit desirable aspects of a particular mouse strain.

The first receptor we chose to inactivate by homologous recombination was the dopamine D_2 receptor. We chose the D_2 receptor gene because an extensive pharmacological literature with D_2 receptor preferring compounds exists, which would aid in behavioral characterization of any putative receptor-deficient mouse. The second dopamine receptor subtype we selected for targeting was the D_4. What attracted us about this subtype was that essentially little was known about its function *in vivo* but its distribution appeared to be unique and interesting. The majority of D_4 receptor mRNA (messenger ribonucleic acid) and immunoreactivity has been detected in the frontal cortex, an area long held as important in impulse control, associative learning, executive function, working memory, and decision making (Deth et al., Chapter 20, this volume; Robbins, 1996; Schultz, 2000).

Appreciative of the fact that the biology of dopamine is complex and has been approached from many levels, we undertook an integrated, multidimensional approach to characterize our genetically engineered, receptor-deficient mice. Beginning with offspring resulting from the mating of F_2 hybrids (Kelly et al., 1997; Rubenstein et al., 1997) and most recently involving their 20th-generation descendants ($n = 20$ on C57Bl/6J), we are analyzing mice that are $n = 5$, $n = 10$, and $n = 20$ on the C57Bl/6J background. We felt that if a phenotype were retained in successive generations, it would constitute support for the interpretation that a given phenotype observed in the initial F_2 generation (the cross between two F_1 mice each with one wildtype and one mutant allele) was, in some direct or indirect way, the consequence of their lacking a functional dopamine receptor subtype. Although much remains to be done, the studies completed to date support the view that the loss of dopamine signaling mediated by D_2 and D_4 receptors affects the neuronal circuitry underlying various aspects of attention.

Dopamine D_2 Receptors and Prepulse Inhibition of the Startle Response

An inability to properly gate differing sensory inputs can result in abnormal or inappropriate behavioral responses such as are often displayed by unmedicated patients with schizophrenia (Geyer, Krebs-Thomson, Braff, & Swedlow, 2001). In an effort to better understand the neurobiology of sensorimotor gating, a cross-species measure has been developed that takes advantage of the observation that the magnitude of the response by a human or mouse to a startling stimulus, such as a loud (80 dB) noise, is significantly reduced in normal subjects if a weaker audible tone (prepulse) is emitted just prior to the startling tone (Geyer et al., 2001).

The ability of the prepulse tone to inhibit the startle response (prepulse inhibition, or PPI) has been shown to be dependent on dopamine signaling. Moreover, direct (apomorphine) and indirect dopamine receptor agonists (e.g., amphetamine) can significantly disrupt normal sensorimotor gating (Dulawa & Geyer, 1996). Furthermore, there is compelling evidence that supports the view that it is the dopamine signaling mediated by the dopamine D_2-like family of receptors (D_2, D_3, & D_4). However, due to the lack of pharmacological tools permitting selective manipulation of individual dopamine receptor subtypes *in vivo*, mice deficient in each receptor subtype of interest could help to establish whether one subtype or another contributed to prepulse inhibition or not.

Wildtype mice and mice that had been genetically rendered partially (+/–; heterozygous) or completely lacking (–/–; homozygous) in one of the dopamine D_2, D_3, or D_4 subtype were collected at a single institution (UC San Diego) where they were allowed to acclimate for at least 1 week prior to behavioral testing (Ralph et al., 1999). After this period, mice from each receptor-subtype-deficient line and their wildtype littermates were evaluated with respect to their baseline acoustic startle response (ASR) and PPI. Three days later their startle reactivity and PPI were evaluated after they received an intraperitoneal injection of saline or amphetamine (10 mg/kg). One week later the mice were tested again to complete a within-subjects design. Baseline PPI, baseline and gender differences in ASR, amphetamine pretreatment effects on PPI, and overall gender and genotype effects were all analyzed across homozygous, heterozygous, and wildtype lines of mice.

This large study, involving three independently generated lines of dopamine receptor-deficient mice and wildtype controls, revealed no phenotypical differences in baseline PPI. However, following exposure to amphetamine, PPI was significantly disrupted in the $D_2^{+/+}$ mice but had no effect in the $D_2^{-/-}$. In contrast, the presence or absence of functional dopamine D_3 or D_4 receptor genes did not prevent amphetamine-induced disruptions of PPI seen in all wildtype mice tested. These findings were interpreted to support the view that amphetamine-induced disruption of PPI involves D_2 receptors and not the D_3 or D_4 subtypes.

Dopamine D_4 Receptors and Novelty Seeking

Healthy primates, including humans, display an innate sense of curiosity and tend to seek situations and environments that are novel (Mesulam, 1998). In contrast, individuals who experienced traumatic brain injury to the prefrontal cortex typically become disinterested in novel aspects of their environment, are unable to respond appropriately when reinforcement contingencies are changed, and become more likely to engage in perseverative, impulsive, and stimulus-bound behaviors than do healthy subjects (Leimkuhler & Mesulam, 1985; Mesulam, 1986). Interestingly, a strong positive correlation between curiosity and longevity in humans has been reported (Swan & Carmelli, 1996).

Although novelty seeking is a complex phenotype and undoubtedly involves numerous brain regions and signaling systems, there are a number of reports that suggest that dopamine signaling plays an important, if not essential, role in the elaboration of appropriate novelty-seeking behavior (Bardo, Donohew, & Harrington, 1996). Interestingly, human genetic studies imply that allelic variants of the dopamine D_4 receptor subtype contribute to the expression of novelty-seeking behavior in a number of contexts and disorders (Ding et al., 2002; Ebstein et al., 1996).

In an effort to establish whether or not the dopamine D_4 receptor subtype plays a role in mouse behaviors related to novelty, wildtype and mutant mice were subjected to three approach–avoidance paradigms: open field, emergence, and novel object tests (Dulawa, Grandy, Low, Paulus, & Geyer, 1999). Each test was carefully chosen because it differed in the extent to which approach or exploratory behavior, avoidance, or anxiety-related behaviors are elicited. The smallest phenotypical effect was observed in the open field test where avoidance behavior is most manifest. However, when the responses of both wildtype and D_4 receptor-deficient mice in all three different paradigms were compared, it was found that the $D_4^{-/-}$ mice responded less to novelty than did their wildtype counterparts. The greatest phenotypical differences were seen during the novel object test and index of approach behavior. These findings were interpreted to suggest, at least in the mouse, that animals lacking a functional D_4 receptor display decreased novelty-related exploration. As such they lend support to the view that D_4 receptor status can influence one's behavioral response to a novel stimulus.

FUTURE DIRECTIONS

If the current excitement can inform future work there is great promise for eventually mapping behavioral aspects of attentional neural networks onto dopamine receptor subtypes. Technological advancements are currently allowing higher resolution *in vivo* imaging of smaller, living brains. The wedding of genetically engineered mice and new imaging technology offers an exciting and powerful new means of describing the exact contributions made by individual receptors and the neuronal circuits they influence.

Progress is also being made with respect to the development of a line of mice in which the expression of a particular dopamine receptor subtype can be turned off selectively in a temporal and regional manner. Although not without their own limitations, spatial and temporal dopamine receptor subtype-deficient mice will be valuable resources in the effort to establish the relationship between a phenotype and the presence or absence of a particular receptor. Interest in knowing where these receptors are in brain tissue remains high, and given the paucity of dopamine receptor antisera, the ability to "knock in" sequences means that it is theoretically possible to tag each dopamine receptor subtype with an immunogenic epitope. An epitope tag is a specific region of protein that an antibody has been directed against. The locations of a specific receptor subtype are then identified with specific antibodies that are radioactive (tagged) or contain some sort of fluorophore. Other reporter systems, such as green fluorescent protein, could be used to determine the exact location of a dopamine receptor subtype in the brain. In addition, the ability to knock in a sequence means that wildtype mouse alleles can be exchanged for human alleles of interest. Knockin lines of both types are in development.

Future studies with currently available dopamine receptor subtype-deficient mice will be used to explore the behavioral actions of methylphenidate that are mediated by D_4 receptors. In addition, studies are in progress to investigate reversal learning in D_2 receptor-deficient mice. The findings to date are so robust that additional studies have been planned that include D_4 receptor-deficient mice. Studies are also under way to investigate the specific involvement of dopamine D_2 and D_4 receptors in the context of behaviors related to impulsivity.

In the not too distant future mice from both the D_2 and D_4 receptor-deficient lines will be examined using positron emission tomography imaging and functional magnetic resonance imaging and eventually it is hoped pharmacological manipulations coupled with imaging will quickly follow. This approach offers the promise of clarifying our understanding of the dynamic and complex roles that the various dopamine receptor subtypes exert in the live functioning brain.

SUMMARY AND CONCLUSIONS

Even though they are simple mammals, mice do respond analogously to pharmacological and environmental stimuli encountered by humans. This is borne out at the molecular level where it is well documented that extensive chromosomal synteny exists between humans and mice and that even at the level of amino acid sequence humans and mice dopamine receptors are highly conserved (Nadeau, 1989).

Mice, in particular those genetically engineered to be deficient in either the dopamine D_2 or D_4 receptor genes, are just beginning to be used to explore the neurobiology of attention. In the future, the ability to selectively ablate or replace a piece of the mouse genome with a genetic sequence of one's own choosing will be exploited as part of a powerful multidimensional, integrated-systems approach to investigate the involvement of a particular receptor gene in highly complex neuronal circuits that mediate the behavioral aspects of attention.

ACKNOWLEDGMENTS

We would like to acknowledge the outstanding technical support provided by Katherine L. Suchland and Audrey Younkin for proofreading the manuscript. This work was supported, in part, by grants from the National Institute on Drug Abuse (Grant No. DA007262 [to Paul J. Kruzich] and Grant No. DA12062 [to David K. Grandy]) and the National Institute of Mental Health (Grant Nos. MH66360 and MH67497 [to David K. Grandy]).

REFERENCES

Bardo, M. T., Donohew, R. L., & Harrington, N. G. (1996). Psychobiology of novelty seeking and drug seeking behavior. *Behavioural Brain Research*, *77*(1–2), 23–43.

Bouthenet, M. L., Souil, E., Martres, M. P., Sokoloff, P., Giros, B., & Schwartz, J. C. (1991). Localization of dopamine D3 receptor mRNA in the rat brain using in situ hybridization histochemistry: Comparison with dopamine D2 receptor mRNA. *Brain Research*, *564*(2), 203–219.

Bunzow, J. R., Van Tol, H. H., Grandy, D. K., Albert, P., Salon, J., Christie, M., et al. (1988). Cloning and expression of a rat D_2 dopamine receptor cDNA. *Nature*, *336*, 783–787.

Bush, G., Luu, P., & Posner, M. I. (2000). Cognitive and emotional influences in anterior cingulate cortex. *Trends in Cognitive Science*, *4*(6), 215–222.

Capecchi, M. R. (1994). Targeted gene replacement. *Scientific American*, *270*, 52–59.

Civelli, O., Bunzow, J. R., & Grandy, D. K. (1993). Molecular diversity of the dopamine receptors. *Annual Review of Pharmacology and Toxicology*, *33*, 281–307.

Cools, A. R., & Van Rossum, J. M. (1976). Excitation-mediating and inhibition-mediating dopamine-receptors: A new concept towards a better understanding of electrophysiological, biochemical, pharmacological, functional and clinical data. *Psychopharmacologia*, *45*(3), 243–254.

Ding, Y. C., Chi, H. C., Grady, D. L., Morishima, A., Kidd, J. R., Kidd, K. K., et al. (2002). Evidence of positive selection acting at the human dopamine receptor D4 gene locus. *Proceedings of the National Academy of Sciences USA*, *99*(1), 309–314.

Dulawa, S. C., & Geyer, M. A. (1996). Psychopharmacology of prepulse inhibition in mice. *Chinese Journal of Physiology*, *39*(3), 139–146.

Dulawa, S. C., Grandy, D. K., Low, M. J., Paulus, M. P., & Geyer, M. A. (1999). Dopamine D_4 receptor-knock-out mice exhibit reduced exploration of novel stimuli. *Journal of Neuroscience*, *19*, 9550–9556.

Ebstein, R. P., Novick, O., Umansky, R., Priel, B., Osher, Y., Blaine, D., et al. (1996). Dopamine D_4 receptor (D4DR) exon III polymorphism associated with the human personality trait of novelty seeking. *Nature Genetics*, *12*(1), 78–80.

Geyer, M. A., Krebs-Thomson, K., Braff, D. L., & Swerdlow, N. R. (2001). Pharmacological studies of prepulse inhibition models of sensorimotor gating deficits in schizophrenia: A decade in review. *Psychopharmacology (Berlin)*, *156*(2–3), 117–154.

Grandy, D. K., Zhang, Y. A., Bouvier, C., Zhou, Q. Y., Johnson, R. A., & Allen, L. (1991). Multiple human D5 dopamine receptor genes: A functional receptor and two pseudogenes. *Proceedings of the National Academy of Sciences USA*, *88*, 9175–9179.

Graybiel, A. M. (1990). Neurotransmitters and neuromodulators in the basal ganglia. *Trends in Neuroscience*, *13*, 244–254.

Kebabian, J. W., & Calne, D. B. (1979). Multiple receptors for dopamine. *Nature*, *277*, 93–96.

Kelly, M. A., Rubinstein, M., Asa, S. L., Zhang, G., Saez, C., Bunzow, J. R., et al. (1997). Pituitary lactotroph hyperplasia and chronic hyperprolactinemia in dopamine D_2 receptor-deficient mice. *Neuron*, *19*(1), 103–113.

Lachowicz, J. E., & Sibley, D. R. (1997). Molecular characteristics of mammalian dopamine receptors. *Pharmacology and Toxicology*, *81*(3), 105–113.

Leimkuhler, M. E., & Mesulam, M. M. (1985). Reversible go-no go deficits in a case of frontal lobe tumor. *Annals of Neurology*, *18*(5), 617–619.

Mesulam, M. M. (1986). Frontal cortex and behavior. *Annals of Neurology*, *19*(4), 320–325.

Mesulam, M. M. (1998). From sensation to cognition. *Brain*, *121*, 1013–1052.

Mrzljak, L., Bergson, C., Pappy, M., Huff, R., Levenson, R., & Goldman-Rakic, P. S. (1996). Localization of dopamine D_4 receptors in GABAergic neurons of the primate brain. *Nature*, *381*(6579), 245–248.

Nadeau, J. H. (1989). Maps of linkage and synteny homologies between mouse and man. *Trends in Genetics*, *5*(3), 82–86.

Neve, K. A., & Neve, R. L. (Eds.). (1997). *The dopamine receptors*. Totowa, NJ: Humana Press.

Nieoullon, A. (2002). Dopamine and the regulation of cognition and attention. *Progress in Neurobiology*, *67*(1), 53–83.

Phillips, T. J., Belknap, J. K., Hitzemann, R. J., Buck, K. J., Cunningham, C. L., & Crabbe, J. C. (2002). Harnessing the mouse to unravel the genetics of human disease. *Genes, Brain and Behavior, 1*(1), 14–26.

Pickel, V. M., Garzon, M., & Mengual, E. (2002). Electron microscopic immunolabeling of transporters and receptors identifies transmitter-specific functional sites envisioned in Cajal's neuron. *Progress in Brain Research, 136*, 145–155.

Ralph, R. J., Varty, G. B., Kelly, M. A., Wang, Y. M., Caron, M. G., Rubinstein, M., et al. (1999). The dopamine D_2, but not D_3 or D_4, receptor subtype is essential for the disruption of prepulse inhibition produced by amphetamine in mice. *Journal of Neuroscience, 19*, 4627–4633.

Robbins, T. W. (1996). Dissociating executive functions of the prefrontal cortex. *Philosophical Transactions of the Royal Society of London on B (Biological Sciences), 351*, 1463–1470.

Robbins, T. W. (2002). The 5-choice serial reaction time task: behavioural pharmacology and functional neurochemistry. *Psychopharmacology (Berlin), 163*(3–4), 362–380.

Rubinstein, M., Phillips, T. J., Bunzow, J. R., Falzone, T. L., Dziewczapolski, G., Zhang, G., et al. (1997). Mice lacking dopamine D_4 receptors are supersensitive to ethanol, cocaine, and methamphetamine. *Cell, 90*(6), 991–1001.

Schultz, W. (2000). Multiple reward signals in the brain. *Nature Reviews Neuroscience, 1*(3), 199–207.

Smith, A. G. (2001). Embryo-derived stem cells: Of mice and men. *Annual Review of Cell and Developmental Biology, 17*, 435–462.

Swan, G. E., & Carmelli, D. (1996). Curiosity and mortality in aging adults: A 5-year follow-up on the Western Collaborative Group Study. *Psychology and Aging, 11*, 449–453.

Van Tol, H. H., Bunzow, J. R., Guan, H. C., Sunahara, R. K., Seeman, P., Niznik, H. B., et al. (1991). Cloning of the gene for a human dopamine D_4 receptor with high affinity for the antipsychotic clozapine. *Nature, 350*, 610–614.

Zhou, Q. Y., Grandy, D. K., Thambi, L., Kushner, J. A., Van Tol, H. H., Cone, R., et al. (1990). Cloning and expression of human and rat D1 dopamine receptors. *Nature, 347*, 76–80.

20

Attention-Related Signaling Activities of the D$_4$ Dopamine Receptor

Richard C. Deth, Anna Kuznetsova, and Mostafa Waly

Attention is the higher-order cognitive ability to selectively amplify a subset of information for the purpose of detailed interrogation and learning. Attended information can arise from either current experience or from memory. While all animals have the capacity for attention, humans are distinguished by their highly developed ability to link attention to learning, providing us with remarkable powers of adaptation. The capacity for attention derives from the molecular actions of neurotransmitters and their receptors, in the context of interconnected neural networks that carry information.

Among neurotransmitters, dopamine plays a particularly important role in attention, and dopamine receptor function is closely linked to attention and to normal cognitive function. Since its initial cloning and characterization (Van Tol et al., 1991), the human D$_4$ dopamine receptor (D$_4$R) subtype has been the subject of extensive research, prompted in part by the unique effectiveness of the D$_4$R-selective drug clozapine in treating schizophrenia and by extraordinary diversity in the primate D$_4$R gene. Among several distinctive polymorphisms in the D$_4$R gene is a 48 base-pair, variable number tandem repeat (VNTR) with more than 35 different possible repeat sequences (Ding et al., 2002). In the D$_4$R protein, these repeats create multiple proline-rich segments that allow the receptor to bind other signaling proteins. Individuals expressing the 7-repeat allele exhibit greater risk-taking and novelty-seeking behaviors (Benjamin et al., 1996; Ebstein et al., 1996) and have a higher risk of attention-deficit/hyperactivity disorder (ADHD) (LaHoste et al., 1996; Swanson et al., 2000), suggesting a role for the D$_4$R in attention.

As first reported by our lab, dopamine activation of the D$_4$R stimulates the receptor-mediated transfer of methyl groups from the single-carbon folate pathway to membrane phospholipids (Sharma et al., 1999). The rate of methyl transfer is robust, reaching 20–50 methylations/receptor/second, implying that D$_4$Rs are capable of rapidly modifying their local membrane environment in response to dopamine. Phospholipid methylation (PLM) causes a decrease in membrane packing density (i.e., increases fluidity), and this unique ability of the D_4R can affect the activity of other membrane proteins in the local environment, an action we describe as "solid-state signaling" (Deth, 2003).

This chapter describes the molecular basis for solid-state signaling and proposes a specific mechanism by which it may contribute to attention. In addition, we examine the factors that regulate the efficiency of solid-state signaling and explore links between this novel neuromodulatory mechanism and psychiatric conditions in which impaired attention is a prominent symptom.

THE STRUCTURAL BASIS FOR SOLID-STATE SIGNALING

The D_4R is a member of a large "superfamily" of receptors that transfer the concentration-dependent neurotransmitter signal across the cell membrane, leading to the activation of intracellular GTP-binding G-proteins. Like other G protein-coupled receptors (and receptors in general) the D_4R exists in alternative shapes, inactive and active, designated as R and R^*, respectively. The transmembrane portion of the receptor consists of seven helices, and the dopamine-induced R to R^* transition is associated with a rotational movement of helix #6 (Figure 20.1). This agonist-induced conformational movement triggers activation of G proteins, which are able to only bind to the rotated helix #6. Dopamine promotes rotation by forming a bond with an amino acid sidechain (PHE331) on this helix exclusively when in the R^* position.

At the inner membrane terminus of helix #6 is a methionine residue (MET313 in the $D_4.4R$ containing four repeats), uniquely present in the D_4R. Located directly below PHE331, MET313 is exposed during the R^* state but hidden in the R state. Dopamine binding promotes a four-step biochemical cycle of PLM (Figure 20.2) by allowing adenosine

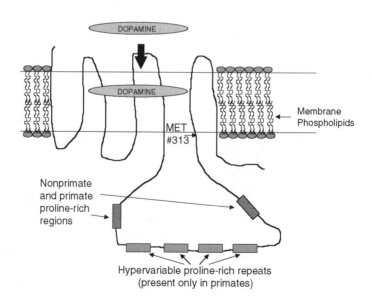

FIGURE 20.1. Structural features of the human dopamine D_4 receptor. MET#313 is located on helix #6, close to the inner membrane surface. Proline-rich regions allow for SH3 domain interactions with other proteins. Humans and other primates have anywhere from two to eleven hypervariable repeated proline-rich regions in their D_4 receptors. From Deth (2003). Copyright 2003 by Kluwer Academic Publishers. Reprinted by permission.

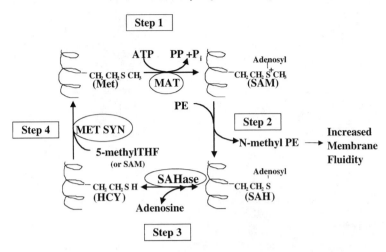

FIGURE 20.2. The four-step cycle of D_4 receptor-mediated PLM. In step 1 MET313 is adenosylated in an ATP-dependent reaction carried out by methionine adenosyltransferase (MAT). In step 2 the methyl group from MET313 is transferred to the phospholipid PE creating increased membrane fluidity. In step 3 the adenosyl group is released to form adenosine in a reversible reaction catalyzed by S-adenosylhomocysteine hydrolase (SAHase). In step 4 MET313 is re-formed by the action of methionine synthase (MET SYN), using 5-methyltetrahydrolfolate (5-methylTHF) as the primary methyl group donor. From Deth (2003). Copyright 2003 by Kluwer Academic Publishers. Reprinted by permission.

triphosphate–dependent adenosylation of the MET313 sidechain, activating its methyl group for transfer to the headgroup of neighboring phospholipids, particularly to phosphatidylethanolamine (PE). MET313 in the D_4R can participate in the methylation of phospholipids, since it is located directly adjacent to their headgroups (Figure 20.1) but cannot donate methyl groups to other methyltransferase reactions. The D_4R PLM cycle is completed by removal of the adenosyl group in a reversible reaction catalyzed by S-adenosylhomocysteine hydrolase (SAHase), and the addition of a new methyl group from the folate pathway, catalyzed by the Vit.B12-requiring enzyme methionine synthase (Met Syn). These steps involve the sidechain of MET313 in reactions that are analogous to the well-described methionine cycle of methylation.

Proline-rich segments in the D_4R allow it to bind other signaling proteins containing SH3 domains, including RasGAP, linker proteins Grb2 and Crk, and the synapse-associated scaffolding protein SAP-97 (Deth, Mehta, Tan, Liu, & Marshall, 1999; Oldenhof et al., 1998). Thus the D_4R serves as an organizing center for signaling activity, and membrane proteins directly or indirectly bound to the receptor are candidates for modulation by dopamine-stimulated solid-state signaling. For example, SAP-97 binds glutamate receptors, Ca^{2+} ATPase, and voltage-dependent K^+ channels (Sheng, 2001) (Figure 20.3). The activity of each of these proteins is highly sensitive to changes in the membrane environment, suggesting that D_4R-mediated PLM could regulate their activity. In support of this concept, D_4R activation has been shown to inhibit the activity of N-methyl-D-aspartate (NMDA) receptors on CA1 cells in hippocampal slice preparations (Kotecha et al., 2002; Otmakhova & Lisman, 1999). Interestingly, the level of SAP-97 is reduced in schizophrenia (Toyooka et al., 2002). The unique ability of the D_4R to carry out dopamine-stimulated PLM and its ability to create a local cluster of membrane fluidity-sensitive proteins suggests that solid-state signaling is a key activity of the D_4R.

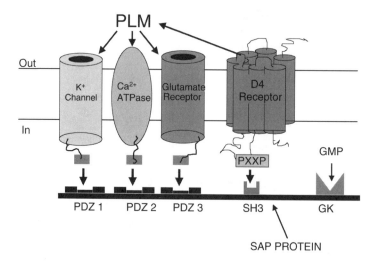

FIGURE 20.3. Synapse-associated proteins (SAPs) provide for clustering of membrane proteins via PDZ domain and SH3 domain interactions and also possess a guanylate kinase (GK) domain. Proteins that co-associate with the D4 receptor are subject to regulation by solid-state signaling via dopamine-stimulated PLM. From Deth (2003). Copyright 2003 by Kluwer Academic Publishers. Reprinted by permission.

A ROLE FOR SOLID-STATE SIGNALING IN ATTENTION

Dopaminergic neurons from the ventral tegmental area (VTA) extensively innervate the frontal cortex, and their activation is thought to play a central role in attention (Horvitz, Stewart, & Jacobs, 1997). Within the frontal cortex, D_4Rs are preferentially located on GABA-ergic interneurons, particularly those expressing the calcium-binding protein parvalbumin (Mrzljak et al., 1996). Calcium-binding proteins exert an important influence on the firing kinetics of interneurons, and different calcium-binding proteins (parvalbumin, calbindin, and calretinin) are differentially expressed in populations of interneurons. Neuronal networks containing GABA-ergic interneurons exhibit synchronized oscillations in their firing pattern and the presence of parvalbumin-expressing interneurons is associated with oscillatory firing in the gamma frequency range (e.g., 30–80 Hz) (Chrobak & Buzsaki, 1998).

During episodes of attention, the magnitude of 40-Hz (i.e., gamma frequency) synchronized oscillations is increased in the cortex (Tiitinen et al., 1993). Magnetoencephalography (MEG) studies have noted particularly strong increases in the temporoparietal region, and the administration of D_4R-blocking drugs reduces the amplitude of the attention-related increase and also reduces the capacity for attention (Ahveninen et al., 2000). Thus it appears that activation of D_4R-like receptors is essential for attention and for the closely associated phenomenon of increased synchronized activity at 40 Hz.

Because D_4Rs are localized on the very cells giving rise to 40-Hz oscillations, it is possible that dopamine-stimulated solid-state signaling may be an important mechanism for promoting attention. Synchronized neuronal firing provides temporal coordination of information content and promotes the formation of complex percepts from elemental information. An increase in the amplitude of synchronized information implies that the particular amplified information content will be more dominant within circuits that give rise to consciousness, providing attention to that specific information. We propose that D$_4$R-mediated solid-state signaling promotes attention by modulating the activity of SAP-97-associated proteins in parvalbumin-expressing GABA-ergic interneurons, resulting in an increased probability that neuronal networks containing these interneurons will exhibit synchronized firing at 40 Hz.

Figure 20.4 provides a simplified schematic view of how D$_4$R activation could promote synchronized oscillations. As illustrated, information-carrying pyramidal cells activate excitatory glutamatergic receptors on parvalbumin-expressing inhibitory GABA-ergic interneurons that feed back upon the pyramidal cells, as well as onto adjacent cells. In such a local loop circuit, the onset of sensory experience initiates an increase of pyramidal cell firing, which activates interneurons, increasing their inhibitory output onto the very same pyramidal cells. The resultant lower firing rate of pyramidal cells reduces excitation of interneurons, reducing negative feedback and causing a rise in pyramidal cell firing rate. Thus local negative-feedback circuits give rise to an oscillatory cycle of mutual excitation and inhibition. By activation of D$_4$R-mediated PLM within postsynaptic densities, dopamine can alter interneuron response such that it fires at the resonance frequency of 40 Hz. By promoting 40-Hz oscillations in multiple networks, dopamine can increase the amplitude of synchronized activity, as is observed during attention (Figure 20.4).

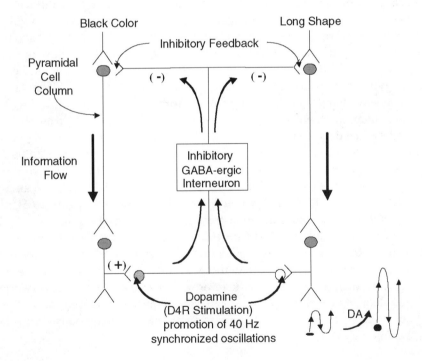

FIGURE 20.4. Synchronized oscillations in firing rate arise from cortical circuits containing pyramidal cells and inhibitory interneurons. Arriving sensory information increases pyramidal cell firing leading to activation of interneurons which inhibit pyramidal cell firing in a feedback manner. Lower pyramidal cell activity in turn reduces interneuron stimulation which restores pyramidal cell firing and creates an oscillatory pattern. Dopamine, acting at the pyramidal cell/interneuron synapse, can increase the amplitude of 40-Hz oscillations by modulating the activity of synapse-associated proteins (lower right). From Deth (2003). Copyright 2003 by Kluwer Academic Publishers. Reprinted by permission.

A prominent role for 40-Hz synchronized neuronal activity in attention and consciousness has been previously suggested in a model advanced by Niebur, Koch, and Rosin (1993). Using hierarchical transfer of visual information from V1 to V4 as an example, they proposed that synchronized oscillations arising from network properties could provide "temporal tagging" of related information in a percept, and that attention could be accomplished by selective inhibition of nontarget information, allowing target information to become dominant. Using similar concepts, we propose that dopamine-stimulated PLM modulates the activation/inactivation properties of membrane proteins regulating oscillatory behavior, such as voltage-gated and ligand-gated ion channels. More specifically, we propose that changes in membrane fluidity may alter the behavior of the gating mechanisms in these channels, which involve rotation and repositioning of transmembrane helices. Fluidity-induced changes in bonding forces between these helices and surrounding phospholipids can alter the kinetics and probability of achieving the active open state, with consequences for exhibiting 40-Hz oscillations. It is important to point out that synchronized oscillations in neuronal activity can occur without changing the net firing rate averaged over a longer time interval and therefore do not disturb information content inherent in the discharge rate.

We have adopted and extended the computational model of Niebur and colleagues (1993) to illustrate how dopamine could promote 40 Hz synchronized firing in neuronal networks. The oscillatory circuit illustrated in Figure 20.5A contains C, R, R_L and L elements, which may correspond to discrete membrane proteins under the influence of dopamine-stimulated PLM. For example, inductance may reflect a contribution of voltage-gated potassium channels, whose gating is controlled by movement of positively charged elements within the membrane, triggering the movement of other helices that allow opening of the channel (Jiang et al., 2003). Dopamine-induced changes in membrane fluidity could influence the energy barrier governing movement of these helices, thereby affecting L and R_L, with accompanying changes in the circuit's oscillatory behavior.

Dopamine-induced changes of R_L (from 300 to 3,300 Ω) and L (from 100 to 34 H) were modeled as time-dependent sigmoidal functions (Figure 20.5B), reflecting the influence of D4R-mediated PLM, while values of C and R were fixed at 1 μF and 2,000 Ω. These changes in R_L and L shifted the resonance frequency (f_{max}) for the circuit from an initial value of 17 Hz to 40 Hz (Figure 20.5B, second from bottom), associated with an increase of impedance at 40 Hz from 1,780 to 2,210 Ω (Figure 20.5B, bottom). Figure 20.5C shows the relationship between impedance and input frequency under basal conditions ($t_1 = 25$ msec) and during dopamine-stimulated PLM ($t_2 = 100$ msec), illustrating the increase at 40 Hz and decrease at lower frequencies. Thus modulation of synaptic proteins by dopamine-stimulated PLM could promote synchronized firing of specific neuronal networks at 40 Hz, thereby increasing attention to the specific information arising from those networks. Dopamine-induced changes in oscillatory circuit behavior in our model closely parallel the experimentally observed effect of attention on gamma frequency oscillations (Fries, Reynolds, Rorie, & Desimone, 2001).

AWARENESS VERSUS ATTENTION

Awareness of sensory information is distinct from attention. For example, awareness facilitates rapid scanning of an array of information, while attention is associated with a higher probability of learning and memory encoding. Awareness is frequently a precursor to atten-

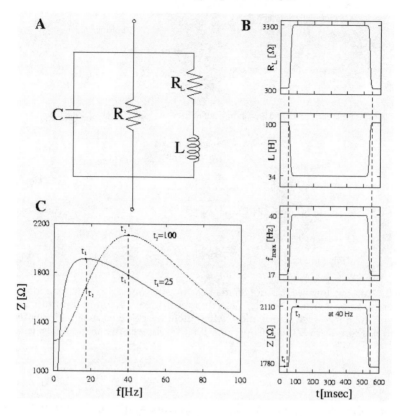

FIGURE 20.5. Computational model of the influence of dopamine-stimulated PLM on oscillatory circuit behavior. (A) Values of C, R, R$_L$, and L in the circuit were set as described by Niebur et al. (1993) at 1 μF, 2000 Ω, 300 Ω, and 100 H, which correspond to a resonance frequency of 17 Hz. (B) The influence of dopamine, starting at 50 msec, was modeled as a sigmoidal increase in R$_L$ from 300 to 3,300 Ω, and a sigmoidal decrease in L from 100 to 34 H (upper panels) lasting for 500 msec. Resonance frequency increased to 40 Hz and impedance increased from 1,780 to 2,110 Ω (lower panels). (C) Dopamine increased resonance frequency to 40 Hz and decreased membrane impedance at 17 Hz (timepoint t_2; 100 msec), as compared to initial conditions (timepoint t_1; 25 msec). Thus in the period from 50 to 75 msec after stimulus onset, membrane impedance at 17 Hz was reduced by 12% due to attention, whereas impedance at 40 Hz was increased by 19%, in good agreement with the experimental results of Fries et al. (2001).

tion, as selected information is prioritized. Because awareness and attention are obviously closely related processes, they may share a common neuronal and biochemical basis. We suggest that the molecular mechanisms of attention and awareness are indeed closely related and that there is room for differences in the intensity of attention within the D$_4$R-based PLM mechanism.

In PLM studies we found that epinephrine was essentially equal in potency to dopamine, and norepinephrine was only fivefold less potent (Sharma et al., 1999), indicating that D$_4$R-mediated PLM is responsive to all three catecholamines. Norepinephrine-releasing neurons are very widely distributed in the cerebral cortex, significantly more so than dopamine-releasing neurons. Noradrenergic neurons originate from the reticular activating system, whose activity is closely associated with our state of wakefulness and awareness. Thus

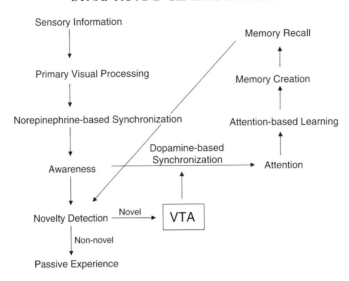

FIGURE 20.6. Norepinephrine and dopamine-based synchronization can function sequentially to provide awareness and attention. Novelty detection results from a comparison of current awareness information with memory-based information. After attention-based learning, information is no longer detected as novel. From Deth (2003). Copyright 2003 by Kluwer Academic Publishers. Reprinted by permission.

norepinephrine is poised to stimulate D_4Rs in the cortex, although at equal concentrations its effect would be weaker than dopamines and would result in a more modest degree of 40-Hz synchronization. Such a moderate degree of synchronization might provide a level of awareness that was less intense than a dopamine-activated episode of attention. The promiscuity of D_4Rs is, therefore, well suited for producing multiple levels of PLM and graded levels of synchronization in response to different neurotransmitters.

From the aforementioned relationship we can further suggest that initial norepinephrine-based awareness information may guide subsequent development of dopamine-based attention, as illustrated in Figure 20.6. Thus activity of norepinephrine releasing nerves would promote synchronization of incoming information, leading to a low-level, rough-draft type of awareness. Such synchronization would be continuous and seamless, rather than episodic and focused like attention, facilitating scanning of the environment and unburdened by attachment to anything. During awareness we constantly make comparisons with prior experience-based expectations. If this vigilance reveals a lack of harmony or is somehow incongruent with memory-based expectations, the presence of novelty is recognized, which can be the basis for activation of dopamine-dependent attention. This hypothetical sequence of events implies that neurons involved in novelty detection are somehow able to initiate dopamine release, presumably by stimulating neurons arising from the VTA, the primary source of dopaminergic neurons in the cortex. The proposed relationship also implies that dopamine-mediated attention involves a second, more intense synchronization of at least a subset of the very same neuronal ensembles that norepinephrine originally acted on. Thus dopamine reenters and interrogates the identical neuronal field, ensuring a seamless transition from unattended awareness to episodes of focused attention and learning.

ATTENTION-RELATED LEARNING

There is more to attention than merely turning up the volume knob for particular sensory experiences. Attention is a time-structured episode that includes both the initial prioritization of specific information and the subsequent activation of learning processes that accompany this prioritization, leading to memory formation. In fact the relationship between attention and learning is so intimate that in general we only learn the particular information we attend to. Nonattended information is experienced, but not necessarily learned, and the more frequently we attend to something the more likely we are to learn it. Conversely, it is clear that deficits in attention lead to deficits in learning.

Learning is associated with formation of new synapses and remodeling of existing synapses, involving both pyramidal cells and interneurons, and the signaling activity of dopamine receptors, including D_4Rs, contributes to these events. Via G protein activation, D_4Rs initiate signals through cAMP and MAP kinase pathways (Oak, Lavine, & Van Tol, 2001), which can lead to altered gene expression and new synapse formation. In addition, proline-containing repeats allow the D_4R to bind other signaling molecules and initiate additional signals, including activation of PI3-kinase and NFκB (Zhen, Zhang, Johnson, & Friedman, 2001). A higher number of repeats allows more proteins to bind to the D_4R receptor and therefore allows a greater number of signaling pathways to be coordinated with dopamine-stimulated PLM. However, as described later, the increased number of receptor-associated proteins can limit the capacity for PLM by displacing phospholipids and/or by interfering with the access of enzymes required for PLM.

While the D_4R in lower species has two proline-rich segments, humans have up to 11 additional proline-rich repeats, and more than 35 distinct variations in the gene sequence for the repeats have been identified (Ding et al., 2002). In contrast, the elements required for dopamine-stimulated PLM are similar in both nonprimates and primates. This implies that while the capacity for attention is shared by all species, the capacity for attention-related learning has been extensively enhanced in primates by increasing the number and variety of signaling pathways that are coordinated with D_4R-mediated PLM.

REGULATION OF METHYLATION BY IGF-1 AND DOPAMINE

Methionine synthase activity is critical to D_4R-mediated PLM, remethylating the homocysteine sidechain at position 313 with 5-methyltetrahydrofolate serving as the methyl-donating co-factor (Figure 20.2). We found that insulin-like growth factor-1 (IGF-1) and dopamine both increase the enzymatic activity of methionine synthase, via activation of the PI3-kinase signaling pathway. Indeed, in neuroblastoma cells, inhibitors of PI3-kinase reduce enzyme activity to zero and block folate-dependent D_4R-mediated PLM, while IGF-1 and dopamine increase activity up to fivefold (Waly et al., 2004). This remarkable finding implies that the efficacy of methionine synthase, and, by extension, its role in attention, are subject to regulation by these two very important signaling molecules. Furthermore, it implies that factors adversely affecting this signaling pathway may cause deficits in attention and in attention-related learning.

We experience prominent changes in our capacity for attention and attention-related learning across the lifespan. Infants and children absorb new information "like a sponge," while in old age our capacity wanes to levels that can become disabling. Interestingly, levels of IGF-1 mirror these age-dependent changes. Under the influence of growth hormone, IGF-1 levels are high during childhood and increase further during pubertal growth until the entry into adulthood. Cognitive decline during later years is accompanied by decreased IGF-1 levels (Rollero et al., 1998). Changes in the capacity for attention across the lifespan presumably reflect changes in the neurochemical pathways that support attention, and we propose that IGF-1 plays an important role in supporting D_4R-mediated attention by promoting methionine synthase activity.

Neurotoxic and neurodevelopmental effects of heavy metals, including lead and mercury, are well described, and a reduced capacity for attention and attention-related learning are prominent features of their exposure syndromes (e.g., lead poisoning). Likewise, acute ethanol exposure impairs attention, while exposure during pregnancy produces a neurodevelopmental disorder (i.e., fetal alcohol syndrome). We found that acute treatment with each of these agents exerts a profound and potent inhibitory effect on methionine synthase, reducing activity to zero, similar to the effect of PI3-kinase inhibitors. Thus impaired methylation (e.g., DNA methylation) may play a role in developmental disorders.

ATTENTION-RELATED DISORDERS

An impaired capacity for attention is associated with a number of neuropsychiatric disorders including, for example, ADHD, autism, and schizophrenia.

As noted previously, a higher incidence of ADHD is observed in individuals carrying a 7-repeat allele of the D_4R (LaHoste et al., 1996; Swanson et al., 2000), and the 7-repeat form of the receptor is complexed with a high number of signaling proteins (Oldenhof et al., 1998). These additional proteins displace membrane phospholipids in the region around the receptor, which can limit the efficiency of dopamine-stimulated PLM. We measured folate-dependent PLM in cells transfected to express D_4Rs containing 2, 4, or 7 repeats (i.e., $D_{4.2}R$, $D_{4.4}R$, or $D_{4.7}R$). As illustrated in Figure 20.7, the maximal level of dopamine-stimulated PLM was significantly lower for cells expressing the $D_4R.7R$ as compared to the $D_{4.2}R$ or $D_{4.4}R$. This result suggests that seven repeats in the D_4R introduces a constraint in dopamine-stimulated PLM that brings an increased risk of ADHD. Thus the potential benefits of recruiting additional signaling pathways to the D_4R is at least partially offset by the risk of

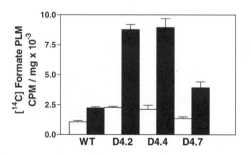

FIGURE 20.7. Dopamine-stimulated PLM is reduced in the D_47 receptor. Folate-dependent PLM was measured in cells expressing D_4Rs with 2-, 4-, or 7-repeats or in wild-type cells (WT) with no D_4Rs. Dopamine (10 (M; solid bars) increased PLM to a greater extent at $D_{4.2}$ and $D_{4.4}$ receptors.

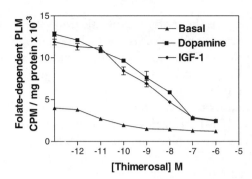

FIGURE 20.8. The vaccine preservative thimerosal potently inhibits folate-dependent PLM stimulated by either dopamine or IGF-1. From Deth (2003). Copyright 2003 by Kluwer Academic Publishers. Reprinted by permission.

impaired attention. Impaired methionine synthase activity, as caused by heavy metal exposure, for example, could combine with the 7-repeat allele to increase the risk of ADHD.

It has been suggested that the recent rise in the incidence of autism may be caused, at least in part, by administration of vaccines containing the ethylmercury derivative thimerosal (Bernard, Enayati, Redwood, Roger, & Binstock, 2001). We tested the effect of thimerosal and found that it inhibited IGF-1 and dopamine-stimulated PLM with extraordinary potency (Waly et al., 2004). Inhibition was clearly evident at concentrations as low as 0.1 nM, while a single vaccination produces blood levels of mercury in the range of 10–100 nM. Assays of methionine synthase after pretreatment of neuroblastoma cells with thimerosal showed a parallel inhibition of enzyme activity. While further studies are needed, these findings lend mechanistic support to the proposal that vaccines containing the preservative thimerosal may impair attention and attention-related learning in a subgroup of sensitive individuals.

Several metabolic abnormalities that have previously been associated with autism can synergize with a decrease in methionine synthase activity (Stone et al., 1992; Stubbs et al., 1982), and these may contribute to the risk of developing heavy metal-induced autism. Vitamin B$_{12}$ (cobalamin) is an essential co-factor for methionine synthase, participating directly in its transfer of folate-derived methyl groups to homocysteine and to the D$_4$R. In a remarkable intersection of clinical and basic science findings, physicians specializing in the treatment of autism have found that injections of the methyl-form of vitamin B$_{12}$ (methylcobalamin) produce significant and sometimes dramatic improvement in approximately 75% of children in autism (J. Neubrander, personal communication, May 2003). An increased capacity for attention was among symptoms showing the most marked improvement.

Impaired attention is a prominent symptom of schizophrenia, and people with schizophrenia have a reduced capacity to produce 40-Hz synchronized oscillations in response to an auditory stimulus (Kwon et al., 1999). The occurrence of hallucinations may reflect the pathological dominance of internally derived representations when attention to external events is impaired. There are numerous reports of abnormal methylation activity in schizophrenia, including the exacerbation of psychosis by methionine administration (Cohen, Nichols, Wyatt, & Pollin, 1974) and a high prevalence of elevated homocysteine levels, particularly in males (Levine et al., 2002). The latter observation strongly suggests impaired methionine synthase activity. Furthermore, neuroleptic drugs used to treat schizophrenia are antagonists at D_4-like receptors, and a portion of their benefit may derive from decreasing the demand for methyl groups. Taken together, these findings suggest that D_4R-mediated PLM may play a role in schizophrenia. The typical age of onset for classical schizophrenia is between 18 and 25 years in males and slightly later in females. This time period corresponds to the early stages of adulthood when growth hormone and IGF-1 signaling undergoes down-regulation. Because IGF-1 is critical for maintaining the activity of methionine synthase, the onset of schizophrenia may commonly be triggered by a loss of IGF-1 stimulation, revealing limitations in D_4R-mediated PLM and/or homocysteine methylation that were latent when IGF-1 activity was high during juvenile years.

SUMMARY

Our studies outline a novel biochemical action of dopamine, involving the D_4 dopamine receptor subtype, that appears integral to the molecular mechanism of attention. While additional studies are needed, particularly in intact animal models of attention, there is mounting evidence that D_4R-mediated PLM modulates the synchronized firing activity of neuronal networks, thereby promoting attention. Moreover, D_4Rs may also play an important role in the formation and refinement of these networks during attention-related learning. Impairment of dopamine-stimulated PLM can arise from genetic or environment factors, including from the ethylmercury-containing vaccine preservative thimerosal. Recent increases in the incidence of ADHD and autism could reflect the adverse consequences of impaired methylation. Our findings underscore the importance of limiting heavy metal exposure, particularly during early development, in order to ensure a normal capacity for attention.

REFERENCES

Ahveninen, J., Kahkonen, S., Tiitinen, H., Pekkonen, E., Huttunen, J., Kaakkola, S., et al. (2000). Suppression of transient 40-Hz auditory response by haloperidol suggests modulation of human selective attention by dopamine D2 receptors. *Neuroscience Letters*, 292, 29–32.

Benjamin, J., Li, L., Patterson, C., Greenberg, B. D., Murphy, D. L., & Hamer, D. H. (1996). Population and familial association between the D_4 dopamine receptor gene and measures of Novelty Seeking. *Nature Genetics*, 12, 81–84.

Bernard, S., Enayati, A., Redwood, L., Roger, H., & Binstock, T. (2001). Autism: A novel form of mercury poisoning. *Medical Hypotheses*, 56, 462–471.

Chrobak, J. J., & Buzsaki, G. (1998). Gamma oscillations in the entorhinal cortex of the freely behaving rat. *Journal of Neuroscience*, 18, 388–398.

Cohen, S. M., Nichols, A., Wyatt, R., & Pollin, W. (1974). The administration of methionine to chronic schizophrenic patients: A review of ten studies. *Biological Psychiatry*, 8, 209–225.

Deth, R. C. (2003). *Molecular origins of human attention: The dopamine–folate connection.* Boston: Kluwer Academic.

Deth, R. C., Mehta, S., Tan, W., Liu, Y. F., & Marshall, J. (1999). D_4 dopamine receptors co-localize with the synaptic scaffolding protein SAP-97 and glutamate receptors in rat brain extracts. *Society for Neuroscience Abstracts*, 25, 2214.

Ding, Y. C., Chi, H. C., Grady, D. L., Morishima, A., Kidd, J. R., Kidd, K. K., et al. (2002). Evidence of positive selection acting at the human dopamine receptor D_4 gene locus. *Proceedings of the National Academy of Sciences USA*, 99, 309–314.

Ebstein, R. P., Novick, O., Umansky, R., Priel, B., Osher, Y., Blaine, D., et al. (1996). Dopamine D_4 receptor (D$_4$DR) exon III polymorphism associated with the human personality trait of Novelty Seeking. *Nature Genetics, 12,* 78–80.

Fries, P., Reynolds, J. H., Rorie, A. E., & Desimone, R. (2001). Modulation of oscillatory neuronal synchronization by selective visual attention. *Science, 291,* 1560–1563.

Horvitz, J. C., Stewart, T., & Jacobs B. L. (1997). Burst activity of ventral tegmental dopamine neurons is elicited by sensory stimuli in the awake cat. *Brain Research, 759,* 251–258.

Jiang, Y., Lee, A., Chen, J., Ruta, V., Cadene, M., Chait, B. T., et al. (2003). X-ray structure of a voltage-dependent K+ channel. *Nature, 423,* 33–41.

Kotecha, S. A., Oak, J. N., Jackson, M. F., Perez, Y., Orser, B. A., Van Tol, H. H., et al. (2002). A D$_2$ class dopamine receptor transactivates a receptor tyrosine kinase to inhibit NMDA receptor transmission. *Neuron, 35,* 1111–1122.

Kwon, J. S., O'Donnell, B. F., Wallenstein, G. V., Greene, R. W., Hirayasu, Y., Nestor, P. G., et al. (1999). Gamma frequency-range abnormalities to auditory stimulation in schizophrenia. *Archives of General Psychiatry, 56,* 1001–1005.

LaHoste, G. J., Swanson, J. M., Wigal, S. B., Glabe, C., Wigal, T., King, N., et al. (1996). Dopamine D4 receptor gene polymorphism is associated with attention deficit hyperactivity disorder. *Molecular Psychiatry, 1,* 121–124.

Levine, J., Stahl, Z., Sela, B. A., Gavendo, S., Ruderman, V., & Belmaker, R. H. (2002). Elevated homocysteine levels in young male patients with schizophrenia. *American Journal of Psychiatry, 159,* 1790–1792.

Mrzljak, L., Bergson, C., Pappy, M., Huff, R., Levenson, R., Goldman-Rakic, P. S. (1996). Localization of dopamine D$_4$ receptors in GABAergic neurons of the primate brain. *Nature, 381,* 245–248.

Niebur, E., Koch, C., & Rosin, C. (1993). An oscillation-based model for the neuronal basis of attention. *Vision Research, 33,* 2789–2802.

Oak, J. N., Lavine, N., & Van Tol, H. H. (2001) Dopamine D(4) and D(2L) receptor stimulation of the mitogen-activated protein kinase pathway is dependent on trans-activation of the platelet-derived growth factor receptor. *Molecular Pharmacology, 60,* 92–103.

Oldenhof, J., Vickery, R., Anafi, M., Oak, J., Ray, A., Schoots, O., et al. (1998). SH3 binding domains in the dopamine D$_4$ receptor. *Biochemistry, 37,* 15726–15736.

Otmakhova, N. A., & Lisman J. E. (1999). Dopamine selectively inhibits the direct cortical pathway to the CA1 hippocampal region. *Journal of Neuroscience, 19,* 1437–1445.

Rollero, A., Murialdo, G., Fonzi, S., Garrone, S., Gianelli, M. V., Gazzerro, E., et al. (1998). Relationship between cognitive function, growth hormone and insulin-like growth factor I plasma levels in aged subjects. *Neuropsychobiology, 38,* 73–79.

Sharma, A., Kramer, M. L., Wick, P. F., Liu, D., Chari, S., Shim, S., et al. (1999). D$_4$ dopamine receptor-mediated phospholipid methylation and its implications for mental illnesses such as schizophrenia. *Molecular Psychiatry, 4,* 235–246.

Sheng, M. (2001). Molecular organization of the postsynaptic specialization. *Proceedings of the National Academy of Sciences USA, 98,* 7058–7061.

Shi, L., & Javitch J. A. (2002). The binding site of aminergic G protein-coupled receptors: The transmembrane segments and second extracellular loop. *Annual Reviews of Pharmacology and Toxicology, 42,* 437–467.

Stone, R. L., Aimi, J., Barshop, B. A., Jaeken, J., Van den Berghe, G., Zalkin, H., et al. (1992). A mutation in adenylosuccinate lyase associated with mental retardation and autistic features. *Nature Genetics, 1,* 59–63.

Stubbs, G., Litt, M., Lis, E., Jackson, R., Voth, W., Lindberg, A., et al. (1982). Adenosine deaminase activity decreased in autism. *Journal of the American Academy of Child Psychiatry, 21,* 71–74.

Swanson, J., Oosterlaan, J., Murias, M., Schuck, S., Flodman, P., Spence, M. A., et al. (2000). Attention deficit/hyperactivity disorder children with a 7-repeat allele of the dopamine receptor D$_4$ gene have extreme behavior but normal performance on critical neuropsychological tests of attention. *Proceedings of the National Academy of Sciences USA, 97,* 4754–4759.

Tiitinen, H., Sinkkonen, J., Reinikainen, K., Alho, K., Lavikainen, J., & Naatanen, R. (1993). Selective attention enhances the auditory 40-Hz transient response in humans. *Nature, 364,* 59–60.

Toyooka, K., Iritani, S., Makifuchi, T., Shirakawa, O., Kitamura, N., Maeda, K., et al. (2002). Selective reduction of a PDZ protein, SAP-97, in the prefrontal cortex of patients with chronic schizophrenia. *Journal of Neurochemistry, 83,* 797–806.

Van Tol, H. H., Bunzow, J. R., Guan, H. C., Sunahara, R. K., Seeman, P., Niznik, H. B., et al. (1991). Cloning of the gene for a human dopamine D$_4$ receptor with high affinity for the antipsychotic clozapine. *Nature, 350,* 610–614.

Waly, M., Olteanu, H., Banerjee, R., Choi, S.-W., Mason, J., Parker, B., et al. (2004). PI3-kinase regulates methionine synthase: Activation by IGF-1 or dopamine and inhibition by ethanol, heavy metals and thimerosal. *Molecular Psychiatry, 9,* 358–370.

Zhen, X., Zhang, J., Johnson, G. P., & Friedman, E. (2001). D$_4$ dopamine receptor differentially regulates Akt/nuclear factor-kappa b and extracellular signal-regulated kinase pathways in D(4)MN9D cells. *Molecular Pharmacology, 60,* 857–864.

21

Neuropharmacology of Attention

Trevor W. Robbins, Jean A. Milstein, and Jeffrey W. Dalley

The study of the neuropsychopharmacology of attention has received impetus from advances in clinical, as well as cognitive, neuroscience. For example, attention-deficit/hyperactivity disorder is treated with psychomotor stimulant drugs (e.g., Ritalin [methylphenidate]) that affect catecholamine (dopamine and noradrenaline) function; patients with Alzheimer's disease or Lewy body dementia exhibit impairments in attention and reaction time performance that are especially amenable to treatment with cholinergic agents such as acetylcholinesterase inhibitors (Sahakian & Coull, 1993) and nicotine (Sahakian, Jones, Levy, Warburton, & Gray, 1989), and patients with schizophrenia have been suggested to have core deficits in sensorimotor gating that are readily modeled in experimental animals, responding to treatment with antipsychotic drugs that block dopamine D_2 receptors (Geyer, Krebs-Thomson, Braff, & Swerdlow, 2001).

Such clinical observations stimulate theoretical thinking about how attentional function is controlled by a variety of mechanisms, including the ascending chemically defined arousal systems. For example, what *uniquely* do these systems normally contribute to the modulation of attention? Under *which circumstances* are these effects observed? How do these systems *interact* to optimize performance? What are the *costs* as well as benefits for cognitive performance? In practical terms, we can then ask how and to what extent it is feasible to improve performance—in normal as well as brain-damaged or psychiatrically disordered patients. While it is often assumed that a treatment corrects some biological deficit, as in the case of insulin for diabetes, it may often be the case that cognitive enhancement may be achieved simply by optimizing the performance of other, intact systems. For example, the underlying neurotransmitter pathology that is presumably "treated" by Ritalin, is still not known, and the beneficial effects of nicotine on attention in Alzheimer's disease may stem more from the availability of intact nicotine receptors than from the restoration of lost cholinergic function. We believe that assessing the costs and benefits of medication on cognitive performance in both normal and impaired individuals will grow in importance in the next period, especially with the advent of functional genomics. It will be especially important to understand the mechanisms of such costs and benefits, as well as precise knowledge of the environmental conditions under which they are obtained.

There is thus a continuing need to investigate novel therapeutic possibilities, as well as the mechanistic basis of existing therapeutic effects, and we argue that this often can only be done in experimental animals. Despite the increasing availability of sophisticated imaging technology in understanding the neural substrates of the psychopharmacology of attention (e.g., see Coull, Nobre, & Frith, 2001), it is still not feasible to study how specific neurotransmitter fluxes or depletions in particular brain regions may cause attentional effects in human subjects. This is because of ethical constaints imposed, for example, by the need to administer drugs systemically, rather than locally into the brain, and also to avoid doses that produce long-lasting or toxic effects. It is often difficult to use agents with specific neuropharmacological actions in humans, such as selective neurotoxins or drugs with specific receptor actions as tools for modeling pathological states—approaches that are feasible in experimental animals. Here, we illustrate our own approach, including the use of sophisticated behavioral tests that simulate in many ways the essential components of human tests of selective, sustained, and divided attention. By studying humans and animals in parallel it is also often possible to obtain invaluable converging evidence, and also to gain some idea of the evolutionary significance of the mechanisms involved.

One of the essential prerequisites is to use tasks that have a reliable baseline level of performance, so that both perturbations and enhancements of performance can be measured reliably. This is also important in the context of using models that depress performance in a defined way, such as an excitotoxic lesion, and then performance is recovered by means of a chronic treatment such as a neural transplant (see, e.g., Muir Dunnett, Everitt, & Robbins, 1992). It is also important for comparing the efficacy of a range of treatments, for example, effects of DA receptor blocking drugs on the deficits in performance produced by a lesion of the medial prefrontal cortex, as a possible model for some of the cognitive impairments in schizophrenia (Passetti, Levita, & Robbins, 2003). It is also important to have many internal controls for nonspecific changes in performance, and to use several distinct outcome variables that may reflect different aspects of attention, which also enables the experiments to be economical as well as illuminating.

Many of the human paradigms for measuring attention now have analogues for experimental animals, for example, Posner's test of covert orienting (Witte & Marrocco, 1997; Beane & Marrocco, Chapter 23, this volume), the five-choice serial reaction time task (5CSRTT; see Figure 21.1) as an analogue of the human continuous performance test (Robbins, 2002), tests of divided attention involving cross-modal integration (McGaughy, Kaiser, & Sarter, 1996), and the human and animal versions of the prepulse inhibition test of sensory gating (Geyer et al., 2001). Tests of attention for humans have also derived from animal learning theory; for example, latent inhibition, the phenomenon whereby learning is retarded about stimuli that have previously been unpredictive of reinforcement; extradimensional shifting between perceptual dimensions which is at the core of the clinical Wisconsin Card Sorting test (see Robbins, 1998, for a review), and trace conditioning (see Han, O'Tuathaigh, & Koch, Chapter 22, this volume). In general, it is necessary to employ several different tests of attention in order to reach firm conclusions, although this is often difficult in practice. In our 5CSRTT for rats, there are multiple measures and behavioral challenges and manipulations that extend the scope and power of the test for individual animals.

The most intensively investigated neurotransmitter systems have been the ascending cholinergic and monoamine projections (dopamine, noradrenaline, and serotonin [5-HT]) that innervate diverse areas of the forebrain. These systems are classically implicated in arousal and behavioral activation, but it is assumed that their activity and control by de-

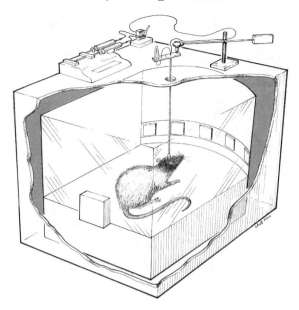

FIGURE 21.1. Schematic diagram of the five-choice serial reaction time (5CSRTT) task and the *in vivo* microdialysis perfusion system. Rats are trained to detect brief flashes of light presented randomly at one of the five apertures, in order to earn food presented at the opposite wall. Errors of commission and omission and premature and perseverative repsonses are all punished by brief periods of darkness. The intertrial interval is generally set at 5s. A session usually comprises 100 trials. Concentric-design microdialysis probes were implanted in the medial prefrontal cortex (prelimbic subregion). Animals were tethered to the apparatus with a head-mounted spring, which was connected to a counterbalanced arm and dual-channel liquid swivel positioned outside the testing chamber. Samples were collected into inverted microvials on a custom-made holder located below the rotational plane of the swivel (see Dalley et al., 2001; McGaughy et al., 2002, for more details).

scending forebrain influences represents an important modulatory mechanism by which signal-to-noise parameters may be adjusted for complex information processing in their terminal domains, often as a function of changes in arousal state. We focus on acetylcholine as a model system and then briefly compare findings using analogous methodology for the catecholamine systems, noradrenaline, and dopamine in order to discern specific functions for these systems.

ACETYLCHOLINE

Our research into the neuropharmacology of cholinergic mechanisms in attention has focused on the cholinergic neurons located in the nucleus basalis magnocellularis (nBM), which provide the major source of cholinergic innervation to the cerebral cortex (Mesulam, Mufson, Warner, & Levey, 1983), although the brain stem cholinergic system probably also has an important role that has not yet been adequately investigated in behavioral terms. Early studies of the nBM focused a great deal on its possible role in the memory and learning deficits seen in patients with Alzheimer's disease (see review by Everitt & Robbins, 1997). However, two sets of independent findings highlighted the attention modulating functions of this cholinergic system. Studies in rats began to show that performance on tests loading on attentional function produced more convincing deficits than in tests of learning or memory (see Everitt & Robbins, 1997). Second, a study by Voytko and colleagues (1994) in monkeys showed convincingly that cholinergic lesions of the nBM had their greatest impact on a test of spatial selective attention that was modeled on the covert orienting test employed by Posner and colleagues to measure attentional deficits in patients with various forms of brain damage.

A major subsequent methodological advance has been the introduction of the highly efficacious cholinergic immunotoxin 192 IgG-saporin (Heckers et al., 1994; Wiley, Oeltmann, & Lappi, 1991), which destroys selectively nerve growth factor–bearing cholinergic neurons in the nBM while sparing GABA-ergic and other noncholinergic neurons in the ventral pallidum and substantia innominata (see Everitt & Robbins, 1997, for review). In particular, recent findings with 192 IgG-saporin have provided important new insights into the nature of attentional processes supported by cholinergic neurotransmission. Thus, cholinergic activity within the nBM can be shown to be *necessary* for performance on tasks that explicitly tax sustained and divided attentional processes (McGaughy et al., 1996; Turchi & Sarter, 1997), including spatially divided visual attention as assessed by the 5CSRTT (McGaughy, Dalley, Morrison, Everitt, & Robbins, 2002; Muir, Everitt, & Robbins, 1994; Risborough, Bontempi, & Menzaghi, 2002). In addition, the capacity to increment attentional capabilities in response to unpredictable cues also requires an intact cholinergic innervation of the nBM (Chiba, Bucci, Holland, & Gallagher, 1995).

Moreover, it is now also possible to measure neurotransmitter fluxes in the behaving animal in discrete regions of the brain, using *in vivo* microdialysis, to provide another, correlative source of evidence for the putative role of acetylcholine in attentional function (see Figure 21.2). For *in vivo* cerebral microdialysis, a probe cannula perfused by an appropriate medium samples the extracellular fluid for molecules that can diffuse into it via the dialysis membrane; the concentration of these molecules is then measured with specific neurochemical methods such as high-performance liquid chromatography, with electrochemical detection. Using this technique, we and others have established that performance on various sustained visual attentional tasks is *sufficient* to increase acetylcholine (ACh) release in the

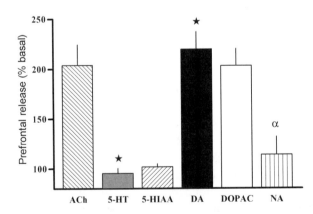

FIGURE 21.2. Differential recruitment of the principal neuromodulatory systems of the medial prefrontal cortex during sustained response-contingent performance on the 5-CSRTT. Performance-related changes (averaged over 1 hour) were greatest with respect to ACh and the DA metabolite DOPAC, but there no significant effects on NA release or the 5-HT metabolite 5-HIAA. *, DA release, but not 5-HT release, increased on a variant of the five-choice task, namely, a one-choice paradigm (Dalley et al., 2002; α, NA release increased to 174 ± 23 % when the predictive relationship between instrumental responding and food reinforcement was abolished (Dalley et al., 2001).

frontal cortex (Dalley et al., 2001; Himmelheber, Sarter, & Bruno, 2000; McGaughy et al., 2002; Passetti, Dalley, O'Connell, Everitt, & Robbins, 2000). Therefore, our evidence, as well as that of others using a different behavioral approach, with monkeys as well as rats, and focusing on more posterior cortical sites such as the lateral intraparietal cortex (see Beane & Marrocco, Chapter 23, this volume) is certainly compatible with the notion that the cortically projecting cholinergic neurons of the nBM contribute in some way to attentional processes.

However, only recently have attempts been made to understand the functional significance of cholinergic inputs in specific areas of frontal cortex to which nBM neurons more or less discretely project. It is relevant that many of the behavioral deficits observed on the five-choice attentional task following nBM lesions, including reduced-choice accuracy, increased impulsiveness, and perseveration, not only resemble qualitatively those produced by excitotoxic lesions of the medial prefrontal cortex itself (Muir, Everitt, & Robbins, 1996; Passetti, Chudasama, & Robbins, 2002) but also that they can be ameliorated by cholinesterase inhibitors such as physostigmine and cholinergic rich neural grafts injected directly into the cortex (Muir et al., 1992; Muir, Robbins, & Everitt, 1995). Therefore, it is logical to consider that some or all of these effects may have resulted from a disruption in the modulation of prefrontal cortex function by cholinergic afferents arising from the nBM.

We have tested this hypothesis further by examining the effects of the muscarinic receptor antagonist scopolamine infused directly into the medial prefrontal cortex (Robbins et al., 1998). The main findings were that scopolamine produced deficits that qualitatively resembled the effects of nBM lesions, with reduced attentional accuracy and overall slower latencies to respond correctly. More recently, we have also assessed the effects of the 192 IgG-saporin toxin itself infused directly into the prefrontal cortex (Dalley et al., in press). Although lesioned animals were generally unaffected under baseline testing conditions, they were impaired when the event rate was increased. Specifically, when the target frequency was increased over a large number of trials, which took significantly longer to complete, frontal saporin-lesioned rats exhibited a significant *decrement* in sustained attention compared to the sham-operated controls. There was also evidence for a disruption in inhibitory response control with increased premature responding and perseveration when the event rate was decreased. Our interpretation of these data is that cholinergic projections from the nBM to the prefrontal cortex support a continuum of cognitive functions relevant to the attentional control of behavior, especially in settings in which attentional resources need to be *maintained* on a continuous basis, as, for example, during a high event rate manipulation (Parasuraman & Giambra, 1991). The idea that prefrontal cholinergic mechanisms contribute to the maintenance of established attentional performance is consistent with evidence that cholinergic afferents in the prefrontal cortex mediate the increases in neuronal activity associated with increased attentional demand (Gill, Sarter, & Givens, 2000).

Further clues to the nature of attentional processes mediated by the cholinergic systems derive from neuropharmacological studies in humans and laboratory animals using selective muscarinic and nicotinic receptor ligands, as well as acetylcholinesterase inhibitors such as neostigmine and physostigmine, to augment cholinergic neurotransmission. Although the effects of systemically administered cholinergic drugs are sometimes hard to interpret, this approach is clearly highly relevant to clinical settings such as normal aging and Alzheimer's disease where disturbances in cholinergic function are implicated. In this regard, the cholinesterase inhibitor tacrine improves attentional performance on a human analogue of the 5CSRTT in patients with probable Alzheimer's disease (Sahakian & Coull, 1993), thus representing one example by which experiments with animals have led directly to clinical application.

Nicotine also enhances sustained attention in normal and elderly volunteers as well as Alzheimer's patients, on a more demanding test of rapid visual information processing (Sahakian et al., 1989; Wesnes & Revill, 1984). This result may also be relevant to suggestions that patients with schizophrenia attempt to self-medicate with nicotine through smoking. Similarly, nicotine improves response accuracy in rats with lesions of the nBM on the 5CSRTT (Muir et al., 1995) or in the presence of distracting auditory stimuli in normal rats, the latter suggestive of effects on selective attention (Hahn, Shoaib, & Stolerman, 2002). The antimuscarinic receptor agent scopolamine generally impairs performance on the 5CSRTT, but its effects are variable and often difficult to obtain in the absence of effects on omissions and other behavioral variables (Jakala et al., 1992; Jones & Higgins, 1995; however, see Mirza & Stolerman, 2000). However, there is some evidence that scopolamine increases distractibility on this task (Jones & Higgins, 1995), which again encourages the speculation that cholinergic mechanisms contribute to the active maintenance of attention, possibly by optimizing the distribution of attentional capacity (Dunne & Hartley, 1986).

A more complete understanding of cholinergic mechanisms in attention may well be forthcoming from a systematic evaluation of newly developed cholinergic compounds, for example, those exhibiting high subunit specificity for nicotinic ACh receptors (see, e.g., Hahn, Sharples, Wonnacott, Shoaib, & Stolerman, 2003)—and this may also lead to more illuminating findings in human studies of attention, as well as to clinical applications.

NORADRENALINE

A role for the coeruleocortical noradrenergic system (or the dorsal noradrenergic ascending bundle [DNAB]) in attention was also suggested from several early lines of evidence, including electrophysiological observations often involving the microiontophoresis (local application) of noradrenaline, and behavioral effects of profound depletion of the DNAB by the neurotoxin 6-hydroxydopamine (see Aston-Jones, Rajkowski, & Cohen, 1999; Robbins & Everitt, 1995b). The latter evidence suggests that reducing cortical noradrenaline (NA) to less than 5% of its normal levels leads to a broadened span of attention to environmental stimuli. This conclusion seems more accurate than simply reduced arousal level. For example, unlike the effects of cholinergic manipulations described earlier, performance on the basic 5CSRTT task is relatively unaffected, unless the task conditions are altered. For example, accuracy was disproportionately impaired in DNAB-lesioned rats when the presentation of the visual targets was made less temporally predictable (Carli, Robbins, Evenden, & Everitt, 1983; Cole & Robbins, 1992). Moreover, when loud bursts of white noise were interpolated just prior to the visual targets, the accuracy of the DNAB-lesioned rats in detecting the visual targets was drastically impaired, suggesting that the coeruleocortical NA system may normally function to preserve attentional selectivity under conditions of elevated arousal. The possible importance of the level of arousal or stress comes from two further lines of evidence that also support the conclusion of enhanced attentional lability of DNAB-lesioned rats in aversive learning situations where the animal's attention may be engaged by relatively proximal or distal cues, often competing with one another (see Selden, Cole, Everett, & Robbins, 1990; Selden, Robbins, & Everitt, 1990).

The evidence is also broadly consistent with studies by other investigators in other species, for example, in electrophysiological studies of the phasic and tonic activity of the noradrenergic locus coeruleus in monkeys (Aston-Jones et al., 1999) and in human psycho-pharmacological experiments (e.g., Clark, Geffen, & Geffen, 1986), including those using functional imaging (Coull et al., 2001). However, there is also evidence that enhanced tonic activity of the locus coeruleus can also lead to attentional lability, and thus the effects of NA depletion on phasic versus tonic modes of activity need further assessment. What can be agreed is that there is probably an optimum level of phasic activity of the locus coeruleus for selective attention (Aston-Jones et al., 1999).

The recent study of 5CSRTT performance using *in vivo* microdialysis in rats also measured NA activity directly in the prefrontal cortex (Dalley et al., 2001). The results contrasted those obtained for acetylcholine at the same time. Extracellular NA levels did not deviate very far from normal during performance of the baseline task, as might have been predicted from the lack of effects of the DNAB lesions described previously. However, when rats were subjected to a shift in contingencies, in which it was no longer necessary to respond to the visual targets in order to obtain food, NA levels showed a significant increase, which was however limited to the first of two sessions of measurement. This result implies that the locus coeruleus neurons are more readily activated by novelty, or (as in this case) altered environmental contingencies, than by the attentional demands of the task. In contrast, the overflow of acetylcholine was *reduced* under these attentionally less demanding but altered conditions in the same rats, showing clear evidence of different functions of these neurotransmitter systems within the prefrontal cortex.

DOPAMINE

The central dopamine systems are most readily associated with motor, motivational (reinforcement; see also Holroyd, Nieuwenhuis, Mars, & Coles, Chapter 16, this volume) and working-memory functions, mediated, respectively, by mesostriatal, mesolimbic, and mesocortical arms of the mesencephalic projections, than in attentional processes per se. However, some forms of attentional functions may be implicated in the phenomenon of prepulse inhibition and the notion of incentive salience, associated with mesolimbic function, as well as in the "sensorimotor neglect" resulting from unilateral striatal dopamine loss, and working memory itself (see Robbins & Everitt, 2002; Sawaguch & Goldman-Rakic, 1991).

In the case of effects of dopaminergic manipulations on 5CSRTT performance, bilateral mesostriatal dopamine depletion produces only a minor tendency to impair the accuracy of detection of targets, and only under certain conditions. More prominent are impairments in the executive control of behavior, such as the inhibition of premature and perseverative responses that interfere with task performance (Baunez & Robbins, 1999). Enhancing dopamine activity in the nucleus accumbens, by central infusions of amphetamine, increases impulsive (premature responses) and only impairs accuracy at high doses (Cole & Robbins, 1989). However, effects of the manipulation of specific dopamine D_1 or D_2 receptors in this region have not yet been determined.

Within the prefrontal cortex, there is evidence that the mesofrontal dopamine system is engaged by tasks such as the 5CSRTT. Thus, in a modified test procedure, (Dalley, Theobald, Eagle, Passetti, & Robbins, 2002) found evidence of increased dopamine overflow in the rat prefrontal cortex. This is consistent with evidence that dopamine D_1 receptors participate in response selection functions. For example, Granon and colleagues (2000) showed that infusions of the D_1 receptor partial agonist SKF 38393 could produce significant improvements in the ability to detect brief visual targets in the 5CSRTT in rats with relatively poor baseline accuracy scores, though without major effect on other parameters of performance. These findings were complemented by the finding of impaired accuracy following infusions of the D_1 receptor antagonist SCH-23390 (but not a D_2 receptor antagonist) in rats with relatively superior baseline accuracy scores. The results were interpreted as showing that activity in the mesofrontal dopamine projection can be recruited to optimize attentional performance. It can be speculated that the cortical D_1 receptors are implicated in the same basic selection functions that may also be engaged to maintain short-term memory traces over delays ("working memory," as defined by electrophysiological researchers).

CONCLUSION

In this brief survey, many of the problems involved in characterizing the functions of the chemically defined systems of the reticular core of the brain in attentional processes have been highlighted, primarily for the cholinergic, and secondarily for the monaminergic, systems. Clearly, global manipulations of these systems can be shown to produce different patterns of performance on a single task under specified test conditions (see Robbins & Everitt, 1995a). However, the more critical issue is now to discriminate possibly distinct functions of the monoamines and acetylcholine in a cortical region to which they each project; thus, it is apparent that attentional accuracy on the 5CSRTT can be influenced by manipulations that affect each of the neurotransmitter systems described, although in different ways. In future work, it will be necessary to elucidate the *interactions* of these systems in optimizing the outputs of the pyramidal cells located there. Thus, the next stage of the analysis will be to examine how these systems combine to modulate discrete neural networks within regions such as the prefrontal cortex that depend on the fast signaling glutamatergic and GABAergic transmitter systems. We also have to be aware of possible contributions of the more recently described ascending systems, such as histamine and orexin (Mignot, Taheri, & Nishino, 2002). Finally, it will continue to be important to perform parallel investigations of the human attentional systems, so that reciprocal, and mutually beneficial, interactions between the research performed in humans and experimental animals may continue to be fruitful.

ACKNOWLEDGMENTS

This work was supported by a Wellcome Trust Programme Grant and by the MRC Centre in Behavioural and Clinical Neuroscience. Jean A. Milstein is an NIH–Cambridge scholar.

REFERENCES

Aston-Jones, G., Rajkowski, J., & Cohen, J. (1999). Role of locus coeruleus in attention and behavioural flexibility. *Biological Psychiatry, 46,* 1309–1320.

Baunez, C., & Robbins, T. W. (1999). Effects of dopamine depletion of the dorsal striatum and further interaction with the subthalamic nucleus lesions in an attentional task in the rat. *Neuroscience, 92,* 1343–1356.

Carli, M., Robbins, T. W., Evenden, J. L., & Everitt, B. J. (1983). Effects of lesions to ascending noradrenergic neurons on performance of a 5-choice serial reaction task in rats: Implications for theories of dorsal noradrenergic bundle function based on selective attention and arousal. *Behavioural Brain Research*, 9, 361–380.

Chiba, A., Bucci, D. J., Holland, P. C., & Gallagher, M. (1995). Basal forebrain cholinergic lesions disrupt increments but not decrements in conditioned stimulus processing. *Journal of Neuroscience*, 15, 7315–7322.

Clark, C. R., Geffen, G. M., & Geffen, L. B. (1986). Catecholamines and the covert orienting of attention. *Neuropsychologia*, 27, 131–140.

Cole, B. J., & Robbins, T. W. (1989). Effects of 6-hydroxydopamine lesions of the nucleus accumbens septi on performance of a 5-choice serial reaction time task in rats: Implications for theories of selective attention and arousal. *Behavioural Brain Research*, 33, 165–179.

Cole, B. J., & Robbins, T. W. (1992). Forebrain norepinephrine: Role in controlled information processing in the rat. *Neuropsychopharmacology*, 7, 129–141.

Coull, J. T., Nobre, A. C., & Frith, C. D. (2001). The noradrenergic alpha-2 agonist clonidine modulates behavioural and neuroanatomical correlates of human attentional orienting and alerting. *Cerebral Cortex*, 11, 73–84.

Dalley, J. W., McGaughy, J., O'Connell, M. T., Cardinal, R. N., Levita, L., & Robbins, T. W. (2001). Distinct changes in cortical acetylcholine and noradrenaline efflux during contingent and non-contingent performance of a visual attentional task. *Journal of Neuroscience*, 21, 4908–4914.

Dalley, J. W., Theobald, D. E., Bouger, P., Chudasama, Y., Cardinal, R. N., & Robbins, T. W. (in press). Cortical cholinergic function and deficits in visual attentional performance in rats following 192 IgG-saporin-induced lesions of the medial prefrontal cortex. *Cerebral Cortex*.

Dalley, J. W., Theobald, D. E., Eagle, D. M., Passetti, F., & Robbins, T. W. (2002). Deficits in impulse control associated with tonically elevated serotonergic function in rat prefrontal cortex. *Neuropsychopharmacology*, 26, 716–728.

Dunne, M. P., & Hartley, L. R. (1986). Scopolamine and the control of attention in humans. *Psychopharmacology*, 89, 94–97.

Everitt, B. J., & Robbins, T. W. (1997). Central cholinergic systems and cognition. *Annual Review of Psychology*, 48, 649–684.

Geyer, M. A., Krebs-Thomson, K., Braff, D. L., & Swerdlow, N. R. (2001). Pharmacological studies of prepulse inhibition models of sensorimotor gating deficits in schizophrenia: A decade in review. *Psychopharmacology*, 156, 117–154.

Gill, T. M., Sarter, M., & Givens, B. (2000). Sustained visual attention performance-associated prefrontal neuronal activity: Evidence for cholinergic modulation. *Journal of Neuroscience*, 20, 4745–4757.

Granon, S., Passetti, F., Thomas, K. L., Dalley, J. W., Everitt, B. J., & Robbins, T.,W. (2000). Enhanced and impaired attentional performance after infusion of D_1 dopaminergic receptor agents into rat prefrontal cortex. *Journal of Neuroscience*, 20, 1208–1215.

Hahn, B., Sharples, C. G., Wonnacott, S., Shoaib, M., & Stolerman, I. P. (2003). Attentional effects of nicotinic agonists in rats. *Neuropsychopharmacology*, 44, 1054–1067.

Hahn, B., Shoaib, M., & Stolerman, I. P. (2002). Nicotine-induced enhancement of attention in the five-choice serial reaction time task: The influence of task demands. *Psychopharmacology*, 162, 129–137.

Heckers, S., Ohtake, T., Wiley, R. G., Lappi, D. A., Geula, C., & Mesulam, M. M. (1994). Complete and selective cholinergic denervation of rat neocortex and hippocampus but not amygdala by an immunotoxin against p75 NGF receptor. *Journal of Neuroscience*, 14, 1271–1289.

Higgins, G. A., Ballard, T. M., Huwyler, J., Kemp, J. A., & Gill, R. (2003). Evaluation of the NR2B-selective NMDA receptor antagonist Ro 63–1908 on rodent behaviour: Evidence for an involvement of NR2B NMDA receptors in response inhibition. *Neuropharmacology*, 44, 324–341.

Himmelheber, A. M., Sarter, M., & Bruno, J. P. (2000). Increases in cortical acetylcholine release during sustained attentional performance in rats. *Brain Research: Cognitive Brain Research*, 9, 313–325.

Jakala, P., Sirvio, J., Jolkkonen, J., Riekkinen, P. Jr., Acsady, L., & Riekkinen, P. (1992). The effects of p-chlorophenylalanine-induced serotonin synthesis and muscarinic blockade on the performance of rats in a 5-choice serial reaction time task. *Behavioural Brain Research*, 51, 29–40.

Jones, D. N. C., & Higgins, G. A. (1995). Effects of scopolamine on visual attention in rats. *Psychopharmacology*, *120*, 142–149.

McGaughy, J., Dalley, J. W., Morrison, C. H., Everitt, B. J., & Robbins, T. W. (2002). Selective behavioral and neurochemical effects of cholinergic lesions produced by intrabasalis infusions of 192 IgG-saporin on attentional performance in a five-choice serial reaction time task. *Journal of Neuroscience*, *22*, 1905–1913.

McGaughy, J., Kaiser, T., & Sarter, M. (1996). Behavioral vigilance following 192 IgG-saporin into the basal forebrain: Selectivity of the behavioral impairment and relation to cortical AChE-positive fiber density. *Behavioural Neuroscience*, *110*, 247–265.

Mesulam, M.-M., Mufson, E. J., Wainer, B. H., & Levey, A. I. (1983). Central cholinergic pathways in the rat: An overview based on alternative nomenclature. *Neuroscience*, *10*, 1185–1201.

Mignot, E., Taheri, S., & Nishino, S. (2002). Sleeping with the hypothalamus: Emerging therapeutic targets for sleep disorders. *Nature Neuroscience*, *5*, 1071–1075.

Mirza, N., & Stolerman, I. P. (2000). The role of nicotinic and muscarinic acetylcholine receptors in attention. *Psychopharmacology*, *107*, 541–550.

Muir, J. L., Dunnett, S. B., Robbins, T. W., & Everitt, B. J. (1992). Attentional functions of the forebrain cholinergic systems: Effects of intraventricular hemicholinium, physostigmine, basal forebrain lesions and intracortical grafts on a multiple-choice serial reaction time task. *Experimental Brain Research*, *89*, 611–622.

Muir, J. L., Everitt, B. J., & Robbins, T. W. (1994). AMPA-induced excitotoxic lesions of the basal forebrain: A significant role for the cortical cholinergic system in attentional function. *Journal of Neuroscience*, *14*, 2313–2326.

Muir, J. L., Everitt, B. J., & Robbins, T. W. (1996). The cerebral cortex of the rat and visual attentional function: Dissociable effects of mediofrontal, cingulate, anterior dorsolateral and parietal cortex on a five choice serial reaction time task. *Cerebral Cortex*, *6*, 470–481.

Muir, J. L., Robbins, T. W., & Everitt, B. J. (1995). Reversal of visual attentional dysfunction following lesions of the cholinergic basal forebrain by physostigmine and nicotine but not the 5-HT3 antagonist, ondansetron. *Psychopharmacology*, *118*, 82–92.

Parasuraman, R., & Giambra, L. (1991). Skill development in vigilance: Effects of event rate and age. *Psychology and Aging*, *6*, 155–169.

Passetti, F., Chudasama, Y., & Robbins, T. W. (2002). The frontal cortex of the rat and visual attentional performance: Dissociable functions of distinct medial prefrontal regions. *Cerebral Cortex*, *12*, 1254–1268.

Passetti, F., Dalley, J. W., O'Connell, M. T., Everitt, B. J., & Robbins, T. W. (2000). Increased acetylcholine release in the rat medial prefrontal cortex during performance of a visual attentional task. *Psychology and Aging*, *12*, 3051–3058.

Passetti, F., Levita, L., & Robbins, T. W. (2003). Sulpiride alleviates the attentional impairments of rats with medial prefrontal lesions. *Behavioural Brain Research*, *138*, 59–79.

Risbrough, V., Bontempi, B., & Menzaghi, F. (2002). Selective immunolesioning of the basal forebrain cholinergic neurons in rats: Effect on attention using the 5-choice serial reaction time task. *Psychopharmacology*, *164*, 71–81.

Robbins, T. W. (1998). Arousal and attention: The psychopharmacology and neuropsychology of attention in experimental animals. In R. Parasuraman (Ed.), *The attentive brain* (pp. 189–220). Cambridge, MA: MIT Press.

Robbins, T. W. (2002). The 5-choice serial reaction time task: Behavioral pharmacology and functional neurochemistry. *Psychopharmacology*, *163*, 362–380.

Robbins, T. W., & Everitt, B. J. (1995a). Arousal systems and attention. In M. S. Gazzaniga (Ed.), *The cognitive neurosciences* (pp. 703–720). Cambridge, MA: MIT Press.

Robbins, T. W., & Everitt, B. J. (1995b). Central norepinephrine neurons and behavior. In F. E. Bloom & D. Kupfer (Eds.), *Psychopharmacology: The fourth generation of progress* (pp. 363–372). New York: Raven Press.

Robbins, T. W., & Everitt, B. J. (2002). Dopamine—its role in behaviour and cognition in experimental animals and humans. In G. Di Chiara (Ed.), *Handbook of experimental pharmacology*, Vol. *154.II: Dopamine in the CNS II* (pp. 173–211). Heidelberg: Springer-Verlag.

Robbins, T. W., Granon, S., Muir, J. L., Durantou, F., Harrison, A., & Everitt, B. J. (1998). Neural systems underlying arousal and attention: Implications for drug abuse. *Annals of the New York Academy of Science, 846,* 222–237.

Sahakian, B. J., & Coull, J. T. (1993). Tetrahydroaminoacridine (THA) in Alzheimer's disease: an assessment of attentional and mnemonic function using CANTAB. *Acta Neurologica Scandinavica Supplementum, 149,* 29–35.

Sahakian, B. J., Jones, G., Levy, R., Warburton, D., & Gray, J. (1989). The effects of nicotine on attention, information processing, and short term memory in patients with dementia of the Alzheimer type. *British Journal of Psychiatry, 154,* 797–800.

Sawaguchi, T., & Goldman-Rakic, P. S. (1991). D_1 DA receptors in prefrontal cortex: Involvement in working memory. *Science, 251,* 947–950.

Selden, N. R. W., Robbins, T. W., & Everitt, B. J. (1990). Enhanced behavioral conditioning to context and impaired behavioral and neuroendocrine responses to conditioning stimuli following ceruleo-cortical noradrenergic lesions: Support for an attentional hypothesis of central noradrenergic function. *Journal of Neuroscience, 10,* 531–539.

Selden, N. R. W., Cole, B. J., Everitt, B. J., & Robbins, T. W. (1990). Damage to ceruleocortical noradrenergic projections impairs locally cued but enhances spatially cued water maze acquisition. *Behavioural Brain Research, 39,* 29–52.

Turchi, J., & Sarter, M. (1997). Cortical aceylcholine and processing capacity: Effects of cortical cholinergic deafferentation on crossmodal divided attention in rats. *Cognitive Brain Research, 6,* 147–158.

Voytko, M., Olton, D. S., Richardson, D. T., Gorman, L. K., Tobin, J. R., & Price, D. J. (1994). Basal forebrain lesions in monkeys disrupt attention but not learning and memory. *Journal of Neuroscience, 14,* 167–180.

Wesnes, K., & Revell, A. (1984). The separate and combined effects of scopolamine and nicotine on human information processing. *Psychopharmacology, 84,* 5–11.

Wiley, R. G., Oeltmann, T. N., & Lappi, D. A. (1991). Immunolesioning: Selective destruction of neurons using immunotoxin to rat NGF receptor. *Brain Research, 562,* 149–153.

Witte, E. A., & Marrocco, R. T. (1997). Alteration of brain noradrenergic activity in rhesus monkeys affects the alerting component of covert orienting. *Psychopharmacology, 132,* 315–323.

22

A Practical Assay for Attention in Mice

C. J. Han, Colm M. O'Tuathaigh, and Christof Koch

Our laboratory has been involved for many years in trying to understand the function and properties of selective visual attention as well as the underlying neuronal mechanisms in human and nonhuman primates using a variety of psychophysical, physiological, and computational techniques (Itti & Koch, 2000; Koch & Ullman, 1985; Kreiman, Fried, & Koch, 2002; Li, Van Rullen, Koch, & Perona, 2002; for a synthesis, see Koch, 2004). For reasons outlined later, we think it is important to also develop animal models of selective attention that are more amenable to interventionist strategies. It is only by intervening delicately, reversibly, selectively, and deliberately with the brain that the gap between correlation and causation can be breached. In this chapter, we describe our efforts to develop a robust and practical model of selective attention in mice that implicates the anterior cingulate cortex in its expression or control.

ATTENTION AND MICE

In the search for the neural substrates mediating attention, nonhuman animal models are of crucial importance. Among the animal models, efforts have been concentrated in the primate visual system (Braun, Koch, & Davis, 2001; Parasuraman, 1998). While extremely useful for identifying neural correlates of attention, primates offer limited accessibility for tests of causation, which involves more invasive perturbations. Various types of attention have also been studied in species such as rats (Mishima et al., 2002; O'Tuathaigh & Moran, 2002; Passetti, Chudasama, & Robbins, 2002; Robbins, 2002), cats (Delagrange et al., 1990; Lomber, Payne, & Cornwell, 2001; Piazza et al., 1988), marmosets (Collins, Wilkinson, Everitt, Robbins, & Roberts, 2000; Crofts et al., 2001), rabbits (Gabriel & Taylor, 1998; Hernandez & Watson, 1997; Kang & Gabriel, 1998), pigeons (Fremouw, Herbranson, & Shimp, 2002; Lemmonds, Williams, & Wenger, 2002; Weiss & Panlilio, 1999) and *Drosophila* (Heisenberg & Wolf, 1984; Tang & Guo, 2001; van Swinderen & Greenspan, 2003). Among these species, mice have gained a prominent position as a model organism for several reasons. First, the mouse is much more closely related to humans than the fruit fly is, a standard biological model organism. This is particularly relevant as the cortex has been heavily implicated in the control and expression of attention. Second, mice are easy to keep and breed all year round, with a short generation time (10–12 weeks), and they are relatively cost-effective. Unlike many other species, inbreeding is well tolerated, and many highly inbred strains have been established during the past century, which allows a variety of comparisons to be performed with subsequent rigorous genetic analysis. Third, the mouse has the most amenable genetics of all mammals. It is one of the rare, if not the only, species for which embryonic stem cells can be isolated and maintained *in vitro* and reliably transmitted through the germ line to produce genetically modified individuals such as transgenics, knockouts, and knockins. Stem cells can be genetically engineered, allowing the production of an almost unlimited number of genetic "custom mice" with loss or gain of function mutations in specific genes of biological or medical interest. Furthermore, not only can these techniques be used to alter the genes of interest, but they can potentially be combined with exogenous genes to reversibly inactivate genetically identifiable populations of neurons (Lechner, Lein, & Calloway, 2002; Slimko, McKinney, Anderson, Davidson, & Lester, 2002; Yamamoto et al., 2003). Recent progress in the refinement of inducible systems such as tTA and rtTA (tetracycline transactivator and reverse tetracycline transactivator) and region- or tissue-specific manipulations driven by specific promoters have greatly increased spatial and temporal control (Mansuy et al., 1998). Fourth, the completion of the initial phase of the human genome project and the rapid sequencing of the genome of other organisms will most definitely revolutionize the field of neurobiology. Among the model organisms (chimpanzee, mouse, rat, chicken, pig, pufferfish, and zebrafish, to name a few), the most advanced sequence analysis of a mammalian model organism is in the mouse, for which a high-quality sequence of the entire genome is targeted for completion by 2005. The availability of the mouse genome sequence will both speed the design of such constructs and reduce the likelihood of unfortunate choices (Lindblad-Toh et al., 2001; Waterston et al., 2002). Beane and Marrocco (Chapter 23, this volume) provides an excellent example of taking advantage of mouse genetics to study attention by using DRD_4 knockout mice (lacking the D_4 dopamine receptor) to probe the neural basis of attention-deficit disorder.

MODELS OF ATTENTION IN MICE

A few paradigms are presently used to assess attention in mice.

- The *orienting paradigm* involves presenting the animals with a stimulus and measuring the head-orienting movement or the direction of its gaze. This tests for nonselective sensory arousal (Vallone et al., 2002).
- As a test of selective attention, the *latent inhibition* task is thought to measure the decrease in attention to stimuli which predict no significant outcome (Moser, Hitchcock, Lister, & Moran, 2000). It has been studied in mice in a number of behavioral assays including the conditioned avoidance response (Kline, Decena, Hitzemann, & McCaughran, 1998), conditioned fear (Restivo, Passino, Middei, & Amassari-Teule, 2002) and conditioned emotional response (Gould, Collins, & Wehner, 2001; Gould & Wehner, 1999).
- The *five-choice serial reaction time task* (5CSRTT) tests for both selective and sustained attention and is well described in rats (Carli, Robbins, Evenden, & Everitt, 1983). The protocol has the animal attending to a series of visual cues (lamps) to detect a discriminative cue and make the correct response (nose poke) into one of the five holes in the training apparatus. Manipulations of the temporal and spatial parameters vary the attentional load. Existing research in mice has revolved around simply adapting and modify-

ing where necessary the structural and procedural parameters of the rat task, including reducing the holes from five to two or one (Humby, Laird, Davies, & Wilkinson, 1999; Lee, Tumu, & Paul, 2002; Marston, Spratt, & Kelly, 2001).

• The *five-arm maze* represents a modified murine analogue of the 5CSRTT. It combines the basic procedure of the 5CSRTT and the structural features of the radial maze, the latter used as a standard test of spatial memory in rodents. Here, mice are trained on a simple visual discrimination task to make a rapid decision among the five open arms of a maze, entering the arm lit by a cue light to receive food reinforcement. After a performance criterion is reached, manipulations of cue light duration, or the introduction of a variable cued trial order, may be used to alter the sustained attentional load (Durkin, Beaufort, Leblond, & Maviel, 2000; Leblond, Beaufort, Delerve, & Durkin, 2002).

All the aforementioned paradigms test different aspects of attention with their particular strengths and weaknesses. The orienting paradigm suffers from problems of interpretation and quantification. Orientation to the direction of the stimulus may not reflect attention to that stimulus and quantification of rapid changes in direction may be difficult (Bushnell, 1998). The decrement in associating the previously unreinforced stimulus in latent inhibition has been explained in terms of a reduction in attention to the conditioned stimulus (CS) (Mackintosh, 1975) or a learning of "inattention" to the CS (Lubow, 1997). However, a number of recent theoretical accounts have argued in favor of a framework that views latent inhibition (and related effects such as Kamin blocking) in terms of associative rather than attentional changes (Escobar, Arcediano, & Miller, 1994; Grahame, Barnet, Gunther, & Miller, 1994). Hence, the construct validity of latent inhibition as reflecting attentional processes is currently in question. The major problem with using powerful operant methods such as the 5CSRTT to measure attention is the length of time taken (up to several months) to train the animals. We were interested in establishing a more rapid, and therefore practical, means of manipulating the attentional state of mice. Such a procedure should be robust enough to allow large-scale automated evaluation of mice for relevant medical applications (e.g., screening for genes or compounds of therapeutic benefit for attention-deficit/hyperactivity disorder).

HOW TO ESTABLISH A FAST AND PRACTICAL MODEL
OF SELECTIVE ATTENTION IN MICE

Studies in humans have suggested that selective attention is required for certain forms of Pavlovian conditioning (Clark, Manns, & Squire, 2002). Two commonly used variants of this procedure are delay and trace conditioning. In delay conditioning, a CS, such as a bell ring, is immediately followed by an unconditioned stimulus (US), such as food. In trace conditioning, a time gap is introduced between the end of the CS and the start of the US. Although this difference seems minute, attention appears to be required for trace but not delay conditioning. In human eyeblink conditioning, in which the CS is a tone and the US is an airpuff to the cornea, distracting stimuli interfere with trace but not delay conditioning, suggesting that attention is necessary for the former but not latter type of learning (Clark et al., 2002; Clark & Squire, 1998, 1999; Manns, Clark, & Squire, 2000a, 2000b; Manns et al., 2002). In human fear conditioning, in which the CS is a tone and the US is an electric shock, the situation appears somewhat more complex. A mild task designed to distract the subjects interferes with trace conditioning but not delay conditioning. However, a very demanding task (such as the two-back memory task, in which the subjects have to answer if the digit shown on the computer screen is the same as the digit shown before the last presentation) can also interfere with delay conditioning (Carter, Hofstötter, Tsuchiya, & Koch, 2003). Pavlovian fear conditioning provides a great advantage over operant conditioning in that mice rapidly learn in a matter of minutes (Kim & Fanselow, 1992). Therefore, we used trace and delay fear conditioning to investigate neural substrates of attention in mice. We show that a visual distractor selectively interferes with trace but not delay fear conditioning, suggesting an attentional requirement for this type of learning in mice, as in humans.

Distraction Disrupts Trace But Not Delay Conditioning

Adult C57BL/6N male mice received six trials of delay, trace, or shock-only conditioning, using a 2-kHz tone as the CS and a footshock as the US (Figure 22.1A, 22.1B). The extent of conditioning was assessed the next day on the basis of freezing (total immobility except for breathing) following presentation of the tone (Figure 22.1E). In control animals, both delay

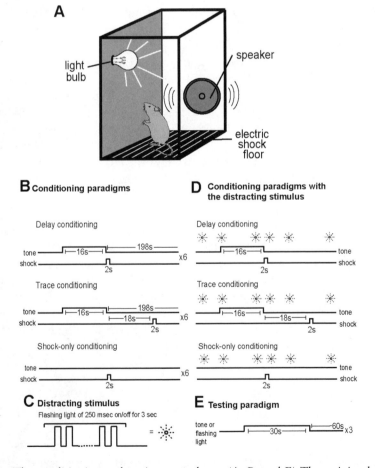

FIGURE 22.1. The conditioning and testing procedures. (A, B, and E) The training box, the conditioning paradigms, and the testing paradigm. (C) A light presentation served as the distractor. (D) For animals in the distraction conditions, the distractor—flashing bright lights—is presented with a random interstimulus interval of 5, 10, 15, or 20 seconds.

and trace conditioning were successfully observed, as shown by a significantly higher level of freezing elicited by the tone, compared with the shock-only conditioning ($p < .05$) (Figure 22.2A; no distractor). Next, we sought to distract the mice by randomly flashing a light in the cage as the distractor (Figure 22.1C) during conditioning (Figure 22.1D). Details of the procedures can be seen elsewhere (Han et al., 2003). The flashing light disrupted freezing in the trace conditioning group, as indicated by a significant reduction in the percent time spent freezing to the tone, compared with the control mice that did not receive the distractor ($p < .05$) (Figure 22.2A). No significant effect of the flashing light in either the delay or shock-only conditions was observed. In control animals, both delay and trace conditioning were observed, as shown by a significantly higher level of freezing elicited by the tone, compared with the shock-only conditioning ($p < .05$) (Figure 22.2A; no distractor).

We attribute the effects of the distractor to a disruption of the attentional processes necessary for trace conditioning. However, it is also known that multiple stimuli compete with each other for the relative strength of association with the US (Rescorla & Wagner, 1972). It does not seem that this associative competition accounts for our results for the following reasons. First, if associative competition did occur, it would be expected that delay conditioning would also be affected by the presentation of the flashing light, which is not the case (Figure 22.2A). Second, animals that received the flashing light during training showed low freezing levels, comparable to those that did not receive the flashing light, when exposed to the light as a test stimulus (Figure 22.2B). This suggests that the flashing light did not compete with the tone as a CS. In addition, we examined the disruptive effect of the flashing light at different time points of the trace conditioning trials. No differences in freezing to the flashing light were observed across any of the six tone-shock pairings, compared with mice that received no flashing light (Figure 22.2C). Therefore, it is unlikely that the flashing light became associated with the shock at the expense of the tone-shock association in the first few training trials in trace conditioning, but that this light-shock association was extinguished in later training trials. The presentation of the flashing light also did not increase contextual freezing (Figure 22.2D), ruling out the possibility that the flashing light increases the saliency of the context, which in turn competes with learning to the tone.

Taken together, these results provide evidence that the distracting effect of the flashing light on trace conditioning is not due to associative competition at any point of training. In addition, locomotor activity, as assessed by the number of crossing and rearing events (i.e., number of times the animal moved across the midline of the cage and reared its upper body above its shoulders per minute), was not significantly different between the light-exposed and nonexposed groups (Figure 22.2E), arguing against the possibility that the decreased freezing level in trace conditioning is due to hyperactivity. The most reasonable alternative explanation is that the flashing light interferes with trace conditioning by distracting the animals' attention during the acquisition phase.

THE ANTERIOR CINGULATE CORTEX ACTIVITY
IS CORRELATED WITH AND REQUIRED FOR ATTENTION

Functional imaging has identified potential neural substrates of attention in humans. For example, attention has been correlated with increased activity in the anterior cingulate cortex (ACC) in humans (Bush et al., 1998, 2002; Bush, Luu, & Posner, 2000; Davis, Hutchison, Lozano, Tasker, & Dostrovsky, 2000a; Devinsky, Morrell, & Vogt, 1995; Jovicich et al., 2001). Furthermore, the human ACC is preferentially activated during presentation of the

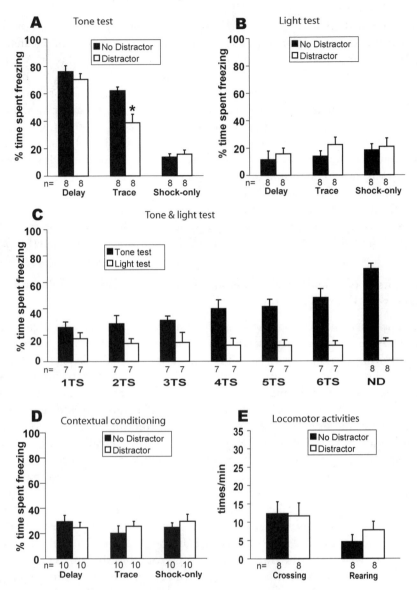

FIGURE 22.2. Animals received either a distractor or no distractor during training. On the testing day, animals were presented with the tone and the light, or vice versa. (A) Percent time spent freezing during tone testing. The distractor during conditioning selectively disrupts trace learning, without affecting delay learning. * indicates significant reduction in time spent freezing for the distractor group compared with the non-distractor group of trace conditioning training ($p < .05$). Both delay and trace conditioning are significantly different from the shock-only conditioning for the non-distracted animals (black bars, $p < .05$). Error bars indicate *SEM*. (B) For light testing, there is no difference in percent time spent freezing between the animals that did and those that did not receive the distractor during training. (C) Six groups of mice received one, two, three, four, five, or six tone-shock (TS) pairings and the flashing light as the distractor during trace conditioning. One group of mice received standard 6 tone-shock pairings and no distractor (ND) during trace conditioning. There is no difference in freezing to the flashing light for any of the six tone-shock pairings, compared with mice that received no flashing light. As a positive control, ND group shows high level of freezing in the tone test. (D) No difference was observed between the distractor and no distractor groups, indicating that the distractor did not affect contextual fear conditioning. (E) No difference was found in locomotor activity, as assessed by the number of crossing and rearing events between the distractor and no distractor groups.

CS, compared with that of a meaningless stimulus, during aversive trace conditioning (Büchel, Dolan, Armony, & Friston, 1999). The ACC has also been implicated in tasks requiring visual attention in rats (Bussey, Everitt, & Robbins, 1997; Bussey, Muir, Everitt, & Robbins, 1996; Muir, Everitt, & Robbins, 1996; Robbins, 2002; Rogers, Baunez, Everitt, & Robbins, 2001). Lesion studies have shown that the medial prefrontal cortex, including the ACC, is critical for trace but not for delay eyeblink conditioning in rabbits (Kronforst-Collins & Disterhoft, 1998; Weible, McEchron, & Disterhoft, 2000). However, a direct link between trace conditioning and attention has not been established in mice.

We show that the acquisition of trace conditioning is associated with increased activation of ACC, as determined using the induction of c-fos mRNA. c-fos has been widely used as a surrogate marker of neuronal activity (Bahu et al., 2001; Chaudhuri, Zangenehpour, Rahbar-Dehgan, & Ye, 2000; Dragunow & Faull, 1989). To extend these correlational studies to a test of causation, we specifically lesioned the ACC prior to training using excitotoxins. Such lesions produced selective deficits in trace but not delay conditioning.

Higher Density of c-fos-Positive Cells in the ACC after Trace Conditioning Compared with Delay Conditioning

To determine whether trace fear conditioning in mice is associated with higher neuronal activity in the ACC compared with delay conditioning, we performed *in situ* hybridization to detect c-fos mRNA, a marker of neuronal activation. This allows us to directly count the number of neurons that were active within the last 2 hours before the animals were killed. After training, a subset of the mice was sacrificed for c-fos analysis, and the rest were saved for tone testing on the next day. The contours of the ACC (divided into subregions Cg1 and Cg2) and primary motor cortex (M1) were fitted electronically on the section with reference to a mouse brain atlas (Paxinos & Franklin, 2001) and were calibrated in relation to relevant anatomical landmarks such as the corpus callosum. Mice that received trace conditioning showed, on average, approximately 50% more c-fos positive cells in the Cg1 subregion of the ACC than mice that received delay conditioning ($t(6)=3.24$, $p < .05$) (Figure 22.3). In each pair of brains (trace vs. delay) from four separate *in situ* hybridization experiments, the Cg1 of the mouse that received trace conditioning had more c-fos positive cells than the Cg1 of the mouse that received delay conditioning. In the Cg2 subregion, there was a trend of more c-fos positive cells in the trace conditioning group but the difference was not significant at the 5% level. No differences were detected between the trace conditioning and delay conditioning groups in the primary motor cortex (Figure 22.3B, M1). Therefore, the increased number of the c-fos-positive cells in the Cg1 subregion in the trace conditioning group does not simply reflect a general increase in activity across all cortical areas. Among mice that were saved for tone testing, animals that received trace conditioning exhibited a significantly higher percent time freezing than those that received the shock-only training (Figure 22.3C; $p < .05$), suggesting that the mice sacrificed for c-fos mRNA *in situ* hybridization were also successfully conditioned. These data suggest that the ACC in mice is more activated during the acquisition of trace fear conditioning compared to delay conditioning.

The ACC Is Required for Trace But Not Delay Conditioning

To assess the requirement of an intact ACC for trace fear conditioning in mice, we used an excitotoxin, NMDA, to lesion the ACC prior to the conditioning procedure. We also included two control groups. One group received sham surgery to control for the effect of the

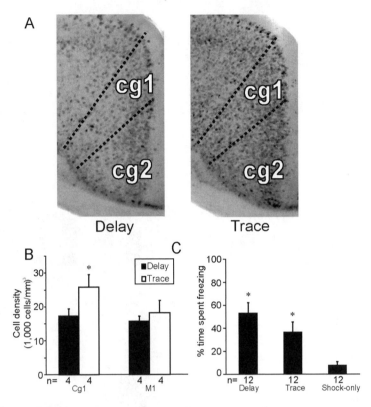

FIGURE 22.3. *c-fos* positive cell counts after trace or delay conditioning. Each grain corresponds to a *c-fos* positive neuron. (A) Representative *c-fos in situ* hybridization expression in the ACC during delay and trace conditioning. Darker dots are *c-fos* positive cells stained by BCIP/NBT. (B) *c-fos* positive cell density in the Cg1 and M1. Mice that received trace conditioning have significantly more *c-fos* positive cells in the ACC compared with mice that received delay conditioning (*$p < .05$). There is no such difference in M1. (C) Percent time spent freezing during the tone test of the mice trained simultaneously with the mice sacrificed for *c-fos* mRNA in situ hybridization. Mice trained on delay and trace conditioning exhibit significantly more freezing than the shock-only group (*$p < .05$).

general surgical procedure, and another group received lesions to the primary visual cortex (V1) to control for the effect of general cortical damage. The extent of the lesion was verified after the experiment for each mouse by histology. Animals received trace, delay, or shock-only training. Mice that received sham operations exhibited both successful delay and trace conditioning, in comparison to the control shock-only group ($p < .05$) (Figure 22.4A). In contrast, animals that received ACC lesions showed significant reduction in trace conditioning by comparison to the sham group and the V1 group ($p < .05$) (Figure 22.4A). Indeed, the level of freezing in the ACC-lesioned animals was not significantly different from freezing in animals that only received the shock. There was no difference in trace conditioning between the sham and V1 groups, suggesting that the impairment in the ACC group was not due to general cortical damage. Importantly, all the lesion groups exhibited successful delay conditioning in comparison to shock-only controls (Figure 22.4A, $p < .05$). That is, removing the ACC on both sides subsequently disrupts trace but not delay fear conditioning in mice. To delineate at what point during testing the impairment of the ACC group first became evident, the time spent freezing was analyzed separately at each of the three consecu-

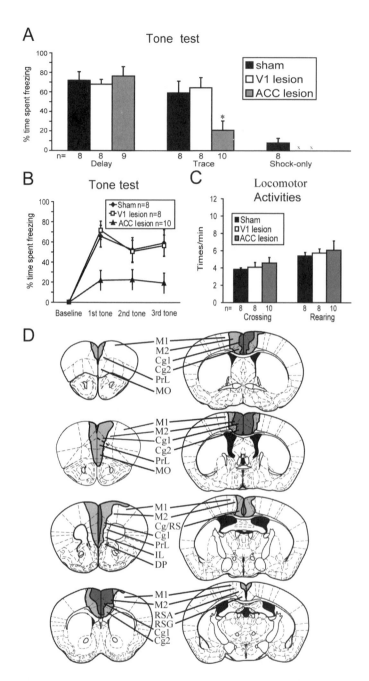

FIGURE 22.4. The effects of the bilateral ACC lesion on trace and delay conditioning. (A) Tone test. The ACC lesion group show impaired freezing performance in trace conditioning but not in delay conditioning, compared with sham control group. There is no difference between the V1 lesion group and the sham group in either delay or trace group.* identifies significantly lower time spent freezing of ACC lesioned animals compared with sham operation and V1 lesions in trace conditioning ($p < .05$). x means the corresponding V1 and ACC groups did not exist. (B) Percent time spent freezing as a function of trial number during testing for trace conditioning. The impairment of the ACC lesions can be seen as early as the first trial. (C) Locomotor activities. No difference is found between the ACC, V1, and sham lesion groups trained in trace, assessed by crossing and rearing activities. (D) The sagittal (upper panel) and coronal (lower panel) view of the ACC in a mouse brain with superimposed lesion sites. Cg, anterior cingulate cortex; M1, primary motor cortex; M2, secondary motor cortex; RS, retrosplenial cortex (posterior cingulate cortex); PrL, prelimbic cortex. Data from Paxinos and Franklin (2001).

tive tone-testing trials for trace conditioning (Figure 22.4B). The ACC lesion group displayed significantly less freezing as early as the first trial, compared with the sham group ($p < .01$) or the V1 lesion group ($p < .01$), suggesting that the lower freezing level of the ACC lesion group is likely caused by learning impairment but not by faster extinction. No difference was found between the ACC lesion and control groups in locomotor activity by measures of crossing and rearing (Figure 22.4C). For contextual conditioning, the percent time freezing for the ACC lesion group and sham group was 37% ± 9% and 36% ± 8% (mean ± *SEM*), respectively. No significant difference was found. However, due to the decreasing size of the ACC toward its anterior tip, and the relatively large domain of excitotoxic cell killing, it was difficult to lesion this region of the ACC without including parts of the prelimbic and the infralimbic cortex. Lesions that spared these latter two areas also spared the anterior tip of the ACC. Nevertheless, when the ACC lesion group was separated into two subgroups, one including and one excluding those subjects with lesions spanning the prelimbic/infralimbic/anterior tip of the ACC, no significant performance difference between these two subgroups was detected, arguing that the effect of our lesions on trace conditioning indeed reflects a requirement for the ACC. Our *c-fos* analysis suggested enhanced activity in the Cg1 subdomain of ACC during trace conditioning, while Cg2 did not show a significant difference. Anatomically, Cg1 projects to the insular cortex, another brain area that was shown to be activated during aversive trace conditioning (Büchel, Dolan, Armony, & Friston, 1999), but Cg2 does not (Zilles & Wree, 1995). Firm conclusions about the subregions of the ACC necessary for trace conditioning will demand a more refined method of functional perturbation, such as a lesion or inactivation driven by specific gene promoters.

NOVEL OBJECT PARADIGM

Novelty is known to attract attention (Anderson, 1994; Daffner et al., 1998; Posner, Rothbart, & DiGirolamo, 1999; Tiitinen, May, Reinikainen, & Näätänen, 1994). We attempted to use novelty detection to establish a second attentional probe for mice. Rodents naturally investigate their environment by demonstrating general exploratory behaviors such as rearing and digging. When a novel object is presented in a familiar environment, mice exhibit object-oriented exploratory behaviors such as touching and sniffing the object. Normal mice immediately start to investigate the object when it is presented, and they spend about half the time exploring the object and half the time exploring the environment. We hypothesized that the ACC is involved in attending to and detecting a novel object in the environment, and we predicted that the ACC would be activated during the presentation of a novel object and that ACC lesions would diminish the object-oriented exploratory behaviors while keeping the sum of all exploratory behaviors constant (i.e., no motor activity deficit).

We proceeded to carry out pilot experiments to test this hypothesis. Naïve male C57B6/N mice were brought into the testing room in their home cages. The nest was removed the day before for better viewing of the behaviors. After a 5-minute baseline video recording, a novel object was dropped into the cage. The mice were videotaped for 5 minutes and the behaviors were analyzed using *The Observer* software (Noldus, VA). Behaviors were categorized into (1) object-oriented exploratory behaviors (e.g., moving toward the object and sniffing at the object), (2) non-object-oriented exploratory behaviors (e.g., climbing the cage lid and rearing not toward the object), and (3) nonexploratory behaviors (e.g., eating and sleeping). In selecting the novel object, we decided on a 15-ml corning tube (diameter: 3.4 cm, length: 11.5 cm, weight: 13 g; see Figure 22.5A) because it has the advantages of being

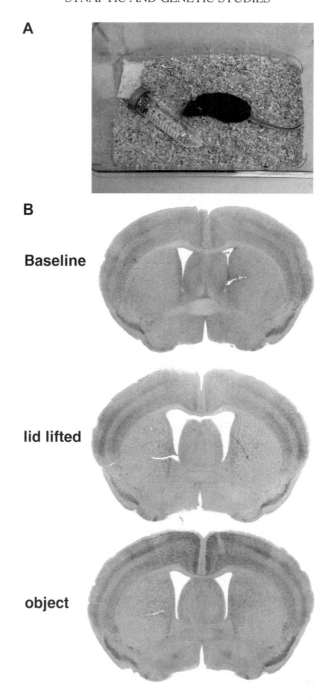

FIGURE 22.5. Exploratory and orienting behaviors in response to a novel object (A) Mice investigate novel objects such as this corning tube. (B) Representative *c-fos in situ* hybridization expression of three mice; each from one of the three groups: baseline, lid lifted, and object presentation. Darker dots are *c-fos* positive cells stained by BCIP/NBT.

transparent (not obstructing the view), stable (too heavy to be dragged around by the mouse weighing about 20 g; this makes it therefore easier to score directional behaviors such as "walking toward the object"), and not taller than the mouse (taller objects tend to evoke neophobia in mice). *c-fos* mRNA *in situ* hybridization was conducted on three groups—the novel object group (object), no object group (baseline), and a group of mice in which the cage lid was lifted but no object was introduced (lid lifted). Each group had two mice for these pilot experiments. We performed the ACC lesions in eight mice (one was later excluded after histology due to lesions in the hippocampus), and included four nonoperated mice as control.

Higher Density of *c-fos*-Positive Cells in the ACC after Receiving a Novel Object Compared with No Object or Cage-Lid-Lifted Groups

Differences discernible by the naked eye are found in the following brain areas (Figure 22.5B): more in the novel object group compared with the other two groups (ACC, motor cortex I and II, claustrum, preoptic area, dorsal caudate putamen, stria medullaris of thalamus); less in the novel object group compared with the other two groups (ventral caudate putamen). This is not an exhaustive list as the quantification of the *c-fos* positive cells for this experiment is an ongoing process. Numerous studies in humans and nonhuman primates, using a variety of indices of brain activity, have implicated the ACC and its surrounding areas in novelty tests (Berns, Cohen, & Mintun, 1997; Bush et al., 2002; Opitz, Mecklinger, Friederici, & von Cramon, 1999). That is, the ACC is known to respond preferentially to novel, as opposed to familiar, objects, regardless of the modality in which the novel stimulus is presented (Downar, Crawley, Mikulis, & Davis, 2002; Kiehl, Laurens, Duty, Forster, & Liddle, 2001; Kirino, Belger, Goldman-Rakic, & McCarthy, 2000). Similarly in rodents, strong ACC activation in the presence of a novel stimulus (Montag-Sallaz, Welzl, Kuhl, Montag, & Schachner, 1999; Zhu, Brown, McCabe, & Aggleton, 1995) or context (Kabbaj & Akil, 2001; Noguchi, Yoshida, & Chiba, 2001) is observed, using a number of markers of immediate early gene expression. The present results are consistent with such accounts, as the introduction of the novel object evoked considerable neural activation in the ACC.

The ACC Is Not Required for Detecting the Novel Object

However, despite the ACC activation, lesioning this structure did not produce behavioral changes measured by our test. The percent time spent in object-oriented exploratory behavior and general exploratory behavior for the ACC lesion group is 55.4 ± 7.3 and 36.9 ± 9.3, respectively (mean $\pm$ *SEM*, $n = 7$). The percent time spent for the nonoperated mice is 47.8 ± 7.9 and 44.7 ± 6.6 ($n = 4$). To our considerable surprise, the ACC lesions did not impair the detection of the novel object. It is clear from these data that the behavioral expression of novelty detection is not functionally dependent on the integrity of the ACC. It is known that insult of the ACC tends to produce performance deficits in attentionally demanding tasks in animals (Bussey et al., 1996; Bussey, Everitt, et al., 1997; Bussey, Muir, et al., 1997), and that ACC activation in humans is pronounced during tasks measuring analogous processes (e.g., Davis et al., 2000). It may be that the effects of ACC manipulations on novelty-related processes can only be observed under conditions of greater task complexity, and that the present paradigm, being relatively simple, is therefore not demanding enough to detect the effects. It is also possible that while the ACC maybe involved in the detection or behavioral response toward a novel object, such processes may be subserved by other structures in its absence, without any decrement of function.

CONCLUSION

Our results showed that a sensory distractor can selectively interfere with trace but not delay or contextual fear conditioning. Furthermore, the *c-fos* positive cell density is higher (by 50% on average) in parts of the ACC in those animals that received trace fear conditioning compared with brains that received delay fear conditioning. We also showed that the lesions of the ACC impair trace but not delay or contextual fear conditioning. In contrast, V1 and sham lesions did not affect either trace or delay conditioning, demonstrating the relative specificity of the ACC lesions. These data suggest that trace conditioning can be a useful model of attention in mice, and that the correlation between increased neuronal activity in the ACC and trace conditioning indeed reflects a functional requirement for the ACC in trace conditioning. We also demonstrated that novel objects elicit more *c-fos* positive cell signals in the ACC and other brain areas compared to baseline. Yet, in an apparent paradox, ACC lesions did not seem to affect exploratory and orienting behaviors directed at the novel object. It is possible that exploring a new object does not require the full resources of the ACC, even though ACC neurons are activated during this behavior. For readers interested in other brain areas involved in novelty detection, Shulman, Astafiev, and Corbetta (Chapter 9, this volume) offer great insight.

Because ACC activity is implicated in attentionally demanding tasks in humans (Bush et al., 1998, 2000, 2002; Davis et al., 2000; Devinsky et al., 1995; Jovicich et al., 2001) and animals (Bussey et al., 1996; Bussey, Everitt, et al., 1997; Bussey, Muir, et al., 1997; Muir et al., 1996; Robbins, 2002; Rogers et al., 2001), and attention to the tone–airpuff contingency is necessary for trace but not delay eyeblink conditioning (Clark & Squire, 1998, 1999), it is possible that the ACC lesions disrupt attention to the tone-shock contingency. The ACC lesion group displayed significantly less freezing as early as the first trial, compared with the sham group or the V1 lesion group (Figure 22.4B). This indicates that the impairment likely lies in early learning stages such as acquisition, when attending to the tone-shock contingency takes place. Whether the ACC is involved in extinction will need to be verified by posttraining lesions. Note that it has been shown in humans that extinction is slower when the shift of contingency from CS–US to CS–nothing is masked, suggesting attention and awareness to the new contingency during extinction correlates with the rate of extinction (Spence, 1963, 1966). The ACC is also known to have an important role in motor functions (Devinsky et al., 1995). In principle, ACC lesions might cause hyperactivity, which lowers the freezing level, and/or interfere with learning. Mice receiving the ACC lesions showed no difference in locomotor activity (Figure 22.4C), arguing that the impairment in freezing seen in the ACC lesion group is unlikely to reflect simply motor hyperactivity.

Previous studies have indicated that the hippocampus is required for trace but not delay conditioning (Clark & Squire, 1998; James, Hardiman, & Yeo, 1987; McEchron, Bouwmeester, Tseng, Weiss, & Disterhoft, 1998; McEchron, Tseng, & Disterhoft, 2000; Moyer, Deyo, & Disterhoft, 1990; Port, Romano, Steinmetz, Mikhail, & Patterson, 1986; Quinn, Oommen, Morrison, & Fanselow, 2002; Solomon, Vanderschaaf, Thompson, & Weisz, 1986). Hippocampal lesions also impair contextual conditioning (Anagnostaras, Gale, & Fanselow, 2001; Bast, Zhang, & Feldon, 2001; Kim & Fanselow, 1992; McEchron et al., 1998, 2000). Because the hippocampal formation and the ACC have bidirectional connections (Kang & Gabriel, 1998), it is possible that the ACC lesions impair trace conditioning by disrupting hippocampal functions. We performed contextual conditioning experiments and found no difference between the ACC lesion group and the sham-operated group. Therefore, it is unlikely that the ACC lesions impair trace conditioning by affecting hippocampal functions. In addition, it is thought that the ACC is involved in emotion (Allman, Hakeem, Erwin, Nimchinsky, & Hof, 2001; Bussey, Everitt, et al., 1997). The lack of effects of the ACC lesions on delay and contextual conditioning argues against a general effect on fear.

Our data provide evidence that the pretraining lesions of the ACC impair trace but not delay fear conditioning, but it is unclear whether the acquisition, consolidation, and/or retrieval processes of trace conditioning is affected. To reveal at which stage the ACC is required, posttraining lesions will be necessary. If the posttraining lesions impair trace conditioning, the ACC is likely involved in the expression stage. In this case, some method of reversible inactivation will be required to determine whether the ACC is required during the acquisition phase.

We show that a visual distractor can selectively interfere with auditory trace but not delay fear conditioning. Such disruption does not reflect competition between the distractor and the tone for association with the shock, suggesting that trace fear conditioning in mice, as in humans (Carter et al., 2003), requires some form of attention. Our data therefore establish a correlation between a requirement for attention and for the ACC in trace fear conditioning in mice but do not yet prove that the ACC is required for attention. Nevertheless, the ability to model an attentionally demanding task in mice opens up the problem to genetic manipulations. Finally, we wish to point out that awareness of the tone–airpuff contingency relationship has been implicated as being necessary for trace but not delay eyeblink conditioning in humans (Clark & Squire, 1998, 1999; Manns et al., 2000a, 2000b). The murine system described here may, therefore, shed light on some processes relevant to the neuronal basis of awareness (Crick & Koch, 2003; Koch, 2004).

ACKNOWLEDGMENTS

We thank E. Chiang, W. Lerchner, R.M. Carter, J.J. Quinn, H. Lester, M.A. MacIver, G. Mosconi, M.R. Tinsley, David J. Anderson, and L. van Trigt for support and assistance throughout the development of this work. This research was supported by Caltech, Moore Discovery Award, the Keck Foundation, the National Institute of Mental Health, and the National Science Foundation under Award Numbers EEC-9402726 and IBN-0091487. Most of the work reported here was carried out jointly with David J. Anderson.

REFERENCES

Allman, J. M., Hakeem, A., Erwin, J. M., Nimchinsky, E., & Hof, P. (2001). The anterior cingulate cortex—The evolution of an interface between emotion and cognition. *Unity of Knowledge: The Convergence of Natural and Human Science, 935,* 107–117.

Anagnostaras, S. G., Gale, G. D., & Fanselow, M. S. (2001). Hippocampus and contextual fear conditioning: Recent controversies and advances. *Hippocampus, 11,* 8–17.

Anderson, B. (1994). The volume of the cerebellar molecular layer predicts attention to novelty in rats. *Brain Research, 641,* 160–162.

Bahu, S. J., Kaltenbach, J. A., Zhang, J. S., Khariwala, S. S., Afman, C. E., & Hnatiuk, M. (2001).

Tonotopic mapping of *c-fos* expression in the dorsal cochlear nucleus of the hamster. *Neuroscience Research Communications, 29,* 107–117.

Bast, T., Zhang, W. N., & Feldon, J. (2001). Hippocampus and classical fear conditioning. *Hippocampus, 11,* 828–831.

Berns, G. S., Cohen, J. D., & Mintun, M. A. (1997). Brain regions responsive to novelty in the absence of awareness. *Science, 276,* 1272–1275.

Braun, J., Koch, C., & Davis, J. L. (2001). *Visual attention and cortical circuits.* Cambridge, MA: MIT Press.

Büchel, C., Dolan, R. J., Armony, J. L., & Friston, K. J. (1999). Amygdala–hippocampal involvement in human aversive trace conditioning revealed through event-related functional magnetic resonance imaging. *Journal of Neuroscience, 19,* 10869–10876.

Bush, G., Luu, P., & Posner, M. I. (2000). Cognitive and emotional influences in anterior cingulate cortex. *Trends in Cognitive Sciences, 4,* 215–222.

Bush, G., Vogt, B. A., Holmes, J., Dale, A. M., Greve, D., Jenike, M. A., et al. (2002). Dorsal anterior cingulate cortex: A role in reward-based decision making. *Proceedings of the National Academy of Sciences USA, 99,* 523–528.

Bush, G., Whalen, P. J., Rosen, B. R., Jenike, M. A., McInerney, S. C., & Rauch, S. L. (1998). The counting stroop: An interference task specialized for functional neuroimaging—Validation study with functional MRI. *Human Brain Mapping, 6,* 270–282.

Bushnell, P. J. (1998). Behavioral approaches to the assessment of attention in animals. *Psychopharmacology, 138,* 231–259.

Bussey, T. J., Everitt, B. J., & Robbins, T. W. (1997). Dissociable effects of cingulate and medial frontal cortex lesions on stimulus–reward learning using a novel Pavlovian autoshaping procedure for the rat: Implications for the neurobiology of emotion. *Behavioral Neuroscience, 111,* 908–919.

Bussey, T. J., Muir, J. L., Everitt, B. J., & Robbins, T. W. (1996). Dissociable effects of anterior and posterior cingulate cortex lesions on the acquisition of a conditional visual discrimination: Facilitation of early learning vs. impairment of late learning. *Behavioural Brain Research, 82,* 45–56.

Bussey, T. J., Muir, J. L., Everitt, B. J., & Robbins, T. W. (1997). Triple dissociation of anterior cingulate, posterior cingulate, and medial frontal cortices on visual discrimination tasks using a touchscreen testing procedure for the rat. *Behavioral Neuroscience, 111,* 920–936.

Carli, M., Robbins, T. W., Evenden, J. L., & Everitt, B. J. (1983). Effects of lesions to ascending noradrenergic neurons on performance of a 5-choice serial reaction task in rats—Implications for theories of dorsal noradrenergic bundle function based on selective attention and arousal. *Behavioural Brain Research, 9,* 361–380.

Carter, R. M., Hofstötter, C., Tsuchiya, N., & Koch, C. (2003). Working memory and fear conditioning. *Proceedings of the National Academy of Sciences USA, 100,* 1399–1404.

Chaudhuri, A., Zangenehpour, S., Rahbar-Dehgan, F., & Ye, F. C. (2000). Molecular maps of neural activity and quiescence. *Acta Neurobiologiae Experimentalis, 60,* 403–410.

Clark, R. E., & Squire, L. R. (1998). Classical conditioning and brain systems: The role of awareness. *Science, 280,* 77–81.

Clark, R. E., & Squire, L. R. (1999). Human eyeblink classical conditioning: Effects of manipulating awareness of the stimulus contingencies. *Psychological Science, 10,* 14–18.

Clark, R. E., Manns, J. R., & Squire, L. R. (2002). Classical conditioning, awareness, and brain systems. *Trends in Cognitive Sciences, 6,* 524–531.

Collins, P., Wilkinson, L. S., Everitt, B. J., Robbins, T. W., & Roberts, A. C. (2000). The effect of dopamine depletion from the caudate nucleus of the common marmoset (*Callithrix jacchus*) on tests of prefrontal cognitive function. *Behavioral Neuroscience, 114,* 3–17.

Crick, F., & Koch, C. (2003). A framework for consciousness. *Nature Neuroscience, 6,* 119–126.

Crofts, H. S., Dalley, J. W., Collins, P., Van Denderen, J. C., Everitt, B. J., Robbins, T. W., et al. (2001). Differential effects of 6-OHDA lesions of the frontal cortex and caudate nucleus on the ability to acquire an attentional set. *Cerebral Cortex, 11,* 1015–1026.

Daffner, K. R., Mesulam, M. M., Scinto, L. F. M., Cohen, L. G., Kennedy, B. P., West, W. C., et al. (1998). Regulation of attention to novel stimuli by frontal lobes: an event-related potential study. *Neuroreport, 9,* 787–791.

Davis, K. D., Hutchison, W. D., Lozano, A. M., Tasker, R. R., & Dostrovsky, J. O. (2000). Human anterior cingulate cortex neurons modulated by attention-demanding tasks. *Journal of Neurophysiology, 83,* 3575–3577.

Delagrange, P., Bouyer, J. J., Montaron, M. F., Durand, C., Mocaer, E., & Rougeul, A. (1990). Action of tianeptine on focalization of attention in cat. *Psychopharmacology, 102,* 227–233.

Devinsky, O., Morrell, M. J., & Vogt, B. A. (1995). Contributions of anterior cingulate cortex to behavior. *Brain, 118,* 279–306.

Downar, J., Crawley, A. P., Mikulis, D. J., & Davis, K. D. (2002). A cortical network sensitive to stimulus salience in a neutral behavioral context across multiple sensory modalities. *Journal of Neurophysiology, 87,* 615–620.

Dragunow, M., & Faull, R. (1989). The use of *c-fos* as a metabolic marker in neuronal pathway tracing. *Journal of Neuroscience Methods, 29,* 261–265.

Durkin, T. P., Beaufort, C., Leblond, L., & Maviel, T. (2000), A 5-arm maze enables parallel measures of sustained visuo-spatial attention and spatial working memory in mice. *Behavioral Brain Research, 116,* 39–53.

Escobar, M., Arcediano, F., & Miller, R. R. (2002). Latent inhibition and contextual associations. *Journal of Experimental Psychology: Animal Behavior Processes, 28,* 123–136.

Fremouw, T., Herbranson, W. T., & Shimp, C. P. (2002). Dynamic shifts of pigeon local/global attention. *Animal Cognition, 5,* 233–243.

Gabriel, M., & Taylor, C. (1998). Prenatal exposure to cocaine impairs neuronal coding of attention and discriminative learning. *Annals of the New York Academy of Sciences, 846,* 194–212.

Gould, T. J., Collins, A. C., & Wehner, J. M. (2001). Nicotine enhances latent inhibition and ameliorates ethanol-induced deficits in latent inhibition. *Nicotine and Tobacco Research, 3,* 17–24.

Gould, T. J., & Wehner, J. M. (1999). Genetic influences on latent inhibition. *Behavioral Neuroscience, 113,* 1291–1296.

Grahame, N. J., Barnet, R. C., Gunther, L. M., & Miller, R. R. (1994). Latent inhibition as a performance deficit resulting from CS- context associations. *Animal Learning and Behavior, 22,* 395–408.

Han, C. J., O'Tuathaigh, C. M., van Trigt, L., Mongeau, R., Quinn, J. J., Fanselow, M. S., et al. (2003). Trace but not delay fear conditioning requires attention and the anterior cingulate cortex. *Proceedings of the National Academy of Sciences USA, 100,* 13087–13092.

Heisenberg, M., & Wolf, R. (1984). Vision in *Drosophila*: Genetics of microbehavior. Berlin: Springer-Verlag.

Hernandez, L. L., & Watson, K. L. (1997). Opioid modulation of attention-related responses: Delta-receptors modulate habituation and conditioned bradycardia. *Psychopharmacology (Berlin), 131,* 140–147.

Humby, T., Laird, F. M., Davies, W., & Wilkinson, L. S. (1999). Visuospatial attentional functioning in mice: Interactions between cholinergic manipulations and genotype. *European Journal of Neuroscience, 11,* 2813–2823.

Itti, L., & Koch, C. (2000). A saliency-based search mechanism for overt and covert shifts of visual attention. *Vision Research, 40,* 1489–1506.

James, G. O., Hardiman, M. J., & Yeo, C. H. (1987). Hippocampal lesions and trace conditioning in the rabbit. *Behavioural Brain Research, 23,* 109–116.

Jovicich, J., Peters, R. J., Koch, C., Braun, J., Chang, L., & Ernst, T. (2001). Brain areas specific for attentional load in a motion-tracking task. *Journal of Cognitive Neuroscience, 13,* 1048–1058.

Kabbaj, M., & Akil, H. (2001). Individual differences in novelty-seeking behavior in rats: A *c-fos* study. *Neuroscience, 106,* 535–545.

Kang, E., & Gabriel, M. (1998). Hippocampal modulation of cingulo-thalamic neuronal activity and discriminative avoidance learning in rabbits. *Hippocampus, 8,* 491–510.

Kiehl, K. A., Laurens, K. R., Duty, T. L., Forster, B. B., & Liddle, P. F. (2001). Neural sources involved in auditory target detection and novelty processing: An event-related fMRI study. *Psychophysiology, 38,* 133–142.

Kim, J. J., & Fanselow, M. S. (1992). Modality-specific retrograde amnesia of fear. *Science, 256,* 675–677.

Kirino, E., Belger, A., Goldman-Rakic, P., & McCarthy, G. (2000). Prefrontal activation evoked by infrequent target and novel stimuli in a visual target detection task: An event-related functional magnetic resonance imaging study. *Journal of Neuroscience, 20,* 6612–6618.

Kline, L., Decena, E., Hitzemann, R., & McCaughran, J. (1998). Acoustic startle, prepulse inhibition, locomotion, and latent inhibition in the neuroleptic–responsive (NR) and neuroleptic-nonresponsive (NNR) lines of mice. *Psychopharmacology, 139,* 322–331.

Koch, C. (2004). *The quest for consciousness: A neurobiological approach.* Denver, CO: Roberts.

Koch, C., & Ullman, S. (1985). Shifts in selective visual attention: Towards the underlying neural circuitry. *Human Neurobiology, 4,* 219–227.

Kreiman, G., Fried, I., & Koch, C. (2002). Single-neuron correlates of subjective vision in the human medial temporal lobe. *Proceedings of the National Academy of Sciences USA, 99,* 8378–8383.

Kronforst-Collins, M. A., & Disterhoft, J. F. (1998). Lesions of the caudal area of rabbit medial prefrontal cortex impair trace eyeblink conditioning. *Neurobiology of Learning and Memory, 69,* 147–162.

Leblond, L., Beaufort, C., Delerue, F., & Durkin, T. P. (2002). Differential roles for nicotinic and muscarinic cholinergic receptors in sustained visuo-spatial attention? A study using a 5-arm maze protocol in mice. *Behavioural Brain Research, 128,* 91–102.

Lechner, H. A., Lein, E. S., & Callaway, E. M. (2002). A genetic method for selective and quickly reversible silencing of Mammalian neurons. *Journal of Neuroscience, 22,* 5287–5290.

Lee, B., Tumu, P., & Paul, I. A. (2002). Effects of LP-BM5 murine leukemia virus infection on errors and response time in a two-choice serial reaction time task in C57BL/6 mice. *Brain Research, 948,* 1–7.

Lemmonds, C. A., Williams, D. K., & Wenger, G. R. (2002). Effect of pentobarbital, d-amphetamine, and nicotine on two models of sustained attention in pigeons. *Psychopharmacology (Berlin), 163,* 391–398.

Li, F. F., VanRullen, R., Koch, C., & Perona, P. (2002). Rapid natural scene categorization in the near absence of attention. *Proceedings of the National Academy of Sciences USA, 99,* 9596–9601.

Lindblad-Toh, K., Lander, E. S., McPherson, J. D., Waterston, R. H., Rodgers, J., & Birney, E. (2001). Progress in sequencing the mouse genome. *Genesis, 31,* 137–141.

Lomber, S. G., Payne, B. R., & Cornwell, P. (2001). Role of the superior colliculus in analyses of space: Superficial and intermediate layer contributions to visual orienting, auditory orienting, and visuospatial discriminations during unilateral and bilateral deactivations. *Journal of Comparative Neurology, 441,* 44–57.

Lubow, R. E. (1997). Latent inhibition as a measure of learned inattention: Some problems and solutions. *Behavioural Brain Research, 88,* 75–83.

Mackintosh, N. J. (1975). Blocking of conditioned suppression: Role of the first compound trial. *Journal of Experimental Psychology: Animal Behavior Processes, 1,* 335–345.

Manns, J. R., Clark, R. E., & Squire, L. R. (2000a). Awareness predicts the magnitude of single-cue trace eyeblink conditioning. *Hippocampus, 10,* 181–186.

Manns, J. R., Clark, R. E., & Squire, L. R. (2000b). Parallel acquisition of awareness and trace eyeblink classical conditioning. *Learning and Memory, 7,* 267–272.

Manns, J. R., Clark, R. E., & Squire, L. R. (2002). Standard delay eyeblink classical conditioning is independent of awareness. *Journal of Experimental Psychology: Animal Behavior Processes, 28,* 32–37.

Mansuy, I. M., Winder, D. G., Moallem, T. M., Osman, M., Mayford, M., Hawkins, R. D., et al. (1998). Inducible and reversible gene expression with the rtTA system for the study of memory. *Neuron, 21,* 257–265.

Marston, H. M., Spratt, C., & Kelly, J. S. (2001). Phenotyping complex behaviours: Assessment of circadian control and 5-choice serial reaction learning in the mouse. *Behavioural Brain Research, 125,* 189–193.

McEchron, M. D., Bouwmeester, H., Tseng, W., Weiss, C., & Disterhoft, J. F. (1998). Hippocampectomy disrupts auditory trace fear conditioning and contextual fear conditioning in the rat. *Hippocampus, 8,* 638–646.

McEchron, M. D., Tseng, W., & Disterhoft, J. F. (2000). Neurotoxic lesions of the dorsal hippocampus disrupt auditory-cued trace heart rate (fear) conditioning in rabbits. *Hippocampus, 10,* 739–751.

Mishima, K., Fujii, M., Aoo, N., Yoshikawa, T., Fukue, Y., Honda, Y., et al. (2002). The pharmacological characterization of attentional processes using a two-lever choice reaction time task in rats. *Biology and Pharmacology Bulletin, 25,* 1570–1576.

Montag-Sallaz, M., Welzl, H., Kuhl, D., Montag, D., & Schachner, M. (1999). Novelty-induced increased expression of immediate-early genes *c-fos* and arg 3.1 in the mouse brain. *Journal of Neurobiology, 38,* 234–246.

Moser, P. C., Hitchcock, J. M., Lister, S., & Moran, P. M. (2000). The pharmacology of latent inhibition as an annual model of schizophrenia. *Brain Research Reviews, 33,* 275–307.

Moyer, J. R., Deyo, R. A., & Disterhoft, J. F. (1990). Hippocampectomy disrupts trace eye-blink conditioning in rabbits. *Behavioural Neuroscience, 104,* 243–252.

Muir, J. L., Everitt, B. J., & Robbins, T. W. (1996). The cerebral cortex of the rat and visual attentional function: Dissociable effects of mediofrontal, cingulate, anterior dorsolateral, and parietal cortex lesions on a five-choice serial reaction time task. *Cerebral Cortex, 6,* 470–481.

Noguchi, T., Yoshida, Y., & Chiba, S. (2001). Effects of psychological stress on monoamine systems in subregions of the frontal cortex and nucleus accumbens of the rat. *Brain Research, 916,* 91–100.

Opitz, B., Mecklinger, A., Friederici, A. D., & von Cramon, D. Y. (1999). The functional neuroanatomy of novelty processing: Integrating ERP and fMRI results. *Cerebral Cortex, 9,* 379–391.

O'Tuathaigh, C. M., & Moran, P. M. (2002). Evidence for dopamine D(1) receptor involvement in the stimulus selection task: Overshadowing in the rat. *Psychopharmacology (Berlin), 162,* 225–231.

Parasuraman, R. (1998). *The attentive brain.* Cambridge, MA: MIT Press.

Passetti, F., Chudasama, Y., & Robbins, T. W. (2002). The frontal cortex of the rat and visual attentional performance: Dissociable functions of distinct medial prefrontal subregions. *Cerebral Cortex, 12,* 1254–1268.

Paxinos, G., & Franklin, K. B. J. (2001). *The mouse brain, in stereotaxic coordinates* (2nd ed.). San Diego, CA: Academic Press.

Piazza, P. V., Ferdico, M., Russo, D., Crescimanno, G., Benigno, A., & Amato, G. (1988). Facilitatory effect of ventral tegmental area A10 region on the attack behaviour in the cat: Possible dopaminergic role in selective attention. *Experimental Brain Research, 72,* 109–116.

Port, R. L., Romano, A. G., Steinmetz, J. E., Mikhail, A. A., & Patterson, M. M. (1986). Retention and acquisition of classical trace conditioned responses by rabbits with hippocampal lesions. *Behavioural Neuroscience, 100,* 745–752.

Posner, M. I., Rothbart, M. K., & DiGirolamo, G. J. (1999). Development of brain networks for orienting to novelty. *Zhurnal Vysshei Nervnoi Deyatel'nosti Imeni I. P. Pavlova, 49,* 715–722.

Quinn, J. J., Oommen, S. S., Morrison, G. E., & Fanselow, M. S. (2002). Post-training excitotoxic lesions of the dorsal hippocampus attenuate forward trace, backward trace, and delay fear conditioning in a temporally specific manner. *Hippocampus, 12,* 495–504.

Rescorla, R. A., & Wagner, A. R. (1972). A theory of Pavlovian conditioning: Variations in the effectiveness of reinforcement and nonreinforcement. In A. H. Black & W. F. Prokasy (Eds.), *Classical conditioning II: current research and theory* (pp. 64–99). New York: Appleton-Century-Crofts.

Restivo, L., Passino, E., Middei, S., & Ammassari-Teule, M. (2002). The strain-specific involvement of nucleus accumbens in latent inhibition might depend on differences in processing configural- and cue-based information between C57BL/6 and DBA mice. *Brain Research Bulletin, 57,* 35–39.

Robbins, T. W. (2002). The 5-choice serial reaction time task: Behavioural pharmacology and functional neurochemistry. *Psychopharmacology, 163,* 362–380.

Rogers, R. D., Baunez, C., Everitt, B. J., & Robbins, T. W. (2001). Lesions of the medial and lateral striatum in the rat produce differential deficits in attentional performance. *Behavioral Neuroscience, 115,* 799–811.

Slimko, E. M., McKinney, S., Anderson, D. J., Davidson, N., & Lester, H. A. (2002). Selective electrical silencing of mammalian neurons in vitro by the use of invertebrate ligand-gated chloride channels. *Journal of Neuroscience, 22,* 7373–7379.

Solomon, P. R., Vanderschaaf, E. R., Thompson, R. F., & Weisz, D. J. (1986). Hippocampus and trace conditioning of the rabbit's classically conditioned nictitating membrane response. *Behavioural Neuroscience, 100,* 729–744.

Spence, K. W. (1963). Cognitive factors in the extinction of the conditioned eyelid response in humans. *Science, 140,* 1224–1225.

Spence, K. W. (1966). Cognitive and drive factors in the extinction of the conditional eye blink in human subjects. *Psychology Review, 73,* 458.

Tang, S., & Guo, A. (2001). Choice behavior of *Drosophila* facing contradictory visual cues. *Science, 294,* 1543–1547.

Tiitinen, H., May, P., Reinikainen, K., & Näätänen, R. (1994). Attentive novelty detection in humans is governed by pre-attentive sensory memory. *Nature, 372,* 90–92.

Vallone, D., Pignatelli, M., Grammatikopoulos, G., Ruocco, L., Bozzi, Y., Westphal H., et al. (2002). Activity, non-selective attention and emotionality in dopamine D2/D3 receptor knock-out mice. *Behavioural Brain Research, 130,* 141–148.

van Swinderen, B., & Greenspan, R. J. (2003). Salience modulates 20–30 Hz brain activity in *Drosophila. Nature Neuroscience, 6,* 579–586.

Waterston, R. H., Lindblad-Toh, K., Birney, E., Rogers, J., Abril, J. F., Agarwal, P., et al. (2002). Initial sequencing and comparative analysis of the mouse genome. *Nature, 420,* 520–562.

Weible, A. P., McEchron, M. D., & Disterhoft, J. F. (2000). Cortical involvement in acquisition and extinction of trace eyeblink conditioning. *Behavioural Neuroscience, 114,* 1058–1067.

Weiss, S. J., & Panlilio, L. V. (1999). Blocking a selective association in pigeons. *Journal of Experimental and Animal Behavior, 71,* 13–24.

Yamamoto, M., Wada, N., Kitabatake, Y., Watanabe, D., Anzai, M., Yokoyama, M., et al. (2003). Reversible suppression of glutamatergic neurotransmission of cerebellar granule cells *in vivo* by genetically manipulated expression of tetanus neurotoxin light chain. *Journal of Neuroscience, 23,* 6759–6767.

Zhu, X. O., Brown, M. W., McCabe, B. J., & Aggleton, J. P. (1995). Effects of the novelty or familiarity of visual stimuli on the expression of the immediate early gene *c-fos* in rat brain. *Neuroscience, 69,* 821–829.

Zilles, K., & Wree, A. (1995). Cortex area and laminar structure. In G. Paxinos (Ed.), *The rat nervous system* (pp. 375–415). Sidney: Academic Press.

23

Cholinergic and Noradrenergic Inputs to the Posterior Parietal Cortex Modulate the Components of Exogenous Attention

Melinda Beane and Richard Marrocco

Advances in cellular neuroscience in the past decade now allow us to specify key neuronal operations underlying the selection and exclusion of information. Our goals are to use these data to identify the structure and function of the major reflexive and voluntary components of attention, understand how they are modulated by other structures, and work in an integrated fashion. In this chapter, we document recent advances from our lab and others that offer some insights into the mechanisms underlying reflexive attention and its interaction with voluntary attention. We also interpret new data on attention deficits in light of these advances.

Four objectives motivate our studies. First, we seek to understand attention in its simplest form, reflexive covert orienting. We practice the comparative approach, using the Posner covert target detection (CTD) task and attention network task (ANT) to study the orienting of rodents and primates (e.g., Marrocco & Davidson, 1998). There are two behavioral components to reflexive attention, orienting and alerting, and we find that an improved CTD task best assesses both components (Witte, Villareal, & Marrocco, 1996). Second, we use pharmacological means to uncover the neurotransmitters that mediate the components of reflexive attention. Third, we localize the structures controlling reflexive attention through the use of local drug infusion and electrical microstimulation. Fourth, we seek to understand attention deficits in humans and animal models within the framework of normal, reflexive attention. It should be appreciated that this chapter is highly selective and not a general summary of the field. Interested readers should refer to several comprehensive reviews (Colby & Goldberg, 1999; Parasuraman, 1998).

VISUAL REFLEXIVE ATTENTION

Behavioral Measurement

The abrupt appearance of a visual stimulus away from the focus of the gaze is detected first by the peripheral retina, which then signals the brain to move attention to the new target location. Ignoring its particular attributes, the new stimulus contains explicit information about its location in space and time. Both types of information may engage attention, and their benefits (or costs) for orienting may be measured individually using recent versions of the CTD task. As practiced in our lab and elsewhere (e.g., Festa-Martino, Ott, & Handel, 2004; Stewart, Burke, & Marrocco, 2001; Tales, Muir, Bayer, & Snowden, 2002; Witte & Marrocco, 1997), the benefit of the spatial information is measured by cueing the subsequent target location (valid cue) and asking how the cue facilitates target detection or discrimination. In contrast, the costs of misorienting can be judged by placing the cue and target at different locations (invalid cue). Subjects react more quickly to the former condition than to the latter and the difference is termed *the validity effect*.

To study the benefits of temporal cues, two locations are cued simultaneously and the target appears subsequently at only one of them. These cues lack explicit spatial information and the subject does not orient to them. However, their onset may cause the subject to estimate when the target will appear or to prepare a response. We compare the reaction time to the double cue with a target presentation that is uncued (i.e., has neither spatial nor temporal information to guide attention) and the difference we term *the alerting effect*. The most recent version of this test (ANT) incorporates spatial and temporal cues and others to measure stimulus conflict (Fan, Wu, Fossella, & Posner, 2001). While the evidence shows that the validity and alerting effects are separable through cue manipulation (Fernandez-Duque & Posner, 1997; Witte et al., 1996) or drug administration (see later), they are usually additive in their effects on reaction times (Clark, Geffen, & Geffen, 1989).

Behavioral responses to the spatial and temporal components of cued stimuli seem to be well conserved across species, at least for the mammals. For example, with a 4:1 ratio of valid to invalid trials (cue validity = 80%), rats, rhesus monkeys, and humans show a validity effect of about 40 msec (Figure 23.1A). In addition, all species show a decline in overall response time of about 10 msec for each 100-msec increase in the interval between the cue and target (Figure 23.1B). This suggests that the evolutionary pressures to develop covert attention may have been similar in these animals.

Pharmacology

The orienting and alerting components of reflexive attention are mediated by different neurotransmitters. Increasing the brain levels of acetylcholine (ACh) through parenteral injections of nicotine generally decreases reaction times, increases accuracy, specifically reduces reaction times for invalid cues, and decreases the validity effect (Phillips, McAlonan, Robb, & Brown, 2000; Stolerman, Mirza, Hahn, & Shoaib, 2000; Witte, Davidson, & Marrocco, 1997). In a complementary fashion, reduced levels of acetylcholine produced by injections of antagonist drugs (e.g., mecamylamine or scopolamine) or those occurring in association with Alzheimer's disease increase response times and increase the validity effect (Festa-Martino et al., 2004; Hahn, Shoaib, & Stolerman, 2002; Phillips et al., 2000; Stewart et al., 2001; Tales et al., 2002). The cholinergic modulation of response time is only found where orienting is necessary. Changes that must be detected at the fixation point are unaffected by cholinergic blockers (Davidson, Cutrell, & Marrocco, 1999).

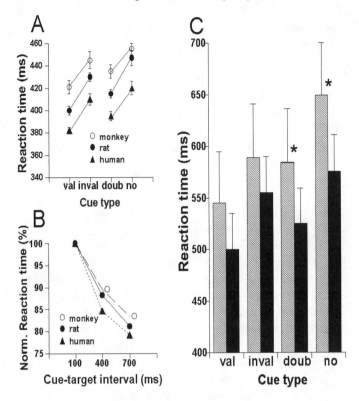

FIGURE 23.1. (A) Comparison of the reaction times of three species to different cue types of the cued target detection task. In each case, there were four times as many valid as invalid (and double- and no-cue) trials. The slopes of the curves are not significantly different from each other). (B) Comparison of reaction time facilitation with increasing cue-target interval for monkey (open circles), rat (filled circles) and human (filled triangles). Data have been normalized to facilitate slope comparisons. (C) Reaction times of subjects with ADHD ($n = 40$) to different cue types of the attention network task. The spatial cue is located either above or below the fixation point. The central cue is at the fixation point. The double cues are above and below the fixation point. The no cue lacks a cue. Hatched columns, "off" stimulant medication; filled columns, "on" stimulant medication. See text for details. Asterisks above double- and no-cue columns represent significant differences, $p < .05$.

Interestingly, systemic administration of cholinergic agonists tend to alter the validity effect with little or no compensatory changes in alerting (Murphy & Klein, 1998; Witte et al., 1997). This result is unexpected because nicotinic cholinergic receptors are distributed broadly in the brain. One explanation is that ACh innervation of locus coeruleus neurons is less potent, perhaps due to inputs located on distal dendrites (Kawahara, Kawahara, & Westerink, 1999; Ruggiero, Giuliano, Anwar, Stornetta, & Reis, 1990). Another is that nicotinic receptors are sparsely expressed in locus coeruleus neurons (Vincler & Eisenach, 2003). In either case, systemic nicotine would be behaviorally effective only in very large doses, as has been observed (Witte et al., 1997). In contrast, disease-related changes affect both orienting and alerting (Festa-Martino et al., 2004), perhaps due to degeneration of both the cholinergic and noradrenergic circuitry.

The alerting effect is mediated by norepinephrine (Coull et al., 2001; Witte & Marrocco, 1997). Selective α-2 noradrenergic drugs such as guanfacine and partially selective drugs such as clonidine have a general slowing effect on all responding and produce a selective slowing of double-cue reaction times. Alpha-2 antagonists (e.g., idazoxan and yohimbine) may have either antagonistic or synergistic effects on double-cue reaction times, depending on dosage (Davidson, Villareal, & Marrocco, 1994). Validity effect magnitudes are unaltered in the presence of these drugs. To date, the pharmacology of reflexive attention appears the same in the three species we have studied.

Dopamine appears to play little role in reflexive attention using peripheral cues (Ward & Brown, 1996; Witte, 1994; Yamaguchi & Kobatashi, 1998). However, high cue validities (i.e., a valid cue to invalid cue ratio greater than 4:1) may increase the predictability of the target and engage frontal, dopaminergic activity (Yamaguchi & Kobatashi, 1998).

Several lines of evidence suggest that the orienting and alerting behaviors reside in separate but overlapping networks of brain structures (Fan et al., 2001; Mesulam, 1990). The posterior attention system consists of the inferior parietal cortex (IPC), the pulvinar in the thalamus, and the superior colliculus (Posner & Petersen, 1990). When subjects orient, the intraparietal cortex (IPC) and other areas show increased blood flow (Beauchamp, Petit, Ellmore, Ingeholm, & Haxby, 2001; Corbetta, Miezen, Shulman, & Petersen, 1993; Corbetta et al., 1998; Mesulam, 1999; Wojciulik, Kanwisher, & Driver, 1998). Using event-related functional magnetic resonance imaging (fMRI), Corbetta and colleagues have been able to demonstrate that target detection and the orienting of attention to the cue is processed in the intraparietal sulcus, whereas the detection of the target occurs later and in the temporoparietal junction (Corbetta, Kincade, Ollinger, McAvoy, & Shulman, 2000). When subjects are alerted by cues, the prefrontal cortex and parts of the parietal cortex become more active, although the time course of this change is less certain (Coull, Nobre, & Frith, 2001). Interestingly, both cholinergic and noradrenergic receptors are found in high density in these areas (Morrison & Foote, 1986).

Structural Localization of the Sources of Reflexive Attention

The second major goal of our work is to localize the sources of attention and we do so by intracranial drug infusion or electrical microstimulation in behaving animals. Inferior parietal cortex infusions of cholinergic drugs reproduce the effects seen through systemic administration of the same agents (Beane, Drew, Massey, & Marrocco, 2002a; Davidson & Marrocco, 2000). Nicotine reduces overall reaction times, the nicotinic antagonist mecamylamine increases them, and validity effects are reduced. Scopolamine's effects were more complex, causing an increase in overall response times, but an increase in valid cue reaction times and a decrease in invalid cue times. The result is mainly due to central nervous system effects because we coadminister neostigmine to offset ACh reduction in the peripheral nervous system. Although the local infusion data are quite similar to what we found with systemic administration of scopolamine (Davidson et al., 1999), they suggest a more complicated pattern than that seen at the nicotinic receptor. To test whether the differences between mecamylamine and scopolamine are due to the properties of the muscarinic receptor, we are currently examining the antagonism between scopolamine and oxotremorine on reflexive attention in rats. It should be stated that, contrary to our findings, Brown and her colleagues (Phillips et al., 2000) found that scopolamine produced a greater slowing of invalid than valid response times and an increase of the validity effect in rats performing the CTD task. Currently, the reasons for this difference are not understood.

We also find a parallel between systemic and central administration of noradrenergic drugs. Beane, Drew, Massey, and Marrocco (2002b) bilaterally infused guanfacine into the posterior parietal cortex of hooded rats. They found a dose-dependent decrease in the alerting effect but no significant change in the validity effect, quite similar to data obtained for systemic injections in rats (unpublished results) and monkeys (Witte & Marrocco, 1997). In addition, overall response times increased in a similar, dose-dependent fashion.

Superficially, the similarities between the systemic and local infusion data are impressive. Spatial analyses of the injection sites show that the effects are localized in the lateral IPC and nearby areas. However, overall reaction times for local infusions were substantially longer than those for systemic administrations, despite similar dose–response relationships. In addition, we conducted the studies in only one attention-related area and cannot eliminate the possibility that these same effects might occur at upstream locations.

Because the application of cholinergic agents suggested that the IPC is at least *necessary* for reflexive attention, we tested the hypothesis that it might be *sufficient* to activate attention shifting. Brief (100 msec), trial-linked electrical microstimulation of IPC induces a substantial facilitation of orienting (valid cue reaction times decrease by 10 msec, invalid cue trials decrease by 50 msec) only when the targets were contralateral to the site stimulated. The current needed to produce the changes is smaller than that required to evoke overt movements of the eye. The size of the facilitation varies with stimulation site and is related to the amplitude of the saccadic eye movements that can be elicited at those sites with higher current. In addition, a bilateral facilitation of alerting is also found in the absence of overall changes in response time and overt movements of the eyes or face. These results are consistent with the idea that electrical stimulation activates IPC neurons and axons of cells originating in the cholinergic basal forebrain and locus coeruleus (Cutrell & Marrocco, 2002). Moore and Armstrong (2003) have produced findings similar to ours. They stimulated frontal eye field (FEF) and were able to show attention-related changes in visually evoked neuronal activity in area V4. This could happen if stimulation of FEF activates the IPC, which then provided top-down facilitation of area V4, or if FEF directly activated V4. In any case, IPC provides direct input into FEF, and it may be responsible for the similarity of the downstream effects. Electrical stimulation could be useful for mapping the structures downstream from the parietal cortex and FEF to determine additional circuitry for covert attention. Will these data be relevant to human attention?

In contrast to the typical single-cell electrophysiology/histological reconstruction methods, key brain regions for human attention are identified using bloodflow measurements (fMRI) and correlated with structural information gleaned from tiny topographical differences in water concentration (MRI). Integrating the data from the very different approaches used in monkeys and humans requires solutions to significant computational problems in topography and topology and the reconcilliation of conflicting systems of nomenclature. The newest studies in this area have largely succeeded in doing so. Van Essen and colleagues (2001), in particular, have published several elegant papers that compare the anatomy of visual structures in monkey and human brains (see also Astafiev et al., 2003). Using surface-based atlases, they show that attention, saccadic eye movements, and pointing in humans induces blood flow in the IPC. In monkeys, similar behaviors lead to increased cellular activity in these same parietal areas (Bisley & Goldberg, 2003; Colby & Goldberg, 1999; Davidson & Marrocco, 2000; Snyder, Batista, & Andersen, 1997). Thus, at least for attention-related activities, there is substantial correspondence between cellular responses and local blood flow in the IPCs of human and nonhuman primates.

OVERLAP BETWEEN MECHANISMS
OF REFLEXIVE AND SUSTAINED ATTENTION

Sustained attention may be defined as the volitional maintainance of the current focus of attention. This may mean awaiting the change from red to green in traffic stoplights or it could mean the search for the appearance of one target letter in a stream of others. In the latter case, sustained attention may interact with working memory to accomplish the task. While the duration of the maintenance is context and motivation dependent, it is, by definition, longer than the dwell time of reflexive orienting. Reflexive and sustained attention may act together in the service of visual exploration but in some instances must be mutually antagonistic. That is, sustained attention to a relevant target is successful to the extent that it inhibits distractors, which may cause orienting to nonrelevant stimuli. Sustained, voluntary fixation on the known target location requires frontocortical activity (Anderson et al., 1994; Hanes, Patterson, & Schall, 1998; Petit et al., 1995) while the posterior parietal cortex is important for attention shifting (e.g., Corbetta, Shulman, Miezen, & Petersen, 1995). This suggests that frontoparietal interconnections may be important for switching between sustained attention and reflexive orienting.

Because the goals of sustained attention and automatic orienting are different, comparisons of their properties may not reveal much about their underlying mechanisms. Nonetheless, the pharmacology of the two tasks is remarkably similar. Using a classic vigilance (oddball) task, Aston-Jones and colleagues (Rajkowski, Kubiak, & Aston-Jones, 1999; Usher, Cohen, Servan-Schreiber, Rajkowski, & Aston-Jones, 1999) report that neuronal activity in the locus coeruleus (LC) is correlated with behavioral performance. The highest accuracy (hits vs. correct rejections) occurs when LC activity is moderate, and performance decreases with either lower or higher cellular discharge rates. Drugs such as clonidine that decrease LC discharge rates are detrimental to task performance (Ivanova, Rajkowski, Silakov, Watanabe, & Aston-Jones, 1997).

Sarter and colleagues take a similar approach to sustained attention. They study how activation or blockade of neurons of the rat cholinergic basal forebrain (CBF) alters stimulus detection performance. They find that cholinergic agonists increase performance accuracy by increasing the number of correct stimulus detections and reducing the number of false alarms (McGaughy, Decker, & Sarter, 1999). The effects are monotonically related to drug dose and, presumably, basal forebrain neuronal activity. Cholinergic blockers or lesions of the basal forebrain reduce response accuracy (Burk & Sarter, 2001).

What is the relationship between the cholinergic and noradrenergic systems in sustained attention? Connections from the locus coeruleus contact β-adrenergic receptors on the CBF neurons (Berridge, Manley, & Foote, 1996), suggesting an excitatory pathway. Thus, increases in LC activity with general arousal (Aston-Jones, Chen, Zhu, & Oshinsky, 2001) or frontal corticofugal activity (Aston-Jones, Chiang, & Alexinsky, 1991; Sara & Herve-Minvielle, 1995) will modulate CBF activity and attention. Low levels of LC activity engender low levels of CBF excitation and attention (orienting, detecting) is slower and inaccurate. As LC activity increases, CBF activity is facilitated even more, causing optimal increases in performance levels. At high activity levels, norepinephrine must begin to disfacilitate the CBF, perhaps by activating γ-aminobutyric acid interneurons in the CBF or adrenergic receptors that cause a net inhibition of CBF neurons.

This model also could explain features of behaviors mediated by the parietal cortex. The components of reflexive attention cooperatively facilitate reaction times (Clark et al.,

1989), which could be an outcome of noradrenergic facilitation. It suggests that moderate, but not high, doses of drugs that increase norepinephrine should facilitate the orienting of attention. This is observed and is highly dose dependent (Davidson et al., 1994). Also consistent with this prediction is the finding that degeneration of noradrenergic circuits in Alzheimer's disease causes a compensatory slowing of orienting (Festa-Martino et al., 2004).

PROPERTIES OF REFLEXIVE ATTENTION
IN ATTENTION-DEFICIT/HYPERACTIVITY DISORDER

Modern research on attention-deficit/hyperactivity disorder (ADHD) began in the early 1980s with the birth of the term *attention-deficit disorder*. The first investigation to use the CTD task was published in 1991 (Swanson et al., 1991). Using valid, invalid, and no-cue trials, they reported that children with ADHD show slower overall reaction times (RTs) and slower left visual field RTs with invalid cues (i.e., increased validity effect). Nigg, Swanson, and Hinshaw (1997) confirmed that both children with ADHD and their biological parents had slower left visual field RTs which were reversed in children by methylphenidate. However, in children and adults, Chen and colleagues (2002) and Epstein, Conners, Erhardt, March, and Swanson (1997) showed invalid cue slowing but in the right visual field. RT asymmetries are typically absent in those without the deficit. Thus, these results point to a faulty orienting mechanism as the cause of inattentiveness in ADHD, although its hemispheric location is unclear. In addition, those with ADHD sometimes show faster RTs to targets when the cue-target interval is long. This is taken to be the indirect result of alerting, but it is not always statistically different than that for controls (e.g., Swanson et al., 1991). The use of double cues, a pure measure of alerting, is preferable.

It is quite possible that the increased validity effect in ADHD is due to a deficit in cholinergic function. This would explain why the incidence of tobacco use is so high among those afflicted: They self-medicate to "normalize" the brain levels of ACh. This would also explain the benefits derived from nicotine patches (Levin, Conners, Silva, Canu, & March, 2001). On the other hand, there is little evidence from genetic studies that abnormal cholinergic receptors are a risk for ADHD, nor is there evidence that cholinergic metabolism is defective in this group (e.g., see Castellanos & Tannock, 2002). Perhaps the benefits of cholinergic agents are indirect, causing increases in the release of the catecholamines (e.g., Clarke & Reuben, 1996). It also difficult to know whether a change in the validity effect is due to actual deficits in orienting or compensatory deficits in alerting. As previously mentioned, the two components of reflexive attention are interdependent and without explicit measurement of each, the real deficit is elusive. To see the problem, it is instructive to review briefly the history of research into the attention deficits found in dementia of the Alzheimer's type. Early work (Parasuraman, Greenwood, Haxby, & Grady, 1992) showed orienting deficits, but no measurements of alerting were made. When both are measured in very recent work, the deficits in invalid cue response times, while present, can be completely explained by the absence of alerting effects in patients that speed invalid cue response times in age-matched controls (Festa-Martino et al., 2004).

On the basis of these data, we (Beckstead & Marrocco, 2003; Oberlin & Marrocco, 2003) reinvestigated the reflexive attention of adults with ADHD using the attention network task (Fan et al., 2001) in over 80 subjects (40 with ADHD, 40 controls). While those with ADHD are slower and make more errors than do controls, their validity effects are not significantly different than those of controls. In contrast, both double- and no-cue trials have very long response times and their alerting effects are significantly larger than controls. Nearly all subjects with ADHD were medicated with stimulants. When we compare the data acquired just after they took their medications with those just before they did so (usually an 11-hour difference), the former showed significantly smaller alerting effects than the latter (Figure 23.1C). Thus, our data support the idea that the alerting mechanism, but not the orienting mechanism, is abnormal in adult ADHD and that the stimulants tend to shorten the abnormally long response times. Long response times to targets in the absence of cues is also seen in young children and patients with lesions of the right parietal area. Neither group appears to be able to maintain the alert state as well as more mature, intact individuals.

Because the alerting effect is mediated by norepinephrine, the improvement is probably due to inhibition of the uptake of norepinephrine into presynaptic terminals. Similarly, nicotine's benefit on attention may be due to the indirect stimulation of norepinephrine as well. This interpretation is consistent with the recent hypotheses of Biederman (Biederman & Spencer, 1999) and Zametkin (Zametkin & Rapoport, 1987). However, it is unlikely to be the whole story because, at least in rats, drugs that lower norepinephrine slow double-cue response times much more than no-cue response times. Of course, the animal data are acute changes to a neuroactive agent, while the human data represent adaptation to chronic states with many potential causes.

ANIMAL MODELS OF ATTENTION DEFICITS

Worldwide, ADHD affects between 3 and 9% of the human population and its prevalence is generating intense interest in this disorder, especially in its genetic determinants (Comings, 2001). There is substantial evidence that the 7-repeat allele polymorphism of the D_4 dopamine receptor gene is a risk factor for acquiring ADHD (Swanson et al., 2000). To explore these issues at the molecular level, an appropriate animal model is required. To date, no realistic primate model exists. Several rat models have been proposed, but attention in these animals has been inferred from the open field test, rather than more rigorous tests that isolate attention from arousal changes and motor behavior (see also Davids, Zhang, Kula, Tarazi, & Baldessarini, 2002). Mice lacking the D_4 receptor have been bred and there is hope that these mice may elucidate the biological cause of ADHD. However, direct quantitative measures of attention in wild and knockout mice are also lacking.

A key issue in deciding whether the DRD_4 knockout model is appropriate is the degree to which the ADHD behavioral phenotype is captured in the animal's behavior. Of primary interest to us are the *inattentive* symptoms, arguably the most important features of the ADHD phenotype. Based on our data and others from humans, we would expect the DRD_4 knockout to have an abnormally large alerting effect and slower overall response times.

Somewhat less straightforward, however, is why a defect in a dopamine receptor should reveal itself in stimulus alerting, mediated by norepinephrine. Deleting the D_4 receptor appears to be associated with lower levels of norepinephrine release. Perhaps other dopamine receptors upregulate their activity, leading to lower dopamine levels and norepinephrine synthesis. Whether the mechanism is correct or not, dopamine or its metabolites are often reduced in humans with ADHD.

This research is an important test of the utility of the knockout model and is currently under way in our laboratory. If the behaviors are comparable with the ADHD phenotype, the work will validate the mouse as a useful subject for understanding the reflexive, and perhaps voluntary, attention in ADHD. If the behaviors are quite different, the DRD$_4$ knockout model may be appropriate for studying the motoric components of the disease only. Given the increasingly large number of studies that support a noradrenergic deficit in ADHD, it would be most interesting to develop a viable noradrenergic receptor knockout. Given the connection we have established between norepinephrine and alerting, the a priori predictions for reflexive attention deficits seem much more straightforward than for dopamine.

CONCLUSION

We have used both comparative and multilevel neuroscientific approaches to study reflexive attention. In all mammals tested, we find that cholinergic and noradrenergic neurotransmission mediate the spatial and nonspatial components of this behavior, respectively. There is good evidence from other labs that these same neuroactive substances mediate voluntary attention as well. Alteration of the activity of the components, either by reversible drug infusions or by disease processes, produces a pattern of deficits consistent with the cholinergic/noradrenergic model and point to the pivotal roles of the LC, CBF, and IPC in reflexive attention.

We also present evidence that supports the conclusion that the IPC integrates intrinsic circuitry with inputs from the LC and CBF to control exogenous attention. These computations include the initiation of the attention shift, its direction and amplitude, and activation of the alerting component. The challenge for systems neuroscience will be to apply similar analyses to voluntary attention and the circuits that link the reflexive and voluntary attention systems to specify the circuits that permit rapid switching between the two.

In light of these findings, we describe new studies of reflexive attention deficits in adult human subjects. The data suggest that in ADHD, the alerting, but not the orienting, component is deficient. This finding presents a more consistent view of reflexive attention deficits in adult ADHD than is currently available. That is, stimulants improve the attentive, not just the motoric, component of ADHD by elevating the deficient levels of brain norepinephrine and improving the subjects ability to be alerted by environmental events. The results also provide further support for the use of noradrenergic-specific stimulants in treating attention deficits. They also imply that animal models of attention deficits that are based on noradrenaline dysfunction could provide a better fit to the human phenotype.

ACKNOWLEDGMENT

This chapter was prepared with support from Grant Nos. 1RO1 DA 12765 and 1 T32-GM 07257 from the National Institutes of Health.

REFERENCES

Anderson, T., Jenkins, L., Brooks, D., Hawken, M., Frackowiak, R., & Kennard, C. (1994). Cortical control of saccades and fixation in man: A PET study. *Brain, 117,* 1073–1084.

Astafiev, S. V., Shulman, G. L., Stanley, C. M., Snyder, A. Z., Van Essen, D. C., & Corbetta, M. (2003). Functional organization of human intraparietal and frontal cortex for attending, looking, and pointing. *Journal of Neuroscience, 23,* 4689–4699.

Aston-Jones, G., Chiang, C., & Alexinsky, T. (1991). Discharge of noradrenergic locus coeruleus neurons in behaving rats and monkeys suggests a role in vigilance. *Progress in Brain Research*, *88*, 501–520.

Aston-Jones, G., Chen, S., Zhu, Y., & Oshinsky, M. L. (2001). A neural circuit for circadian regulation of arousal. *Nature Neuroscience*, *4*, 732–738.

Beane, M., Drew, A., Massey, K., & Marrocco, R. (2002a). Infusion of cholinergic and noradrenergic agents into rat posterior parietal cortex modifies orienting and alerting components of covert visual attention, respectively. *Neuroscience Abstracts*, *28*.

Beane, M., Drew, A., Massey, K., & Marrocco, R. (2002b). *Local infusion of cholinergic and noradrenergic agents into rat posterior parietal cortex modifies orienting and alerting components of covert attention, respectively.* Manuscript in preparation.

Beauchamp, M. S., Petit, L., Ellmore, T. M., Ingeholm, J., & Haxby, J. V. (2001). A parametric fMRI study of overt and covert shifts of visuospatial attention. *NeuroImage*, *14*, 310–321.

Beckstead, M., & Marrocco, R. T. (2003). *Nicotinic effects on reflexive orienting and alerting in adult ADHD.* Manuscript in preparation.

Berridge, C. W., Bolen, S. J., Manley, M. S., & Foote, S. L. (1996). Modulation of forebrain electroencephalographic activity in halothane-anesthetized rat via actions of noradrenergic beta-receptors within the medial septal region. *Journal of Neuroscience*, *16*, 7010–7020.

Biederman, J., & Spencer, T. (1999). Attention-deficit/hyperactivity disorder (ADHD) as a noradrenergic disorder. *Biological Psychiatry*, *46*, 1234–1242.

Bisley, J. W., & Goldberg, M. E. (2003). Neuronal activity in the lateral intraparietal area and spatial attention. *Science*, *299*, 81–86.

Burk, J. A., & Sarter, M. (2001). Dissociation between the attentional functions mediated via basal forebrain cholinergic and GABA-ergic neurons. *Neuroscience*, *105*, 899–909.

Castellanos, F. X., & Tannock, R. (2002). Neuroscience of attention-deficit/hyperactivity disorder: The search for endophenotypes. *Nature Reviews Neuroscience*, *3*, 617–628.

Chen, C. Y., Chen, C. L., Wu, C. Y., Chen, H. C., Tang, F. T., & Wong, M. K. (2002). Visual spatial attention in children with attention deficit hyperactivity disorder. *Chang Gung Medical Journal*, *25*, 514–521.

Clark, C. R., Geffen, G. M., & Geffen, L. B. (1989). Catecholamines and the covert orientation of attention in humans. *Neuropsychologia*, *27*, 131–139.

Clarke, P. B., & Reuben, M. (1996). Release of [^{3}H]-noradrenaline from rat hippocampal synaptosomes by nicotine: Mediation by different nicotinic receptor subtypes from striatal [^{3}H]-dopamine release. *British Journal of Pharmacology*, *117*, 595–606.

Colby, C., & Goldberg, M. (1999). Space and attention in parietal cortex. *Annual Review of Neuroscience*, *22*, 319–349.

Comings, D. E. (2001). Clinical and molecular genetics of ADHD and Tourette syndrome. Two related polygenic disorders. *Annals of the New York Academy of Sciences*, *931*, 50–83.

Corbetta, M., Akbudak, E., Conturo, T. E., Snyder, A. Z., Ollinger, J. M., Drury, H. A., et al. (1998). A common network of functional areas for attention and eye movements. *Neuron*, *21*, 761–773.

Corbetta, M., Kincade, J. M., Ollinger, J. M., McAvoy, M. P., & Shulman, G. L. (2000). Voluntary orienting is dissociated from target detection in human posterior cortex. *Nature Neuroscience*, *3*, 292–297.

Corbetta, M., Miezen, F. M., Shulman, G. L., & Petersen, S. E. (1993). A PET study of visuospatial attention. *Journal of Neuroscience*, *13*, 1202–1226.

Corbetta, M., Shulman, G. L., Miezin, F. M., & Petersen, S. E. (1995). Superior parietal cortex activation during spatial attention shifts and visual feature conjunction. *Science*, *270*, 802–805.

Coull, J. T., Nobre, A. C., & Frith, C. D. (2001). The noradrenergic alpha2 agonist clonidine modulates behavioural and neuroanatomical correlates of human attentional orienting and alerting. *Cerebral Cortex*, *11*, 73–84.

Cutrell, E. B., & Marrocco, R. T. (2002). Electrical microstimulation of primate posterior parietal cortex initiates orienting and alerting components of covert attention. *Experimental Brain Research*, *144*, 103–113.

Davids, E., Zhang, K., Kula, N. S., Tarazi, F. I., & Baldessarini, R. J. (2002). Effects of norepinephrine and serotonin transporter inhibitors on hyperactivity induced by neonatal 6-hydroxydopamine lesioning in rats. *Journal of Pharmacology and Experimental Therapeutics*, *301*, 1097–1102.

Davidson, M. C., Cutrell, E. B., & Marrocco, R. T. (1999). Scopolamine slows the orienting of attention in primates to cued visual targets. *Psychopharmacology (Berlin)*, *142*, 1–8.

Davidson, M. C., & Marrocco, R. T. (2000). Local infusion of scopolamine into intraparietal cortex slows covert orienting in rhesus monkeys. *Journal of Neurophysiology*, *83*, 1536–1549.

Davidson, M., Villareal, M., & Marrocco, R. (1994). Pharmacological manipulation of noradrenaline activity influences covert orienting in rhesus monkey. *Neuroscience Abstracts*, *20*, 829.

Epstein, J. N., Conners, C. K., Erhardt, D., March, J. S., & Swanson, J. M. (1997). Asymmetrical hemispheric control of visual–spatial attention in adults with attention deficit hyperactivity disorder. *Neuropsychology*, *11*, 467–473.

Fan, J., Wu, Y., Fossella, J. A., & Posner, M. I. (2001). Assessing the heritability of attentional networks. *BMC Neuroscience*, *2*, 14–20.

Fernandez-Duque, D., & Posner, M. I. (1997). Relating the mechanisms of orienting and alerting. *Neuropsychologia*, *35*, 477–486.

Festa-Martino, E., Ott, B., & Heindel, W. (2004). Interactions between phasic alerting and spatial orienting: Effects of normal aging and Alzheimer's disease. *Neuropsychologia*, *18*, 258–268.

Hahn, B., Shoaib, M., & Stolerman, I. P. (2002). Nicotine-induced enhancement of attention in the five-choice serial reaction time task: The influence of task demands. *Psychopharmacology (Berlin)*, *162*, 129–137.

Hanes, D. P., Patterson, W. F. II, & Schall, J. D. (1998). Role of frontal eye fields in countermanding saccades: Visual, movement, and fixation activity. *Journal of Neurophysiology*, *79*, 817–834.

Ivanova, S., Rajkowski, J., Silakov, V., Watanabe, R., & Aston-Jones, G. (1997). Local chemomanipulations of locus coeruleus (LC) activity in monkeys alter cortical event-related potentials (ERP) and task performance. *Society for Neuroscience Abstracts*, *23*, 1587.

Kawahara, Y., Kawahara, H., & Westerink, B. H. (1999). Tonic regulation of the activity of noradrenergic neurons in the locus coeruleus of the conscious rat studied by dual-probe microdialysis. *Brain Research*, *823*, 42–48.

Levin, E. D., Conners, C. K., Silva, D., Canu, W., & March, J. (2001). Effects of chronic nicotine and methylphenidate in adults with attention deficit/hyperactivity disorder. *Experimental and Clinical Psychopharmacology*, *9*, 83–90.

Marrocco, R. T., & Davidson, M. C. (1998). Neurochemistry of attention. In R. Parasuraman (Ed.), *The attentive brain* (pp. 35–50). Cambridge, UK: Cambridge University Press.

McGaughy, J., Decker, J., & Sarter, M. (1999). Enhancement of sustained attention performance by the nicotinic acetylcholine receptor agonist ABT-418 in intact but not basal forebrain-lesioned rats. *Psychopharmacology*, *144*, 175–182.

Mesulam, M. M. (1990), Large-scale neurocognitive networks and distributed. *Annals of Neurology*, *28*, 597–613.

Mesulam, M. M. (1999). Spatial attention and neglect: Parietal, frontal and cingulate contributions to the mental representation and attentional targeting of salient extrapersonal events. *Philosophical Transactions of the Royal Society London, Series B, Biological Sciences*, *354*, 1325–1346.

Moore, T., & Armstrong, K. M. (2003). Selective gating of visual signals by microstimulation of frontal cortex. *Nature*, *421*, 370–373.

Morrison, J., & Foote, S. (1986). Noradrenergic and serotonergic innervation of cortical, thalamic, and tectal regions in old and new world monkeys. *Neuropsychologia*, *243*, 117–138.

Murphy, F., & Klein, R. (1998). The effects of nicotine on spatial and non-spatial expectancies in a covert orienting task. *Journal of Cognitive Neuroscience*, *36*, 1103–1114.

Nigg, J., Swanson, J., & Hinshaw, S. (1997). Covert visual spatial attention in boys with attention deficit hyperactivity disorder: Lateral effects, methylphenidate response and results for parents. *Neuropsychologia*, *35*, 165–176.

Oberlin, B., & Marrocco, R. T. (2003). *ADHD: Normal orienting but impaired alerting during reflexive attention in human adults.* Manuscript in preparation.

Parasuraman, R. (1998). *The attentive brain.* Cambridge, MA: Bradford Books.

Parasuraman, R., Greenwood, P. M., Haxby, J. V., & Grady, C. L. (1992). Visuospatial attention in dementia of the Alzheimer type. *Brain, 115,* 711–733.

Petit, L., Tzourio, N., Orssaud, C., Pietrzyk, U., Berthoz, A., & Mazoyer, B. (1995). Functional neuroanatomy of the human visual fixation system. *European Journal of Neuroscience, 7,* 169–174.

Phillips, J. M., McAlonan, K., Robb, W. G., & Brown, V. J. (2000). Cholinergic neurotransmission influences covert orientation of visuospatial attention in the rat. *Psychopharmacology, 150,* 112–116.

Posner, M., & Petersen, S. (1990). The attention system of the human brain. *Annal Review of Neuroscience, 13,* 25–42.

Rajkowski, J., Kubiak, P., & Aston-Jones, G. (1994). Locus coeruleus activity in monkey: Phasic and tonic changes are associated with altered vigilance. *Brain Research Bulletin, 35,* 607–616.

Ruggiero, D. A., Giuliano, R., Anwar, M., Stornetta, R., & Reis, D. J. (1990). Anatomical substrates of cholinergic autonomic regulation in the rat. *Journal of Comparative Neurology, 292,* 1–53.

Sara, S. J., & Herve-Minvielle, A. (1995). Inhibitory influence of frontal cortex on locus coeruleus neurons. *Proceedings of the National Academy of Sciences, 92,* 6032–6036.

Snyder, A. Z., Batista, A. P., & Andersen, R. A. (1997). Coding of intention in the posterior parietal cortex. *Nature, 386,* 167–170.

Stewart, C., Burke, S., & Marrocco, R. (2001). Cholinergic modulation of covert attention in the rat. *Psychopharmacology, 155,* 210–218.

Stolerman, I. P., Mirza, N. R., Hahn, B., & Shoaib, M. (2000). Nicotine in an animal model of attention. *European Journal of Pharmacology, 393,* 147–154.

Swanson, J. M., Flodman, P., Kennedy, J., Spence, M. A., Moyzis, R., Schuck, S., et al. (2000). Dopamine genes and ADHD. *Neuroscience and Biobehavioral Reviews, 24,* 21–25.

Swanson, J. M., Posner, M., Potkin, S., Bonforte, S., Youpa, D., Fiore, C., et al. (1991). Activating tasks for the study of visual-spatial attention in ADHD children: A cognitive anatomic approach. *Journal of Child Neurology, 6*(Suppl.), S119–127.

Tales, A., Muir, J. L., Bayer, A., & Snowden, R. J. (2002). Spatial shifts in visual attention in normal ageing and dementia of the Alzheimer type. *Neuropsychologia, 40,* 2000–2012.

Usher, M., Cohen, J. D., Servan-Schreiber, D., Rajkowski, J., & Aston-Jones, G. (1999). The role of locus coeruleus in the regulation of cognitive performance. *Science, 283,* 549–554.

Van Essen, D. C., Lewis, J. W., Drury, H. A., Hadjikhani, N., Tootell, R. B. H., Bakircioglu, M., et al. (2001). Mapping visual cortex in monkeys and humans using surface-based atlases. *Vision Research, 41,* 1359–1378.

Vincler, M. A., & Eisenach, J. C. (2003). Immunocytochemical localization of the alpha3, alpha4, alpha5, alpha7, beta2, beta3 and beta4 nicotinic acetylcholine receptor subunits in the locus coeruleus of the rat. *Brain Research, 974,* 25–36.

Ward, N. M., & Brown, V. J. (1996). Covert orienting of attention in the rat and the role of striatal dopamine. *Journal of Neuroscience, 16,* 3082–3088.

Witte, E. A. (1994). *The effects of pharmacological changes in the catecholaminergic and cholinergic systems on arousal and covert orienting.* Eugene: University of Oregon, Department of Psychology.

Witte, E. A., Davidson, M. C., & Marrocco, R. T. (1997). Effects of altering brain cholinergic activity on covert orienting of attention: Comparison of monkey and human performance. *Psychopharmacology (Berlin), 132,* 324–334.

Witte, E. A., & Marrocco, R. T. (1997). Alteration of brain noradrenergic activity in rhesus monkeys affects the alerting component of covert orienting. *Psychopharmacology (Berlin), 132,* 315–323.

Witte, E. A., Villareal, M., & Marrocco, R. (1996). Visual orienting and alerting in Rhesus monkeys: comparison with humans. *Behavioural Brain Research, 82,* 103–112.

Wojciulik, E., Kanwisher, N., & Driver, J. (1998). Covert visual attention modulates face-specific activity in the human fusiform gyrus: fMRI Study. *Journal of Neurophysiology, 79,* 1574.

Yamaguchi, S., & Kobatashi, S. (1998). Contributions of the dopaminergic system to voluntary and automatic orienting of visuospatial attention. *Journal of Neuroscience, 18,* 1869–1878.

Zametkin, A., & Rapoport, J. (1987). Noradrenergic hypothesis of attention deficit disorder with hyperactivity: A critical review. In H. Meltzer (Ed.), *Psychopharmacology: The third generation* (pp. 837–842). New York: Raven Press.

V

DEVELOPMENT
OF ATTENTION

24

Visual Attention in Infancy

Process and Product in Early Cognitive Development

John Colombo

The systematic study of cognitive function in the human infant emerged with the use of the corneal reflection technique in the late 1950s and 1960s (Fantz, 1956, 1958, 1961). Initial demonstrations of the habituation of infants' visual responses to repetitive stimulus presentations and selective looking to novel stimulus presentations (e.g., Fantz, 1964) provided a noninvasive behavioral technology that fueled unprecedented growth in the field of developmental psychology over the course of four decades. In the years that followed, the distribution of infants' attention to visual stimuli was used widely as a tool for documenting important perceptual and cognitive capacities (e.g., pattern and form perception, visual discrimination, recognition memory, and category formation) in infancy. However, with only a few notable exceptions (e.g., Cohen, 1972, 1973) the topic of attention per se in infancy was not a primary or fundamental focus of systematic investigation in this literature and has only recently begun to be investigated in earnest (Richards, 1998; Ruff & Rothbart, 1996; see also Colombo, 2002). We have elsewhere (Colombo & Mitchell, 1988, 1990) characterized the neglect of attention as a primary topic of study in favor of the study of perceptual–cognitive capacities as an emphasis on the *products* of early cognitive function over the *process* through which such products are attained.

Given that a true understanding of the nature of cognitive function can only be derived from an understanding of its underlying mechanisms, an overarching theme of our research program has been to focus on the processes of attention in infancy, and the relationship of those processes to more general cognitive products (e.g., perception, learning, recognition, discrimination, and categorization). In doing this, we have also adopted Underwood's (1975) framework for the role of individual differences in theory development, which has in turn led us to investigate both developmental and individual differences in attention during infancy and early childhood. This work has taken several forms—for example, longitudinal studies examining the predictive validity of attentional constructs for later cognitive function (Colombo, Mitchell, Dodd, Coldren, & Horowitz, 1989; Colombo, Shaddy, Richman, Maikranz, & Blaga, in press; Saxon, Colombo, Robinson, & Frick, 2000), experimental studies of perceptual–attentional effects (e.g., Colombo, Ryther, Frick, & Gifford, 1995), the interface between attention and higher-order cognitive functions (Coldren & Colombo, 1994; Colombo, McCollam, Coldren, Mitchell, & Rash, 1990; Colombo, Mitchell, Coldren, & Atwater, 1990), and the role of arousal in early attention (Colombo, Frick, & Gorman, 1997; Maikranz, Colombo, Richman, & Frick, 2000). Our research strategies and assumptions are perhaps best explicated in a description of our program of work on identifying those subtypes of attention that contribute to or influence common measures of visual cognition across the first year. In the sections that follow, we briefly review those assumptions and strategies in the conduct of this program. We end with a discussion of what we believe are promising paths for discovery in the future.

DEVELOPMENTAL AND INDIVIDUAL DIFFERENCES IN LOOKING

For the last three decades, the primary method for the study of infant cognition has been visual habituation, and the primary dependent variable for the study of infant attention has been looking (i.e., its duration, direction, and movement). In visual habituation, an infant's looking to a visual stimulus is recorded while the stimulus is repeatedly exposed over a series of discrete trials. The resulting decline in look duration across trials has generally been interpreted as a decrease in the strength or magnitude of the orienting reflex, which in turn is thought to reflect the formation of an internal representation of the stimulus (Sokolov, 1963). When we began our research program, little was known about (1) how best to quantify the habituation curve, (2) the developmental course of habituation performance, or (3) the degree to which such performance reflected valid measures of individual differences in early cognitive activity. Our initial studies using the infant-controlled habituation procedure (Horowitz, Paden, Bhana, & Self, 1972) quickly established that much of the variance in the parameters of the habituation curve across the first year (i.e., 3–9 months of age) was directly attributable to the duration of infant looking at the start of the sequence (Colombo, Mitchell, O'Brien, & Horowitz, 1987a).

Furthermore, the duration of infant looking changed most robustly with age, showing a sharp decline in the first half of the first year (Colombo & Mitchell, 1990; Mayes & Kessen, 1989; see Figure 24.1). Our initial belief that look duration followed a simple course of linear decline across the first year has been recently challenged by several reports of increases in looking in both early and later periods during infancy. As a result, we conducted a comprehensive survey of the literature on the developmental course of infant looking (Colombo, Harlan, & Mitchell, 1999; see also Colombo, 2002; Colombo et al., 2004), and have found evidence that suggests a course composed of three distinct phases: brief looking that increases to 8–10 weeks of age (e.g., Hood et al., 1996; Slater, Brown, Mattock, & Bornstein, 1996), a sharp decline from that point to some point after 6 months of age (Colombo & Mitchell, 1990; Mayes & Kessen, 1989), and then a plateau or perhaps a gradual increase thereafter (Kagan, 1971; Saxon, Frick, & Colombo, 1997).

Finally, measures of the duration of looking provided the most reliable indices of individual differences within and across ages (Colombo et al., 1987a, 1987b). Test–retest correlations for look duration generally range from .40 to .50, although cross-age correlations are more modest.

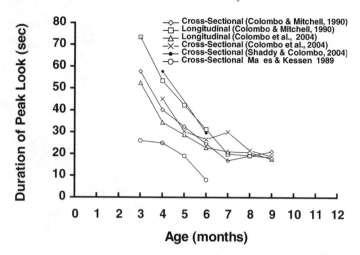

FIGURE 24.1. Compilation of longitudinal and cross-sectional studies of infant look duration during the first year. All show evidence of a drop in look duration from early infancy to the middle of the first year. Most studies reflect curves for static visual stimuli, although Shaddy and Colombo (in press) used dynamic displays.

Infant Looking and Encoding Efficiency

If the theory most often invoked to explain visual habituation (Sokolov, 1963) was accurate, then these findings suggested that look duration likely reflected the rapidity with which infants' encoded visual stimuli. This certainly fit the developmental trends; it explained why looking declined over age, as older infants were presumably more efficient at encoding than were younger infants. Furthermore, the data on within-age reliability suggested that reliable individual differences in encoding could be accessed through this variable.

We examined these hypotheses in a series of follow-up studies with infants 4–7 months of age (e.g., Colombo, Mitchell, & Horowitz, 1988) using a procedure consisting of two phases. In the first phase, we assess infants' looking time; in the second phase, we administer a separate task to test for infants' discrimination/recognition. We then examine the degree to which infants' look duration predicts success on the subsequent discrimination/recognition task.

In look-duration assessments, we present one or more stimuli to the infant and obtain some index of the infant's characteristic look duration to these. This can be done in a number of ways. Most often the assessment is independent of the subsequent discrimination/recognition task, and we use a pretest (or set of pretests) in which stimuli are presented until the infant accumulates some amount of looking time (Colombo, Mitchell, Coldren, & Freeseman, 1991; Freeseman, Colombo, & Coldren, 1993; but see Colombo et al., 1988) or fully habituates to a stimulus (Colombo, Frick, Ryther, & Gifford, 1996). Once the look-duration assessment is complete, we administer a discrimination/recognition task. In such tasks, the infant is familiarized for some predetermined amount of time with another visual stimulus, and then that familiarized stimulus is simultaneously paired with a novel one. If the infant has been given sufficient familiarization with the first stimulus, discrimination or recognition is manifest through increased looking to the novel one (i.e., a "novelty preference").

It should be noted that in the discrimination/recognition tasks, infants' speed of encoding can be ascertained by manipulating the amount of familiarization. Infants who encode more quickly will be successful at such tasks under conditions of less familiarization; infants who encode more slowly will be successful only if more familiarization is provided. In addition, by carefully controlling the characteristics of the familiarized and novel stimulus, it is possible to precisely determine the perceptual basis on which infants successfully discriminate or recognize stimuli.

Using these methods, our basic hypotheses about look duration were generally confirmed. Older infants (who looked for briefer durations than younger infants) needed less familiarization time to encode visual stimuli than did younger infants (Colombo et al., 1988). Furthermore, with infants from the same-age cohort, those who looked for briefer durations needed less familiarization time to encode visual stimuli than those who looked for more prolonged durations (Colombo et al., 1991; Freeseman et al., 1993).

Infant Looking and Attention to Visual Stimulus Properties

These initial results were encouraging, but they did not directly address the specific nature of the relationship between the duration of infant attention and the rapidity or efficiency of encoding. Given extant data suggesting more limited and less active visual scanning in younger infants relative to older infants (Bronson, 1982, 1990; Salapatek, 1975), we hypothesized that perhaps those younger infants (and those who looked for prolonged periods, relative to their same-age peers) were processing more slowly because they were less likely to engage in wide-ranging inspection of stimulus features. If this were true, we should see major differences in the several aspects of visual stimulus processing among infants who varied in their duration of looking: Such differences should emerge in the encoding of global and local visual properties, and in the response to visual symmetry (see Figure 24.2).

We began working on studies of local and global properties using hierarchical stimulus arrangements (Colombo et al., 1991; Freeseman et al., 1993; see also Frick, Colombo, & Allen, 2000). We eventually obtained data from both 3- and 4-month-olds in support of the hypothesis that the tendency to show longer durations of looking in infancy was associated with a bias for processing local features over global configurations. For example, in Colombo, Freeseman, Coldren, and Frick (1995), we familiarized both long- and short-looking infants with a hierarchical display and then placed the global and local properties in competition with one another on the test trials of the recognition task. Infants with briefer looking patterns showed evidence of a global-to-local shift in attention as familiarization increased; however, infants with patterns of prolonged look duration remained focused on local visual elements. In Colombo and colleagues (1996; see also Frick & Colombo, 1996) we examined infants' performance on a task in which we familiarized with a shape that was missing 50% of its contour. On the test trials, we asked whether infants would recognize that shape if the other half of its contour were presented; one cannot be successful at this task if relying on local visual properties for recognition. In keeping with the hypothesis, infants with briefer look durations were successful on the task; infants with longer durations performed at chance. Finally, based on the assumption that the advantage in encoding vertically symmetrical stimuli is attributable to a global-processing strategy, we tested whether long- and short-looking infants would show such an advantage. Again consistent with the hypothesis, infants with short look durations were quicker (i.e., needed less familiarization) to encode symmetrical stimuli than asymmetrical stimuli; infants with longer look durations did not show this typical advantage for symmetrical stimuli (Stoecker, Colombo, Frick, & Ryther, 1998).

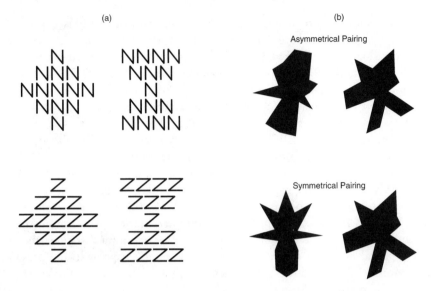

FIGURE 24.2. Examples of visual properties examined in the context of infant look duration. Figure 24.2a shows hierarchical stimuli used in Freeseman et al. (1993) and Colombo et al. (1995). "Global" properties are represented by low-spatial frequency configuration (diamond or hourglass), "local" properties are represented by high-spatial frequency features (N's or Z's). The recognition performance of infants with long look durations supports the hypothesis that they are biased toward encoding using local features; the performance of infants with briefer look durations suggests an adult-like global-to-local encoding sequence. Figure 24.2b shows vertically symmetrical and asymmetrical stimuli from Stoecker et al. (1998); advantages for processing symmetrical stimuli are observed for infants with brief look durations but not for infants with prolonged look durations.

Our findings were corroborated by research from other laboratories, which also observed shorter looking to be associated with wider inspection of visual stimuli using both corneal reflection techniques (Jankowski & Rose, 1997) and eye-tracking methodology (Krinsky-McHale, 1996). Longer looking was found to be associated with success at discrimination of finer visual details (Orlian & Rose, 1998). Finally, an intervention that encouraged long-looking infants to shift their attention around a stimulus display was effective in eliminating deficits in recognition/discrimination performance (Jankowski, Rose, & Feldman, 2001).

Infant Looking and the Disengagement of Attention

These lines of work suggested that individual and developmental differences in look duration (i.e., the characteristic indication of attentional maturity in human infants) were likely related to different modes of operation in visual processing. Behavioral studies consistently linked shorter look durations with a rapid encoding, which were likely attributable to the tendency for broader visual inspection of stimuli. Prolonged looking was consistently linked with slower encoding, and results suggested that this was attributable to the tendency for infants to become "stuck" on local visual features and rely on them for visual discrimination and processing. We next wondered what might be the underlying mechanism through which infants might become visually "stuck" on particular parts of stimulus displays. For some time, the looking of very young infants had been characterized as being somewhat dissociated from active stimulus processing, and more a function of stimulus capture. As such, terms such as *obligatory looking* (Stechler & Latz, 1966) or *tropistic fixation* (Caron, Caron, Minichiello, Weiss, & Friedman, 1977) had been used to describe it (see also Greenberg & Weizmann, 1971; Hopkins & Van Wulfften-Palthe, 1985). More recently, this phenomenon has been recast or reinterpreted in light of the phenomenon of disengagement of attention (Hood & Atkinson, 1993; Johnson, Dziurawiec, Ellis, & Morton, 1991), a function of the posterior attention network (e.g., Posner & Petersen, 1990; Posner, Rothbart, & Thomas-Thrapp, 1997). As such, our own focus turned to study the relationship between look duration and disengagement of attention.

The initial study in this line of work (Frick, Colombo, & Saxon, 1999) was conducted using a variant of the gap/overlap paradigm (Atkinson, Hood, Wattam-Bell, & Braddick, 1992; Johnson, Posner, & Rothbart, 1991). In this paradigm, infants' attention is drawn to a central fixation stimulus prior to the presentation of a stimulus in the visual periphery, and the dependent variable is the latency of the infant's ocular movement toward the peripheral target. If the central stimulus is removed prior to the presentation of peripheral stimulus (gap condition), latencies are short. However, if the central stimulus remains when the peripheral stimulus appears (overlap condition), the infant must disengage attention from the central stimulus before moving attention and eyes to the peripheral target. As with previous work, an initial set of pretests were administered to assess look duration in a characteristic sample of 3- and 4-month-olds. As expected, latencies were slower for both age groups in the overlap condition (i.e., which required disengagement of attention), but 3-month-olds were significantly more impaired by the presence of the midline stimulus than were 4-month-olds. In addition, strong positive correlations were observed between look duration and ocular latency in the overlap (but not the gap) condition, even when age was partialed.

A second set of studies in this line of work used simultaneous measurement of heart rate (HR) during infant looking. HR has been used as an indicant of infant attention for over 40 years (Bridger, 1962), although its precise relation to discrete attentional processes in the infant has been described and explored by Richards (e.g., 1985). Colombo, Frick, Gorman, and Casebolt (1997) examined the course of 4-month-olds' HR during a standard infant-controlled habituation procedure, and analysis of infants' HR during the peak look provided further evidence for the role of disengagement to look duration. Figure 24.3 presents the results of HR change (relative to a prestimulus baseline) of 1-second epochs taken at three points: (1) immediately after the onset of the look, (2) at the lowest/deepest point of deceleration during the look, and (3) immediately prior to the infant's termination of the look. We divided infants into long-looking and short-looking groups based on a median split on the duration of the longest look. There were no differences between the groups on the first two points of analysis but strong differences on the last. Specifically, infants with brief look durations tended to terminate their looking while HR was at, or below, the prestimulus baseline HR levels. Infants with longer look durations, however, did not release their look until HR was well above the baseline. This finding was reminiscent of Richards and Casey's (1992) description of three distinct phases of infant attention through the measurement of HR taken while infants looked at visual stimuli: orienting (a brief and initial reaction to stimulus content), sustained attention (an extended period of encoding and processing), and attention termination (a period during which processing has ended, but during which the look continues; similar to the construct of disengagement). The pattern of results we observed here strongly suggested to us that prolonged looking might reflect an extended period of attention termination, and thus difficulty with disengagement.

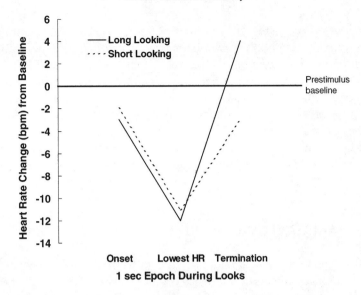

FIGURE 24.3. Results from Colombo et al. (1997). During the peak (longest) look from an infant-controlled habituation session, 4-month-olds' HR was measured during in the 1-second epochs (1) just after onset, (2) at its lowest point, and (3) then just prior to termination. Infants differed significantly ($p < .01$) only on the last epoch: infants who looked for briefer durations released the look while HR was at or just below prestimulus levels, while infants who looked for long durations released the look only after HR had exceeded prestimulus levels. Prolonged fixations may reflect difficulty in disengagement of attention.

We next asked whether the association between look duration and attention termination/disengagement could be directly demonstrated, and whether this relationship might bear on the propensity for infants with prolonged fixation to perform less optimally on recognition/discrimination tasks (Colombo, Richman, Shaddy, Maikranz, & Greenhoot, 2001). To do this, we chose a task in which the discrimination was based on global visual properties (Colombo et al., 1991) and set the familiarization at a level that would just barely allow recognition by 4-month-olds. We then pretested infants for look duration and administered the task in question. Infant HR was measured across both parts of the session. As we expected, infants' look duration (measured both in the pretest and during the familiarization period of the recognition task) predicted task performance; briefer looking was significantly associated with a higher likelihood of recognition. Furthermore, look duration was significantly and positively correlated with both sustained attention and attention termination. Finally, we entered these two phases into a regression to determine whether either mediated the relationship between look duration and performance, and the results confirmed our suspicions that attention termination (and thus, disengagement of attention) significantly mediated this relationship.

Summary and Cautions

We have by no means come to a comprehensive understanding of developmental and individual differences in visual attention in infancy. The line of work described previously is limited to a particular age range (3–9 months of age), and with particular types of stimuli (generally two-dimensional static displays). We have good reason to believe that different attentional processes predominate in later infancy (see Colombo, 2001) and that the encoding of different types of stimuli may well be mediated by different types of attention (e.g., sustained attention vs. attention termination; see Richards & Cronise, 2000; Shaddy & Colombo, in press). What we have established, however, is that processes other than traditional Sokolovian encoding make significant contributions to attentional measures during the first year, and that these processes bear on infants' cognitive performance and likely on developmental outcomes (see Colombo et al., in press). These alternate processes are drawn directly from the literature on the cognitive neuroscience of attention (e.g., Posner & Petersen, 1990) and thus hold great promise for the identification of the developmental course of those brain pathways and structures that are particularly critical for cognitive development.

EARLY ATTENTION AND COGNITIVE OUTCOME

The study of attention within the developmental context holds great promise for the behavioral sciences, and for the integration of basic cognitive neuroscience with the fields of education, clinical practice, and developmental disabilities. The realization of such promise will come in part through the identification of the underlying bases of early attentional functions, as described in our program of work, as well as in the programs of other scientists, some of whom are also represented in this volume. However, this realization also requires an understanding of how those early functions relate to meaningful cognitive-developmental outcomes. It has been well known for 40 years that postnatal experience plays a critical role in determining the structure and function of the central nervous system and that early experience tends to have a disproportionate degree of influence on mature function (Bornstein, 1989; Colombo, 1982; Gottlieb, 1976). Most of this work has focused on the role of visual input in structuring various aspects of development in the visual system as an exemplar (e.g., Hubel & Wiesel, 1965; Wiesel & Hubel, 1963); thus, it is reasonable to propose here that early differences in attention may play a similar role in structuring the central nervous system and long-term development. After Watson and Ewy (1983), we can delineate three different ways in the relationship that attention in infancy and early childhood to mature cognitive function can be conceptualized (see Figure 24.4).

First, early attention may be taken as a manifestation of later function. This has been the path most widely investigated to this point; indeed, individual differences in attention during infancy have been used as an indicant of general intellectual function in predicting developmental outcome (see Colombo, 1993). However, given the limitation of this approach that have become evident over the past decade (e.g., Colombo & Saxon, 2002), the pursuit of more process-oriented mechanisms seems in order.

Second, attention may affect the development of mature cognition by mediating the roles of experience and environment on brain development. Clearly, attention mediates the types of experience that organisms will have (e.g., NICHD Early Child Care Research Network, 2003). As obvious as this is, it is worth noting that the degree to which early attentional skills interact with environmental conditions or situations to produce particular developmental outcomes has been investigated in only a handful of studies (see, e.g., Colombo & Saxon, 2002, for a review).

A third and less obvious potential role of attention in long-term cognitive outcome lies in the direct effects that attention exerts on the brain per se. The evidence strongly suggests that the act of attending changes brain activity; for example, it modulates synchronous neural firing (e.g., Niebur, Hsiao, & Johnson, 2002; Steinmetz et al., 2000), and it enhances the

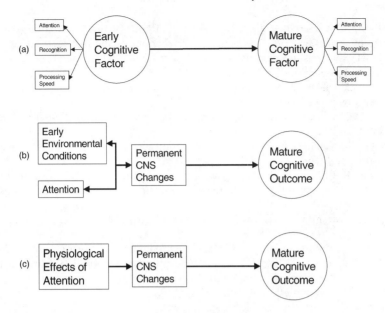

FIGURE 24.4. Schematic theoretical paths through which attention in infancy and early childhood can theoretically affect or influence the long-term development of the central nervous system and mature cognitive function. The horizontal dimension represents time. The top pathway (Figure 24.4a) represents early attention as merely manifestation of an underlying latent general cognitive/intellectual factor; there is simple continuity in the underlying latent factor. The middle pathway (Figure 24.4b) shows an indirect effect in which attention modulates or interacts with environmental conditions in order to produce changes in the brain. The bottom pathway (Figure 24.4c) represents the direct effects of attention on the brain, such that the effects of attention experienced during early periods of plasticity and may permanently affect central nervous system structure and function.

neural activity of areas that correspond to the object or object properties being attended to (Alais & Blake, 1999; McAdams & Maunsell, 1999; Reynolds & Desimone, 2003). It is possible that these direct, physical, and typically short-term consequences of attention may have disproportionate effects on the structure and function of the brain when they occur repetitively or for extended durations during early development. This pathway of influence has not been widely considered, much less directly investigated to this point, but seems to deserve some discourse within the broader discussion of the development of attention.

ACKNOWLEDGMENTS

Preparation of this chapter was supported by Grant No. HD35903 from the National Institutes of Health (NIH) and Grant No. 0318072 from the National Science Foundation. Research described in this review was supported by NIH Grant Nos. MH41395, MH43246, HD29960, and HD35903. I thank Kathleen Kannass, Jill Shaddy, Christa Anderson, and Dominie Writt-Haas for comments on an earlier draft of the manuscript, and Andrea Greenhoot for commentary on Figure 24.4.

REFERENCES

Alais, D., & Blake, R. (1999). Neural strength of visual attention gauged by motion adaptation. *Nature Neuroscience, 2,* 1015–1018.

Atkinson, J., Hood, B., Wattam-Bell, J., & Braddick, O. (1992). Changes in infants' ability to switch visual attention in the first three years of life. *Perception, 21,* 643–653.

Bornstein, M. H. (1989). Sensitive periods in development: Structural characteristics and causal interpretations. *Psychological Bulletin, 105,* 179–197.

Bridger, W. H. (1962). Sensory discrimination and autonomic function in the newborn. *Journal of the American Academy of Child Psychiatry, 1,* 67–91.

Bronson, G. W. (1982). *The scanning patterns of human infants: Implications for visual learning.* Norwood, NJ: Ablex.

Bronson, G. W. (1990). Changes in infants' visual scanning across the 2- to 14-week age period. *Journal of Experimental Child Psychology, 49,* 101–125.

Caron, A. J., Caron, R. F., Minichiello, C., Weiss, S., & Friedman, S. E. (1977). Constraints on the use of the familiarization-novelty method in the assessment of infant discrimination. *Child Development, 48,* 747–762.

Cohen, L. B. (1972). Attention-getting and attention-holding processes of infant visual preferences. *Child Development, 43,* 869–879.

Cohen, L. B. (1973). A two-process model of infant attention. *Merrill-Palmer Quarterly, 19,* 157–180.

Coldren, J. T., & Colombo, J. (1994). The nature and processes of preverbal learning: Implications from nine-month-old infants' discrimination problem solving. *Monographs of the Society for Research in Child Development, 59*(4, Whole No. 249).

Colombo, J. (1982). The critical period concept: Research, methodology, and conceptual issues. *Psychological Bulletin, 92,* 260–275.

Colombo, J. (1993). *Infant cognition: Predicting later intellectual functioning.* Newbury Park, CA: Sage.

Colombo, J. (2001). The development of visual attention in infancy. *Annual Review of Psychology, 52,* 337–367.

Colombo, J. (2002). Infant attention grows up: The emergence of a developmental cognitive neuroscience perspective. *Current Directions in Psychological Science, 11,* 196–199.

Colombo, J., Freeseman, L. J., Coldren, J. T., & Frick, J. E. (1995). Individual differences in infant visual fixation: Dominance of global and local stimulus properties. *Cognitive Development, 10,* 271–285.

Colombo, J., Frick, J. E., & Gorman, S. A. (1997). Sensitization during visual habituation sequences: Procedural effects and individual differences. *Journal of Experimental Child Psychology, 67,* 223–235.

Colombo, J., Frick, J. E., Gorman, S. A., & Casebolt, K. (1997). *Heart rate patterns during infant-controlled habituation sessions.* Paper presented at the biennial meeting of the Society for Research in Child Development, Washington, DC.

Colombo, J., Frick, J. E., Ryther, J. S., & Gifford, J. J. (1996). Individual differences in infant visual attention: Four-month-olds' recognition of forms connoted by complementary contour. *Infant Behavior and Development, 19,* 113–119.

Colombo, J., Harlan, J. E., & Mitchell, D. W. (1999). *The development of look duration in infancy: Evidence for a triphasic course.* Paper presented at the biennial meeting of the Society for Research in Child Development, Albuquerque, NM.

Colombo, J., McCollam, K., Coldren, J. T., Mitchell, D. W., & Rash, S. J. (1990). Form categorization in 10-month-old infants. *Journal of Experimental Child Psychology, 49,* 173–188.

Colombo, J., & Mitchell, D. W. (1988). Infant visual habituation: In defense of an information-processing analysis. *European Bulletin of Cognitive Psychology/Cahiers de Psychologie Cognitive, 8,* 455–461.

Colombo, J., & Mitchell, D. W. (1990). Individual and developmental differences in infant visual attention: Fixation time and information processing. In J. Colombo & J.W. Fagen (Eds.), *Individual differences in infancy: Reliability, stability, and prediction* (pp. 193–227). Hillsdale, NJ: Erlbaum.

Colombo, J., Mitchell, D. W., Coldren, J. T., & Atwater, J. D. (1990). Discrimination learning during the first year of life: Stimulus and positional cues. *Journal of Experimental Psychology: Learning, Memory, and Cognition, 16,* 98–109.

Colombo, J., Mitchell, D. W., Coldren, J. T., & Freeseman, L. J. (1991). Individual differences in infant attention: Are short lookers faster processors or feature processors? *Child Development, 62,* 1247–1257.

Colombo, J., Mitchell, D. W., Dodd, J. D., Coldren, J. T., & Horowitz, F. D. (1989). Longitudinal correlates of infant attention in the paired comparison paradigm. *Intelligence, 13,* 33–42.

Colombo, J., Mitchell, D. W., & Horowitz, F. D. (1988). Infant visual behavior in the paired-comparison paradigm: Test–retest and attention–performance relations. *Child Development, 59,* 1198–1210.

Colombo, J., Mitchell, D. W., O'Brien, M., & Horowitz, F. D. (1987a). Stability of infant visual habituation during the first year. *Child Development, 58,* 474–489.

Colombo, J., Mitchell, D. W., O'Brien, M., & Horowitz, F. D. (1987b). Stimulus and motoric influences on visual habituation at three months. *Infant Behavior and Development, 10,* 173–181.

Colombo, J., Richman, W. A., Shaddy, D. J., Greenhoot, A. F., & Maikranz, J. (2001). HR-defined phases of attention, look duration, and infant performance in the paired-comparison paradigm. *Child Development, 72,* 1605–1616.

Colombo, J., Shaddy, D. J., Richman, W. A., Maikranz, J. M., & Blaga, O. (in press). Developmental course of visual habituation and preschool cognitive and language outcome. *Infancy.*

Colombo, J., Ryther, J. S., Frick, J. E., & Gifford, J. J. (1995). A visual "pop-out" effect in infants: Evidence for preattentive search in 3- and 4-month-olds. *Psychonomic Bulletin and Review, 2,* 266–268.

Colombo, J., & Saxon, T. (2002). Infant attention and the development of cognition: Does the environment moderate continuity? In H. Fitzgerald, K. Karraker, & T. Luster (Eds.), *Infant development: Ecological perspectives* (pp. 35–60). Washington, DC: Garland Press.

Fantz, R. L. (1956). A method for studying early visual development. *Perceptual and Motor Skills, 6,* 13–15.

Fantz, R. L. (1958). Pattern vision in young infants. *Psychological Record, 8,* 43–47.

Fantz, R. L. (1961). The origin of form perception. *Scientific American, 204,* 66–72.

Fantz, R. L. (1964). Visual experience in infants: Decreased attention to familiar patterns relative to novel ones. *Science, 146,* 668–670.

Freeseman, L. J., Colombo, J., & Coldren, J. T. (1993). Individual differences in infant visual attention: Discrimination and generalization of global and local stimulus properties. *Child Development, 64,* 1191–1203.

Frick, J. E., & Colombo, J. (1996). Individual differences in infant visual attention: Recognition of degraded visual forms by 4-month-olds. *Child Development, 67,* 188–204.

Frick, J.E., Colombo, J., & Allen, J. R. (2000). The temporal sequence of global-local processing in 3-month-olds. *Infancy, 1,* 375–386.

Frick, J. E., Colombo, J., & Saxon, T. F. (1999). Individual and developmental differences in disengagement of fixation in early infancy. *Child Development, 70,* 537–548.

Gottlieb, G. (1976). Conceptions of prenatal development: Behavioral embryology. *Psychological Review, 83,* 215–234.

Greenberg, D. J., & Weizmann, F. (1971). The measurement of visual attention in infants: A comparison of two methodologies. *Journal of Experimental Child Psychology, 11,* 234–243.

Haith, M. M. (1980). *Rules that babies look by.* Hillsdale, NJ: Erlbaum.

Hood, B. M., & Atkinson, J. (1993). Disengaging visual attention in the infant and adult. *Infant Behavior and Development, 16,* 405–422

Hood, B. M., Murray, L., King, F., Hooper, R., Atkinson, J., & Braddick, O. (1996). Habituation changes in early infancy: Longitudinal measures from birth to 6 months. *Journal of Reproductive and Infant Psychology, 14,* 177–185.

Hopkins, B., & Van Wulffthen-Palthe, T. (1985). Staring in infancy. *Early Human Development, 12,* 261–267.

Horowitz, F. D., Paden, L. Y., Bhana, K., & Self, P. (1972). An infant-control procedure for studying infant visual fixations. *Developmental Psychology, 7,* 90.

Hubel, D. H., & Wiesel, T. N. (1965). Binocular interaction in striate cortex of kittens reared with artificial squint. *Journal of Neurophysiology, 28,* 1041–1059.

Jankowski, J. J., & Rose, S. A. (1997). The distribution of visual attention in infants. *Journal of Experimental Child Psychology, 65,* 127–140.

Jankowski, J. J., Rose, S. A., & Feldman, J. F. (2001). Modifying the distribution of attention in infants. *Child Development, 72,* 339–351.

Johnson, M. H., Dziurawiec, S., Ellis, H., & Morton, J. (1991). Newborns' preferential tracking of face-like stimuli and its subsequent decline. *Cognition, 40,* 1–19

Johnson, M. H., Posner, M. I., & Rothbart, M. K. (1991). Components of visual orienting in early infancy: Contingency learning, anticipatory looking, and disengaging. *Journal of Cognitive Neuroscience, 3,* 335–344.

Kagan, J. (1971). *Change and continuity in infancy.* New York: Wiley.

Krinsky-McHale, S. J. (1996). Visual scanning during information processing in infancy. *Dissertation Abstracts International Section B: The Sciences and Engineering, 56,* 5796.

Maikranz, J. M., Colombo, J., Richman, W. A., & Frick, J. E. (2001). Autonomic indicators of sensitization and look duration in infancy. *Infant Behavior and Development, 23,* 137–151.

Mayes, L. C., & Kessen, W. (1989). Maturational changes in measures of habituation. *Infant Behavior and Development, 12,* 437–450

McAdams, C. J., & Maunsell, J. H. R. (1999). Effects of attention on the reliability of individual neurons in monkey visual cortex. *Neuron, 23,* 765–773.

NICHD Early Child Care Research Network. (2003). Do children's attention processes mediate the link between family predictors and school readiness? *Developmental Psychology, 39,* 581–593.

Niebur, E., Hsiao, S., & Johnson, K. O. (2002). Synchrony: A neuronal mechanism for attentional selection? *Current Opinion in Neurobiology, 12,* 190–194.

Orlian, E. K., & Rose, S. A. (1998). Speed vs. thoroughness in infant visual information processing. *Infant Behavior and Development, 20,* 371–381.

Posner, M. I., & Petersen, S. E. (1990). The attention system of the human brain. *Annual Review of Neuroscience, 13,* 25–42

Posner, M. I., Rothbart, M. K., & Thomas-Thrapp, L. (1997). Functions of orienting in early infancy. In P. J. Lang & R. F. Simons (Eds.), *Attention and orienting: Sensory and motivational processes* (pp. 327–345). Mahwah, NJ: Erlbaum.

Reynolds, J. H., & Desimone, R. (2003). Interacting roles of attention and visual salience in V4. *Neuron, 37,* 853–863.

Richards, J. E. (1985). Respiratory sinus arrhythmia predicts heart rate and visual responses during visual attention in 14 and 20 week old infants. *Psychophysiology, 22,* 101–109

Richards, J. E. (Ed.). (1998). *Cognitive neuroscience of attention: Developmental perspectives.* Mahwah, NJ: Erlbaum.

Richards, J. E., & Casey, B. J. (1992). Development of sustained visual attention in the human infant. In B. A. Campbell, H. A. Hayne, & R. Richardson (Eds.), *Attention and information processing in infants and adults: Perspectives from human and animal research* (pp. 30–60). Hillsdale, NJ: Erlbaum.

Richards, J. E., & Cronise, K. (2000). Extended visual fixation in the early preschool years: Look duration, heart rate changes, and attentional inertia. *Child Development, 71,* 602–620.

Ruff, H. A., & Rothbart, M. K. (1996). *Attention in early development: Variations and themes.* New York: Oxford University Press.

Salapatek, P. (1975). Pattern perception and early infancy. In L. Cohen & P. Salapatek (Eds.), *Infant perception, from sensation to cognition* (Vol. 2, pp. 133–248). New York: Academic Press.

Saxon, T. F., Colombo, J., Robinson, E., & Frick, J. E. (2000). Dyadic interaction profiles in infancy and preschool intelligence. *Journal of School Psychology, 38,* 9–25.

Saxon, T. F., Frick, J. E., & Colombo, J. (1997). Individual differences in infant visual fixation and maternal interactional styles. *Merrill-Palmer Quarterly, 43,* 48–66.

Shaddy, D. J., & Colombo, J. (in press). Developmental change in attention: Dynamic and static stimuli. *Infancy.*

Slater, A., Brown, E., Mattock, A., & Bornstein, M. H. (1996). Continuity and change in habituation in the first 4 months from birth. *Journal of Reproductive and Infant Psychology, 14,* 187–194.

Sokolov, E. (1963). *Perception and the conditioned reflex.* New York: Pergamon Press.

Stechler, G., & Latz, E. (1966). Some observations on attention and arousal in the human infant. *Journal of the American Academy of Child Psychiatry, 5*, 517–525.

Steinmetz, P. N., Roy, A., Fitzgerald, P. J., Hsiao, S. S., Johnson, K. O., & Niebur, E. (2000). Attention modulates synchronized neuronal firing in primate somatosensory cortex. *Nature, 187*, 187–190.

Stoecker, J. J., Colombo, J., & Frick, J. E., & Ryther, J. S. (1998). Long- and short-looking infants' recognition of symmetrical and asymmetrical visual forms. *Journal of Experimental Child Psychology, 71*, 63–78.

Underwood, B. J. (1975). Individual differences as a crucible in theory construction. *American Psychologist, 30*, 128–134.

Watson, J. S., & Ewy, R. D. (1983). Early learning and intelligence. In M. Lewis (Ed.), *Origins of intelligence* (2nd ed., pp. 225–254). New York: Plenum Press.

Wiesel, T. N., & Hubel, D. H. (1963). Single-cell responses in striate cortex of kittens deprived of vision in one eye. *Journal of Neurophysiology, 26*, 1002–1017.

25

The Development of Sustained Attention in Infants

John E. Richards

Attention may be characterized by its selectivity and intensity. The selective aspect of attention narrows the focus of information processing from a wide range of available stimuli, thoughts, and responses to a single aspect of the environment, or a selected set of stimulus–response activities. The intensity aspect of attention improves the quality of information-processing once the information processing focus is narrowed, which results in improvements in the quality of the cognitive activities involved in the attentive behavior. Researchers interested in infant attention have used behavioral measures during toy play to distinguish between periods when attention is intensified, "focused attention," and periods when the infant is inattentive, "casual attention" (Lansink & Richards, 1997; Oakes & Tellinghuisen, 1994; Ruff, 1986; Ruff & Capozzoli, 2003; Ruff & Rothbart, 1997). These behavioral measures, however, are applicable only after infants are capable of manipulating toys (e.g., after 6 months). Psychophysiological measures may be used with young infants as a noninvasive measure of attentiveness. Heart rate (HR) changes to environmental changes also may index periods of attentiveness and inattentiveness in young infants (Graham, 1979; Graham, Anthony, & Ziegler, 1983; Porges, 1976, 1980; Richards, 2001; Richards & Casey, 1991).

One type of attention that may be measured with HR changes is sustained attention. Sustained attention is indicated by a large deceleration of HR and an extended lowered HR. Sustained attention measures the alertness/arousal function of the brain (Richards, 2001). The broad range of influence that the arousal system has on cortical activity is consistent with the role that sustained attention plays in a wide variety of infant cognitive processes. For example, the modulation of blink reflexes by attention, and the development of the modulation, is revealed through measurements of HR-defined sustained attention (Richards, 1998, 2000; see review in Richards, 2001). The characteristics of eye movements and developmental changes in eye movements in young infants are mediated by sustained attention (e.g., Hunter & Richards, 2003; McKinney & Richards, 2004; Richards & Holley, 1999; Richards & Hunter, 1997; see reviews in Richards & Hunter, 1998, 2002). Sustained attention plays an important role in the development of extended looking to television programs in young children (Richards & Anderson, in press; Richards & Cronise, 2000; Richards & Gibson, 1997; Richards & Turner, 2001).

This chapter does two things. First, I review evidence showing how HR may be used as a measure of sustained attention. This section also shows the important changes occurring in sustained attention in the first year. Second, two areas of work are briefly reviewed that show how sustained attention affects infant cognitive processes. The first shows that attention to a central stimulus attenuates infants' responsiveness to peripheral stimuli. The second shows that developmental changes in the event-related potential response to briefly presented stimuli are mediated by infant attentiveness.

HEART RATE CHANGES AS A PSYCHOPHYSIOLOGICAL MEASURE OF INFANT ATTENTION

Infant attention has often been measured with HR. The first use of HR as a measure of attention was motivated by Sokolov's (1963) theory of the orienting reflex. The orienting reflex is the first response of an organism to a stimulus. Sokolov believed that this response was the first sign of a decrease in sensory thresholds and was mediated by peripheral sensory receptivity changes and central brain function activity. This response is composed of behavioral reactions and changes in autonomic nervous system activity. Graham and Clifton (1966) hypothesized that HR deceleration was a component of the orienting reflex and could be used as a sensitive measure of orienting in many species and at several ages.

The first studies of infant attention using HR examined the orienting reflex. Infants over a wide variety of ages were presented with brief (~2 seconds) visual or auditory stimuli and HR was measured. Newborn infants appeared to show only heart rate acceleration to such stimuli, implying that the orienting response did not function well at birth (Chase, 1965; Davis, Crowell, & Chun, 1965; Keen, Chase, & Graham, 1965). Infants were more likely to show heart rate decelerations to such brief stimuli at later ages. Figure 25.1 shows a graph summarizing several studies of the heart rate responses to a 2-second tone as a function of testing age (Graham et al., 1970, 1983). The heart rate deceleration increases in magnitude from birth to 16 weeks of age (about 3 months). This deceleration occurs to a wide variety of auditory, visual, and audiovisual stimuli from this age through the first year of life. The HR responses to such stimuli in adults are dissimilar to that of young infants. Adults show a brief deceleration at the onset of stimulus presentation and show larger HR decelerations only when presented with extended stimuli or in other procedures (e.g., foreperiod of a fixed-foreperiod reaction time task; van der Veen, Lange, van der Molen, Mulder, & Mulder, 2000).

I began my work in the study of HR changes by presenting infants with extended stimulus presentations. The HR changes to briefly presented stimuli represent a subcortically mediated orienting reflex or an automatic interrupt component of attention (Graham, 1979). Although these attention components are interesting and important, the information processing occurring during complex cognitive behavior goes beyond simple stimulus orienting. In one of my first studies I presented infants with complex visual stimuli, such as checkerboards, moving objects, and face-like stimuli (Richards, 1985). The infants in this study were 14, 20, or 26 weeks of age (3, 4½, 6 months). Figure 25.2 presents the HR responses that occurred during uninterrupted looking ("C") or when a peripheral stimulus was presented to distract looking ("S"). The HR change revealed two interesting patterns. First,

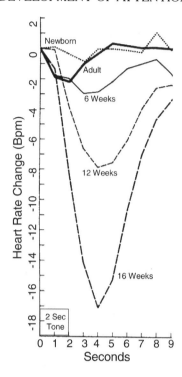

FIGURE 25.1. Changes in HR response as a function of age to a 2-second 75-dB, 1,000-Hz tone. Data from Graham et al. (1970).

there were no age differences in the HR occurring in the first few seconds of fixation, the stimulus orienting phase (cf. Figure 25.1). Second, there were no age changes in the pattern of the heart rate response during uninterrupted looking ("C"). But, when infants were paying attention to the center pattern and ignoring the distractor ("S"), there were age changes in the sustaining of the HR deceleration as the infant continued to look at this stimulus. From 14 to 26 weeks, there was an increasingly sustained deceleration of HR. I labeled this HR change "sustained attention."

Based on the findings that HR changes index short latency responses during stimulus orienting and longer latency sustained deceleration during sustained attention, I developed a model showing how HR changes index four attention phases (Richards & Casey, 1992; also see Graham, 1979; Graham et al., 1983; Porges, 1976, 1980). Figure 25.3 presents the changes in HR that occur in 3-, 4½-, and 6-month-old infants while viewing interesting computer-generated geometric patterns (Richards & Casey, 1991). The preattention period represents inattentiveness in the infant. At the beginning of stimulus presentation, there is a brief automatic interrupt that detects transient changes in environmental stimulation (Graham, 1979). This phase results in a brief biphasic deceleration–acceleration in HR (not labeled on Figure 25.3). The second phase, stimulus orienting, represents the activation by the automatic interrupt system of a preliminary processing of stimulus information (i.e., novelty, information value) and is identical to the orienting reflex studied by Sokolov (1963; Graham & Clifton, 1966). A large deceleration in HR occurs during this phase (Figure 25.3). Sustained attention is the third phase. Sustained attention involves voluntary, subject-controlled cognitive processing (Richards, 2001; Richards & Casey, 1992; Richards &

Hunter, 1998). It represents the activation of the alertness/arousal system of the brain (Richards, 2001). Heart rate shows a sustained decrease from baseline, this lowered HR continues (Figure 25.3; cf. Figure 25.2) with decreased HR variability, and sustained attention is accompanied by other bodily changes facilitating attentiveness. The final HR attention phase is attention termination, during which the infant continues to look at the stimulus but no longer processes information in the stimulus and is resistant for 5 to 6 seconds to new stimulation (Casey & Richards, 1991; Richards, 1988b; Richards & Casey, 1990). Heart rate during this phase returns to its prestimulus level and variability (Figure 25.3). Following attention termination, the infant may continue to gaze at the stimulus without further information-processing engagement, a period of inattentiveness.

The most recent studies we have done on sustained attention have examined sustained attention in a number of ways. The observations of the extended HR deceleration to simple geometric patterns (Figure 25.2) have been extended to children viewing complex visual–auditory stimuli such as *Sesame Street* television programs (Richards & Anderson, in press; Richards & Cronise, 2000; Richards & Gibson, 1997; Richards & Turner, 2001). Figure 25.4 shows the interbeat–interval changes in 3- to 6-month-old infants when viewing a *Ses-*

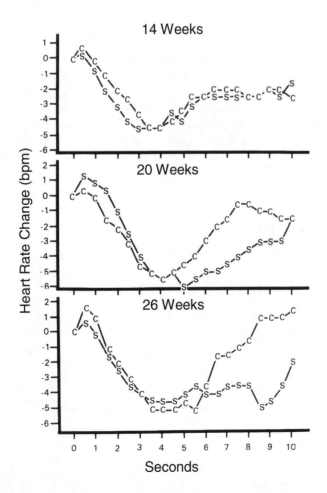

FIGURE 25.2. Change in HR response as a function of age to interesting geometric patterns in 14-, 20-, and 26-week-old infants. Data from Richards (1985).

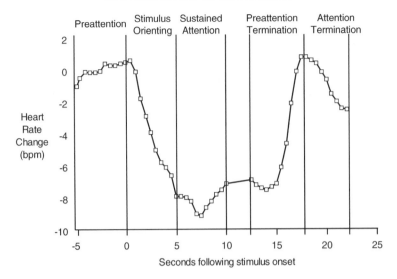

FIGURE 25.3. Average HR change as a function of seconds following stimulus onset during the HR-defined attention phases. Data from Richards and Casey (1991, 1992).

ame Street movie for up to 100 seconds. This figure shows short latency changes associated with short looks, an increasingly sustained HR change for longer looks (40 seconds, "4"), and continued sustained HR change for the extremely long looks (up to 100 seconds, "5"). Complex stimuli extend the HR deceleration change that is found for relatively simple stimuli. As with the response to the brief stimulus presentation (Figure 25.1), adults show a dissimilar pattern of HR changes during sustained attention. At stimulus onset, HR decelerates only briefly and then returns to prestimulus level (e.g., Figure 25.1). Subsequently, adult

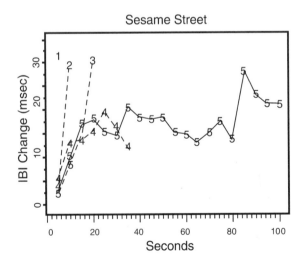

FIGURE 25.4. Increases in interbeat interval (IBI) length (HR deceleration) as a function of the duration of fixation on a *Sesame Street* movie for the same-age infants (Richards & Gibson, 1997). The lines represent IBI changes occurring for looks that lasted 5 seconds ("1"), 6 to 10 seconds ("2"), 11 to 20 seconds ("3"), 21 to 40 seconds ("4"), and greater than 40 seconds ("5").

TABLE 25.1. HR Changes in Attention Phases from 2 to 6 Months of Age and for High- and Low-RSA Infants, and Baseline HR and RSA in Full-Term Infants from 3 to 6 Months of Age

	HR changes in attention phases from 2 to 6 months			
	8 weeks	14 weeks	20 weeks	26 weeks
Stimulus orienting	−3.7	−4.2	−5.2	−4.7
Sustained attention	−6.9	−6.9	−8.5	−11.0
Attention termination	−1.7	−2.8	0.3	0.3
	HR changes in attention phases for high- and low-RSA infants			
	Low RSA		High RSA	
Stimulus orienting	−4.8		−5.2	
Sustained attention	−7.9		−11.5	
Attention termination	−1.3		−0.5	
	Baseline HR and RSA in full-term infants from 3 to 6 months of age			
	14 weeks		20 weeks	26 weeks
Baseline HR	152		148	142
Baseline RSA	0.78		0.86	0.92

Note. From Richards (1995). Copyright 1995 by Plenum Press. Adapted by permission.

beat-to-beat HR variability is suppressed during sustained attention in proportion to the intensity of the cognitive processing (Hansen, Johnsen, & Thayer, 2003; Mulder & Mulder, 1981, 1987; Redondo & Del Valle-Inclán, 1992).

We also have studied the development of sustained attention and heart rate changes in a number of studies. Table 25.1 contains the mean HR changes during attention compiled from a number of studies. There is an increase in the level of the HR deceleration in response to interesting stimuli from 8 weeks to 26 weeks of age. This increase is accompanied by decreasing levels of resting HR and increasing levels of respiratory sinus arrhythmia (RSA), both of which reflect developmental changes in cardiovascular control (Bar-Haim, Marshall, & Fox, 2000; Frick & Richards, 2001; Harper, Hoppenbrowers, Sterman, McGinty, & Hodgman, 1976; Harper et al., 1978; Katona, Frasz, & Egbert, 1980; Richards, 1985, 1987; Richards & Casey, 1991; Watanabe, Iwase, & Hara, 1973).

Several studies in my laboratory have investigated the characteristics of these attention phases, focusing primarily on the development of sustained attention. My colleagues and I have reviewed these studies in several places (Reynolds & Richards, in press; Richards, 1988a, 1995, 2001, 2002, in press; Richards & Anderson, in press; Richards & Casey, 1992; Richards & Hunter, 1998, 2002; Richards & Lansink, 1998). In the rest of the chapter I focus on two areas of work showing the role that sustained attention plays in infant behavior.

SUSTAINED ATTENTION AND PERIPHERAL STIMULUS RESPONSIVITY

The first area of work that I review are studies demonstrating that infants presented with stimuli in focal stimulus locations will be less likely to shift fixation to peripheral stimuli (see Richards & Lansink, 1998). The first interpretations of this work suggested that central stimuli restrict the infant's visual field. The most recent work has shown that it is only when central stimuli engage infant attention that peripheral stimulus localization is attenuated.

The first studies of infant's response to visual stimuli presented in the periphery were done to determine the extent of the visual field with "localization perimetry" (Aslin & Salapatek, 1975; de Schonen, McKenzie, Maury, & Bresson, 1978; Harris & MacFarlane, 1974; MacFarlane, Harris, & Barnes, 1976; Tronick, 1972; see review by Maurer & Lewis, 1998). Localization perimetry defined the infant's effective visual field as the eccentricity at which an infant will shift fixation from a center location to a peripheral location. A procedure used in these early studies was to attract the infant's fixation to the central visual field with a stimulus in the center of the visual field. If the stimulus in the center was left on, the "effective visual field" seemed to decrease. One- and 2-month old infants, for example, make directionally appropriate eye movements toward a peripheral stimulus at 40 degrees more than 50% of the time without a central stimulus, but less than 20% of the time in the focal central stimulus's presence (e.g., Aslin & Salapatek, 1975). The focal stimulus' presence increases the latency to make a directionally appropriate eye movement if the focal stimulus remains on long enough for the infant to make an eye movement to the peripheral stimulus (Aslin & Salapatek, 1975; Atkinson, Hood, Braddick, & Wattam-Bell, 1988; Atkinson, Hood, Wattam-Bell, & Braddick, 1992; Hood & Atkinson, 1993; Richards, 1987, 1997b).

The best interpretation of these results is that attention to the central stimulus is the cause of the attenuation of peripheral stimulus localization. Finlay and Ivinskis (1982, 1984, 1987) and Richards (1987, 1997b) have interpreted the longer latencies to shift fixation toward the peripheral stimulus as an indication of the attention level to the central stimulus. In this interpretation, the presence of a central stimulus engages attention. As long as attention to the center stimulus is occurring, there is decreased responsiveness to the peripheral stimulus. In contrast, at times infants will continue to look at the center stimulus in the absence of active attention engagement. In this case, localization percentage of a fixed-duration peripheral stimulus is likely (Finlay & Ivinskis, 1982, 1984, 1987; Hunter & Richards, 2003; Richards, 1997b; Richards & Hunter, 1997), or localization of a continuing stimulus occurs quickly (Richards, 1987). Focal stimulus attention results in a spatial selectivity for fixation, with fixation being directed primarily toward the location in which the attended stimulus occurs.

The role of attentiveness on infant peripheral stimulus localization is illustrated by a study of infants of 14, 20, and 26 weeks of age (Richards, 1997b). The infants were presented with interesting visual stimuli in the center. These stimuli were known to elicit HR changes such as those shown in Figure 25.3. A small peripheral stimulus was presented for 2 seconds. The dependent variable for the study was whether the infant looked toward the peripheral stimulus when it was presented and localization percentage (hits) was calculated. The peripheral stimuli were presented at delays from the onset of the center pattern defined by fixed time intervals (e.g., 2 seconds after stimulus onset, 4 seconds after stimulus onset) or by changes in HR (e.g., significant HR deceleration and return of HR to prestimulus level). Thus, the probability of localizing the peripheral stimulus when it was presented could be examined either by the fixed delays or by delays defined by HR changes.

Figure 25.5 shows some results from this study. This figure shows the percentage of localization of the peripheral stimulus as a function of the delays. The "Prestim" condition was the peripheral stimulus presented before the center stimulus—that is, the baseline level of localization for this peripheral stimulus (about 82%). The "Immed" delay was a presen-

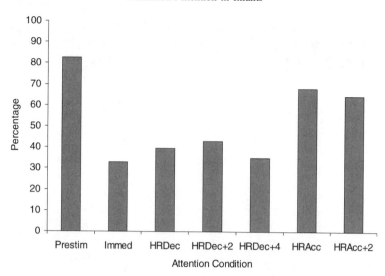

FIGURE 25.5. Percentages of peripheral stimulus localization as a function of the HR changes occurring during distractor presentations. No central stimulus was present during the prestimulus period (Prestim). The immediate period (Immed) refers to stimulus onset. Sustained attention coincides with all of the HR deceleration periods (HRDec), and attention termination is represented by HR accelerations (HRAcc).

tation of the peripheral stimulus about 100 msec following the central stimulus, the "HRDec" (HRDec, HRDec + 2 seconds, HRDec + 4 seconds) delays were defined by the occurrence of a deceleration in HR following by 0, 2, or 4 seconds, and the "HRReturn" (HRReturn, HRReturn + 2) delays were defined as occurring when HR returned to its prestimulus level. The immediate and HR deceleration conditions represent a period when sustained attention is directed toward the central pattern. These resulted in a very low percentage of localization. The return of HR to its prestimulus level represented a period of inattentiveness, even though the infants continued to look toward the central stimulus. When the peripheral stimulus was presented it was localized more frequently in this condition. When infants show by sustained lowered HR that sustained attention to the central stimulus is engaged, a peripheral stimulus presented for a fixed interval is missed (cf. Finlay & Ivinskis, 1984), or the latency to localize a continuing peripheral stimulus is very long (Richards, 1987). Unresponsiveness to the peripheral stimulus indicates an enhanced attention level for the central stimulus. In contrast, when infants show by lack of a significant HR response that attention is not engaged, then a stimulus presented for a fixed interval is more likely to be localized, or localized with a shorter latency than during sustained attention.

The effect of attention on peripheral stimulus localization is general across a wide range of testing situations, testing ages, and measures of attentiveness (Richards & Lansink, 1998). For example, young children age 6, 12, 18, or 24 months when engaged in viewing television programs will be less likely to look away toward peripheral events when showing HR or behavioral signs of attentiveness (Richards & Turner, 2001). This is true also for older-age children (e.g., 3 to 5 years) when watching television programs (Anderson, Choi, & Lorch, 1987; Lorch & Castle, 1997). Infants playing with small toys during periods showing facial expressions consistent with focused attention will continue to look toward and play with the toys, compared to periods when they do not show attentiveness (Doolittle

& Ruff, 1998; Lansink & Richards, 1997; Oakes & Tellinghuisen, 1994; Ruff & Capozzoli, 2003; Ruff, Capozzoli, & Saltarelli, 1996; Tellinghuisen & Oakes, 1997). A similar pattern of indistractibility during engaged toy play is found in older children (3 and 5 years; Choi & Anderson, 1991).

SUSTAINED ATTENTION AND OTHER COGNITIVE PROCESSES

The second area of work that is reviewed are studies demonstrating that infant recognition memory is enhanced during sustained attention (see Reynolds & Richards, in press; Richards, 2001, 2002). This work is part of a larger context of work that shows that infant sustained attention affects a wide variety of cognitive processes (e.g., peripheral stimulus responsivity, eye movement control, and extended television viewing). A typical procedure for measuring infant recognition memory is the familiarization/paired-comparison test procedure. This procedure presents an interesting visual stimulus for several seconds until the infant is familiar with it. Following familiarization, the infant is presented with the exposed stimulus and a novel stimulus not previously seen. A novelty preference indicates recognition of the familiar stimulus.

Several studies have shown the role that sustained attention plays in this procedure. Richards (1997a; also see Frick & Richards, 2001) presented infants between 3 and 6 months of age with a *Sesame Street* video that elicited the HR-defined attention phases (Figure 25.3). The infants were exposed to the familiarization stimulus for only 5 seconds during stimulus orienting, sustained attention, and attention termination, or 5 seconds following attention termination. Following the exposure, a paired-comparison test procedure was done. Trials on which the familiarization stimulus was presented during sustained attention resulted in a significant novelty preference for 20- and 26-week-old infants. Trials on which the familiar stimulus was presented 5 seconds after attention termination and HR had significantly decelerated again (reengaged sustained attention) also resulted in a significant novelty preference. Novelty preference on these two trials types was at similar levels to a 20-second accumulated fixation familiarization trial, a procedure commonly used in research studies using the paired-comparison method. The younger infants, and all infants presented with the familiar stimulus during stimulus orienting or attention termination, did not show the novelty preference. Thus, familiarization during sustained attention results in greater levels of recognition memory than during inattentiveness. The results for the different ages in this procedure show the increasing level of sustained attention across this age range. Other studies have shown similar roles that sustained attention plays in the familiarization and test phases of this infant recognition memory procedure (Colombo, Richman, Shaddy, Greenhoot, & Maikranz, 2001; Frick & Richards, 2001; Maikranz, Colombo, Richman, & Frick, 2000; Richards & Casey, 1990).

Another procedure that has been used to show the effect of sustained attention on recognition memory is a modified oddball procedure and the measurement of scalp-recorded event-related potentials (ERPs). The "oddball" procedure has been used in adults to measure response to low-probability stimuli, particularly the P300 (P3). This procedure presents a standard stimulus repeatedly and frequently and occasionally presents an "oddball" stimulus. The P300 amplitude is larger to the oddball than to the standard stimulus. This procedure was first tested in infants by Courchesne (1977, 1978). He found a large negative ERP component occurring about 400–800 msec after stimulus onset located primarily in the frontal and central electroencephalographic (EEG) leads, labeled the "Nc" (Negative central). It is plausible that the Nc represents a general orienting of attention and the late slow waves represent processes akin to recognition memory (see review by Nelson & Monk, 2001).

The association between sustained attention and the Nc has been addressed in two recent studies (Reynolds & Richards, 2003; Richards, 2003) with 4½-, 6-, and 7½-month-old infants. The oddball procedure was modified in the following manner. During the brief stimulus presentations, a *Sesame Street* stimulus was used to elicit the HR-defined attention phases (as in Frick & Richards, 2001; Richards, 1997a). The presentation of the test stimuli were done at the very beginning of the trial (stimulus orienting), when HR had decelerated below its prestimulus level (sustained attention), or when the infant was inattentive (attention termination, or after attention termination). There were two interesting findings related to the attention phases (Richards, 2003). First, the Nc amplitude was much larger during sustained attention and stimulus orienting than during inattentiveness. Second, the Nc amplitude increased over the three testing ages, but this change was confined to ERP amplitude measured during sustained attention. Figure 25.6 shows the ERP changes during attention separately for the infants age 4½, 6, or 7 months. The ERP changes (left panels, Fz and Cz) showed an increasing level of the negative ERP response over the three testing ages at about 500–600 msec following stimulus onset (i.e., the Nc). The topographical maps show the Nc at the maximal response. A clear increase occurred over the three testing ages in the magnitude and extent of the Nc. These age differences suggest that the developmental changes in sustained attention known to occur over this age are shown in the Nc and suggest that the Nc is predominantly an indicator of the cortical processes involved in stimulus orienting and arousal. The changes in the Nc over these testing ages reflects developmental changes in sustained attention rather than changes in recognition memory or associated memory processes.

The most recent work we are doing (Reynolds & Richards, 2003) uses high-density (124 channel) EEG recordings. This study involves the estimation of cortical sources of the ERP data with equivalent current dipole analysis. Preliminary findings indicate that the cor-

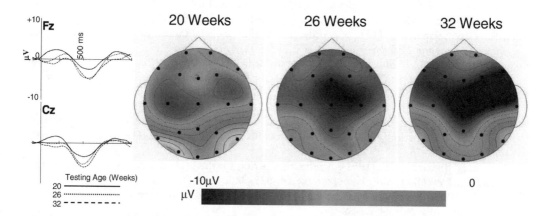

FIGURE 25.6. Development of the Nc component during attention. The ERP recording from 100 msec prior to stimulus onset through 1 second following stimulus onset is shown for the Fz and Cz electrodes for attentive (top figures) and inattentive (bottom figures) periods, separately for the three testing ages. The topographical maps represent an 80-msec average of the ERP for the Nc component at the maximum point of the ERP response. From Richards (2003). Copyright 2003 by Blackwell. Reprinted by permission.

tical source of the Nc component is in areas of prefrontal cortex including the anterior cingulate. This implies that the prefrontal cortex may mediate initial stimulus responsivity in young infants. This finding is consistent with some recent work with adults (Critchley et al., 2003). This work showed that changes in HR variability in adults during cognitive tasks involving controlled processing were closely associated with functional magnetic resonance imaging activity located in the anterior cingulate cortex. A decrease in HR variability is the primary indicator of sustained attention in adult participants (Hansen et al., 2003; Mulder & Mulder, 1981, 1987; Redondo & del Valle-Inclán, 1992).

SUMMARY AND CONCLUSION

The chapter has reviewed work showing that sustained attention may be measured in young infants with HR, that sustained attention develops in the first few months of infancy, and that several cognitive processes in young infants are enhanced by sustained attention. The intensity aspect of attention represents the enhancement of cognitive processing that occurs when alertness and arousal are functioning. Sustained attention in young infants represents this type of arousal and thus enhances processes selected by attention resulting in improvements in infant cognitive processing.

ACKNOWLEDGMENT

This research was supported by Grant No. R01-HD18942 from the National Institute of Child Health and Human Development.

REFERENCES

Anderson, D. R., Choi, H. P., & Lorch, E. (1987). Attentional inertia reduces distractibility during young children's television viewing. *Child Development, 58,* 798–806.

Aslin, R. N., & Salapatek, P. (1975). Saccadic localization of visual targets by the very young human infant. *Perception and Psychophysics, 17,* 293–302.

Atkinson, J., Hood, B., Braddick, O. J., & Wattam-Bell, J. (1988). Infants' control of fixation shifts with single and competing targets: Mechanisms for shifting attention. *Perception, 17,* 367–368.

Atkinson, J., Hood, B., Wattam-Bell, J., & Braddick, O. J. (1992). Changes in infants' ability to switch visual attention in the first three months of life. *Perception, 21,* 643–653.

Bar-Haim, Y., Marshall, P. J., & Fox, N. A. (2000). Developmental changes in heart period and high-frequency heart period variability from 4 months to 4 years of age. *Developmental Psychobiology, 37,* 44–56.

Casey, B. J., & Richards, J. E. (1991). A refractory period for the heart rate response in infant visual attention. *Developmental Psychobiology, 24,* 327–340.

Chase, H. H. (1965). *Habituation of an acceleratory cardiac response in neonates.* Unpublished master's thesis, University of Wisconsin.

Choi, H. P., & Anderson, D. R. (1991). A temporal analysis of free toy play and distractibility in young children. *Journal of Experimental Child Psychology, 52,* 41–69.

Colombo, J., Richman, W. A., Shaddy, D. J., Greenhoot, A. F., & Maikranz, J. M. (2001). Heart rate-defend phases of attention, look duration, and infant performance in the paired-comparison paradigm. *Child Development, 72,* 1605–1616.

Courchesne, E. (1977). Event-related brain potentials: Comparison between children and adults. *Science, 197,* 589–592.

Courchesne, E. (1978). Neurophysiological correlates of cognitive development: Changes in long-latency event-related potentials from childhood to adulthood. *Electroencephalography and Clinical Neurophysiology, 45,* 468–482.

Critchley, H. D., Mathias, C. J., Josephs, O., O'Doherty, J., Sanini, S., Dewar, B., et al. (2003). Human cingulate cortex and autonomic control: Converging neuroimaging and clinical evidence. *Brain, 126,* 2139–2152.

Davis, C. M., Crowell, D. H., & Chun, B. J. (1965). Monophasic heart rate accelerations in human infants to peripheral stimulation. *American Psychologist, 20,* 478.

de Schonen, S., McKenzie, B., Maury, L., & Bresson, F. (1978). Central and peripheral object distances as determinants of the effective visual field in early infancy. *Perception, 7,* 499–506.

Doolittle, E. J., & Ruff, H. A. (1998). Distractibility during infants' examining and repetitive rhythmic activity. *Developmental Psychobiology, 32,* 275–283.

Finlay, D., & Ivinskis, A. (1982). Cardiac and visual responses to stimuli presented both foveally and peripherally as a function of speed of moving stimuli. *Developmental Psychology, 18,* 692–698.

Finlay, D., & Ivinskis, A. (1984). Cardiac and visual responses to moving stimuli presented either successively or simultaneously to the central and peripheral visual fields in 4-month-old infants. *Developmental Psychology, 20,* 29–36.

Finlay, D., & Ivinskis, A. (1987). Cardiac change responses and attentional mechanisms in infants. In B. E. McKenzie & R. H. Day (Eds.), *Perceptual development in early infancy* (pp. 45–63). Hillsdale, NJ: Erlbaum.

Frick, J. E., & Richards, J. E. (2001). Individual differences in recogntion of briefly presented stimuli. *Infancy, 2,* 331–352.

Graham, F. K. (1979). Distinguishing among orienting, defense, and startle reflexes. In H. D. Kimmel, E. H. van Olst, & J. F. Orlebeke (Eds.), *The orienting reflex in humans* (pp. 137–167). Hillsdale, NJ: Erlbaum.

Graham, F. K., Anthony, B. J., & Ziegler, B. L. (1983). The orienting response and developmental processes. In D. Siddle (Ed.), *Orienting and habituation: Perspectives in human research* (pp. 371–430). Sussex, UK: Wiley.

Graham, F. K., Berg, K. M., Berg, W. K., Jackson, J. C., Hatton, H. M., & Kantowitz, S. R. (1970). Cardiac orienting response as a function of age. *Psychonomic Science, 19,* 363–365.

Graham, F. K., & Clifton, R. K. (1966). Heart-rate change as a component of the orienting response. *Psychological Bulletin, 65,* 305–320.

Graham, F. K., & Jackson, J. C. (1970). Arousal systems and infant heart rate responses. In H. W. Reese & L. P. Lipsitt (Eds.), *Advances in child development and behavior* (Vol. 5, pp. 59–17). New York: Academic Press.

Hansen, A. L., Johnsen, B. H., & Thayer, J. F. (2003). Vagal influence on working memory and attention. *International Journal of Psychophysiology, 48,* 263–274.

Harper, R. M., Hoppenbrouwers, T., Sterman, M. B., McGinty, D. J., & Hodgman, J. (1976). Polygraphic studies of normal infants during the first six months of life. I. Heart rate and variability as a function of state. *Pediatric Research, 10,* 945–961.

Harper, R. M., Walter, D. O., Leake, B., Hoffman, H. J., Sieck, G. C., Sterman, M. B., et al. (1978). Development of sinus arrhythmia during sleeping and waking states in normal infants. *Sleep, 1,* 33–48.

Harris, P., & MacFarlane, A. (1974). The growth of the effective visual field from birth to seven weeks. *Journal of Experimental Child Psychology, 18,* 340–348.

Hood, B. M., & Atkinson, J. (1993). Disengaging visual attention in the infant and adult. *Infant Behavior and Development, 16,* 405–422.

Hunter, S. K., & Richards, J. E. (2003). Peripheral stimulus localization by 5- to 14-week-old infants during phases of attention. *Infancy, 4,* 1–25.

Katona, P. G. Frasz, A., & Egbert, J. R. (1980). Maturation of cardiac control in full-term and preterm infants during sleep. *Early Human Development, 4,* 145–159.

Keen, R. E., Chase, H. H., & Graham, F. K. (1965). Twenty-four hour retention by neonates of an habituated heart rate response. *Psychonomic Science, 2,* 265–266.

Lansink, J. M., & Richards, J. E. (1997). Heart rate and behavioral measures of attention in 6-, 9-, and 12-month-old infants during object exploration. *Child Development, 68,* 610–620.

Lorch, E. P., & Castle, V. J. (1997). Preschool children's attention to television: Visual attention and probe response times. *Journal of Experimental Child Psychology, 66,* 111–127.

MacFarlane, A., Harris, P., & Barnes, I. (1976). Central and peripheral vision in early infancy. *Journal of Experimental Child Psychology, 21,* 532–538.

Maikranz, J. M., Colombo, J., Richman, W. A., & Frick, J. E. (2000). Autonomic correlates of individual differences in sensitization and look duration during infancy. *Infant Behavior and Development, 23,* 137–151.

Maurer, D., & Lewis, T. L. (1998). Overt orienting toward peripheral stimuli: Normal development and underlying mechanisms. In J. E. Richards (Ed.), *Cognitive neuroscience of attention: A developmental perspective* (pp. 51–102). Hillsdale, NJ: Erlbaum.

McKinney, B., & Richards, J. E. (2004). *Developmental changes in the main sequence using interesting visual stimuli.* Manuscript submitted for publication.

Mulder, G., & Mulder, L. J. M. (1981). Information processing and cardiovascular control. *Psychophysiology, 18,* 392–402.

Mulder, L. J. M., & Mulder, G. (1987). Cardiovascular reactivity and mental workload. In O. Rompelman & R. I. Kitney (Eds.), *The beat-by-beat investigation of cardiovascular function* (pp. 216–253). Oxford, UK: Oxford University Press.

Nelson, C. A., & Monk, C. S. (2001). The use of event-related potentials in the study of cognitive development. In C. A. Nelson & M. Luciana (Eds.), *Handbook of developmental cognitive neuroscience* (pp. 125–136). Cambridge, MA: MIT Press.

Oakes, L. M., & Tellinghuisen, D. J. (1994). Examining in infancy: Does it reflect active processing? *Developmental Psychology, 30,* 748–756.

Porges, S. W. (1976). Peripheral and neurochemical parallels of psychopathology: A psychophysiological model relating autonomic imbalance in hyperactivity, psychopathology, and autism. In H. Reese (Ed.), *Advances in child development and behavior* (Vol. 11, pp. 35–65). New York: Academic Press.

Porges, S. W. (1980). Individual differences in attention: A possible physiological substrate. In *Advances in special education* (Vol. 2, pp. 111–134). Greenwich, CT: JAI Press.

Redondo, M., & del Valle-Inclán, F. (1992). Decrements in heart rate variability during memory search. *International Journal of Psychophysiology, 13,* 29–35.

Reynolds, G. D., & Richards, J. E. (2003). *Infant attention and cortical sources of ERP for recognition of briefly presented visual stimuli.* Poster presented at the biennial meeting of the Society for Research in Child Development, Tampa, FL.

Reynolds, G. D., & Richards, J. E. (in press). Infant heart rate: A developmental psychophysiological perspective. In L. A. Schmidt & S. J. Segalowitz (Eds.), *Developmental psychophysiology.* Cambridge, UK: Cambridge University Press.

Richards, J. E. (1985). The development of sustained attention in infants from 14 to 26 weeks of age. *Psychophysiology, 22,* 409–416.

Richards, J. E. (1987). Infant visual sustained attention and respiratory sinus arrhythmia. *Child Development, 58,* 488–496.

Richards, J. E. (1988a). Heart rate changes and heart rate rhythms, and infant visual sustained attention. In P. K. Ackles, J. R. Jennings, & M. G. H. Coles (Eds.), *Advances in psychophysiology* (Vol. 3, pp. 189–221). Greenwich, CT: JAI Press.

Richards, J. E. (1988b). Heart rate offset responses to visual stimuli in infants from 14 to 26 weeks of age. *Psychophysiology, 25,* 278–291.

Richards, J. E. (1995). Infant cognitive psychophysiology: Normal development and implications for abnormal developmental outcomes. In T. H. Ollendick & R. J. Prinz (Eds.), *Advances in clinical child psychology* (Vol. 17, pp. 77–107). New York: Plenum Press.

Richards, J. E. (1997a). Effects of attention on infants' preference for briefly exposed visual stimuli in the paired-comparison recognition-memory paradigm. *Developmental Psychology, 33,* 22–31.

Richards, J. E. (1997b). Peripheral stimulus localization by infants: Attention, age and individual differences in heart rate variability. *Journal of Experimental Psychology: Human Perception and Performance, 23,* 667–680.

Richards, J. E. (1998). Development of selective attention in young infants. *Developmental Science, 1,* 45–51.

Richards, J. E. (2000). Development of multimodal attention in young infants: Modification of the startle reflex by attention. *Psychophysiology, 37,* 65–75.

Richards, J. E. (2001). Attention in young infants: A developmental psychophysiological perspective. In C. A. Nelson & M. Luciana (Eds.), *Handbook of developmental cognitive neuroscience* (pp. 321–338). Cambridge, MA: MIT Press.

Richards, J. E. (2002). Development of attentional systems. In M. De Haan & M. H. Johnson (Eds.), *The cognitive neuroscience of development.* East Sussex, UK: Psychology Press

Richards, J. E. (2003). Attention affects the recognition of briefly presented visual stimuli in infants: An ERP study. *Developmental Science, 6,* 312–328.

Richards, J. E. (in press). Development of covert orienting in young infants. In L. Itti, G. Rees, & J. Tsotsos (Eds.), *Neurobiology of attention.* New York: Academic Press/Elsevier.

Richards, J. E., & Anderson, D. R. (in press). Attentional inertia in children's extended looking at television. *Advances in child development and behavior* (Vol. 32).

Richards, J. E., & Casey, B. J. (1990). Infant visual recognition memory performance as a function of heart rate defined phases of attention. *Infant Behavior and Development, 13,* 585.

Richards, J. E., & Casey, B. J. (1991). Heart rate variability during attention phases in young infants. *Psychophysiology, 28,* 43–53.

Richards, J. E., & Casey, B. J. (1992). Development of sustained visual attention in the human infant. In B. A. Campbell, H. Hayne, & R. Richardson (Eds.), *Attention and information processing in infants and adults: Perspectives from human and animal research* (pp. 30–60). Hillsdale, NJ: Erlbaum.

Richards, J. E., & Cronise, K. (2000). Extended visual fixation in the early preschool years: look duration, heart rate changes, and attentional inertia. *Child Development, 71,* 602–620.

Richards, J. E., & Gibson, T. L. (1997). Extended visual fixation in young infants: Look distributions, heart rate changes, and attention. *Child Development, 68,* 1041–1056.

Richards, J. E., & Holley, F. B. (1999). Infant attention and the development of smooth pursuit tracking. *Developmental Psychology, 35,* 856–867.

Richards, J. E., & Hunter, S. K. (1997). Peripheral stimulus localization by infants with eye and head movements during visual attention. *Vision Research, 37,* 3021–3035

Richards, J. E., & Hunter, S. K. (1998). Attention and eye movement in young infants: Neural control and development. In J. E. Richards (Ed.), *Cognitive neuroscience of attention: A developmental perspective* (pp. 131–162). Hillsdale, NJ: Erlbaum.

Richards, J. E., & Hunter, S. K. (2002). Testing neural models of the development of infant visual attention. *Developmental Psychobiology, 40,* 226–236.

Richards, J. E., & Lansink, J. M. (1998). Distractibility during visual fixation in young infants: The selectivity of attention. In C. Rovee-Collier (Ed.), *Advances in infancy research* (Vol. 13, pp. 407–444). Stamford, CT: Ablex.

Richards, J. E., & Turner, E. D. (2001). Distractibility during extended viewing of television in the early preschool years. *Child Development, 72,* 963–972.

Ruff, H. A. (1986). Components of attention during infants' manipulative exploration. *Child Development, 57,* 105–114.

Ruff, H. A., & Capozzoli, M. C. (2003). Development of attention and distractibility in the first 4 years of life. *Developmental Psychology, 39,* 877–890.

Ruff, H. A., Capozzoli, M., & Saltarelli, L. M. (1996). Focused visual attention and distractibility in 10-month old infants. *Infant Behavior and Development, 19,* 281–293.

Ruff, H. A., & Rothbart, M. K. (1997). *Attention in early development.* New York: Oxford University Press.

Sokolov, E. N. (1963). *Perception and the conditioned reflex.* New York: Macmillan.

Tellinghuisen, D. J., & Oakes, L. M. (1997). Distractibility in infancy: The effects of distractor characteristics and type of attention. *Journal of Experimental Child Psychology, 64,* 232– 254.

Tronick, E. (1972). Stimulus control and growth of the infants' effective visual field. *Perception and Psychophysics, 11,* 373–376.

van der Veen, F. M., Lange, J. J., van der Molen, M. W., Mulder, G., & Mulder, L. J. M. (2000). Event-related brain potential and heart rate manifestations of visual selective attention. *Psychophysiology, 37,* 677–682.

Watanabe, K., Iwase, K., & Hara, K. (1973). Heart rate variability during sleep and wakefulness in low-birthweight infants. *Biology of the Neonate, 22,* 87–98.

26

Attention, Emotion, and the Development of Psychopathology

Seth D. Pollak and Stephanie Tolley-Schell

A promising venue for understanding the association between early emotional experience and the development of behavioral problems may lie in the developmental plasticity of attentional and perceptual systems. Neurodevelopmental changes in attentional abilities clearly influence the adaptiveness and success of children's behavioral regulation (Pollak, 2004; Pollak, Cicchetti, & Klorman, 1998; Posner & Rothbart, 2000; Ruff & Rothbart, 1996). As the anatomy and circuitry of attentional networks contributing to orienting and disengagement matures (Richards, Chapter 25, and Ridderenkof, van den Wildenberg, Wijnen, & Burle, Chapter 27, this volume), children are provided with increasingly elaborate and flexible mechanisms for self-regulation. However, appearance of higher-level regulation abilities may depend on a child first acquiring some strategic control of attention, such as looking away from distressing stimuli and sustaining attention in pleasurable situations such as play (Johnson, Posner, & Rothbart, 1991; Rothbart, Ziaie, & O'Boyle, 1992).

The development of abused children provides a compelling clue about where to begin looking for answers to questions about how early experience can influence aspects of brain development associated with regulatory processes. The maltreatment of children is a horrific psychosocial phenomenon in which young infants and children do not receive the protection, care, nurturance, and interactions that are typical of how humans (and many other species) care for their young. More than 2 million children are victims of child maltreatment in the United States each year (U.S. Department of Health and Human Services, 2000). Maltreated children often evince unusual patterns in their abilities to recognize, express, and regulate emotional states (Camras et al., 1990; Camras, Sachs-Alter, & Ribordy, 1996; Pollak, Cichetti, Hornung, & Reed, 2000). Physically abused children, in particular, often display both withdrawal and aggression (Hoffman-Plotkin & Twentyman, 1984; Jacobson & Straker, 1982; Rogosch, Cicchetti, & Aber, 1995), readily assimilate and remember cues related to aggression (Pollak & Tolley-Schell, 2003; Rieder & Cicchetti, 1989), and tend to attribute hostility to others (Weiss, Dodge, Bates, & Pettit, 1992). As might be expected, such constellations of behaviors often lead to poorly regulated and situationally inappropriate affect and interpersonal difficulties for these children (Klimes-Dougan & Kistner, 1990; Main & George, 1985; Rogosch et al., 1995). To date, the precise mechanisms linking the experience of maltreatment with the development of psychopathology are infrequently examined and largely unknown. Attentional processes appear to play a central role in the ontogenesis of emotional difficulties in these children.

CHILD MALTREATMENT AS A MODEL
OF DEVELOPMENTAL PLASTICITY

In this chapter, we summarize a theoretical framework and empirical evidence supporting the idea that exposure to maltreating environments affects children's perceptual and attentional processing of emotional information. These attentional effects may account for the interpersonal difficulties observed in abused children. To account for such phenomena, we explore the possibility of a general, biologically prepared, perceptual mechanism that becomes tuned to combinations of signals, which, through experience, combine to form affective neural circuitry and categories. Such a learning mechanism might include the ability to parse sensory inputs into meaningful units and to track the regularity, predictiveness, and temporal synchrony of emotional information. We suspect that if such a mechanism exists, it need not be specialized for emotion. Indeed, observations of similar learning mechanisms have been proposed for the emergence of many cognitive abilities such as cross-modal matching, phonetic discrimination, and word segmentation (Kuhl, 1987; Kuhl & Meltzoff, 1982; Saffran, Aslin, & Newport, 1996).

If learning about emotional signals is biologically prepared, how might a history of abusive parenting affect the developmental trajectory of an individual child? Developmental affective learning problems may arise because the emotional signals the maltreated child receives can be disproportionately complicated, inconsistent, poorly conveyed, distressing, limited, threatening, and/or excessive. In other words, there are two possible learning problems. On one view, the nature of the signaling the child receives may be too poor for the child to adequately distill the nuances and underlying structure of emotional discourse. Alternatively, the emotional stimuli that the child receives may be far too powerful or salient, perhaps generating affective responses that undermine effective learning. In such a case, emotion processing differences may arise because abused children learn, first and foremost, to orient and track signs of threat. Such an outcome would reflect both an adaptive ability to effectively pair a signal with a meaningful outcome (Rescorla, 1966), as well as a maladaptive parameter setting in which sensory thresholds for threat detection become too low for healthy social functioning. Future research is needed to examine each of these hypotheses. But both positions are consistent with the idea that in abusive environments, signals of anger are a critical feature of the environment that disproportionately recruits children's attentional resources.

Our view is that the continuing influence of childhood affective experiences across developmental epochs may be understood in terms of the general immaturity and neuroplasticity of sensory and perceptual systems early in development (Bjorklund, 1997; Pollak et al., 1998). The relative immaturity and limited capacity of processing resources available to the young child imposes a maturational limitation on how much stimuli the child can take in and understand. But this same limitation, combined with biological preparedness to track certain associations between stimuli and outcomes, may well help the child to begin to learn about his or her social environment. In short, limited capacity would dictate that some aspects of the environment are privileged and thus filtered or selected over others to facilitate rapid learning. This leaves the developmental organization of emotion systems contingent upon features of input that are most learnable, such as signals that are highly salient, or frequent, or highly predictable or regular. For the abused child, what is salient, frequent, or stochastic in the environment may well be species atypical or culturally aberrant—but these features of the environment are what the child is exposed to and learning from, constituting experience-dependent plasticity.

MALTREATED CHILDREN'S ATTENTION TO EMOTIONAL CUES

The ability to shift attention toward or away from different aspects of the environment is adaptive, allowing the individual to control an emotional response (as when we avert our gaze from something that is disgusting or distract ourselves with mundane or pleasant tasks to avoid worrying about impending concerns). Yet such attentional regulation may at times be in conflict with affective systems, whose adaptive value resides precisely in their drawing attention to salient, unexpected, or potentially threatening aspects of the environment. These conflicting motivations result in reflexive affective systems serving adaptive ends by alerting us to potential danger, while voluntary attentional systems allow us to regulate our encounters with such stimuli. One possibility is that rather than using their attentional resources to attenuate emotional reactivity, physically abused children overly attend to threatening cues, perhaps at the expense of other contextually relevant information (Dodge, Pettit, Bates, & Valente, 1995; Pollak & Tolley-Schell, 2003). Such a proposal is consistent with clinical studies of anxiety, phobia, and trauma patients, suggesting that prior learning about the affective significance of stimuli can strongly influence aspects of attentional orienting (McNally, 1998; Mogg & Bradley, 1998). In this manner, children's prior experience affects how they undertake subsequent learning.

Our starting point for testing and refining our hypothesis has been the phenomenon of emotion recognition: How do signals received from the environment acquire the salience that makes them "emotional," and how do children process such salient cues? Here, we consider both the anterior mechanisms involved in regulating attention and also earlier developing posterior attentional systems which subserve orienting, arousal, and alerting functions.

In one of our earliest studies, we found that physically abused children perceived angry faces as highly salient relative to other emotions (Pollak et al., 2000). A significant aspect of this study was that we were able to contrast children with different types of maltreatment experience. Physically abused children had experienced abuse by commission—they were directly injured by a parent. In contrast, neglected children experienced abuse by omission— lack of care and responsiveness from parents. Neglected children, who purportedly received less parental support and experience in learning about communicative signals, had difficulty differentiating facial expressions of emotion. Rather than showing global deficits in performance, physically abused children performed well, especially when differentiating angry facial expressions. These data suggest that specific kinds of emotional experiences, rather than simply the presence of stress or maltreatment, differentially affect children's emotional functioning (Pollak et al., 2000).

Because the ability to allocate attention to emotional cues in the environment is an important feature of adaptive self-regulation (Posner & Rothbart, 2000), we have used psychophysiological techniques to measure children's selective allocation of attention to emotional signals. Event-related potentials (ERPs) provide an index of central nervous system functioning thought to reflect the underlying neural processing of discrete stimuli, especially those involved in attentional resource allocation (Coles & Rugg, 1995; Kramer & Spinks, 1991; Polich & Kok, 1995). Our ERP studies reveal that whereas nonmaltreated children and adults responded uniformly when attending to happy, fearful, and angry faces, physically abused children displayed relative increases in brain electrical activity only when actively searching for angry faces. Abused children performed identically to controls when attending to other emotional expressions, suggesting that attentional processes directed toward detecting angry cues distinguish maltreated children's emotion processing (Pollak, Cicchetti, Klorman, & Brumaghim, 1997; Pollak, Klorman, Thatcher, & Cicchetti, 2001).

It is adaptive for salient stimuli such as emotions to elicit attention. In fact, a bias to select emotionally arousing stimuli for attention over neutral stimuli is normal early in development, even when such information is task irrelevant (Vasey & MacLeod, 2001). But for children to develop successful regulatory strategies, it is critical for them to achieve some flexibility or control over attentional processes. We consider two ways in which an emotionally aberrant environment can undermine this goal. One possibility is that early experiences of abuse may affect developing perceptual systems in part by shaping the sensory threshold that anger-related stimuli must pass to recruit attentional focus. This would make thresholds so low that any indication of threat initiates a host of cascading defensive systems that are not situationally appropriate. A second possibility is that once perceived, abused children are less able to use attentional control when signals of interpersonal threat have been engaged. In this way, affect generated by certain environmental cues may undermine subsequent cognitive processes. Of course, these two possibilities are not mutually exclusive.

To test the sensory-threshold hypothesis, we reasoned that if abused children are overattending to anger, we might expect to observe differences in how these children perceive angry cues from the environment as compared to other emotional cues. Therefore, we examined abused children's perception of anger. Categorical perception occurs when perceptual mechanisms enhance differences between categories at the expense of perception of incremental changes within a category. Perceiving in terms of categories is adaptive in that it allows an observer to efficiently assess changes between categories that are environmentally important (e.g., to see that a traffic light has changed from green to yellow) at the cost of noticing subtle changes in stimuli that are not important (e.g., such as variations in shades of greens or yellows across individual traffic lights). Children performed a facial discrimination task that required them to distinguish faces that had been morphed to produce a continuum on which each face differed by 20% in signal intensity. To create continua of facial expressions of affect, we used a two-dimensional morphing system to generate stimuli that spanned four emotional categories– happiness, anger, fear, and sadness (Figure 26.1). We found that the experience of abuse was associated with a change in children's perceptual preferences and also altered the discriminative abilities that influence how children categorize angry facial expressions (Pollak & Kistler, 2002). Yet, abused children performed identically to controls when discriminating emotions other than anger. These findings suggest that whatever perceptual capacities infants possess when they enter the world, they need to adjust or tune these mechanisms to process specific, salient aspects of their environments. Thus affective experiences appear to influence perceptual representations of basic emotions.

To further test the hypothesis that children exposed to high levels of threat are especially sensitive to visual cues of anger, we examined whether these children can readily relate visual cues to representations of emotions. The examination of this issue required a technique that could capture the dynamics of emotion recognition, including the sequen-

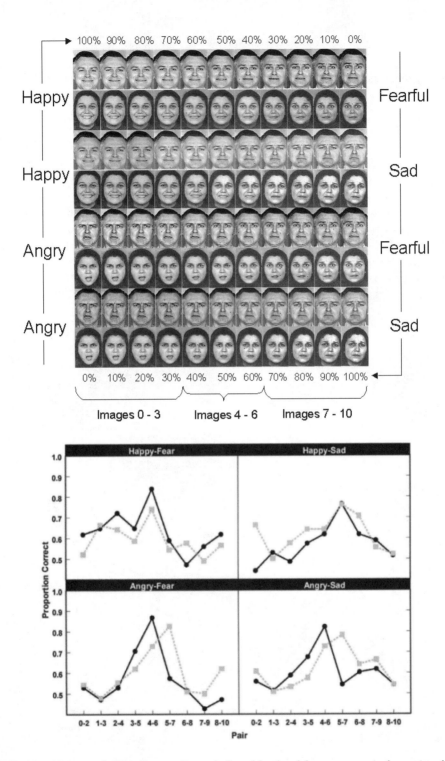

FIGURE 26.1. *Top panel:* Stimuli were "morphs" or blends of four prototypical emotional expressions. Facial images differed by 10% in pixel intensities. *Bottom panel:* Children's discrimination of emotional expressions as proportion correct for sequential pairs of faces along each continuum. Chance performance (0.5) indicates children had difficulty discriminating between stimuli. Control children (solid line) showed best discrimination of emotions at the center of the continua. Perceptual category boundaries for abused children (dashed line) differed from controls only in continua that involved angry facial expressions. From Pollak and Kistler (2002). Copyright 2002 by the National Academy of Sciences USA. Reprinted by permission.

tial and content-based processes of feature detection involved in emotion recognition. To do so, we presented affective stimuli to children incrementally as sequences of emotional expressions that were initially degraded and asked participants to report what emotion they thought they were seeing (Figure 26.2). As predicted, physically abused children needed less sensory input than did controls to accurately identify facial displays of anger (Pollak & Sinha, 2002).

Our second hypothesis is that the acquired salience of anger- or threat-related signals undermines abused children's attentional control. This position is consistent with data suggesting that problems disengaging from sensory cues are a function of the depth of processing or strength of engagement of that cue (Derryberry & Reed, 2002; Fox, Russo, & Dutton, 2002; Laberge, 1995). Using an adaptation of Posner, Snyder, and Davidson's (1980) spatial selective attention paradigm, we found that abused children demonstrated relative increases in brain electrical activity only when they were required to disengage their attention from angry faces, reflecting increased allocation of cognitive resources (Figure

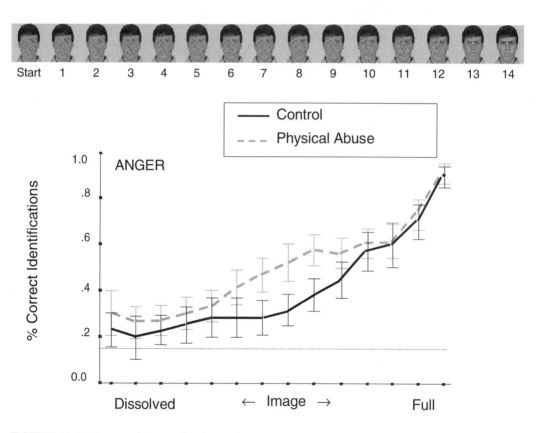

FIGURE 26.2. *Top panel:* Example of a random image structure evolution sequence. Children began each trial viewing an unstructured field that gradually became a clear depiction of a facial expression. *Bottom panel:* Mean identification rates for angry facial expressions as a function of amount of visual information (95% confidence intervals are plotted around each mean). Chance performance is indicated by the horizontal line. Note that abused children accurately recognize anger based upon less perceptual information. From Pollak and Sinha (2002). Copyright 2002 by the American Psychological Association. Reprinted by permission.

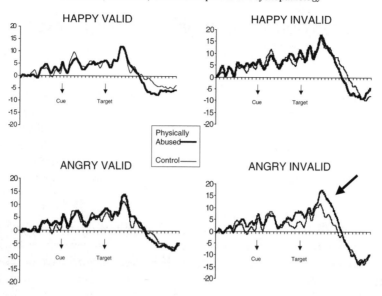

FIGURE 26.3. Grand average waveforms derived from the parietal (Pz) electrode site show that differences between abused and control children emerge only when children are required to disengage attention from angry faces. Topographic maps indicate the magnitude of voltage differences as a function of emotion and validity, reflecting the average event-related potentials (ERPs) of the physically abused minus the average ERP of the control children. From Pollak and Tolley-Schell (2003). Copyright 2003 by the American Psychological Association. Reprinted by permission.

26.3; Pollak & Tolley-Schell, 2003). Indeed, abused children's brain electrical activity did not differ from controls when subjects needed to engage a valid cue, only when they needed to disengage from an invalid cue. Importantly, abused and nonmaltreated children did not differ in other types of trials or in response to happy faces, consistent with the hypothesis that physically abused children have a specific problem involving flexible processing of anger rather than general information-processing deficits. One inconsistency between the physiological and behavioral data, however, was that physically abused children oriented more rapidly than did controls to angry faces (e.g., they showed decreased response times on valid angry trials, with no decrement in accuracy).

To examine the possibility that a difference in initial attentional engagement of angry faces could also contribute to the disengagement problems we observed in abused children, we conducted a second selective attention study. These data suggest that abused and nonabused children also differed in terms of how anger is initially engaged and decoded in the visual stream. First, abused children allocated more resources when engaging attention to angry as opposed to happy faces. For example, the abused children showed increases in P1 and N400 waveforms following presentation of angry faces. Second, abused children produced strikingly different scalp topographies in a later emerging component, the N170, which is associated with configural expertise such as face processing. These differences correlated with magnitude of abuse endured by children (Tolley-Schell & Pollak, 2003). These data provide further evidence that learning leads abused children to allocate more attentional resources signals associated with threat or harm. However, future research is necessary to more precisely parse the relative effects of abused children's engagement and disengagement to signals of threat.

ATTENTION, DEVELOPMENT, AND EXPERIENCE

We have proposed that predispositions to attend and learn about emotionally salient events, in tandem with developmental constraints on perceptual systems, leads children in abusive contexts to overprocess environmental signals associated with harm. Over time, such processes may lead to complex information-processing atypicalities that compromise healthy, adaptive functioning. Preliminary evidence supporting this position includes findings that physically abused children perceive angry faces as more distinctive than other emotions, develop broad perceptual category boundaries for anger, require less visual information to detect the presence of angry facial expressions, devote more attentional resources to detecting anger, display increased brain electrical activity when disengaging attention from anger, and evince early sensory electrophysiological activation to angry faces. In short, based on multimethod studies including electrophysiological, cognitive, and perceptual tasks, it appears that early perceptual and attentional processes directed toward angry cues distinguish maltreated children's emotion processing. Abused children seem to have become experts at anger detection. But at what cost? While it is adaptive for salient environmental stimuli to elicit attention, successful self-regulation includes flexibility and control over these processes. We suspect that failure of regulatory capacities is a proximal link between early experience and abused children's troubles. These studies suggest new ways of understanding the neural mechanisms through which early experience contributes to the organization of attentional systems and to the development of psychopathology.

FUTURE DIRECTIONS

One area of future growth concerns the need for empirically tractable models for the effects of experience on brain development. Recently, compelling examples of nature–nurture interactions with important implications for children's mental health have appeared in the literature (Bennett et al., 2002; Caspi et al., 2002, 2003; Gross et al., 2002). These reports highlight the complex, dynamic interplay between biology and experience in shaping children's behavior. As we advance understanding how biological factors are associated with mental health problems, compelling questions emerge about the processes through which experience shapes biology, necessitating a more fine-grained approach to explaining mechanisms of change and development. Therefore, a critical question about the role of attention and mental health outcomes concerns what mechanisms act in combination with children's experiences to direct or constrain an organism's future interactions and subsequent learning.

In this regard, nonhuman animal studies, in which experiences can be experimentally manipulated, are essential. Although care must be taken in translating animal studies to humans, nonhuman animal maltreatment studies provide important information that can guide future research into the neurodevelopmental processes affected by early experience. As a case in point, the original impetus for isolate rearing in rhesus monkeys was the desire to study learning unfettered by differences in mother–infant interaction (Harlow, Harlow, & Suomi, 1971). However, these socially deprived animals proved difficult to test in the laboratory because of their heightened emotional reactivity, leading researchers to redirect their studies to emotional processes and behavioral regulation (Harlow et al., 1971). Research with monkeys suggested that early experience affects development of the parietal and prefrontal cortices, important anatomical areas in terms of attentional functioning, as well as the limbic–cortical pathways involved in regulating neuroendocrine and behavioral responses to stress (Sanchez, Ladd, & Plotsky, 2001; Siegel et al., 1993). For example, hyperarousal associated with tonic activation of the LC–NE (locus coeruleus-norepinephrine) system in the macaque promotes vigilant, labile, and scanning visual attention (Aston-Jones, Rajkowski, & Cohen, 1999; see also Beane & Marrocco, Chapter 23, this volume). Although complementary human evidence is sparse, it is known that both the hypothalamic–pituitary–adrenal (HPA) axis and sympathetic-adrenomedullary systems in humans undergo reorganization during postnatal life that is associated with the child's social relationships (Gunnar, 2000), and that there is an association between the integrity of the anterior attention system and cortisol regulation (Davis, Bruce, & Gunnar, 2001). In addition, electroencephalographic (EEG) activation, a neural correlate of social withdrawal and avoidance, and ERP activation to emotion, a correlate of attention, have been associated with early social experiences (Davidson, 1994; Pollak, Klorman, Brumaghim, & Cicchetti, 2001). These data suggest that future research needs to focus on the neural substrates of children's emotion–regulatory behavior to better understand the effects of experience on development.

A second area in need of increased research attention concerns understanding the role of context in development. This is a central problem in understanding both child mental health problems and the ways to effectively remediate those problems. One problem inherent in studying children's experiences concerns the difficulty in precisely parametizing the rich, complicated "booming, buzzing, confusion" of sensory experiences to which humans are exposed within moments of birth. A related problem in the area of child psychopathology is that it is not yet clear which aspects of the environment need to be measured. Moreover, although we may be able to link biological similarities across species, it may be more difficult to link affective experiences between human and nonhuman animals. Maternal care in the rat involves licking and abuse in the monkey is operationalized as biting and dragging. How can we best model in nonhuman animals phenomena such as being threatened, criticized, beaten while being blamed, ignored, and other experiences encountered by abused children? Insights from animal learning theory suggesting that processes such as computation of proximity and probability of threat can predict the animal's selection of defensive inhibition, withdrawal, or attack (Fanselow & Lester, 1988) may be particularly useful in attempts to understand how particular patterns of maladaptive behavior emerge.

CONCLUSIONS

Child psychopathology is a field that is dominated by descriptive studies that aim to characterize the ways in which children with psychological disorders look and act differently than those without a particular disorder. However, descriptions of behavioral problems observed in clinical populations of children have not adequately informed our understanding of the neurodevelopmental processes that lead to problem behaviors. What is needed now is a new generation of research aimed at articulating candidate mechanisms believed to cause or maintain mental health difficulties. With specific mechanisms identified, it is likely that clinicians can better develop effective interventions for children that are targeted to correct discrete pathological processes. Treatments not directed at underlying mechanisms may address distal symptoms rather than the etiology of mental illness in children.

Our view is that to trace back the developmental origins of complex emotional behavior requires a focus on developmental mechanisms, not static lesions, diatheses, or deficits. Maladaptive behavioral outcomes emerge from cascading effects (and interactions) over time. To get at these interactions, we need to consider both developmental biology and context, taking into account anatomical and dynamic constraints on the developing brain as well as an understanding of what situations the organisms has had to respond to—not only what is in the genome but what the genome is in. In sum, we believe it is important to consider the emergence of children's regulatory abilities in the context of the give-and-take with the wide welter of signals and sensory inputs the developing brain receives from the outside world.

The patterns of information processing we have described suggest that children who experienced early abuse are processing certain types of emotional information atypically, while appearing to process other types of emotional information similarly to nonmaltreated children. Focusing in more detail on attentional processes may help to excavate the link between these children's early experience and the development of psychopathology later in their lives, as well as create new possibilities for remediation of these difficulties.

ACKNOWLEDGMENT

This chapter was prepared with support from Grant Nos. R01-MH61285 and T32-MH18931 from the National Institutes of Health.

REFERENCES

Aston-Jones, G., Rajkowski, J., & Cohen, J. (1999). Role of locus coeruleus in attention and behavioral flexibility. *Biological Psychiatry, 46,* 1309–1320.

Bennett, A. J., Lesch, K. P., Heils, A., Long, J. C., Lorenz, J. G., Shoaf, S. E., et al. (2002). Early experience and serotonin transporter gene variation interact to influence primate CNS function. *Molecular Psychiatry, 7,* 118–122.

Bjorklund, D. F. (1997). The role of immaturity in human development. *Psychological Bulletin, 122,* 153–169.

Camras, L. A., Ribordy, S., Hill, J., Martino, S., Sachs, V., Spaccarelli, S., et al. (1990). Maternal facial behavior and the recognition and production of emotional expression by maltreated and nonmaltreated children. *Developmental Psychology, 26,* 304–312.

Camras, L. A., Sachs-Alter, E., & Ribordy, S. (1996). Emotion understanding in maltreated children: Recognition of facial expressions and integration with other emotion cues. In M. Lewis & M.Sullivan (Eds.), *Emotional development in atypical children* (pp. 203–225). Hillsdale, NJ: Erlbaum.

Caspi, A., McClay, J., Moffitt, T. E., Mill, J., Martin, J., Craig, I. W., et al. (2002). Role of genotype in the cycle of violence in maltreated children. *Science, 297,* 851–854.

Caspi, A., Sugden, K., Moffitt, T. E., Taylor, A., Craig, I. W., Harrington, H., et al. (2003). Influence of life stress on depression: Moderation by a polymorphism in the 5-HTT gene. *Science, 301,* 386–389.

Coles, M. G., & Rugg, M. D. (1995). Event-related brain potentials: An introduction. In M. Coles & M. Rugg (Eds.), *Electrophysiology of mind: Event-related brain potentials and cognition* (pp. 1–26). Oxford, UK: Oxford University Press.

Davidson, R. J. (1994). Asymmetric brain function, affective style, and psychopathology: The role of early experience and plasticity. *Development and Psychopathology, 6,* 741–758.

Davis, E., Bruce, J., & Gunnar, M. R. (2002). The anterior attention network: Associations with temperament and neuroendocrine activity in 6-year-old children. *Developmental Psychobiology, 40,* 43–56.

Derryberry, D., & Reed, M. A. (2002). Anxiety-related attentional biases and their regulation by attentional control. *Journal of Abnormal Psychology, 111,* 225–236.

Dodge, K. A., Pettit G. S., Bates, J. E., & Valente, E. (1995). Social information-processing patterns partially mediate the effect of early physical abuse on later conduct problems. *Journal of Abnormal Psychology, 104,* 632–643.

Fanselow, M. S., & Lester, L. S. (1988). A functional behavioristic approach to aversively motivated behavior: Predatory imminence as a determinant of the topography of defensive behavior. In R. Bolles & M. Beecher (Eds.), *Evolution and learning* (pp. 185–212). Hillsdale, NJ: Erlbaum.

Fox, E., Russo, R., & Dutton, K. (2002). Attentional bias for threat: Evidence for delayed disengagement from emotional faces. *Cognition and Emotion, 16,* 355–379.

Gross, C., Zhuang, X. X., Stark, K., Ramboz, S., Oosting, R., Kirby, L., et al. (2002). Serotonin (1A) receptor acts during development to establish normal anxiety-like behaviour in the adult. *Nature, 416,* 396–400.

Gunnar, M. R. (2000). Early adversity and the development of stress reactivity and regulation. In C. Nelson (Ed.), *The effects of adversity on neurobehavioral development: Minnesota Symposia on Child Psychology* (Vol. 31, pp. 163–200). Mahwah, NJ: Erlbaum.

Harlow, H. F., Harlow, M. K., & Suomi, S. J. (1971). From thought to therapy: Lessons from a primate laboratory. *American Scientist, 59,* 538–549.

Hoffman-Poltkin, D., & Twentyman, C. T. (1984). A multimodal assessment of behavioral and cognitive deficits in abused and neglected preschoolers. *Child Development, 55,* 794–802.

Jacobson, R. S., & Straker, G. (1982). Peer group interaction of physically abused children. *International Journal of Child Abuse and Neglect, 6,* 327.

Johnson, M. H., Posner, M. I., & Rothbart, M. K. (1991). Components of visual orienting in early infancy: Contingency learning, anticipatory looking and disengaging. *Journal of Cognitive Neuroscience, 3,* 335–344.

Klimes-Dougan, B., & Kistner, J. (1990). Physically abused preschoolers' responses to peers' distress. *Developmental Psychology, 26,* 599–602.

Kramer, A. F., & Spinks, J. (1991). Capacity views of human information processing. In J. Jennings & M. Coles (Eds.), *Handbook of cognitive psychophysiology: Central and autonomic nervous system approaches* (pp. 179–242). New York: Wiley.

Kuhl, P. (1987). The special-mechanisms debate in speech research: Categorization tests on animals and infants. In S. Harnad (Ed.), *Categorical perception: The groundwork of cognition* (pp. 355–386). New York: Cambridge University Press.

Kuhl, P., & Meltzoff, A. N. (1982). The bimodal perception of speech in infancy. *Science, 218,* 1138–1141.

Laberge, D. (1995). *Attentional processing: The brain's art of mindfulness.* Cambridge, MA: Harvard University Press.

Main, M., & George C. (1985). Responses of abused and disadvantaged toddlers to distress in agemates. *Developmental Psychology, 21,* 407–412.

McNally, R. J. (1998). Experimental approaches to cognitive abnormality in posttraumatic stress disorder. *Clinical Psychology Review [Special issue: Memory for trauma: The intersection of clinical psychology and cognitive science], 18,* 971–982.

Mogg, K., & Bradley, B. P. (1998). A cognitive-motivational analysis of anxiety. *Behaviour Research and Therapy, 36,* 809–848.

Polich, J., & Kok, A. (1995). Cognitive and biological determinants of P300: An integrative review. *Biological Psychology, 41,* 103–146.

Pollak, S. D. (2004). Experience-dependent affective learning and risk for psychopathology in children. *Annals of the New York Academy of Sciences, 1008,* 102–111.

Pollak, S. D., Cicchetti, D., Hornung, K., & Reed, A. (2000). Recognizing emotion in faces: Developmental effects of child abuse and neglect. *Developmental Psychology, 36,* 679–688.

Pollak, S. D., Cicchetti, D., & Klorman, R. (1998). Stress, memory, and emotion: Developmental considerations from the study of child maltreatment. *Development and Psychopathology, 10,* 811–828.

Pollak, S. D., Cicchetti, D., Klorman, R., & Brumaghim, J. (1997). Cognitive brain event-related potentials and emotion processing in maltreated children. *Child Development, 68,* 773–787.

Pollak, S. D., & Kistler, D. (2002). Early experience alters the development of categorical representations for facial expressions of emotion. *Proceedings of the National Academy of Sciences USA, 99,* 9072–9076.

Pollak, S. D., Klorman, R., Brumaghim, J., & Cicchetti, D. (2001). P3b reflects maltreated children's reactions to facial displays of emotion. *Psychophysiology, 38,* 267–274.

Pollak, S. D., & Sinha, P. (2002). Effects of early experience on children's recognition of facial displays of emotion. *Developmental Psychology, 38,* 784–791.

Pollak, S. D., & Tolley-Schell, S. (2003). Selective attention to facial emotion in physically abused children. *Journal of Abnormal Psychology, 112,* 323–338.

Posner, M. I., & Rothbart, M. K. (2000). Developing mechanisms of self-regulation. *Development and Psychopathology, 12,* 427–441.

Posner M. I., Snyder, C. R., & Davidson, B. J. (1980). Attention and the detection of signals. *Journal of Experimental Psychology: General, 109,* 160–174.

Rescorla, R. A. (1966). Predictability and number of pairings in Pavlovian fear conditioning. *Psychometric Science 4,* 38–84.

Rieder, C., & Cicchetti, D. (1989). Organizational perspective on cognitive control functioning and cognitive affective balance in maltreated children. *Developmental Psychology, 25,* 382–393.

Rogosch, F. A., Cicchetti, D., & Aber, J. L. (1995). The role of child maltreatment in early deviations in cognitive and affective processing abilities and later peer relationship problems. *Development and Psychopathology, 7,* 591–609.

Rothbart, M. K., Zaie, H., & O'Boyle, C. G. (1992). Self-regulation and emotion in infancy. In N. Eisenberg & R. A. Fabes (Eds.), *Emotion and its regulation in early development. New directions for child development* (Vol. 55, pp. 7–24). San Francisco: Jossey-Bass/Pfeiffer.

Ruff, H. A., & Rothbart, M. K. (1996). *Attention in early development: Themes and variations.* London: Oxford University Press.

Saffran, J. R., Aslin, R. N., & Newport, E. (1996). Statistical learning by 8-month-old infants. *Science, 274,* 1926–1928.

Sanchez, M. M., Ladd, C. O., & Plotsky, P. M. (2001). Early adverse experience as a developmental risk factor for later psychopathology: Evidence from rodent and primate models. *Development and Psychopathology, 13,* 419–450.

Siegel, S. J., Ginsberg, S. D., Hof, P. R., Foote, S. L., Young, W. G., & Draemer, G. W. (1993). Effects of social deprivation in prepubescent rhesus monkeys: Immunohistochemical analysis of the neurofilament protein triplet in the hippocampal formation. *Brain Research, 619,* 299–305.

Tolley-Schell, S., & Pollak, S. D. (2003). *Engagement and disengagement of attention to emotion among physically abused children with and without social anxiety.* Manuscript under review.

U.S. Department of Health and Human Services. (2000). *Trends of well-being of America's children and youth.* Washington, DC: U.S. Government Printing Office.

Vasey, M., & MacLeod, C. (2001). Information processing factors in childhood anxiety: A review and developmental perspective. In M. Vasey & C. MacLeod (Eds.), *The developmental psychopathology of anxiety* (pp. 253–277). London: Oxford University Press.

Weiss, B., Dodge, K. A., Bates, J. E., & Pettit, J. T. (1992). Some consequences of early harsh discipline: Child aggression and a maladaptive social information processing style. *Child Development, 63,* 1321–1335.

27

Response Inhibition in Conflict Tasks Is Revealed in Delta Plots

K. Richard Ridderinkhof, Wery P. M. van den Wildenberg,
Jasper Wijnen, and Borís Burle

Dealing with conflicting response tendencies in human information processing is thought to be an important aspect of goal-directed behavior. In a choice reaction task, one type of stimulus may designate one particular response (e.g., a speeded button press with the left hand) whereas another type of stimulus designates an alternative response (e.g., a speeded button press with the right hand). The term *response inhibition* is used here descriptively to refer to the mechanism or set of processes that results in the containment of prepotent behavioral responses when such responses are reflex-like, premature, inappropriate, or incorrect; thus, response inhibition is a key instrument of executive attention. The exact neural mechanism (in terms of, e.g., the exact paths and projection sites of inhibitory neurons and interneurons) of this form of response inhibition is not entirely understood, but neuroimaging studies and patient work suggest that response inhibition is mediated by structures in (pre)frontal cortex and basal ganglia (e.g., Casey, Tottenham, & Fossella, 2002; Garavan, Ross, Murphy, Roche, & Stein, 2002; for a review, see Band & van Boxtel, 1999). Functional neuroimaging studies have provided support for the alleged role of frontal brain areas in resolving response conflict (e.g., Bench et al., 1993; Bush et al., 1998; Carter, Mintun, & Cohen, 1995; Hazeltine, Poldrack, & Gabriel, 2000; McKeown et al., 1998; Ullsperger & von Cramon, 2001). However, few studies have provided direct evidence for the role of response inhibition in resolving or preventing conflict.

Our main goal in this chapter is to present a method that allows us to examine the proficiency of response inhibition in behavioral (reaction time) data. We review two examples in which we use an analytical technique known as *delta-plot analysis* to highlight the role of response inhibition in resolving response conflict. The first study is on individual differences in resolving response conflict and included subjects in the normal population. In the second experiment, delta plots were used to mark inhibitory deficits in children diagnosed with attention-deficit/hyperactivity disorder (ADHD). First, we briefly introduce the conflict paradigm.

RESPONSE INHIBITION IN CONFLICT TASKS

The choice reaction time (RT) tasks introduced by Stroop (1935), Simon (1990), and Eriksen (Eriksen & Eriksen, 1974) are prototypical representatives of experimental paradigms that induce conflicting responses. Responses are defined here as button presses with either the left or right hand. The signals employed in these tasks typically consist of two dimensions: a relevant one, on which the participant should base his or her response and an irrelevant one, unrelated to the task. In the Stroop task, the subject is asked to name the font color (task-relevant aspect) in which a color word (task-irrelevant aspect) is printed. Responses are slowed when the font color is different from the word itself (e.g., the word *red* printed in blue ink). In the arrow version of the Eriksen task, participants are instructed to issue a discriminative response based on the direction of a target arrow, and to ignore flanking arrows. Responses are typically slower when the flanking arrows point to the other direction as the central arrow, inducing conflict. In the Simon task, participants are instructed to generate a swift button-press response with either the right or the left hand based on the color of a signal (relevant feature)—for example, to press left to a green signal and to press right to a blue one. This signal can appear on the right or on the left side, and this task-irrelevant position-related aspect of the signal automatically activates the response associated with it. The typical observation in the Simon task is that RTs are slowed due to conflict occurring when the irrelevant feature of the stimulus activates the alternative response. When a signal is presented to the right but its color designates a left-hand button press, we speak of *incongruent* trials. Signals that require a left-hand response and are also presented on the left side are referred to as *congruent trials*. RTs are typically slower to incongruent compared to congruent trials, a finding referred to as the *congruency effect or interference effect*.

To account for interference effects in conflict tasks, many authors have invoked a processing model that involves two distinct pathways (e.g., de Jong, Liang, & Lauber, 1994; Eimer, Hommel, & Prinz, 1995; Kornblum, Hasbroucq, & Osman, 1990; Ridderinkhof, van der Molen, & Bashore, 1995). Figure 27.1 shows a schematic representation of this type of model. Most significant, an attention-controlled pathway of stimulus–response transla-

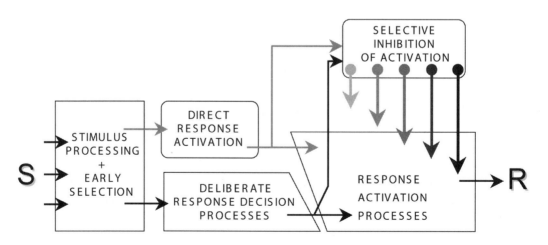

FIGURE 27.1. Elementary architecture of the dual-process model. The inhibition mechanism acts selectively upon reponse-activation processes that are associated with the direct response-activation route. Selective inhibition needs time to develop (represented by the length and shading of the vertical arrows) before it can result in effective reduction of response activation processes.

tion is paralleled by a direct reflex-like route. The two routes converge at the level of re-sponse-activation processes (i.e., at the level where motor programs for specific behavioral responses are initiated and executed). An active response-inhibition mechanism, serving to selectively reduce the activation of specific responses, has often been suggested to keep inappropriate response activations in check (e.g., Eriksen & Schultz, 1979; Kopp, Rist, & Mattler, 1996). This selective response-inhibition mechanism is the focus of this chapter.

THE ACTIVATION–SUPPRESSION HYPOTHESIS: PREDICTIONS AND OBSERVATIONS

In an explicit formulation, *the activation–suppression hypothesis* (Ridderinkhof, 2002a) holds that the behavioral response activated by the irrelevant stimulus features is selectively inhibited. This selective inhibition takes some time to build up and hence becomes effective only after a given amount of time. A separate series of studies support these dynamics. Eimer (e.g., 1999; Eimer & Schlaghecken, 1998) presented masked prime stimuli that could be congruent or incongruent to subsequently presented target stimuli. Faster and more accurate performance was observed for congruent compared to incongruent trials, but only when the interval between prime and target was brief. At longer intervals, responses to congruent targets were slower and more error prone than responses to incongruent targets. Event-related brain potentials suggested that the masked primes initially generated direct activation of the corresponding response, which was subsequently inhibited. If the target was presented soon after the prime, the initial prime-based activation escaped inhibition and thus resulted in rapid responses to congruent trials but slow responses to incongruent trials. Conversely, if presentation of the target was delayed, the initial prime-based response activation was selectively inhibited by the time response activation was elicited by the target. Thus, long delays are detrimental for responses to congruent trials, making them relatively slow and error-prone, as the *correct* response associated with the prime was being inhibited. Equally, responses to incongruent targets benefit from longer delays, such that they are relatively fast and accurate, as the incorrect response elicited by the prime was being inhibited.

The activation–suppression hypothesis has several implications in the Simon task. Because of the same dynamics described previously (in particular the gradual buildup of response inhibition as time progresses across a trial), slower responses will be more affected by selective response inhibition than will faster responses (see also Burle, Possamaï, Vidal, Bonnet, & Hasbroucq, 2002; Eimer, 1999). The automatic route will facilitate the correct response on congruent trials, but it will interfere with the correct response on incongruent trials. While this is true for fast responses, an additional factor comes into play for slower responses: With slower responses, the selective inhibition process has had time to develop, and thus the activation of the incorrect response along the direct route will be reduced. Correct responses to congruent trials will be less facilitated by the position-driven route, whereas correct responses to incongruent trials will be less delayed. Thus, congruency effects are affected by selective response inhibition more in slow then in fast responses.

Like most mental processes, selective response inhibition can be assumed to be subject to variability. The strength, onset time, and buildup rate of selective inhibition of the response activated by the direct route may vary interindividually and with experimental manipulations. If selective inhibition results in a reduction of the congruency effect in slow responses, as argued earlier, then the more effective this selective inhibition, the more pronounced the influence on congruency effects in slow responses. These dynamics point to the need to examine RT distributions. Several tools are available for distributional analyses. Here we focus on *delta plots*. Delta plots are constructed by plotting the congruency effect as a function of response speed (de Jong et al., 1994; Ridderinkhof, 2002a). While delta plots prototypically have a positive slope (i.e., the effects of any experimental factor increases as a function of response speed), the notion that selective inhibition results in a reduction of the congruency effect in slow responses (outlined previously) implies a different delta-plot pattern: The congruency effect should not increase linearly as a function of response speed but instead should level off and become reduced for slow responses. If more effective selective inhibition results in a more pronounced reduction of congruency effects in slow responses, as argued earlier, then the leveling off of the delta plot should be more pronounced in individuals who are more proficient in response inhibition than in those who are less proficient. Likewise, the leveling off of the delta plot should be more pronounced in experimental conditions that require more stringent response inhibition compared to less demanding conditions.

Ridderinkhof (2002a) designed a series of experiments to verify this prediction. The point of divergence between two delta plots (representing two different levels of inhibitory strength) was the critical variable in comparisons between conditions. Each experiment comprised a regular Simon task (that required a two-choice response on the basis of stimulus color) intermixed with a second task in which stimulus position was either irrelevant (Experiment 1) or relevant (Experiment 2). In the majority of trials in Experiment 1, subjects had to perform the regular Simon task. In the remaining trials, subjects responded as a function of stimulus shape. The location-driven information was irrelevant in both tasks and hence could always be inhibited. In the second experiment, which used the same stimuli, the second task required a response on the basis of the location of the stimuli. Thus, in a small subset of trials location-driven information was relevant and should not be inhibited. Therefore, it would be disadvantageous to always inhibit location-driven direct response activation here. The regular Simon task was identical in all respects across the two experiments but nevertheless revealed opposite results depending on the nature of the intermixed task. Delta plots leveled off early and turned negative when location-driven activation could always be inhibited but not when location was relevant in half of the trials.

Inhibitory control in the Simon task, as expressed in negative-going delta plots, is increased after errors (Ridderinkhof, 2002b). Burle and colleagues (2002) used electromyographic recordings to extend this finding and demonstrate that this delta-plot effect in fact reflects an *online* act of inhibitory control. In a regular version of the Simon task, these authors showed that the leveling off and turning negative of the delta plot was most prominent on those trials that contained partial errors (i.e., subthreshold activation of the muscles involved in the incorrect response prior to the threshold activation of the correct response). The operation of response inhibition is most critical on those trials in which the incorrect response is actually activated to the motor level, and this inhibitory engagement is expressed in the prominent deflection in the delta plot.

ILLUSTRATING THE UTILITY OF DELTA-PLOT ANALYSIS

Individual Differences in Response Inhibition

An example that illustrates the usefulness of delta plots in indexing response inhibition is taken from Ridderinkhof (2002a). One set of analyses used the delta-plot techniques to demonstrate that, compared to subjects with larger Simon effects, subjects with smaller Si-

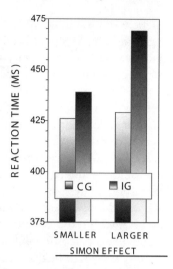

FIGURE 27.2. Mean RTs for congruent (CG) and incongruent (IG) conditions in subjects with relatively small Simon effects and in subjects with relatively large Simon effects.

mon effects displayed stronger inhibition effects, as expressed in the diverging slopes of the delta plots for RT. These patterns are shown in Figures 27.2 and 27.3.

Response Inhibition Deficits in ADHD

Here we aim to point out the merits of delta plots to the study of individual differences, including developmental trends and clinical disorders, by applying them to investigate performance of children diagnosed with ADHD. ADHD is among the most prevalent childhood pathologies and has been studied extensively in various branches of the cognitive neurosciences. Among the different theoretical perspectives in the study of ADHD, several main-

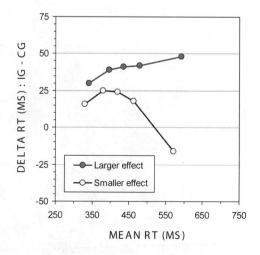

FIGURE 27.3. Delta plots for congruency effects in subjects with relatively small Simon effects and for subjects with relatively large Simon effects.

stream theories of neurocognitive deficits associated with ADHD focus on the role of impulsivity and response inhibition (e.g., Barkley, 1997; Nigg, 2001). Studies that examined response conflict in the Eriksen flanker task have frequently reported ADHD deficits (e.g., Carter, Krener, Chaderjian, Northcutt, & Wolfe, 1995; Crone, Jennings, & van der Molen, 2003; Hooks, Milich, & Lorch, 1994; Jonkman et al., 1999).

Scheres and colleagues (2003) used the arrow version of the Eriksen flanker task to examine the performance of children with ADHD in comparison to matched controls. In this conflict task, participants are instructed to respond based on the direction of a target arrow, and to ignore flanking arrows. Responses are slower to incongruent stimulus displays, in which the flanking arrows point to the other direction as the central arrow. Ridderinkhof and colleagues (in press) applied delta-plot analysis to the data from Scheres and colleagues (2003) to explore differences between children with ADHD and control children (matched carefully in terms of age, gender, and IQ) with respect to the ability to inhibit task-irrelevant response activation. If ADHD does involve a response-inhibition deficit, as hypothesized by current mainstream theories (e.g., Barkley, 1997; Nigg, 2001), then the slopes of (especially the slower segments of) delta plots for RT should level off more prominently for controls than for children with ADHD.

The congruency effect was larger for children with ADHD compared to controls (see Figure 27.4). Thus, overall performance measures suggest that compared to matched controls, children diagnosed with ADHD are more sensitive to interference effects. Closer examination of intraindividual performance variability revealed that the leveling off in the positive-going delta plots for RT was more pronounced and was manifest earlier in the distribution for controls than for children with ADHD (see Figure 27.5). In accordance with the activation–suppression model, these findings can be interpreted to indicate that, compared to normal controls, children with ADHD show a deficiency in the selective inhibition of responses that were activated on the basis of flankers.

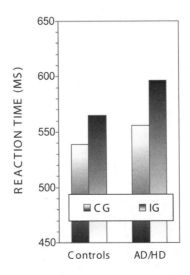

FIGURE 27.4. Mean RTs for congruent (CG) and incongruent (IG) conditions in ADHD versus matched controls.

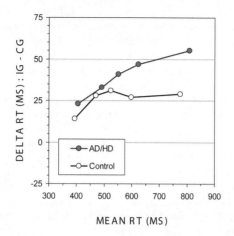

FIGURE 27.5. Delta plots for congruency effects in ADHD versus matched controls.

These findings highlight the usefulness of the delta-plot technique in developmental and clinical research. These results provide unique evidence for theories that emphasize response inhibition as a fundamental neurocognitive deficit in ADHD (e.g., Barkley, 1997; Nigg, 2001). Note that these conclusions could not possibly have been obtained when analyses were confined to overall performance. The delta-plot technique has also been applied successfully to examine the pharmacological effects of alcohol (Ridderinkhof et al., 2002) and methylphenidate (Ridderinkhof, Scheres, Oosterlaan, & Sergeant, in press) on the efficiency of response inhibition in conflict tasks. Preliminary results of currently ongoing research in our lab suggest that these distributional analyses are also useful in the study of eye movements (in particular the inhibition of reflexive saccades).

REFERENCES

Band, G. P. H., & van Boxtel, G. J. M. (1999). Inhibitory motor control in the stop paradigm: Review and reinterpretation of neural mechanisms. *Acta Psychologica, 101*, 179–211.

Barkley, R. A. (1997). Behavioral inhibition, sustained attention, and executive functions: Constructing a unifying theory of AD/HD. *Psychological Bulletin, 121*, 65–94.

Bench, C. J., Frith, C. D., Grasby, P. M., Friston, K. J., Paulesu, E., Frackowiak, R. S. J., et al. (1993). Investigations of the functional anatomy of attention using the Stroop test. *Neuropsychologia, 31*, 907–922.

Burle, B., Possamaï, C.-A., Vidal, F., Bonnet, M., & Hasbroucq, T. (2002). Executive control in the Simon effect: An electromyographic and distributional analysis. *Psychological Research, 66*, 324–339.

Bush, G., Whalen, P. J., Rosen, B. R., Jenike, M. A., Mcinery, S. C., & Rauch, S. L. (1998). The counting Stroop: An interference task specialized for functional neuroimaging. A validation study with functional MRI. *Human Brain Mapping, 6*, 270–282.

Carter, C. S., Krener, P., Chaderjian, M., Northcutt, C., & Wolfe, V. (1995). Abnormal processing of irrelevant information in attention deficit hyperactivity disorder. *Psychiatric Research, 56*, 59–70.

Carter, C. S., Mintun, M., & Cohen, J. D. (1995). Interference and facilitation effects during selective attention: An H2150 PET study of Stroop task performance. *NeuroImage, 2*, 264–272.

Casey, B. J., Tottenham, N., & Fossella, J. (2002). Clinical imaging, lesion, and genetic approaches toward a model of cognitive control. *Developmental Psychobiology, 40,* 237–254.

Crone, E. A., Jennings, J. R., & van der Molen, M. W. (2003). Sensitivity to interference and response contingencies in attention deficit/hyperactivity disorder. *Journal of Child Psychology and Psychiatry and Allied Disciplines, 44,* 214–226.

de Jong, R., Liang, C.-C., & Lauber, E. (1994). Conditional and unconditional automaticity: A dual process model of effects of spatial stimulus–response correspondence. *Journal of Experimental Psychology: Human Perception and Performance, 20,* 731–750.

Eimer, M. (1999). Facilitatory and inhibitory effects of masked prime stimuli on motor activation and behavioral performance. *Acta Psychologica, 101,* 293–314.

Eimer, M., Hommel, B., & Prinz, W. (1995). S-R compatibility and response selection. *Acta Psychologica, 90,* 301–313.

Eimer, M., & Schlaghecken, F. (1998). Effects of masked stimuli on motor activation: Behavioral and electrophysiological evidence. *Journal of Experimental Psychology: Human Perception and Performance, 24,* 1737–1747.

Eriksen, B. A., & Eriksen, C. W. (1974). Effects of noise letters upon the identification of target letters in a non-search task. *Perception and Psychophysics, 16,* 143–149.

Eriksen, C. W., & Schultz, D. W. (1979). Information processing in visual search: A continuous flow conception and experimental results. *Perception and Psychophysics, 25,* 249–263.

Garavan, H., Ross, T. J., Murphy, K., Roche, R. A. P., & Stein, E. A. (2002). Dissociable executive functions in the dynamic control of behavior: Inhibition, error detection, and correction. *NeuroImage, 17,* 1820–1829.

Hazeltine, E., Poldrack, R., & Gabrieli, J. D. E. (2000). Neural activation during response competition. *Journal of Cognitive Neuroscience, 12,* 118–129.

Hooks, K., Milich, R., & Lorch, E. P. (1994). Sustained and selective attention in boys with attention deficit hyperactivity disorder. *Journal of Clinical Child Psychology, 23,* 69–77.

Jonkman, L. M., Kemner, C., Verbaten, M. N., van Engeland, H., Kenemans, J. L., Camferman, G., et al. (1999). Perceptual and response interference in children with attention deficit hyperactivity disorder, and the effects of methylphenidate. *Psychophysiology, 36,* 419–429.

Kopp, B., Rist, F., & Mattler, U. (1996). N200 in the flanker task as a neurobehavioral tool for investigating executive control. *Psychophysiology, 33,* 282–294.

Kornblum, S., Hasbroucq, T., & Osman, A. (1990). Dimensional overlap: Cognitive basis for stimulus–response compatibility—A model and taxonomy. *Psychological Review, 97,* 253–270.

McKeown, M. J., Jung, T. P., Makeig, S., Brown, G., Kindermann, S. S., Lee, T. W., et al. (1998). Spatially independent activity patterns in functional MRI data during the Stroop color naming task. *Proceedings of the National Academy of Science USA, 95,* 803–810.

Nigg, J. T. (2001). Is ADHD a disinhibitory disorder? *Psychological Bulletin, 127,* 571–598.

Ridderinkhof, K. R. (2002a). Activation and suppression in conflict tasks: Empirical clarification through distributional analyses. In W. Prinz & B. Hommel (Eds.), *Common mechanisms in perception and action. Attention and performance* (Vol. XIX, pp. 494–519). Oxford, UK: Oxford University Press.

Ridderinkhof, K. R. (2002b). Micro- and macro-adjustments of task set: Activation and suppression in conflict tasks. *Psychological Research, 66,* 312–323.

Ridderinkhof, K. R., de Vlugt, Y., Bramlage, A., Spaan, M., Elton, M., Snel, J., et al. (2002). Alcohol consumption impairs detection of performance errors in mediofrontal cortex. *Science, 298,* 2209–2211.

Ridderinkhof, K. R., Scheres, A., Oosterlaan, J., & Sergeant, J. A. (in press). Delta plots in the study of individual differences: New tools reveal response inhibition deficits in AD/HD that are eliminated by methylphenidate treatment. *Journal of Abnormal Psychology.*

Ridderinkhof, K. R., van der Molen, M. W., & Bashore, T. R. (1995). Limits on the application of additive factors logic: Violations of stage robustness suggest a dual-process architecture to explain flanker effects on target processing. *Acta Psychologica, 90,* 29–48.

Scheres, A., Oosterlaan, J., Geurts, H., Morein-Zamir, S., Meiran, N., Schut, R., et al. (2003). Executive functioning in boys with ADHD: Primarily an inhibition deficit? *Archives of Clinical Neuro-psychology.*

Simon, J. R. (1990). The effect of an irrelevant directional cue on human information processing. In R. Proctor & T. Reeve (Eds.), *Stimulus–response compatibility: An integrated perspective* (pp. 31–88). Amsterdam: North-Holland.

Stroop, J. (1935). Studies of interference in serial verbal reactions. *Journal of Experimental Psychology, 18,* 643–662.

Ullsperger, M., & von Cramon, D. Y. (2001). Subprocesses of performance monitoring: A dissociation of error processing and response competition revealed by event-related fMRI and ERPs. *NeuroImage, 14,* 1387–1401.

VI

DEFICITS OF ATTENTION

28

Multisensory Integration of Audiovisual Inputs in Individuals with and without Visuospatial Impairment

Elisabetta Làdavas, Nadia Bolognini, and Francesca Frassinetti

Cross-modal spatial integration between auditory and visual stimuli is a common phenomenon in space perception. The principles underlying such integration have been outlined by neurophysiological and behavioral studies in animals (Stein & Meredith, 1993), but little evidence exists proving that similar principles occur also in humans.

In this chapter we explore the integration of visual and auditory stimuli in individuals with and without visuospatial impairment (visual neglect) in order to understand whether the neurophysiological principles found in animal studies can help us understand aspects of cross-modal integration in humans.

Our senses are constantly bombarded by information from multitudinous events occurring in our everyday environment. Events occur at various positions in space and time, and each animal must create perceptual order out of this seemingly array to produce an integrated, comprensive assessment of its external world. This assessment is accomplished by attending to some complexes of stimuli and ignoring other and by determining which stimuli are related to one another and which are not. The coordination and the integration of information derived from different sensory systems is essential for providing an unified perception of our environment, and for directing attention and controlling action within it. The capacity of the central nervous system to combine inputs across the senses can lead to marked improvements in the detection, localization, and discrimination of external stimuli and to faster reactions to those stimuli. However, under certain circumstances, cross-modal interactions may alter, rather than enhance, our perception of events. For instance, althought our ability to comprehend speech is significantly improved when the speaker can be seen as well as heard (Sumby & Pollack, 1954), when the visual and acoustic stimuli are incongruent, as occurs when dubbing one syllable onto a movie showing a person mouthing a different syllable, subjects typically report hearing a third syllable that represents a combination of what was seen and heard (McGurk & MacDonald, 1976).

Much of what we know about the mechanisms involved in combining multisensory signals comes from anatomical and physiological experiments in animals. *Some* of this multisensory integration reflects the intrinsic circuitry of the brain: Certain combinations of stimuli become more salient because neuronal responses to them are enhanced, and other combinations of stimuli remain less salient by producing the opposite effect (i.e., neuronal depression). Stimuli that occur at different times and/or in different places are unlikely to be related and will produce depression. It has been documented that in several brain structures, like the superior colliculus, there are multisensory neurons responding to stimuli in different modalities (e.g., vision and audition). At single-cell level, inputs from different modalities are integrated by the multisensory neurons according to three main principles (Stein & Meredith, 1993): the first concerning the spatial proximity of the stimuli (spatial rule), the second the temporal interval between the stimuli (temporal rule), and the third the nature of the multimodal response (inverse effectiveness) (Stein & Meredith, 1993).

According to the spatial rule, only spatially coincident stimuli from different modalities are integrated, producing neurons' response enhancement, whereas spatially disparate stimuli are not integrated, producing either depression or no interaction at the single-cell level. The spatial property of multisensory integration depends on the organization in zones of excitation and inhibition that define the receptive fields of multisensory neurons. The receptive fields of these neurons are organized in two areas: a central excitatory area, called the best area, surrounded by an inhibitory area. Because of the auditory and the visual receptive fields of bimodal neurons are overlapped (Jay & Sparks, 1987; King & Hutchings, 1987; King & Palmer, 1985; Knudsen, 1982; Middlebrooks & Knudsen, 1984), spatially coincident audiovisual stimuli fall within their excitatory receptive fields and enhance one another's effects. However, if the stimuli are spatially disparate, one may fall within the inhibitory receptive region and depress the effects of the other, or it may be processed as a separate event (Meredith & Stein, 1986a; Stein & Meredith, 1993).

According to the temporal rule, stimuli temporally coincident are integrated, while those separated by intervals are processed as separate events. To ensure an interaction among the responses to stimuli of different modalities, the two inputs should be presented simultaneously, without temporal disparity. The absence of temporal disparity turned out to be the "optimal" interactive period for most multisensory neurons (Meredith, Nemizt, & Stein, 1987), but it is not always the rule. In some neurons, for example, the combination of unimodal auditory and visual stimuli at some intervals (50 msec and 150 msec) also produced response enhancement. But, at longer intervals (200 msec and 300 msec), audiovisual stimulation produced response depression of neuron's activity or no interaction (Meredith, Nemizt, & Stein, 1987; Stein & Meredith, 1993). Finally, according to the inverse effectiveness rule, there is an inverse relationship between the effectiveness of the stimuli and the neural response evoked by the stimuli. The combination of weak unimodal stimuli produces greater response enhancement comparing to combinations of potent stimuli: Combining two seemingly unimodal stimuli (i.e., neither stimulus alone is capable of evoking an obvious effect on the neuron's activity) can dramatically enhance responses in multisensory neurons (Meredith & Stein, 1986b; Stein & Meredith, 1993).

Despite a long tradition of single-cell studies on multimodal neurons in animals, the existence of these integrated systems has been investigated only recently in psychological and neuropsychological domains (Frassinetti, Bolognini, & Làdavas, 2002: Frassinetti, Pavani, & Làdavas, 2002). Such a relatively low (but rapidly increasing) number of studies is surprising given that these multisensory systems can offer a unique opportunity for the recovery from cognitive impairment following brain lesion. For instance, altered performance in a unimodal sensory system can be influenced (e.g., enhanced or degraded) via activation of another modality (Làdavas, 2002). In this respect, it is interesting to study cross-modal effects in patients with impairments in spatial representation, such as extinction or neglect, which is caused by a loss of neurons representing particular locations in space in one or more modalities (Pouget & Sejnowski, 1997). Due to the lesion, stimuli presented in that portion of space are neglected or extinguished (Làdavas, Berti, & Farnè, 2000), whereas stimuli presented in the intact portion of space are detected. Therefore it is possible to postulate that whenever patients' perceptual problems due to extinction or neglect are limited to the impairment of unimodal space representations, detection in these patients could be obtained by the activation of an integrated system coding stimuli presented in the affected space in different modalities.

Before presenting the relevance of cross-modal integration in the remediation of visuospatial deficits, we provide psychophysical evidence about the existence of an integrated acoustic–visual system in normal subjects.

CROSS-MODAL INTEGRATION BETWEEN AUDITION AND VISION IN INDIVIDUALS WITHOUT VISUOSPATIAL IMPAIRMENT

Some authors have investigated the possibility that the exogenous shift of attention in one modality (audition) leads to a corresponding shift of attention in another modality (vision) (Driver & Spence, 1998; Macaluso, Frith, & Driver, 2001; McDonald, Teder-Salerjarvi, & Hillyard, 2000; Spence & Driver, 1997). Spence and Driver (1997) demonstrated that an uninformative auditory cue affected elevation judgments for visual targets (i.e., that is elevation discriminations were faster when the visual target was presented on the cued side). Similar facilitatory effects were found by McDonald and colleagues (2000). They provided psychophysical evidence that a sudden sound improves the detectability of a subsequent flash appearing at the same location when the delay between the cue and the target was less than 300 msec. Because these authors adopted only two spatial positions for both visual and acoustical stimuli, it is possible to interpret their findings either as an evidence for cross-modal consequences of involuntary exogenous shift in spatial attention or for cross-modal integration effects.

To investigate whether the integrative effects observed in animals could also be found in humans, an experiment was conducted by Frassinetti, Bolognini, and Làdavas (2002) considering different spatial positions for visual and auditory stimulation. In this experiment the visual stimuli were presented below threshold and signal detection measures were used. Signal detection measures allow for the separation of perceptual level and decision level, with d' parameter reflecting subjects' accuracy to discern a sensory event from its background (perceptual level) and β parameter reflecting subjectas' decision criterion of response (decision level). Moreover, because multisensory response occurs with weak unimodal stimuli (Stein & Meredith, 1983), the visual target was degraded by using a visual mask.

Subjects were asked to fixate a central point and to detect masked visual targets horizontally displayed at 8, 24, 40, and 56 degrees, in the left visual field (LVF) as well as in the right visual field (RVF) (see Figure 28.1). Subjects were exposed to auditory (white noise burst) and visual (a flash of green LED) stimuli in two conditions: The task was performed either in a unimodal condition (i.e., only visual stimuli were presented) or in cross-modal

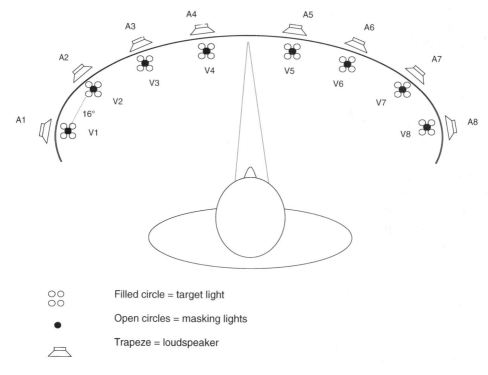

FIGURE 28.1. Bird's-eye schematic view of the position of light displays and loudspeakers. From Frassinetti, Bolognini, and Làdavas (2002). Copyright 2002 by Springer-Verlag. Reprinted by permission.

conditions (i.e., a sound was presented together with the visual target). In the cross-modal conditions, sounds could be presented either at the same spatial position as the visual target (spatially coincident cross-modal condition), or at one of the remaining seven spatial positions (spatially disparate cross-modal conditions). Subjects were instructed to detect the presence of visual stimuli (light) and ignore auditory stimuli. Moreover, to determine the effect of the temporal proximity on auditory–visual interaction, the acoustic and the visual stimuli were presented simultaneously (Experiment 1a) or the acoustic stimulus preceded the visual stimulus by 500 msec (Experiment 1b).

The results, in accordance to the cross-modal integration hypothesis, showed that d' parameter varied with the degree of spatial and temporal correspondence between the acoustic and the visual stimuli: An increased perceptual sensitivity (d') was found by presenting temporally overlapping visual and acoustic stimuli in the same spatial position.

The findings of the Experiment 1 show that an auditory stimulus presented at one spatial location facilitates responses to a visual target at that location. Instead, when the same visual and auditory stimuli were presented at spatially disparate loci, the detectability of the visual stimulus did not improve. Moreover, the capacity of an acoustic stimulus to enhance the detectability of a visual stimulus was evident only when the two stimuli were presented simultaneously (Experiment 1a) (see Figure 28.2). By contrast when the acoustic stimulus preceded the visual stimulus of 500 msec no improvement of visual detectability was found (Experiment 1b).

Moreover, the results from the signal detection analyses showed that a sound influenced vision at early perceptual levels more than at later, decision-related levels. The presentation

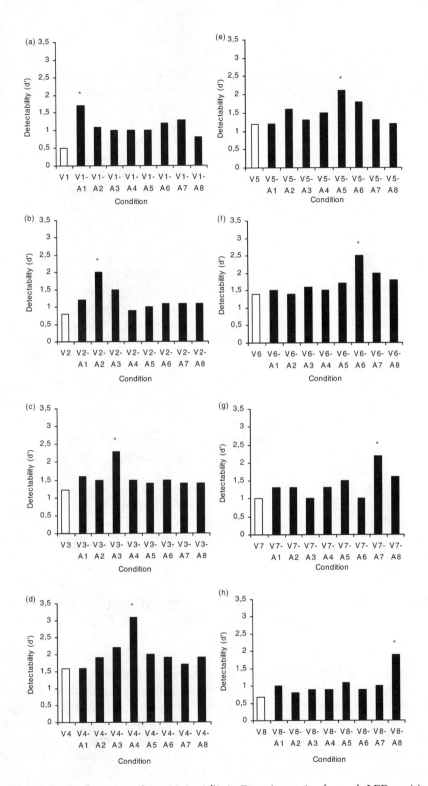

FIGURE 28.2. Means of perceptual sensitivity (d'), in Experiment 1a, for each LED position (Figure 28.2a, 28.2b, 28.2c, 28.2d, 28.2e, 28.2f, 28.2g, and 28.2h for V1, V2, V3, V4, V5, V6, V7 and V8, respectively). Dotted bars represent unimodal visual conditions; black bars represent cross-modal visual–auditory conditions; asterisks indicate significant pairwise comparisons between unimodal and cross-modal conditions. From Frassinetti, Bolognini, and Làdavas (2002). Copyright 2002 by Springer-Verlag. Reprinted by permission.

of temporally overlapping visual and acoustic stimuli in the same spatial position produced an increment of d' parameter (i.e., the ability to discern a sensory event from its background). On the contrary, analysis of response criterion (β) data showed that the presentation of an auditory cue also influenced the participants "willingness" to respond, both in Experiment 1a and 1b, but the effect was not spatially specific.

Neurophysiological studies have found that in some neurons combination of unimodal auditory and visual stimuli at some intervals (50 msec and 150 msec) produced also response enhancement (Meredith, Nemizt, & Stein, 1987; Stein & Meredith, 1993). To verify this possibility in humans, in another study we systematically varied the temporal interval (0, 100, 200, 300, 400, and 500 msec) between the visual and the acoustic stimuli as well as the spatial disparity (0, 16, and 32 degrees) (Bolognini, Frassinetti, & Làdavas, 2004).

The results replicated previous findings, that is, the existence of the audiovisual integrated system and the relevance of spatiotemporal correlation for the integration of the auditory and visual modalities. In particular, we have shown that an auditory stimulus presented at one spatial location facilitates responses to a visual target at that location. Instead, when the auditory stimulus was presented at a spatial disparity of 16 degrees or 32 degrees from the visual stimulus, the detectability of the visual stimulus did not improve. Moreover, the capacity of an acoustic stimulus to enhance the detectability of a visual stimulus depends on the temporal lag between the two events. A visuoperceptual enhancement was found when the two stimuli were presented simultaneously. By contrast, when the acoustic stimulus preceded the visual stimulus of 100 to 500 msec the improvement was not found. In addition, at an interval of 500 msec, visual and acoustic stimuli presented at the same location produced a decrement of visual stimulus detectability. The findings of the present behavioral study confirms in humans the response enhancement due to the integration of the two modalities, and the behavioral effect of the response depression when the temporal interval between the two stimuli was 500 msec. Thus, the combination of spatially and temporally coincident audiovisual stimuli can enhance visual stimulus detection, whereas spatially and/or temporally disparate stimuli can depress response to visual stimulus. These results on normal subjects can be considered evidence of the existence of an integrated acoustic–visual system in humans.

CROSS-MODAL INTEGRATION BETWEEN AUDITION AND VISION IN PATIENTS WITH VISUAL NEGLECT

As already said, another way to explore whether the neurophysiological principles found in animal studies occur also in humans is to study cross-modal effect in patients with impairments in visual modality. Patients with neglect fail to report, respond, or orient to visual stimuli presented contralaterally to the lesioned hemisphere, usually the right hemisphere (for review, see Karnath, Milner, & Vallar, 2002). In the most severe cases, they miss the objects on the left side of the environment, do not interact with people when they are on the left side of the room, and do not even eat the part of meal on the left side of the plate. In addition to the visuospatial deficit, they show an impairment of auditory space perception (Pavani, Làdavas, & Driver, 2003; Pavani, Meneghello, & Làdavas, 2001) as revealed by their inability to discriminate the relative spatial positions of sound presented in the contralesional space. In contrast, their performance is comparable to that of normals when the acoustic stimuli are presented in the ipsilesional space. Because patients with neglect present impairments in both visual and acoustic spatial representations, they seems to be the best candidates to show a beneficial effect of "bimodal" stimulation. The integration of visual and auditory information can potentially enable patients to detect "bimodal" stimuli for which unimodal components are below behavioral threshold. It is worthwhile to remember that according to the inverse effectiveness rule, a greater enhancement of neuron activity is obtained when two weak rather than two potent stimuli are combined.

Therefore, in a recent study we tried to verify whether bimodal presentation of auditory and visual stimuli could improve visual stimulus detection in patients with visual neglect (Frassinetti, Pavani, & Làdavas, 2002). Moreover, consistent with the expectation based on the electrophysiological studies, the magnitude of facilitation was varied with the degree of spatial and temporal correspondence between the acoustic and the visual stimulus. Toward this goal, patients were asked to fixate a central stimulus and to detect visual stimuli horizontally displayed at 8, 24, and 40 degrees, in the LVF as well as in the RVF.

The task was performed either in a unimodal condition (i.e., only visual stimuli were presented) or in cross-modal conditions (i.e., a sound was presented simultaneous to the visual target). In the cross-modal conditions, sounds could be presented either at the same spatial position as the visual target or at one of the remaining five spatial positions. Patients were instructed to detect the presence of visual stimuli (light) and ignore auditory stimuli.

The results of this study showed an improvement of visual stimulus detection in the cross-modal conditions as compared to the unimodal condition. Indeed, acoustic stimuli produced a great increase of visual responses when the two stimuli were spatially coincident, or when they were located near one another in space, at a distance of 16 degrees. In contrast, when the spatial disparity between the two sensory stimuli was larger than 16 degrees, patients' visual performance remained unvaried. Crucially, this pattern of results was particularly evident for the most peripheral stimuli in the LVF where neglect was more severe (see Figure 28.3a and 28.3b).

In contrast, for less peripheral stimuli where neglect was less severe, we were not able to find specific spatial effect (see Figure 28.3c), in accordance with the inverse effectiveness rule, which predicts a greater enhancement when two weak rather than two potent different sensory stimuli are combined. In fact, in animal work (Meredith & Stein, 1986a), the enhancement of correct responses with combined stimuli was observed when single-modality stimuli evoked a poor performance. Visually responsive multisensory neurons show proportionately greater response enhancement with subthreshold (not reported) stimuli and the superadditive feature of this type of interaction reached its extreme when unimodal stimuli were rarely or never responded to.

The finding that an amelioration of neglect is observable only when the two stimuli are presented at the same position, or at a small disparity, cannot be explained as a result of an arousal phenomenon; that is, the presence of two stimuli, instead of one, might have produced greater activity throughout the brain by generally increasing neural sensitivity to all stimuli. Recently, Robertson, Mattingley, Rorden, and Driver (1998) have suggested that nonspatial phasic alerting events (e.g., warning tones) can overcome a neglect patients' spatial bias in visual perceptual awareness. In that study, however, at variance with our results, the beneficial effect of sound on visual perception was not spatially specific. The acceleration of perceptual events on the contralesional side was found both when the warning sound was presented on the left or the right side of space. However, such an arousal effect cannot *alone* explain the pattern of results found in our study (Frassinetti, Pavaini, & Làdavas, 2002b), because by varying the positions of different sensory stimuli and evaluating their effects on visual detection, we found an improvement only when the stimuli followed a rather clear-cut spatial rule.

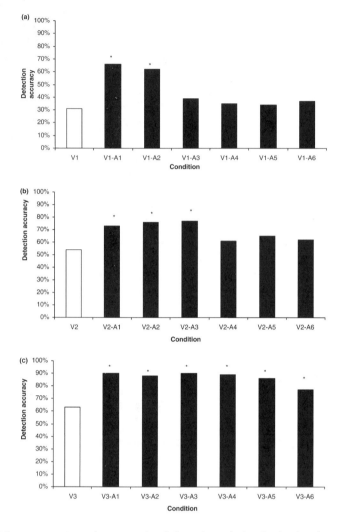

FIGURE 28.3. Mean percentage of correct visual detection of visual stimulus for each LED position in LVF (Figure 28.3a, 28.3b, and 28.3c for V1, V2, and V3, respectively). Dotted bars represent unimodal visual conditions; black bars represent cross-modal auditory–visual conditions; asterisks indicate significant pairwise comparisons between unimodal and cross-modal conditions. From Frassinetti, Pavani, and Làdavas (2002). Copyright 2002 by Springer-Verlag. Adapted by permission.

Thus, the results on neglect patients confirm those obtained on normal subjects under visual subthreshold presentation with the exception of the spatial extension of the beneficial effect of bimodal presentation. In normal subjects, the enhancement of visual responses was found only when the two stimuli were presented on the same position, whereas the amelioration of neglect was observable also at a disparity of 16 degrees. This can be explaining by considering that the angular distance that can separate visual and auditory stimuli and still result in a facilitatory effect depends on the size of the visual and auditory receptive fields. Auditory receptive fields are larger than visual receptive fields (Jay & Sparks, 1987; King & Hutchings, 1987; King & Palmer, 1983; Knudsen, 1982; Middlebrooks & Knudsen, 1984) and, as a consequence, the auditory stimulus will excite neurons over a large region, including the region excited by the visual stimulus. It seems that the functional organization of the auditory and visual fields is enhanced when two single modalities have being damaged by the lesion, as in the case of patients with neglect. Instead, in normal subjects, where only the visual information was rendered less salient, the effect manifest itself only in the condition in which it is expected the maximum of enhancement (i.e., when the stimuli are presented in the "best area" of stimulation).

In conclusion, the results show that the spatially specific combination of auditory and visual stimuli produces an improvement in visual detection accuracy. This beneficial effect is observable only when two multisensory stimuli are presented; by contrast, the occurrence of two unimodal stimuli (i.e., a visual cue followed by a visual target), although presented in the same spatial position, does not produce in an amelioration of visual detection in patients with visual neglect (Làdavas, Carletti, & Gori, 1994). In this study, where a left exogenous noninformative visual cue was presented in the impaired visual field immediately before the visual target, an amelioration of performance in LVF target detection was not found.

Recently, attention has been devoted to the possible neural bases for these and other cross-modal phenomena (Stein, Laurenti, Wallace, & Stanford, 2003). The results of these studies suggest that although a characteristic property of many superior colliculus neurons is their ability to integrate information from different sensory modalities (Stein & Meredith, 1993), the capability to synthesize cross-modal inputs, and thereby produce an enhanced multisensory response, requires functional inputs from cortex.

The possible role of cortex in multisensory integration was recently demonstrated by neurophysiological (Jiang, Wallace, Jiang, Vaughan, & Stein, 2001) and behavioral studies (Jang, Jang, & Stein, 2002; Wilkinson, Meredith, & Stein, 1996) in animals and by using functional magnetic resonance imaging, magnetoencephalographic, and event-related potential techniques in humans (e.g., Calvert, Campbell, & Brammer, 2000; Calvert et al., 1999; Giard & Peronnet, 1999; McDonald, Wolfgang, Teder-Salerjarvi, Di Russo, & Hillyard, 2003). For example, it has been shown that in cat the deactivation of two adjacent "polysensory" cortical areas, AES (anterior ectosylvian sulcus) and rLS (rostral aspect of the lateral suprasylvian sulcus) eliminated the synthesized multisensory responses of nearly all SC neurons and rendered their multisensory responses indistinguishable from those of their nonintegrative counterparts (Jiang et al., 2001).

Besides studies that have demonstrated that "polisensory" areas of cortex are involved in multisensory integration, there is also evidence suggesting that "sensory specific" cortices, such as visual and auditory cortex, may also be involved in cross-modal integration (Calvert et al., 1999; Giard & Peronnet, 1999).

Thus, according to these studies, no cross-modal effects are expected in patients with a cerebral lesion which involves the visual cortex or areas which project to visual cortex—for example, patients with visual field deficit (e.g., hemianopia). To test this hypothesis, an experiment was conducted (Frassinetti, Bottari, Bonora, & Làdavas, 2004), by using a similar paradigm as one used in previous study (Frassinetti, Pavani, & Làdavas, 2002) in two groups of patients: patients with visual neglect with hemianopia and patients with visual neglect without hemianopia.

Cross-modal integration effects similar to those already described were observed only in patients with visual neglect without hemianopia. By contrast, in patients with visual neglect with hemianopia, no improvement was observed in a cross-modal as compared to a unimodal visual condition. Therefore, it seems likely that in patients with visual neglect and hemianopia, audiovisual integration did not occur because a primary visual deficit was associated with visual neglect. A possible explanation of this finding is that lesion location plays an important causal role for cross-modal effects' manifestations.

It is worthwhile to emphasize that in this study the paraventricular occipital area (O06) was involved by the lesion in all patients with visual neglect and hemianopia whereas the same area was only *partially* lesioned in some patients with visual neglect without hemianopia. A lesion of this paraventricular area can damage the optical radiations crossing this area and projecting to the visual cortex, which plays both a direct and an indirect, SC-mediated role in the visuoacustic integrative effects. Thus, a reduction of visual cortex activation also disrupt SC visuoacustic synthesis that, in turn, disables SC-mediated multisensory orientation behaviors.

To understand more deeply the functional relationship between cross-modal integration effects and cerebral structures mediating these effects, it is important to study more extensively the anatomical and physiological characteristics of these damaged areas and their correlations with the behavioral responses of patients with and without visual field deficit.

In conclusion, taken together these results considerably extend our knowledge about the multisensory integration, by showing the existence of an integrated visuoauditory system in humans. Moreover, they document the importance of multisensory integrated systems in the construction of the spatial representation and in the recovery of related disorders, such as visual neglect. In the future, it would be very interesting to verify whether the short-term neglect improvement described in this chapter could be converted into long-term therapeutic improvement. This procedure, based on bottom-up mechanisms, seems to be very promising because it does not require patients' awareness of their difficulties and the capacity to voluntarily maintain attention oriented to the affected field (Làdavas, Menghini, & Umiltà, 1994; Pizzamiglio et al., 1992), which, in everyday life, may result to be difficult for patients with visual neglect.

REFERENCES

Bolognini, N., Frassinetti, F., & Làdavas, E. (2004). *Acoustical vision of below threshold stimuli! Interaction among spatially converging audiovisual inputs.* Manuscript submitted for publication.

Calvert, G. A., Brammer, M. J., Bullmore, E. T., Campbell, R., Iversen, S. D., & David, A. S. (1999). Response amplification in sensory-specific cortices during crossmodal binding. *Neuroreport, 10,* 2619–2623.

Calvert, G. A., Campbell, R., & Brammer, M. J. (2000). Evidence from functional magnetic resonance imaging of crossmodal binding in the human heteromodal cortex. *Current Biology, 10,* 649–657.

Driver, J., & Spence, C. (1998). Crossmodal attention. *Current Opinion in Neurobiology, 8,* 245–253.

Francesca, F., Bottari, D., Bonora, A., & Làdavas, E. (2004). *Effects of hemianopia on audio-visual integration of neglect patients.* Manuscript submitted for publication.

Frassinetti, F., Bolognini, N., & Làdavas, E. (2002). Enhancement of visual perception by crossmodal visuo-auditory interaction. *Experimental Brain Research, 147*(3), 332–343.

Frassinetti, F., Pavani, F., & Làdavas, E. (2002). Acoustic vision of neglected stimuli: Interaction among spatially converging audiovisual inputs in neglect patients. *Journal of Cognitive Neuroscience, 14*(1), 62–64.

Giard, M. H., & Peronnet, F. (1999). Auditory-visual integration during multimodal object recognition in humans: A behavioral and electrophysiological study. *Journal of Cognitive Neuroscience, 11,* 473–490.

Jay, M. F., & Sparks, D. L. (1987). Sensorimotor integration in the primate superior colliculus. II. Coordinates of auditory signals. *Journal of Neurophysiology, 57*, 35–55.

Jiang, W., Jiang, H., & Stein, B. E. (2002). Two corticotectal areas facilitate multisensory orientation behavior. *Journal of Cognitive Neuroscience, 14*(8), 1240–1255.

Jiang, W., Wallace, M. T., Jiang, H., Vaughan, J. W., & Stein, B. E. (2001). Two cortical areas mediate multisensory integration in superior colliculus neurons. *Journal of Neurophysiology, 85*(2), 506–522.

Karnath, H. O., Milner, A. D., & Vallar, G. (Eds). (2002). *Cognitive and neural bases of spatial neglect.* Oxford, UK: Oxford University Press.

King, A. J., & Hutchings, M. E. (1987). Spatial response property of acoustically responsive neurons in the superior colliculus of the ferret: A map of auditory space. *Journal of Neurophysiology, 57*, 596–624.

King, A. J., & Palmer, A. R. (1985). Spatial response proprieties of visual and auditory information in bimodal neurons in the guinea-pig superior colliculus. *Experimental Brain Research, 60*, 492–500.

Knudsen, E. I. (1982). Auditory and visual maps of space in the optic tectum of the owl. *Neuroscience, 2*, 1177–94.

Làdavas, E. (2002). Functional and dynamic properties of visual peripersonal space. *Trends in Cognitive Sciences, 6*(1), 17–22.

Làdavas, E., Berti, A., & Farnè, A. (2000). Dissociation between conscious and non-conscious processing in neglect. In Y. Rossetti & A. Revonsuo (Eds.), *Interaction between dissociated implicit and explicit processing.* Amsterdam/Philadelphia: John Benjamins.

Làdavas, E., Carletti, M., & Gori, G. (1994). Automatic and voluntary orienting of attention in patients with visual neglect: Horizontal and vertical dimensions. *Neuropsychologia, 32*(10), 1195–1208.

Làdavas, E., Menghini, G., & Umiltà, C. (1994). A rehabilitation study of hemispatial neglect. *Cognitive Neuropsychology, 11*, 75–95.

Macaluso, E., Frith, C., & Driver, J. (2001). Multisensory integration and crossmodal attention effects in the human brain. *Science, 292*, 1791a.

McDonald, J. J., Teder-Salerjarvi, W. A., & Hillyard, S. A. (2000). Involuntary orienting to a sound improves visual perception. *Nature, 407*, 906–908.

McDonald, J. J., Wolfgang, A., Teder-Salerjarvi, W. A., Di Russo, F., & Hillyard, S. A. (2003). Neural substrates of perceptual enhancement by crossmodal spatial attention. *Journal of Cognitive Neuroscience, 15*(1), 10–19.

McGurk, H., & MacDonald, J. (1976). Visual influences on speech perception processes. *Perception and Psychophysics, 24*, 253–257.

Meredith, M. A., Nemitz, J. W., & Stein, B. E. (1987). Determinants of multisensory integration in superior colliculus neurons. I. Temporal factors. *Journal of Neuroscience, 10*, 3215–3229.

Meredith, M. A., & Stein, B. E. (1986a). Spatial factors determine the activity of multisensory neurons in cat superior colliculus. *Brain Research, 365*, 350–354.

Meredith, M. A., & Stein, B. E. (1986b). Visual, auditory and somatosensory convergence on cells in superior colliculus results in multisensory integration. *Journal of Neurophysiology, 56*, 640–662.

Middlebrooks, J. C., & Knudsen, E. I. (1984). A neural code for auditory space in the cat's superior colliculus. *Journal of Neuroscience, 4*, 2621–34.

Pavani, F., Làdavas, E., & Driver J. (2003). Auditory and multisensory aspects of visual spatial neglect. *Trend in Cognitive Neurosciences, 7*, 407–414.

Pavani, F., Meneghello, F., & Làdavas, E. (2001). Deficit of auditory space perception in patients with visuospatial neglect. *Neuropsychologia, 39*, 1401–1409.

Pizzamiglio, L., Antonucci, G., Judica, A., Montenero, P., Razzano, C., & Zoccolotti, P. (1992). Cognitive rehabilitation of the hemineglect disorders in chronic patients with unilateral brain damage. *Journal of Clinical Experimental Neuropsychology, 14*, 901–923.

Robertson, I. H., Mattingley, J. B., Rorden, C., & Driver, J. (1998). Phasic alerting of neglect patients overcomes their spatial deficit in visual awareness. *Nature, 395*, 169–172.

Spence, C., & Driver, J. (1997). Audiovisual links in exogenous covert spatial orienting. *Perception and Psychophysics, 59*(1), 1–22.

Stein, B. E., Laurienti, P. J., Wallace, M. T., & Stanford, T. R. (2003). Multisensory integration. In V. S. Ramachandran (Ed.), *Encyclopedia of the human brain.* New York: Academic Press.

Stein, B. E., & Meredith, M. A. (1993). *Merging of the senses.* Cambridge, MA: MIT Press.

Sumby, W. H., & Pollack, I. (1954). Visual contribution to speech intelligibility in noise. *Journal of the Acoustical Society of America, 26,* 212–215.

Wilkinson, L. K., Meredith, M. A., & Stein, B. E. (1996). The role of anterior ectosylvian cortex in cross-modality orientation and approach behavior. *Experimental Brain Research, 112,* 1–10.

29

Focusing on the Anterior Cingulate Cortex

Effects of Focal Lesions on Cognitive Performance

Diane Swick and And U. Turken

Attentional control over behavior is important for flexible and adaptive responding in a complex environment. Automatic, habitual responses are inadequate during situations in which multiple goals and sources of information must be maintained simultaneously, such as during planning and decision making, the avoidance and correction of erroneous responses, novel responding, and the resolution of conflict. These executive control functions, as assessed by neuropsychological tests, are often compromised in individuals with injuries in the frontal lobes (Stuss & Alexander, 2000). The lateral prefrontal cortex (PFC) is thought to play a critical role in executive control processes by exerting top-down influences over other brain regions involved in sensory and motor processing (Miller & Cohen, 2001).

In addition, neuroimaging investigations have highlighted the importance of the anterior cingulate cortex (ACC). Positron emission tomography (PET) and functional magnetic resonance imaging (fMRI) experiments have detected enhanced neural activity in the ACC during the performance of tasks that demand high levels of attentional control (Bush, Luu, & Posner, 2000). The ACC is densely interconnected with other frontal lobe regions, especially the mid-dorsolateral PFC, as well as parietal and motor cortices (Bates & Goldman-Rakic, 1993; Dum & Strick, 1993; Vogt & Pandya, 1987). Meta-analyses of multiple neuroimaging studies have shown that ACC and lateral PFC are coactive in demanding task conditions (Duncan & Owen, 2000; Koski & Paus, 2000). These observations have prompted the suggestion that the ACC is a key component of the neural mechanisms that mediate executive control over thought and behavior (Posner, 1994; Posner & Petersen, 1990). Anatomical and physiological abnormalities in the ACC have been observed in disorders ranging from schizophrenia and Parkinson's disease to clinical depression and obsessive–compulsive disorder. Theoretical accounts of the symptoms in these conditions all indicate a critical role for the ACC in brain function (Benes, 2000; Frith, 1992; Mayberg, 1997), which has yet to be elucidated in a specific manner.

Studying the effects of neurological damage is a powerful method of investigating brain function in humans. By detailing the abilities that are spared and compromised after focal injury to a specific brain area, conclusions can be reached about the role of that region. Further, the functional significance of results from neuroimaging studies can be tested directly in neuropsychological experiments. There have been relatively few reports of focal ACC lesions (e.g., Cohen et al., 1999; Corkin, Twitchell, & Sullivan, 1979; Danckert et al., 2000; Janer & Pardo, 1991; Ochsner et al., 2001), due to the rare occurrence of isolated lesions to this region. Most studies have tested patients who underwent cingulotomy, a psychosurgical procedure occasionally performed on individuals with psychiatric disorders or chronic pain. The occurrence of preexisting, severe, and intractable psychiatric illnesses complicates the interpretation of results in these individuals.

We have tested two patients with focal ACC lesions in a series of experimental tasks designed to assess high-level attentional control over perceptual, cognitive, and motor processes, in the sense originally defined by Norman and Shallice (1986). Our objectives were to investigate the nature of ACC involvement in the control of attention, and to test the validity of conclusions drawn from neuroimaging findings. Patient R.N., a 69-year-old right-handed male, has a left-hemisphere lesion extending from rostral ACC (around the genu of the corpus callosum) to mid-ACC (Figure 29.1A, 29.1B) due to occlusion of the pericallosal

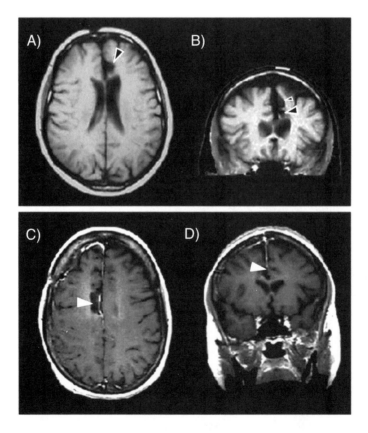

FIGURE 29.1. MRI scans showing the lesions of patient R.N. (A, B) and patient D.L. (C, D). (A) Horizontal section illustrating the lesion in left ACC (black arrowhead). (B) Coronal section with ACC damage. The larger arrowhead shows the damage in the cingulate sulcus, while the smaller arrowhead above it indicates the lesion in the paracingulate sulcus. (C) Horizontal section at the level of the cingulate sulcus. The damaged area in the right hemisphere is indicated by a white arrowhead on the left side of the scan. (D) Coronal section of caudal ACC illustrating the lesion in the cingulate sulcus, while the paracingulate sulcus is intact.

Patient R.N.

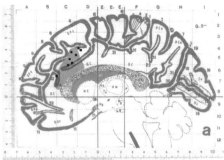

Patient D.L.

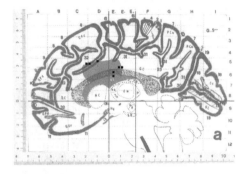

FIGURE 29.2. The sagittal extent of the lesion is represented in gray shading on the Talairach and Tournoux (1988) coordinate system for R.N. (top) and D.L. (bottom). Peaks of activation from neuro-imaging studies of conflict detection are plotted inside, or within close proximity of, the regions of damaged ACC for each patient. The activation foci for D.L.'s lesion are located in the right hemisphere or within 5 mm of the midline. For ease of comparison, R.N.'s left-hemisphere lesion is depicted on the right-hemisphere section, although all activations are located in the left hemisphere or at midline.

branch of the anterior cerebral artery. Patient D.L. is a 35-year-old right-handed female who had a tumor resected from the right ACC. The resulting lesion extends from the mid- to caudal portion of the ACC (Figure 29.1C, 29.1D). Many foci of activation from neuroimaging studies are located within R.N.'s or D.L.'s lesions (Figure 29.2). Behavioral testing in these patients can be informative about the necessity of the ACC for particular executive control functions, and event-related potential (ERP) recordings can enrich our understanding of the temporal parameters underlying any attentional deficits that might be observed. Scalp-recorded ERPs have excellent temporal resolution, but their spatial resolution is relatively poor. However, the plausible neural generators for a given ERP component can be constrained if it is absent or altered in patients with focal brain lesions (Swick & Knight, 1998). Such an approach can also speak to the question whether the contribution of ACC to attentional control occurs only in later stages of performance or if it extends to the sensory domain as well.

Specifically, we sought to investigate whether an intact ACC is necessary to carry out individual cognitive control functions such as conflict detection, error monitoring, response selection, and/or task switching, or whether the ACC subserves a more general control function that can be defined as "responsiveness to task difficulty." In addition, we used the divergence in lesion location in the two patients to test whether anatomical specificity of function can be demonstrated. If the ACC is a nodal point for the large-scale attentional networks in the frontal lobes, then focal ACC damage should result in performance deficits in multiple task domains. If the ACC contributes to some aspects of performance but not others, such dissociations would favor the view of multiple interactive processes, rather than a single control module. Also, such findings would support the notion that the ACC is a functionally heterogeneous structure (Paus, 2001) and is not likely to be the sole locus for executive control mechanisms. The functions under study here include the detection of conflict between competing response alternatives, monitoring for errors in performance, flexible adjustment of performance strategy, and switching attention between stimulus dimensions, all of which are important measures of attentional control. The chapter addresses a series of ongoing controversies in the functional neuroimaging literature over the interpretation of hemodynamic changes that occur within the ACC during the performance of specific cognitive and motor tasks.

CONFLICTS OR ERRORS?

One enduring debate about the role of the ACC in attentional control is whether conflict monitoring and error monitoring can be viewed as unitary (Carter et al., 1998, 2000) or distinct (Coles, Scheffers, & Holroyd, 2001; Falkenstein, Hoormann, Christ, & Hohnsbein, 2000) functions of the ACC. Models postulating that error monitoring can be viewed as separate from conflict monitoring are based on ERP data, although recent fMRI results have lent support to this stance as well (Braver, Barch, Gray, Molfese, & Snyder, 2001; Garavan, Ross, Kaufman, & Stein, 2003; Ullsperger & von Cramon, 2001). The error-related negativity (ERN) component of the ERP is recorded from frontocentral midline electrodes when subjects make errors in speeded reaction-time tasks (Falkenstein, Hohnsbein, Hoorman, & Blanke, 1990; Gehring, Goss, Coles, Meyer, & Donchin, 1993). The ERN is a measure of performance monitoring that seems to be independent of response conflict, because it is observed in very simple tasks without conflicting response alternatives (Falkenstein et al., 2000). Thorough reviews on the ERN, error processing, and the ACC are provided by Holroyd, Niewenhuis, Mars, and Coles (Chapter 16, this volume) and by Luu and Pederson (Chapter 17, this volume).

On the other hand, the conflict-monitoring hypothesis suggests that the primary function of the ACC's cognitive subdivision (as defined by Devinsky, Morrell, & Vogt, 1995) is to detect response conflict, based on imaging results during tasks such as divided attention (Corbetta, Miezin, Dobmeyer, Shulman, & Petersen, 1991), flanker interference (Botvinick, Nystrom, Fissell, Carter, & Cohen, 1999), and the color–word Stroop interference task (Carter et al., 2000; Milham et al., 2002; Pardo, Pardo, Janer, & Raichle, 1990). One such study used the continuous performance test and observed that the same region of dorsal ACC showed increases in activity during error trials as well as correct trials with high levels of conflict (Carter et al., 1998). Because mistakes are more likely to occur when competing response tendencies must be resolved, errors are considered to be a subset of conflict-monitoring processes in this model.

Lesion studies can help to adjudicate between these alternative views. The lesion in Patient R.N. is located in the dorsal ACC region implicated in conflict detection (Carter et al., 1998), with the rostral-most extent impinging upon the affective subdivision, which has been linked to error processing (Bush et al., 2000). The damage in Patient D.L. is more caudally located and includes the caudal cingulate motor area (CMA) involved in controlling

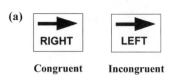

(a)

RIGHT   LEFT

Congruent   Incongruent

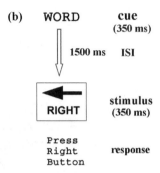

(b)   WORD   cue
(350 ms)

1500 ms   ISI

RIGHT   stimulus
(350 ms)

Press
Right   response
Button

FIGURE 29.3. (a) Examples of the stimuli used in the word–arrow Stroop task. The word and the arrow indicated the same response on congruent trials and the opposite response on incongruent trials. In the blocked version, subjects responded to either the word or the arrow by giving a vocal or a manual response. These four conditions were administered in separate blocks. (b) In the switching version used in the ERP study, only manual responses were given. The attended stimulus dimension was cued on each trial by presentation of the cue word ("arrow" or "word") for 350 msec, followed 1,500 msec later by the word–arrow stimulus display.

the selection of manual responses (Paus, Petrides, Evans, & Meyer, 1993). A recent ERP study tested whether error-related and conflict-related activity within the ACC are separable phenomena (Swick & Turken, 2002). The experiment used a word–arrow variant of the Stroop conflict paradigm designed to investigate the relationship between response modality (manual or vocal) and the compatibility between stimuli and responses (Baldo, Shimamura, & Prinzmetal, 1998). We modified the original design, in which subjects attended to words or arrows in separate blocks, to a switching version, in which the attended stimulus dimension (word or arrow) was cued on each trial (Figure 29.3). First, we examined the status of error monitoring by asking whether the ERN component on incorrect trials, and subsequent compensatory behaviors, were impaired in R.N. Second, we examined whether the N2 component, related to the detection of competing response tendencies (Kopp, Rist, & Mattler, 1996), was diminished, as predicted by the conflict-monitoring hypothesis (Carter et al., 2000). If not, this would suggest that ACC activations might not reflect activity that is strictly time-locked to conflict detection processes.

Figure 29.4A illustrates that control subjects generated a negative potential (the ERN) in the ERP recordings for error trials, which was greater than the response for correct trials. The ERN peaked at ~65 msec after incorrect responses and was largest at the frontocentral midline electrodes (FCz, Cz). In the stimulus-locked ERP averages, controls generated a potential (the N2) that was more negative-going for correct conflict trials than for correct congruent trials (Figure 29.4B). The onset of the N2 component was at ~350 msec and its peak at 450 msec poststimulus. R.N. showed a dissociation between ERPs related to conflict and error processing. Figure 29.4B illustrates that the amplitude of his N2 component to correct incongruent stimuli was enhanced relative to controls. By contrast, R.N. exhibited a reduction in the amplitude of the ERN component to incorrect responses, such that it did not differ from the "correct-related negativity" (or CRN) for accurate responses (Figure 29.4A). Thus, R.N. did not show a difference between response-locked ERP activity on correct and incorrect trials. In addition, R.N. showed a deficit in correcting his erroneous responses, 78% corrected versus 88% for controls.

One viewpoint about action-monitoring processes is that the CRN may signal the outcome of a general, response-related monitoring process, and the ERN reflects this generic monitoring process plus error-specific activity (Ford, 1999). If this is the case, ACC damage eliminated the error-specific activity in R.N. (reduced ERN) but spared the general monitoring process (intact CRN). Some fMRI studies (Kiehl, Liddle, & Hopfinger, 2000; Menon, Adleman, White, Glover, & Reiss, 2001) have reported error-related activity in the ACC that is rostral to the cognitive subdivision. In addition, recent studies have linked the ERN to negative affective responses (Luu, Collins, & Tucker, 2000) and to financial loss in a gambling task (Gehring & Willoughby, 2002). If R.N. showed a dampened affective response to errors, his motivation to self-correct could have been reduced. Because the more rostral and ventral ACC regions are considered part of the affective subdivision, the ERN may largely reflect emotional processing rather than a cognitive operation. This interpretation is supported by the abolition of all ERN activity in patients with lesions of ventromedial PFC that included ventral ACC (Swick et al., 2001).

Along with the enhancement of conflict-detection processes as measured by the N2, R.N.'s behavioral performance in the Stroop task was impaired. He showed elevated interference effects and lower accuracy relative to controls. One explanation for these findings is that R.N. has an impairment in engaging the control processes that reduce the effects of response conflict. It appears that intact brain regions detected the conflict at the same time as controls, as indicated by N2 onset latency, but were recruited for prolonged evaluation and conflict-resolution processes. This observation, combined with his exaggerated behavioral interference effects, suggest a deficit in the recruitment of inhibitory processes under difficult task conditions. We hypothesize that intact regions in lateral PFC and the basal ganglia (BG) are able to represent stimulus–response mappings and detect response conflict, but damage to the dorsal ACC renders him impaired in response inhibition, which may be due to disconnection from cingulate and supplementary motor areas (SMA). Our findings are consistent

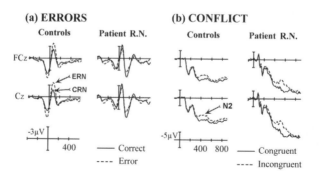

FIGURE 29.4. Dissociation of error-related and conflict-related ERPs in R.N. (a) The ERN and CRN in the response-locked waves at frontocentral midline electrodes (FCz and Cz). Response onset occurs at the vertical bar (time = 0 msec), tic marks are 200 msec, and negative is plotted upward. (b) ERPs related to conflict (N2) in the stimulus-locked waves at FCz and Cz. Stimulus onset occurs at the vertical bar (time = 0 msec).

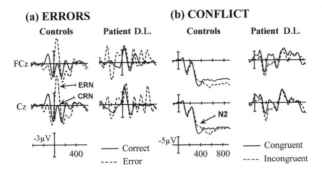

(a) ERRORS **(b) CONFLICT**

FIGURE 29.5. Caudal ACC lesion resulted in reduction of both (a) ERN and (b) N2 in patient D.L. relative to age-matched controls. Details as in Figure 29.4.

with the proposal that PFC and BG detect incompatible response options on incongruent trials and signal conflict-resolution processes, perhaps in caudal ACC and SMA.

Preliminary data from patient D.L. (Swick & Turken, 2004), with damage in the right caudal ACC, revealed a diminution of both ERN and N2 relative to age-matched controls (Figure 29.5). This is supportive of the view that these processes do overlap to some extent but are not entirely co-localized within the ACC (Ullsperger & von Cramon, 2001). Thus, the scalp-recorded ERN is influenced by neural generators in both perigenual ACC extending dorsally into Brodmann area 32 as well as in mid-to-caudal ACC. Conversely, N2 amplitude was diminished only by caudal ACC damage. Previous behavioral results in D.L. demonstrated that she showed significant performance decrements when giving manual responses in the word–arrow Stroop task (Turken & Swick, 1999). However, her performance was comparable to controls when giving vocal responses, even when arbitrary response mappings were used, suggesting that her executive control functions were intact. Those findings demonstrated that caudal ACC is not critical for attentional control processes, because D.L. could produce the correct decisions in each task. Rather, this region is important for manual response control. Taken together, these results support a somatotopic organization of the ACC based on response modality (Paus et al., 1993; Picard & Strick, 1996) and provide neuropsychological evidence for functional specialization within the human ACC.

CONFLICT OR CONTROL?

The N2 results in R.N. indicate that the dorsal ACC does not generate conflict-related activity that occurs prior to the behavioral response. Nevertheless, numerous imaging studies have observed increased ACC activity during incongruent conditions of the Stroop task (reviewed in MacLeod & MacDonald, 2000). The conflict-monitoring hypothesis suggests that the ACC detects response conflict, then signals the dorsolateral PFC to implement the control functions (MacDonald, Cohen, Stenger, & Carter, 2000), such as greater focusing of attention. On the other hand, the executive control view maintains that ACC implements control under difficult conditions where routine behavior must be suppressed (Posner & DiGirolamo, 1998). One missing link is when, exactly, the ACC comes online to implement this control (or to signal other regions to do so).

To evaluate the *necessity* of ACC for conflict detection and attentional control processes, the ACC patients were tested on three versions of the color–word Stroop task with vocal responses (Swick & Jovanovic, 2002). Although many foci of activation from neuro-imaging studies are located within D.L.'s and R.N.'s lesions (Figure 29.2), prior findings of regional specialization within ACC (Turken & Swick, 1999) led us to predict different results in the two patients. In one experiment, mixed blocks of trials (congruent, neutral, incongruent) alternated with uniform blocks of either all congruent or all incongruent trials. The third version was modeled after the study of Carter and colleagues (2000), in which the probabilities of congruent and incongruent trials were manipulated from block to block. This design varied the level of response conflict (high in blocks with mostly congruent trials; low in blocks with mostly incongruent trials) and the degree to which executive control processes were engaged (low in mostly congruent blocks; high in mostly incongruent blocks).

Results in D.L. indicated that damage to caudal ACC was not associated with excessive interference effects for vocal responses, in accord with previous results (Turken & Swick, 1999). Furthermore, her interference was not modulated by the probability manipulation: D.L. exhibited less interference than controls in the high-conflict condition, suggesting equivalently high levels of cognitive control in both conditions. Conversely, damage to dorsal ACC resulted in consistently lower accuracy on incongruent trials, indicating that R.N. showed a deficit in inhibiting the automatic response. R.N. also showed greater interference than did controls in the low-conflict condition, suggesting that dorsal ACC implements the strategic processes engaged here to reduce conflict (Posner, 1994). Thus, subregions of ACC appear to have separable functions, with the caudal area involved in high-level motor control for manual responses and the more rostral and dorsal regions involved in conflict-resolution and attentional-control processes under difficult task conditions.

RESPONSE CONFLICT OR TASK DIFFICULTY?

Another unresolved issue is whether the rubric of "response conflict" is able to account for the totality of the ACC literature, or whether a more general idea such as "task difficulty" is a better fit to the data. In the next experiment, the Eriksen flanker task was used to further investigate selective attention and response competition. In this task, subjects are slower to respond when a central target letter is surrounded by incongruent flanker letters than if the flankers are congruent or neutral (Eriksen & Eriksen, 1974). Neither D.L. nor R.N. showed an increase in flanker interference relative to their age-matched control groups (Turken, 2000). An additional analysis was performed to investigate the effects of the preceding stimulus on the current response. The Gratton effect (Gratton, Coles, & Donchin, 1992) is a reduction in the behavioral costs of interference after response conflict on the previous trial, presumably due to an adjustment in performance strategy, where more weight is put into top-down control processes. For controls, the standard Gratton effect was obtained: Flanker interference was reduced if the preceding trial was incongruent. D.L. showed increased interference when responding with the left (contralesional) hand to incongruent stimuli preceded by a congruent stimulus trial. This suggests that D.L. has compromised control over motor response conflicts, possibly expressed more strongly on the contralesional side, as would be expected from the fact that her lesion includes the caudal CMA region implicated in manual response control (Paus et al., 1993). This is also consistent with our previous report with this patient (Turken & Swick, 1999). That she showed the Gratton effect has two consequences. First, it suggests that she is capable of using strategic control processes to compensate for the effect of her lesion on motor response control. Second, it indicates the caudal CMA is not likely to be the source of the warning signal that would trigger a high-level control process by the lateral PFC.

In contrast, R.N.'s performance was comparable to his controls'. He showed normal interference and Gratton effects in the flanker task, which would argue against a deficit in either manual response control or flexible adjustment of performance strategy. How do we reconcile these seemingly disparate findings with R.N.? He was not impaired in the Eriksen flanker task, yet he showed deficits in the classic color–word Stroop and the cued version of the word–arrow Stroop. Are there differences in the conflict operations tapped by Stroop and flanker tasks (Fan, Flombaum, McCandliss, Thomas, & Posner, 2003)? Could the general construct of "task difficulty" or the recruitment of another attentional control function account for the differences?

ATTENTIONAL SWITCHING

To pursue this latter question, we investigated mental flexibility, as indexed by the ability to switch successfully between stimulus dimensions (Swick & Turken, 2004). Here, we compared the cued word–arrow Stroop (Figure 29.3B) to a version where the attended dimension remained constant throughout a block. Overall performance in the blocked condition was compared to the condition where switches were needed randomly on a trial-by-trial basis. Furthermore, we examined whether R.N. would show large costs in terms of longer reaction times (RTs), lower accuracy, and altered ERPs on trials that require switching versus those that repeat the same attended stimulus. If so, this would suggest that the ACC is critical for switching attention between relevant stimulus dimensions, which is another executive control function.

R.N. performed better than did controls in the blocked version of the task, as he was significantly faster, more accurate, and less affected by conflicting information (Swick & Turken, 2004). Thus, the left dorsal ACC is not essential for response-selection mechanisms or for conflict-monitoring functions. In contrast, R.N. was quite impaired when the stimulus dimension was cued on each trial, requiring rapid, unpredictable switches of attention. This pattern of results suggests that dorsal ACC plays a role in inhibition of the inappropriate response under conditions that require switching between attended stimulus dimensions. In addition, R.N. exhibited exaggerated costs for RT and accuracy on switch relative to no-switch trials. He also showed a prolonged ERP effect on switch trials, lasting until 800 msec poststimulus, compared to only 400 msec poststimulus in controls. Although R.N. can execute the attend word/attend arrow tasks themselves, he cannot easily shift between the two tasks. Advance configuration of task set involves activation of an appropriate schema (Norman & Shallice, 1986) or of a task demand node (Cohen, Dunbar, & McClelland, 1990), both of which can be seen as top-down control functions. Thus, dorsal ACC does not appear to be necessary for conflict monitoring per se, but it is important for unpredictable switches of attention when the task involves response conflict. These results complement an fMRI study in which a reverse Stroop effect was induced by rapid switches between color-naming and word-reading tasks (Ruff, Woodward, Laurens, & Liddle, 2001). Other imaging experiments have reported switching-related activations which overlap with the dorsal ACC region damaged in R.N. (Dove, Pollman, Schubert, Wiggins, & von Cramon, 2000; Kimberg, Aguirre, & D'Esposito, 2000). These findings were not predicted by the conflict-monitoring hypothesis, which postulates that the dorsal ACC's domain is limited to detection of motor conflicts and not conflicts between different task sets.

A related explanation for R.N.'s discrepant performance in the blocked and cued Stroop is the idea that the ACC responds to increased levels of arousal during more cognitively demanding tasks and is recruited under conditions of greater task difficulty (Paus, Koski, Caramanos,

& Westbury, 1998). This hypothesis can also encompass R.N.'s prior results in the classic Stroop task, where he committed more errors than did controls on incongruent trials, indicating a deficit in inhibiting the prepotent word-reading response (Swick & Jovanovic, 2002). In the color–word Stroop, the irrelevant word-reading response is much more automatic than the arrow button-press response in the word–arrow experiment. This account views the dorsal ACC as a bridge between lateral PFC and ventromedial PFC regions. If lateral PFC signals that more cognitive resources need to be recruited, dorsal ACC relays the message to rostral ACC and other ventromedial regions, leading to a general increase in arousal, reflected in enhanced activity in the autonomic nervous system (Critchley et al., 2003) and in brainstem nuclei such as the locus coeruleus (Aston-Jones, Rajkowski, & Cohen, 1999). The alerted brainstem nuclei trigger an increase in cortical arousal (Foote & Morrison, 1987), which results in enhanced concentration, thus improving performance in difficult situations.

ACC, SCHIZOPHRENIA, AND ERROR MONITORING

As cited previously, a number of investigations into neurological and psychiatric disorders have indicated abnormalities in various subregions of the ACC as correlates of these conditions. As a particular example, the neuropsychological deficits associated with schizophrenia have been challenging for researchers to characterize and interpret, and a coherent theoretical framework for explaining them has only begun to evolve over recent years (Frith, 1992). Numerous studies have documented abnormalities in the ACC in patients with schizophrenia (Benes, 2000). Better characterization of how these abnormalities are related to the symptoms of schizophrenia can thus help us make advances in both schizophrenia research and the understanding of ACC function. Our recent work has aimed to follow this approach (Turken, Vuilleumier, Mathalon, Swick, & Ford, 2003). Using a specially designed task, we investigated the relation between disorders in self-monitoring, which have been proposed to be one of the key functions of ACC, and other measures of executive attention (conflict resolution, task set preparation, and task switching). A group of high-functioning patients with schizophrenia showed a specific deficit in monitoring the consequences of their actions, as assessed by their ability to correct their erroneous responses in the absence of external feedback on accuracy. This finding successfully replicated earlier reports demonstrating the same phenomenon (Frith & Done, 1989; Malenka, Angel, Hampton, & Berger, 1982). In contrast, the other measures of executive attention did not show a significant worsening of performance for the patients compared to controls. These findings have two implications. First, one of the primary effects of ACC dysfunction in schizophrenia might be specifically related to the ability to monitor self-initiated cognitive processes and actions, which is crucial for volitional activity, while possibly sparing to some extent other attention control processes. Second, and in a broader sense, such a finding provides further support for the notion that error monitoring and conflict resolution are dissociable processes with distinct neural bases.

CONCLUSIONS

As has been noted, each approach to the study of brain function has unique benefits as well as particular shortcomings. Therefore, converging evidence from parallel lines of research allow us to validate findings produced by a particular area of research and produce novel hypotheses that can be tested using a combination of the existing methods. Our research provides an example of this approach. The question whether error monitoring and conflict resolution might be related but distinct psychological processes, with emphasis on how they relate to ACC function, has primarily been motivated by ERP and functional neuroimaging findings with normal populations. In another vein, the notion that the ACC has multiple anatomically and functionally defined subregions has emerged mostly from animal research (Devinsky et al., 1995), from the analysis of its patterns of connectivity with other regions (Bates & Goldman-Rakic, 1993), and from its differential response to task manipulations and coactivation with other brain regions in neuroimaging studies (Koski & Paus, 2000). Whether ACC activations in cognitive studies reflect the execution of specific cognitive operations or a more general contribution whenever task demands increase is another question motivated by imaging studies.

One approach for future work is to combine fMRI and ERP studies in the same groups of patients to distinguish between direct and distal effects of ACC lesions. Lesions might disrupt the functioning of larger networks, rather than compromise a particular operation carried out by the damaged area itself. Whole brain imaging, together with newer approaches to network analysis, can provide clues. This approach can also reveal the mechanisms of recovery of function after brain damage.

Another tactic for further neuropsychological experimentation is the comparison of different patient groups, such as ventral ACC, dorsal ACC, and lateral PFC, to look for the existence of double dissociations. Along these lines, the use of newer structural mapping techniques, including three-dimensional reconstruction methods (Frank, Damasio, & Grabowski, 1997), diffusion-tensor imaging (Conturo et al., 1999), and voxel-based lesion-symptom mapping (Bates et al., 2003) can refine the ability to quantify and localize the brain lesions. These methods can help to determine which part of the lesion is primarily responsible for a particular behavioral deficit. The combination of anatomically precise structural MRI with ERPs will allow more accurate localization of the neural generators.

Finally, ERP and fMRI studies can be designed to test hypotheses that have emerged from our patient findings. The neuropsychological data provide support for topographic specialization of control functions within the ACC. Furthermore, the lesion results suggest that there is not a single locus for attentional control in the brain.

ACKNOWLEDGMENTS

This work was supported by Grant No. DC03424 from the National Institute on Deafness and Other Communication Disorders and No. 98-47 CNS-QUA.05 from the James S. McDonnell Foundation (Diane Swick), and by Grant No. 5 F32 NS43961-02 from the National Institutes of Health (And U. Turken). Thanks to Robert Knight and Robert Rafal for patient referrals, and Jelena Jovanovic, Jonathan Kopelovich, Jary Larsen, Kim Miller, and Caitlin Roxby for their assistance.

REFERENCES

Aston-Jones, G., Rajkowski, J., & Cohen, J. (1999). Role of locus coeruleus in attention and behavioral flexibility. *Biological Psychiatry, 46*, 1309–1320.

Baldo, J. V., Shimamura, A. P., & Prinzmetal, W. (1998). Mapping symbols to response modalities: Interference effects on Stroop-like tasks. *Perception and Psychophysics, 60*, 427–437.

Bates, E., Wilson, S. M., Saygin, A. P., Dick, F., Sereno, M. I., Knight, R. T., et al. (2003). Voxel-based lesion-symptom mapping. *Nature Neuroscience, 6*, 448–450.

Bates, J. F., & Goldman-Rakic, P. S. (1993). Prefrontal connections of medial motor areas in the rhesus monkey. *Journal of Comparative Neurology, 336,* 211–228.

Benes, F. M. (2000). Emerging principles of altered neural circuitry in schizophrenia. *Brain Research Reviews, 31,* 251–269.

Botvinick, M., Nystrom, L., Fissell, K., Carter, C. S., & Cohen, J. D. (1999). Conflict monitoring versus selection-for-action in anterior cingulate cortex. *Nature, 402,* 179–181.

Braver, T. S., Barch D. M., Gray, J. R., Molfese, D. L., & Snyder, A. (2001). Anterior cingulate cortex and response conflict: Effects of frequency, inhibition and errors. *Cerebral Cortex, 11,* 825–836.

Bush, G., Luu, P., & Posner, M. I. (2000). Cognitive and emotional influences in anterior cingulate cortex. *Trends in Cognitive Sciences, 4,* 215–222.

Carter, C. S., Braver, T. S., Barch, D. M., Botvinick, M. M., Noll, D., & Cohen, J. D. (1998). Anterior cingulate cortex, error detection, and the online monitoring of performance. *Science, 280,* 747–749.

Carter, C. S., Macdonald, A. M., Botvinick, M., Ross, L. L., Stenger, V. A., Noll, D., et al. (2000). Parsing executive processes: Strategic vs. evaluative functions of the anterior cingulate cortex. *Proceedings of the National Academy of Sciences USA, 99,* 1944–1948.

Cohen, J. D., Dunbar, K., & McClelland, J. L. (1990). On the control of automatic processes: A parallel distributed processing model of the Stroop effect. *Psychological Review, 97,* 332–361.

Cohen, R. A., Kaplan, R. F., Zuffante, P., Moser, D. J., Jenkins, M. A., Salloway, S., et al. (1999). Alteration of intention and self-initiated action associated with bilateral anterior cingulotomy. *Journal of Neuropsychology and Clinical Neuroscience, 11,* 444–453.

Coles, M. G. H., Scheffers, M. K., & Holroyd, C. B. (2001). Why is there an ERN/Ne on correct trials? Response representations, stimulus–related components, and the theory of error-processing. *Biological Psychology, 56,* 173–189.

Conturo, T. E., Lori, N. F., Cull, T. S., Akbudak, E., Snyder, A. Z., Shimony, J. S., et al. (1999). Tracking neuronal fiber pathways in the living human brain. *Proceedings of the National Academy of Sciences USA, 96,* 10422–10427.

Corbetta, M., Miezin, F. M., Dobmeyer, S., Shulman, G. L., & Petersen, S. E. (1991). Selective and divided attention during visual discriminations of shape, color, and speed: Functional anatomy by positron emission tomography. *Journal of Neuroscience, 11,* 2383–2402.

Corkin, S., Twitchell, T. E., & Sullivan, E. V. (1979). Safety and efficacy of cingulotomy for pain and psychiatric disorders. In E. R. Hitchcock, H. T. Ballantine, Jr., & B. A. Meyerson (Eds.), *Modern concepts in psychiatric surgery* (pp. 253–271). New York: Elsevier.

Critchley, H. D., Mathias, C. J., Josephs, O., O'Doherty, J., Zanini, S., Dewar, B.-K., et al. (2003). Human cingulate cortex and autonomic control: Converging neuroimaging and clinical evidence. *Brain, 126,* 2139–2152.

Danckert, J., Maruff, P., Ymer, C., Kinsella, G., Yucel, M., de Graaff, S., et al. (2000). Goal-directed selective attention and response competition monitoring: Evidence from unilateral parietal and anterior cingulate lesions. *Neuropsychology, 14,* 16–28.

Devinsky, O., Morrell, M. J., & Vogt, B. A. (1995). Contributions of anterior cingulate cortex to behaviour. *Brain, 118,* 279–306.

Dove, A., Pollman, S., Schubert, T., Wiggins, C. J., & von Carmaon D. Y. (2000). Prefrontal cortex activation in task switching: An event-related fMRI study. *Cognitive Brain Research, 9,* 102–109.

Dum, R. P., & Strick, P. L. (1993). Cingulate motor areas. In B. A. Vogt & M. Gabriel (Eds.), *Neurobiology of cingulate cortex and limbic thalamus: A comprehensive handbook* (pp. 415–441). Boston: Birkhauser.

Duncan, J., & Owen, A. M. (2000). Common regions of the human frontal lobe recruited by diverse cognitive demands. *Trends in Neurosciences, 23,* 475–483.

Eriksen, B. A., & Eriksen, C. W. (1974). Effects of noise letters upon the identification of a target letter in a nonsearch task. *Perception and Psychophysics, 16,* 143–149.

Falkenstein, M., Hohnsbein, J., Hoorman, J., & Blanke, L. (1990). Effects of errors in choice reaction tasks on the ERP under focused and divided attention. In C. H. M. Brunia, A. W. K Gaillard, & A. Kok (Eds.), *Psychophysiological brain research* (pp. 192–195). Tilburg, Netherlands: Tilburg University Press.

Falkenstein, M., Hoormann, J., Christ, S., & Hohnsbein J. (2000). ERP components on reaction errors and their functional significance: A tutorial. *Biological Psychology, 51*, 87–107.

Fan, J., Flombaum, J. I., McCandliss, B. D., Thomas, K. M., & Posner, M. I. (2003). Cognitive and brain consequences of conflict. *NeuroImage, 18*, 42–57.

Foote, S. L., & Morrison, J. H. (1987). Extrathalamic modulation of cortical function. *Annual Review of Neuroscience, 10*, 67–95.

Ford, J. M. (1999). Schizophrenia: The broken P300 and beyond. *Psychophysiology, 36*, 667–682.

Frank, R. J., Damasio, H., & Grabowski, T. J. (1997). Brainvox: An interactive, multimodal visualization and analysis system for neuroanatomical imaging. *NeuroImage, 5*, 13–30.

Frith, C. D. (1992). *The cognitive neuropsychology of schizophrenia.* Hillsdale, NJ: Erlbaum.

Frith, C. D., & Done, D. J. (1989). Experiences of alien control in schizophrenia reflect a disorder in the central monitoring of action. *Psychological Medicine, 19*, 359–363.

Garavan, H. Ross, T. L., Kaufman, J., & Stein, E. A. (2003). A midline dissociation between error-processing and response-conflict monitoring. *NeuroImage, 20*, 1132–1139.

Gehring, W. J., Goss, B., Coles, M. G. H., Meyer, D. E., & Donchin, E. (1993). A neural system for error detection and compensation. *Psychological Science, 4*, 385–390.

Gehring, W. J., & Willoughby, A. R. (2002). The medial frontal cortex and the rapid processing of monetary gains and losses. *Science, 295*, 2279–2282.

Gratton, G., Coles, M. G. H., & Donchin, E. (1992). Optimizing the use of information: Strategic control of activation and responses. *Journal of Experimental Psychology: General, 4*, 480–506.

Janer, K. W., & Pardo, J. V. (1991). Deficits in selective attention following bilateral anterior cingulotomy. *Journal of Cognitive Neuroscience, 3*, 231–241.

Kiehl, K. A., Liddle, P. F., & Hopfinger, J. B. (2000). Error processing and the rostral anterior cingulate: An event–related fMRI study. *Psychophysiology, 37*, 216–223.

Kimberg, D. Y., Aguirre, G. K., & D'Esposito, M. (2000). Modulation of task–related neural activity in task-switching: An fMRI study. *Cognitive Brain Research, 10*, 189–196.

Kopp, B., Rist, F., & Mattler, U. (1996). N200 in the flanker task as a neurobehavioral tool for investigating executive control. *Psychophysiology, 33*, 282–294.

Koski, L., & Paus, T. (2000). Functional connectivity of the anterior cingulate cortex within the human frontal lobe: A brain-mapping meta-analysis. *Experimental Brain Research, 133*, 55–65.

Luu, P., Collins, P., & Tucker, D. M. (2000). Mood, personality, and self–monitoring: Negative affect and emotionality in relation to frontal lobe mechanisms of error monitoring. *Journal of Experimental Psychology: General, 129*, 43–60.

MacDonald, A. W. III, Cohen, J. D., Stenger, V. A., & Carter, C. S. (2000). Dissociating the role of the dorsolateral prefrontal and anterior cingulate cortex in cognitive control. *Science, 288*, 1835–1838.

MacLeod, C. M., & MacDonald, P. A. (2000). Interdimensional interference in the Stroop effect: Uncovering the cognitive and neural anatomy of attention. *Trends in Cognitive Sciences, 4*, 383–391.

Malenka, R. C., Angel, R. W., Hampton, B., & Berger, P. A. (1982). Impaired central error-correcting behavior in schizophrenia. *Archives of General Psychiatry, 39*, 101–107.

Mayberg, H. S. (1997). Limbic–cortical dysregulation: A proposed model of depression. *Journal of Neuropsychiatry and Clinical Neuroscience, 9*, 471–481.

Menon, V., Adleman, N. E., White, C. D., Glover, G. H., & Reiss, A. L. (2001). Error-related brain activation during a Go/NoGo response inhibition task. *Human Brain Mapping, 12*, 131–143.

Milham, M. P., Erickson, K. I., Banich, M. T., Kramer, A. F., Webb, A., Wszalek, T., et al. (2002). Attentional control in the aging brain: insights from an fMRI study of the stroop task. *Brain and Cognition, 49*, 277–296.

Miller, E. K., & Cohen, J. D. (2001). An integrative theory of prefrontal cortex function. *Annual Review of Neuroscience, 24*, 167–202.

Norman, D. A., & Shallice, T. (1986). Attention to action: Willed and automatic control of behavior. In R. J. Davidson, G. E. Schwartz, & D. Shapiro (Eds.), *Consciousness and self-regulation* (Vol. 4, pp. 1–18) New York: Plenum Press.

Ochsner, K. N., Kosslyn, S. M., Cosgrove, G. R., Cassem, E. H., Price, B. H., Nierenberg, A. A., et al. (2001). Deficits in visual cognition and attention following bilateral anterior cingulotomy. *Neuropsychologia, 39*, 219–230.

Pardo, J. V., Pardo, P. J., Janer, K. W., & Raichle, M. E. (1990). The anterior cingulate cortex mediates processing selection in the Stroop attentional conflict paradigm. *Proceedings of the National Academy of Sciences USA, 87,* 256 259.

Paus, T. (2001). Primate anterior cingulate cortex: Where motor control, drive and cognition interface. *Nature Reviews Neuroscience, 2,* 417–424.

Paus, T., Koski, L., Caramanos, Z., & Westbury, C. (1998). Regional differences in the effects of task difficulty and motor output on blood flow response in the human anterior cingulate cortex: A review of 107 PET activation studies. *Neuroreport, 9,* R37–R47.

Paus, T., Petrides, M., Evans, A. C., & Meyer E. (1993). Role of the human anterior cingulate cortex in the control of oculomotor, manual, and speech responses: A positron emission tomography study. *Journal of Neurophysiology, 70,* 453–469.

Picard, N., & Strick, P. L. (1996). Motor areas of the medial wall: A review of their location and functional activation. *Cerebral Cortex, 6,* 342–353.

Posner, M. I. (1994). Attention: The mechanisms of consciousness. *Proceedings of the National Academy of Sciences USA, 91,* 7398–7403.

Posner, M. I., & DiGirolamo, G. J. (1998). Executive attention: Conflict, target detection, and cognitive control. In R. Parasuraman (Ed.), *The attentive brain* (pp. 401–423). Cambridge, MA: MIT Press.

Posner, M. I., & Petersen, S. E. (1990). The attention system of the human brain. *Annual Review of Neuroscience, 13,* 25–42.

Ruff, C. C., Woodward, T. S., Laurens, K. R., & Liddle, P. F. (2001). The role of the anterior cingulate cortex in conflict processing: Evidence from reverse Stroop interference. *NeuroImage, 14,* 1150–1158.

Stuss, D. T., & Alexander, M. P. (2000). Executive functions and the frontal lobes: A conceptual view. *Psychological Research, 63,* 289–298.

Swick, D., & Jovanovich, J. (2002). Anterior cingulate cortex and the Stroop task: Neuropsychological evidence for topographic specificity. *Neuropsychologia, 40,* 1240–1253.

Swick, D., & Knight, R. T. (1998). Cortical lesions and attention. In R. Parasuraman (Ed.), *The attentive brain* (pp. 143–162). Cambridge, MA: MIT Press.

Swick, D., & Turken, A. U. (2002). Dissociation between conflict detection and error monitoring in the human anterior cingulate cortex. *Proceedings of the National Academy of Sciences USA, 99,* 16354–16359.

Swick, D., & Turken, A. U. (2004). Errors can be dissociated from conflict: Implications for theories of performance monitoring. In M. Ullsperger & M. Falkenstein (Eds.), *Errors, conflicts, and the brain: Current opinions on performance monitoring* (pp. 195–204). Leipzig, Germany: MPI.

Swick, D., Turken, A. U., Larsen, J., Roxby, C., Kopelovich, J. C. S., Jovanovic, J., et al. (2001). Anterior cingulate cortex: Error monitoring or conflict monitoring? *Cognitve Neuroscience Society Abstracts, 8,* 72.

Talairach, J., & Tournoux, P. (1988). Co-planar stereotaxic atlas of the human brain. Stuttgart, Germany: Thieme.

Turken, A. U. (2000). *Role of the anterior cingulate cortex in attentional control: A report on two neurological patients.* Doctoral dissertation, University of California, Santa Barbara.

Turken, A. U., & Swick, D. (1999). Response selection in the human anterior cingulate cortex. *Nature Neuroscience, 2,* 920–924.

Turken, A. U., Vuilleumier, P., Mathalon, D. H., Swick, D., & Ford, J. M. (2003). Are impairments of action monitoring and executive control true dissociative dysfunctions in patients with schizophrenia? *American Journal of Psychiatry, 160,* 1881–1883.

Ullsperger, M., & von Cramon, D. Y. (2001). Subprocesses of performance monitoring: A dissociation of error processing and response competition revealed by event-related fMRI and ERPs. *NeuroImage, 14,* 1387–1401.

Vogt, B. A., & Pandya, D. N. (1987). Cingulate cortex of the rhesus monkey: II. Cortical afferents. *Journal of Comparative Neurology, 262,* 271–289.

30

Examining Attentional Rehabilitation

Ian H. Robertson

A CLINICIAN'S BEWILDERMENT

I came to the study of attention from an unusual route—that of trying to rehabilitate it. In retrospect, it was a peculiar activity—trying to rehabilitate something that one could not actually define clearly. I was working as a clinical neuropsychologist in Edinburgh, Scotland, trying to work out what such a lone individual could possibly do with hundreds of people each one suffering from a bewilderingly complex range of brain disorders. This was the early 1980s when we could measure memory, perceptual disorders, language process, and so on, but attention was a mysterious beast that lurked in two equally dark caves. In the first we found backward digit span, serial 7's, Paced Auditory Serial Addition, and the Wisconsin Card Sorting Test. Somewhere we heard vague rumors about continuous performance, but no standardized instruments were easily available. I briefly review some of the work on attention that applied at that time before returning to the question of attentional rehabilitation.

In the dimly lit second cave we could read dense, beautifully crafted articles in *Journal of Experimental Psychology* and similar journals, where attention was dissected into its minutiae in a range of exquisite experimental paradigms. Each paradigm's author had his or her own theory of attention that related only that paradigm and no other. The theories and the paradigms were largely domains not so much of mutual incomprehension as of mutual disinterest. I remember reading Johnston and Dark's (1986) conclusion to their article in *Annual Review of Psychology*, reporting rather bleakly that William James gave up psychology after he tried to study attention. Some Dutch clinical studies on traumatic brain injury coming out around that time were similarly discouraging with respect to attention: van Zomeren and his colleagues in Groningen repeatedly found that when one controlled for speed of processing, the oft-reported attentional deficits that reputedly so characterized closed head injury disappeared (Zomeren & Burg, 1985; Zomeren & Deelman, 1976,

1978). Salthouse (1982) was coming to similar conclusions about the purported attentional deficits in normal aging (Salthouse, 1982). To cap it all, the early 1980s saw an apparent blow to a concept long linked to attention—arousal. The classic studies of Moruzzi and Magoun (1949) suggesting the existence of a single arousal-modulating reticular formation gave way to evidence for the existence of multiple ascending pathways from subcortical nuclei, each linked to different neurotransmitters and different cortical innervation (Olszewski & Baxter, 1982).

Little wonder that cognitive psychologist Alan Allport of Oxford University was able to perform an elegant postmortem on the attentional homunculus at the 14th meeting on attention and performance (Allport, 1993). To him, attention was no more than the emergent property of the interaction of a number of other processes in the brain, particularly inhibitory and motor preparatory processes. How else could we explain the fact—for instance—that it is harder to switch from speaking a less familiar foreign language to one's native language than vice versa, as several of his experiments showed (Allport, 1993)?

"Attention is simply an early form of action," Alan Allport said to me at a conference, citing the beautiful experiments of Giacomo Rizzolatti in Parma, as well as his own work. Rizzolatti had already, in characteristically robust terms, demolished attention as a useful concept in a book I edited with John Marshall (Rizzolatti & Berti, 1993). My own research was strongly influenced by this approach, and I found that—as would indeed be predicted by the premotor theories of attention—left-sided inattention was greatly improved when even small movements were made by the left side of the body on the left side of space (Robertson & North, 1992). I and my colleagues also found that inattention to the left side of a long object greatly diminished when a pincer reaching-to-grasp movement was made to the object, as opposed as a pointing-to-indicate one (Robertson, Nico, & Hood, 1995). But as I worked with these men and women who had suffered strokes leaving them with a diminished attention to the left side of space, I became increasingly aware of other problems of attention that they suffered from that seemed additional to the crippling problems of paying attention to the left side of space. For instance they "drifted off" in midconversation—seeming to lose track of what they were doing—but were readily reengaged with a simple prompt. I found, for instance, that if I cued them to the left side of space, they began to neglect things on their supposedly unimpaired right side (Robertson, 1989).

Resorting to the introspective methods of our discipline's forbears in Germany—it became clear to me that attention could not *only* be an early form of preparatory motor action. Some attention yes—but not all of attention. "How do I manage to pick out the viola in a string quartet and follow that through a movement?" I asked Alan Allport at a conference in the mid-1990s. "What motor actions was I preparing?—I can't play the viola." He could not answer—I doubt that anyone could fully reduce that type of sensory selectivity to an early form of preparation for action. So there I was, a bemused clinician trying to treat something that many denied existed. Did I give up? I would have, had I not met Mike Posner at a conference on consciousness in St. Andrews in Scotland. Through jet lag and a throat-clogging virus, Mike croaked the answer to my bemusement about my patients suffering from unilateral neglect: "The right parietals fall to pieces when they're not cued, irrespective of the side." Perhaps not his exact words, but he handed me a copy of his just-published review with Steve Petersen in *Annual Review of Neuroscience* (Posner & Petersen, 1990) and the direction of my research for the next 13 years was set.

THERE IS NO SUCH THING AS ATTENTION
. . . BUT THERE ARE SEVERAL ATTENTIONS

Mike Posner had been saying it for several years (Posner & Boies, 1971), but somehow the story had not gotten through—to me at least. Now, and this was the really persuasive advance, with the help of new functional brain imaging data he could say more clearly and affirmatively: There are three main functionally and anatomically distinct types of supramodal attentional control systems—*selection, orientation, and alertness,* respectively. This was somewhat different from Posner and Boies's (1971) earlier typology—*selection, capacity, and alertness.* It was, however, close to another typology developed by Raja Parasuraman who proposed the typology of *selection, control, and vigilance* (Parasuraman, Warm, & See, 1998). More recently, Posner and his colleagues have refined the typology to *orienting, alerting, and executive control.* Orienting can be roughly equated with Parasuraman's notion of selection, executive control with Parasuraman's control, and alerting with Parasuraman's vigilance. Eminent attention researchers at the MRC Applied Psychology Unit in Cambridge where I was by then working did not really subscribe to this idea, however: John Duncan in particular was not persuaded about modularity of function in the prefrontal cortex—and he developed a theory of goal neglect theory that led to some beautiful experiments and persuasive data (Duncan, Emslie, Williams, Johnson, & Freer, 1996), and much later the basis for a method of rehabilitating executive deficits following frontal lobe damage that I developed (Levine et al., 2000).

But how did Duncan's view of attention and executive functions map onto Posner's? How did the wandering attention lapses of the neglect patients—so different from the insouciant perseverations of the frankly frontally damaged patients—relate to the executive deficits that John Duncan identified? For a clinician to treat, it is first necessary to assess, and thus I felt obliged to set about finding ways to assess these putatively distinct type of attentional systems, in a way that would be clinically useful. We put together a range of everyday tasks that putatively tapped the different components of Posner's typology—tasks such as searching for symbols in maps, looking up particular entries in the phone book, listening to lottery number announcements, and so on. The resulting Test of Everyday Attention (Robertson, Ward, Ridgeway, & Nimmo-Smith, 1994) yielded in a principal components analysis—to our surprise—a factor structure that was closely compatible with Posner's typology when given to several hundred normal adults (Robertson, Ward, Ridgeway, & Nimmo-Smith, 1996).

Given the post hoc nature of standard principal components analysis, my colleagues Tom Manly and Vicki Anderson and I set ourselves a stringent challenge: Using a completely different set of child-friendly game-type materials, we carried out a prospective confirmatory factor analysis on the attentional performance of some 300 Australian children. If there really was something in Posner's typology, it should be robust enough to reveal itself across the domains of simulated everyday life. Confirmatory factor analysis not only requires us to specify in advance what and how many factors underpin the variance in the data we have collected, it also requires us to specify which of our subtests load on which of these hypothetical factors. This is not a forgiving statistical method. To our further astonishment, our new test—the Test of Everyday Attention for Children (Manly, Robertson, Anderson, & Nimmo-Smith, 1998)—yielded data that completely supported the first analysis on the adult data using quite different material (Manly et al., 2001). The analysis showed that in order to explain the variance in children's performance, it was imperative to have three factors, not one, and furthermore it was necessary to have the kinds of factors that we were measuring and that had been derived from Posner's theories.

VIGILANT ATTENTION

The phenomenon of alerting—Parasuraman's vigilance—seemed to be one that played a major part in many of the clinical conditions I was dealing with, particularly unilateral neglect but also traumatic brain injury. The problem was, it was extremely difficult to get normal individuals off maximum score in most of the currently available tests of this type of attention—these being largely continuous performance tasks. In some of the earliest studies of vigilance, for instance, it was often found that errors, when they did occur, were only observed over relatively long periods of usually more than 30 minutes (Mackworth, 1950). Even in people with traumatic brain injury and consequently impaired frontal lobe/attentional deficits, marginal decrements could only be observed in sustained attention when the visual stimuli were heavily perceptually degraded (Parasuraman, Mutter, & Molloy, 1991).

Why should train drivers frequently miss danger signals, an extremely commonly reported phenomenon, while participants in vigilance experiments show such relatively good performance? A possible answer to this question may be that, unlike the radar operators who must *make* a response to rare targets, train drivers must *inhibit* their ongoing behavior in the context of a rare target—namely, a red or warning signal. When required to make a response, the presentation of the rare target can facilitate performance insofar as (1) the default response in a task such as this is not to respond, thereby providing time to detect the target and make the appropriate response, and (2) the presentation of the rare target can itself serve to orient attention to its presence. Contrast this with the circumstance in which people must inhibit responding to rare stimuli. Here, the ongoing default behavior (responding, or in the case of the train driver, to keep driving forward) is opposite to the desired response (i.e., interrupt the default behavior). Furthermore, the ongoing behavior that engages the person in well-practiced behaviors can create the illusion that the person is attentively engaged in the task at hand. However, the automatic quality of the behavior can be deceptive as it, in fact, requires little vigilant attention. Consequently, the commission error might be committed before the person can countermand it or, as in the train driver, without the person even noticing that the countermand was required. This distinction between responding and inhibiting also rests on whether the vigilant attention for the task must be generated endogenously or is supported by exogenous task demands, an important issue that I address later.

This distinction can be seen clearly when we compare frontally and attentionally impaired patients with traumatic brain injury (TBI) with controls on a task that requires detection of rare targets with one that requires inhibition of response to rare targets—the latter being more closely analogous to the train driver situation (Robertson, Manly, Andrade, Baddeley, & Yiend, 1997). In this study, controls and traumatic brain injured patients made statistically indistinguishable numbers of errors when they had to *detect* rare (11%) targets—ascending or descending trios of digits (e.g., 234 or 987 in an otherwise random stream of one-per-second digits). Yet the frontally impaired patients did show significant impairment—twice the error rate of controls—on a task where they had to *withhold* a response to the number 3, also appearing 11% of the time in the same stream of randomly appearing digits (Sustained Attention to Response Task, or SART). We believe these deficits result from a dynamic interaction between inhibitory abilities and vigilant attention as becomes apparent when we made the sequence of digits entirely predictable—1,2,3,4,5,6,7,8,9,1,2,3 . . . etc. Whereas normal controls make only occasional errors on this task, patients with TBI have considerable difficulty and in one study made more than 7 out of 25 errors—28%—despite there being a totally predictable sequence leading up to the target letter (Manly et al., 2003). Here, the inability to withhold responding is likely due to an inability to maintain a sufficient level of arousal and a sufficiently strong representation of the task goals ("don't respond to 3"): when vigilant attention is poor, the patient defaults to the frequent response.

REHABILITATION OF ATTENTION

The ability to sustain vigilant attention seems to be an important factor in determining recovery of motor and other function following stroke (Blanc-Garin, 1994). Furthermore we have shown that motor recovery in the 2 years following right-hemisphere stroke was significantly predicted by measures of sustained attention taken 2 months after stroke. Specifically, the ability to sustain attention to a tone counting task (a validated measure of sustained attention related to right frontal function (Wilkins, Shallice, & McCarthy, 1987) at 2 months poststroke predicted not only everyday life function 2 years later but also the functional dexterity of the left hand in a pegboard task (Robertson, Ridgeway, Greenfield, & Parr, 1997). Attentional impairment is therefore important not only as a problem in itself but also as a factor in the recovery of other impaired cognitive, sensory and motor functions.

Ever since I began to think about neuropsychological rehabilitation, I had wanted to bind treatments into underlying neurocognitive models in the way that many pharmaceutical agents are based on a clear model of the their effects on underlying physiology. In 1984, however, this was an unrealized dream. Unilateral neglect, thought to represent a disorder of Posner's orientation system, seemed like a good candidate for the development of such a theory–practice rapprochement. And, indeed, in subsequent years a number of counterintuitive but effective rehabilitation methods for unilateral neglect have been devised through the application of basic cognitive neuroscience.

One such example is Limb Activation Training, which induces neglect patients to make small movements with the left side of their body in left hemispace in order to improve their visual attention to the left (Robertson, North, & Geggie, 1992); patients with acute neglect who receive this minimally labor-intensive additional treatment are discharged from the hospital on average 28 days earlier than patients who do not receive it (Kalra, Perez, Gupta, & Wittink, 1997). Limb activation training also significantly improves left-sided motor function in patients with neglect as far as 24 months after the end of brief therapy (Robertson, McMillan, MacLeod, & Brock, 2002). We have also shown that the same principles of limb activation apply in a 7-year-old child with developmental neglect and attention-deficit disorder (ADD) (Dobler, Manly, Verity, Woolrych, & Robertson, 2003). Figure 30.1 shows this child's neglect on the Balloons Test (Edgworth, Robertson, & McMillan, 1998). Figure 30.2 shows the reduction of neglect only with movements of the left hand in left hemispace, a finding identical to that shown in adults with neglect (Robertson & North, 1992), and the basis for Limb Activation Training (Robertson et al., 1992). Figure 30.3 shows the long-term effects of this training on an adult with severe neglect following right-hemisphere stroke (Wilson, Manly, Coyle, & Robertson, 2000).

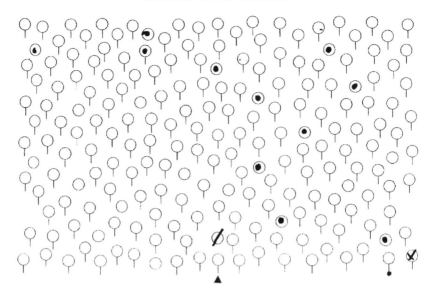

FIGURE 30.1. Child's performance on the Balloons Test. In the Balloons Test (A3 size) the child was asked to find all the circles without a descending line. On this task he showed strong neglect of left-sided targets. From Dobler et al. (2003). Copyright 2003 by MacKeith Press. Reprinted by permission.

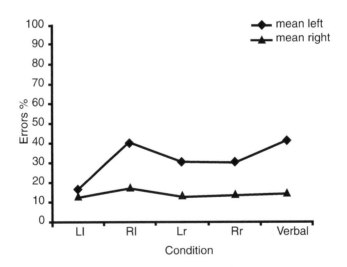

FIGURE 30.2. Child's performance on test of neglect with "limb activation." Using the left hand within the left space (Ll condition) abolished the difference for "left-first" and "right-first" targets. Ll, left hand within left space; Lr, left hand within right space; Rr, right hand within right space; Rl, right hand within left space. From Dobler et al. (2003). Copyright 2003 by MacKeith Press. Reprinted by permission.

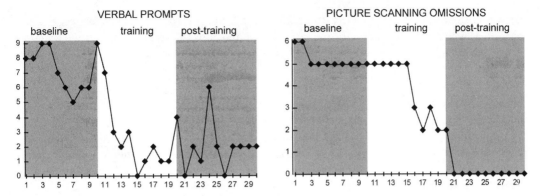

FIGURE 30.3. Improvements in self-care program and performance on a picture scanning task before, during, and after limb activation training in an adult with severe unilateral left neglect. From Wilson et al. (2000). Copyright 2000 by IOS Press. Reprinted by permission.

I have reviewed a number of other counterintuitive but clinically effective treatments for neglect derived from basic cognitive neuroscience elsewhere (Robertson, 2002; Robertson & Murre, 1999).

So, we had made some progress with rehabilitation of unilateral inattention. But what about nonspatial attention: Could we make progress in this domain also, and how? Mike Posner came to the rescue again. In his chapter in Donald Broadbent's *Festschrift*, he spelt out an interesting hypothetical relationship between two of his attentional systems: He proposed that the right frontoparietal vigilant system actually modulated the posterior orientation system (Posner, 1993). This right temperoparietal region is implicated in both unilateral left spatial inattention and detection of targets throughout space and happens also to be specifically involved in vigilant monitoring of the external world for infrequent targets (Pardo, Fox, & Raichle, 1991). Furthermore, this region is brain region most densely innervated by noradrenergic projections from the locus coeruleus known to be implicated in vigilance and arousal (Foote & Morrison, 1987). Heilman and colleagues had already showed the predominance of the right hemisphere in mediating a generalized enhanced responsivity/activation to stimuli (Coslett, Bowers, & Heilman, 1987). Patients with right-hemisphere lesions were hypoaroused relative to patients with left-hemisphere lesion, for example, showing virtually absent galvanic skin response (GSR) to pictures of emotionally arousing scenes (Morrow, Vrtunski, Kim, & Boller, 1981). Similar results were obtained from painful stimuli; again, right temporoparietal lesioned patients showed greatly reduced GSR responses in comparison to either left-brain-damaged patients or controls. Unilateral right temporal lobectomy patients also show basic hypoarousal when compared to left-temporal-lobectomy patients, as measured by GSR (Davidson, Fedio, Smith, Aureille, & Martin, 1992).

The possibility that the spatially nonselective component of attentional deficit in unilateral neglect may be linked to some basic alertness/arousal dysfunction can be examined in the context of monkey research on the role of the locus coeruleus (LC) in target detection. Aston-Jones, Chiang, and Alexinsky (1991) recorded extracellularly from noradrenergic neurons in the nucleus LC of monkeys performing an oddball visual discrimination task. In response to rewarded detection of rare target stimuli (10–20% of trials) intermixed with nontarget visual stimuli, all LC neurons examined were phasically and selectively activated by target cues in this task. Furthermore, LC response magnitudes varied with behavioral performance and were significantly attenuated during periods of poor performance. In addition, there was a positive correlation between the latency of LC responses and the latency of behavioral responses to same target cues, consistent with the possibility that LC responses may have a role in selective attention by facilitating responses to the target stimuli. LC responses became reduced in magnitude over time during prolonged task performance (> 90 minutes), in parallel with a behavioral performance decrement, again supporting the view that these processes may be related to vigilance and arousal.

This study showed that LC neurons are activated selectively by attended stimuli, and that this activation may in turn serve to enhance processing of the attended stimuli. Deficient processing of target stimuli of the type observed in unilateral neglect could therefore be caused by insufficient activation of the LC by parietal neurons responsible for selective attention, by impairment of the LC itself, or by impaired functioning of the upward or downward projections between the LC and the parietal cortex. This argument has particular strength given the evidence for a right-hemispheric predominance in the distribution of noradrenalin (Oke, Keller, Mefford, & Adams, 1978).

We (Robertson, Mattingley, Rorden, & Driver, 1998) tested the hypothesis originally suggested by Mike Posner, that a right-hemisphere alertness system linked to noradrenergic arousal mechanisms should directly and specifically modulate the spatial selection system. The prediction was that phasically increasing the patients' alertness should transiently ameliorate the spatial bias in perceptual awareness, and indeed the results provided the first direct confirmation of this proposal. The task required right-hemisphere patients with neglect to judge whether a left visual event preceded a comparable right event, or vice versa. Neglect patients became aware of left events half a second slower than right events, on average. This dramatic spatial imbalance in the time course of visual awareness could be reversed if a warning sound alerted the patients phasically. Even a sound on the right dramatically accelerated the perception of left visual events in this way. A nonspatial alerting intervention can thus overcome disabling spatial biases in perceptual awareness after brain injury.

In a clinical–experimental corollary (Robertson, Tegner, Tham, Lo, & Nimmo-Smith, 1995) of the aforementioned study, we attempted directly to rehabilitate sustained attention in a group of patients with unilateral left neglect following right-hemisphere lesions. These patients were trained while doing a variety of tasks with no lateralized scanning component: Periodically the patients had their attention drawn to a routine task—for example, a sorting task—by combining a loud noise with an instruction to attend. Patients were then gradually taught to "take over" this alerting procedure using a self-generated verbal cue so that eventually it became a self-alerting procedure. Among this group of eight patients, not only were there improvements in sustained attention but there were also very significant improvements on spatial neglect over and above those expected by natural recovery. This study shows that the spatial bias in unilateral neglect can be briefly reduced using exogenous alerting stimuli, but that it may also be possible to reduce this bias endogenously, using self-initiated alerting mechanisms.

In attempting to rehabilitate unilateral spatial inattention via a semi-independent companion function—vigilant or sustained attention—we had also shown that it was possible to enhance the vigilant attention system itself. Vigilant attention can be impaired through administration of drugs (e.g., clonidine) that inhibit noradrenaline release. One study (e.g., Smith & Nutt, 1996) confirmed that noradrenaline suppression in humans led to vigilant attention lapses, but it also showed that this effect was much attenuated when the participants were exposed to loud white noise while performing the task. This suggests that external stimuli can induce "bottom-up" or exogenous modulation of the cortical systems for vigilant attention. Coull and her colleagues confirmed that this is indeed the case (Coull, 1998) showing that clonidine-induced noradrenergic suppression impaired vigilant attention performance much more when the task was familiar than when it was unfamiliar. This apparently paradoxical effect where the deleterious effect of a drug is reduced by making the task more *difficult* is a key finding in understanding how the vigilant attention system might function. What these findings suggest is that this system can be engaged by both endogenous and exogenous means; furthermore, when exogenous activation takes place, we argue, it considerably reduces the demands on the endogenous components of the system. But do exogenous and endogenous inputs activate the system in the same way? One of our recent studies suggests that this may not be the case.

We carried out a recent functional magnetic resonance imaging (fMRI) study of the SART (O'Connor, Manly, Robertson, Hevenor, & Levine, 2003). In the SART, participants have to respond to all randomly appearing digits but withhold responses to rare targets (number 3) that appear 11% of the time on average. Compared to a rest period, we showed precisely the right frontoparietal activation that we would predict as being needed for a task that placed demands on the vigilant attention system. We had previously shown, however, that performance on SART and on other tasks requiring vigilant attention could be much enhanced by presenting noninformative auditory arousing tones randomly during task performance (Manly et al., 2004). On the basis of these data, we predicted that these exogenous stimuli externally activated vigilant attention, hence reducing the demands on the endogenous components of that system that we argue are based in the right-hemisphere frontoparietal system. What we in fact found was that presenting alerting tones during SART *did* eliminate the right frontal activation but *did not* eliminate the right parietal activation. In other words, it seems as if the parietal component of the right-hemisphere vigilant attention system may be a common pathway for both endogenous and exogenous routes, while the right frontal element may be particularly linked to endogenous activation. We have also shown that increasing the task demand in the SART paradoxically reduces the proportional number of errors of commission. When the inhibit target is relatively rare—11%—proportionately more errors are made than when the target is more common—25%—and the proportional error rate declines linearly as the target rate increases to 50% (Manly, Robertson, Galloway, & Hawkins, 1999). Furthermore, self-reported proneness to everyday attentional slips, such as forgetting why one has walked into a room, are significantly related to the proportion of errors made on the 11% target frequency SART, but not where the targets are more frequent (Manly et al., 1999). We interpret these effects as being due to the repeated targets in the higher-frequency condition providing increased exogenous support for the task through repeated activation of the "inhibit response" motor action and goal representation. We believe that one feature of tasks sensitive to the vigilance system is that this type of exogenous support is absent or relatively weak and consequently the vigilance system must be maintained endogenously, a function for which the right prefrontal areas appear especially important.

This capacity to maintain alert and vigilant responding may cause the breakdown in more complex executive behaviors usually associated with the prefrontal cortex. A number of studies indicate that an adequately represented behavioral goal may become neglected as patients become overly engaged in current activity. On the assumption that impaired vigilant attention may play a part in such impairment, we have studied whether the provision of the type of brief auditory stimuli mentioned previously, would improve performance in more complex tasks. In one study (Manly, Hawkins, Evans, Woldt, & Robertson, 2002), 10 patients with brain injury completed a test of executive function—the Hotel Task—under two conditions.

The Hotel Task was devised by my colleague Tom Manly in Cambridge and comprises six distinct activities that would plausibly need to be completed in the course of running a hotel. The tasks included compiling individual bills, sorting the charity collection, looking up telephone numbers, sorting conference labels, proofreading the hotel leaflet, and opening and closing remotely the garage doors at two predetermined times. In the task, individuals were asked to try and do some of each of five subtasks within 15 minutes. As the total time to complete all the tasks would exceed 1 hour, the measure emphasizes patients' ability to monitor the time, switch between the tasks, and keep track of their intentions.

Using participants as their own controls, we compared performance on this task with and without auditory alerting tones. In the alerting—experimental—condition, six brief 60-dB tones were played from a tape recorder at predetermined times during the task. Without these external auditory cues, the patients performed significantly more poorly than age- and IQ-matched control volunteers, a common error being to continue performing one task to the detriment of beginning or allocating sufficient time to others. When exposed to the interrupting tones, however, their performance was both significantly improved and no longer significantly different from the control group on important variables. Specifically, whereas without the alert they missed out, on average, one entire task, when the alerts were in place their performance normalized, attempting all tasks with a good distribution of time between them.

These results have value in assessment in helping to attribute poor performance to "goal neglect" (Duncan et al., 1996) rather than, for example, poor memory or comprehension. They also suggest that providing environmental support to one aspect of executive function may facilitate monitoring and behavioral flexibility—and therefore the useful expression of other skills that may be relatively intact.

Complex executive behaviors require the active maintenance in working memory of a series of goals, and Duncan (Duncan et al., 2000) has demonstrated that the maintenance and management of these goals may be a key function of the frontal lobes of the brain. While the precise relationship between working memory and Posner's three types of attention is as yet unclear, what does seem clear is that the alerting/vigilant attention system may be one important and separable factor in maintaining the integrity of behavioral goals in working memory. This may be particularly true where the tasks and question are routine and easily automatized—as is, for instance, true for the component tasks of the Hotel task described earlier.

CONCLUSION

I am still bewildered, but a little less so than before. Attention cannot be reduced to premotor processes, nor is it simply the output of competition among other processing domains. But attention is plural, not singular, and in the 18 years since I was a bewildered clinician, we have not only made progress in conceptualizing and measuring different types of attention, but we have also begun to take some steps toward developing theoretically grounded methods for enhancing attentional functions.

REFERENCES

Allport, A. (1993). Attention and control—Have we been asking the wrong questions: A critical review of 25 years. In D. E. Meyer & S. Kornblum (Eds.), *Attention and performance. XIV: Synergies in experimental psychology, artificial intelligence and cognitive neuroscience* (pp. 183–218). Cambridge, MA: MIT Press.

Aston-Jones, G., Chiang, C., & Alexinsky, T. (1991). Discharge of noradrenergic locus coeruleus neurons in behaving rats and monkeys suggests a role in vigilance. In C. D. Barnes & O. Pompeiano (Eds.), *Progress in brain research* (Vol. 88, pp. 501–520). Amsterdam: Elsevier Science.

Blanc-Garin, J. (1994). Patterns of recovery from hemiplegia following stroke. *Neuropsychological Rehabilitation, 4,* 359–385.

Coslett, H. B., Bowers, D., & Heilman, K. M. (1987). Reduction in cerebral activation after right hemisphere stroke. *Neurology, 37,* 957–962.

Coull, J. T. (1998). Neural correlates of attention and arousal: Insights from electrophysiology, functional neuroimaging and psychopharmacology. *Progress in Neurobiology, 55,* 343–361.

Davidson, R. A., Fedio, P., Smith, B. D., Aureille, E., & Martin, A. (1992). Lateralised mediation of arousal and habituation: Differential bilateral electrodermal activity in unilateral temporal lobectomy patients. *Neuropsychologia, 30,* 1053–1063.

Dobler, V. B., Manly, T., Verity, C., Woolrych, J., & Robertson, I. H. (2003). Modulation of spatial attention in a child with developmental unilateral neglect. *Developmental Medicine and Child Neurolology, 45,* 282–288.

Duncan, J., Emslie, H., Williams, P., Johnson, R., & Freer, C. (1996). Intelligence and the frontal-lobe: The organization of goal-directed behavior. *Cognitive Psychology, 30,* 257–303.

Duncan, J., Seitz, R., Kolodny, J., Bor, D., Herzog, H., Ahmed, A., et al. (2000). A neural basis for general intelligence. *Science, 289,* 457–46.

Edgworth, J., Robertson, I. H., & MacMillan, T. (1998). *The Balloons Test: A screening test for visual inattention.* Bury St. Edmunds, UK: Thames Valley Test Company.

Foote, S. L., & Morrison, J. H. (1997). Extrathalamic modulation of cortical function. *Annual Review of Neuroscience, 19,* 67–95.

Johnston, W. A., & Dark, V. J. (1986). Selective attention. *Annual Review of Psychology, 37,* 43–75.

Kalra, L., Perez, I., Gupta, S., & Wittink, M. (1997). The influence of visual neglect on stroke rehabilitation. *Stroke, 28,* 1386–1391.

Levine, B., Robertson, I. H., Clare, L., Carter, G., Hong, J., Wilson, B. A., et al. (2000). Rehabilitation of executive functioning: An experimental–clinical validation of Goal Management Training. *Journal of the International Neuropsychological Society, 6,* 299–312.

Mackworth, N. H. (1950). Researches in the measurement of human performance. In H. W. Sinaiko (Ed.), *Selected papers on human factors in the design and use of control systems.* New York: Dover Publications.

Manly, T., Anderson, V., Nimmo-Smith, I., Turner, A., Watson, P., & Robertson, I. H. (2001). The differential assessment of children's attention: The Test of Everyday Attention for Children (TEACh), normative sample and ADHD performance. *Journal of Child Psychology and Psychiatry, 42,* 1–10.

Manly, T., Hawkins, K., Evans, J., Woldt, K., & Robertson, I. H. (2002). Rehabilitation of Executive Function: Facilitation of effective goal management on complex tasks using periodic auditory alerts. *Neuropsychologia, 40,* 271–281.

Manly, T., Heutink, J., Davison, B., Gaynord, B., Greenfield, E., Parr, A., et al. (2004). An electronic knot in the handkerchief: "Content free cueing" and the maintenance of attentive control. *Neuropsychological Rehabilitation, 14,* 89–116.

Manly, T., Owen, A. M., Datta, A., Lewis, G., Scott, S., Rorden, C., et al. (2003). Enhancing the sensitivity of a sustained attention task to frontal damage. Convergent clinical and functional imaging evidence. *Neurocase, 9,* 340–349.

Manly, T., Robertson, I. H., Anderson, V., & Nimmo-Smith, I. (1998). *Test of Everyday Attention for Children (TEAch).* Bury St. Edmunds, UK: Thames Valley Test Company.

Manly, T., Robertson, I. H., Galloway, M., & Hawkins, K. (1999). The absent mind: Further investigations of sustained attention to response. *Neuropsychologia, 37*, 661–670.

Morrow, L., Vrtunski, K., Kim, Y., & Boller, F. (1981). Arousal responses to emotional stimuli and laterality of lesion. *Neuropsychologia, 19*, 65–71.

Moruzzi, G., & Magoun, H. W. (1949). Brainstem reticular formation and activation of the EEG. *Electroencephalography and Clinical Neurophysiology, 1*, 455–473.

O'Connor, C., Manly, T., Robertson, I. H., Hevenor, S. J., & Levine, B. (2003). Endogenous vs. exogenous engagement of sustained attention: an fMRI study. *The Clinical Neuropsychologist, 17*, 117.

Oke, A., Keller, R., Mefford, I., & Adams, R. (1978). Lateralization of norepinephrine in human thalamus. *Science, 200*, 1411–1413.

Olszewski, J., & Baxter, D. (1982). *Cytoarchitecture of the human brainstem* (2nd ed). New York: Karger.

Parasuraman, R., Mutter, S. A., & Molloy, R. (1991). Sustained attention following mild closed-head injury. *Journal of Clinical and Experimental Neuropsychology, 13*, 789–811.

Parasuraman, R., Warm, J., & See, J. (1998). Brain systems of vigilance. In R. Parasuraman (Ed.), *Varieties of attention* (pp. 221–256). Cambridge, MA: MIT Press.

Pardo, J. V., Fox, P. T., & Raichle, M. E. (1991). Localization of a human system for sustained attention by positron emission tomography. *Nature, 349*, 61–64.

Posner, M. I. (1993). Interaction of arousal and selection in the posterior attention network. In A. Baddeley & L. Weiskrantz (Eds.), *Attention: Selection, awareness and control* (pp. 390–405). Oxford, UK: Clarendon Press.

Posner, M. I., & Boies, S. (1971). Components of attention. *Psychological Review, 78*, 391–408.

Posner, M. I., & Petersen, S. E. (1990). The attention system of the human brain. *Annual Review of Neuroscience, 13*, 25–42.

Rizzolatti, G., & Berti, A. (1993). Neural mechanisms of unilateral neglect. In I. H. Robertson & J. C. Marshall (Eds.), *Unilateral neglect: Clinical and experimental studies.* Hove, Sussex, UK: Erlbaum.

Robertson, I. H. (1989). Anomolies in the lateralisation of omissions in unilateral left neglect. *Neuropsychologia, 27*, 157–165.

Robertson, I. H. (2002). Cognitive neuroscience and brain rehabilitation: A promise kept [Editorial]. *Journal of Neurology, Neurosurgery and Psychiatry, 73*, 357.

Robertson, I. H., Manly, T., Andrade, J., Baddeley, B. T., & Yiend, J. (1997). Oops!: Performance correlates of everyday attentional failures in traumatic brain injured and normal subjects: The Sustained Attention to Response Task (SART). *Neuropsychologia, 35*, 747–758.

Robertson, I. H., Mattingley, J. B., Rorden, C., & Driver, J. (1998). Phasic alerting of neglect patients overcomes their spatial deficit in visual awareness. *Nature, 395*, 169–172.

Robertson, I. H., McMillan, T. M., MacLeod, E., & Brock, D. (2002). Rehabilitation by limb activation training (LAT) reduces impairment in unilateral neglect patients: A single-blind randomised control trial. *Neuropsychological Rehabilitation, 12*, 439–454.

Robertson, I. H., & Murre, J. M. J. (1999). Rehabilitation of brain damage: Brain plasticity and principles of guided recovery. *Psychological Bulletin, 125*, 544–575.

Robertson, I. H., Nico, D., & Hood, B. (1995). The intention to act improves unilateral neglect: Two demonstrations. *Neuroreport, 17*, 246–248.

Robertson, I. H., & North, N. (1992). Spatio-motor cueing in unilateral neglect: The role of hemispace, hand and motor activation. *Neuropsychologia, 30*, 553–563.

Robertson, I. H., North, N., & Geggie, C. (1992). Spatio-motor cueing in unilateral neglect: Three single case studies of its therapeutic effectiveness. *Journal of Neurology, Neurosurgery and Psychiatry, 55*, 799–805.

Robertson, I. H., Ridgeway, V., Greenfield, E., & Parr, A. (1997). Motor recovery after stroke depends on intact sustained attention: A two-year follow-up study. *Neuropsychology, 11*, 290–295.

Robertson, I. H., Tegner, R., Tham, K., Lo, A., & Nimmo-Smith, I. (1995). Sustained attention training for unilateral neglect: Theoretical and rehabilitation implications. *Journal of Clinical and Experimental Neuropsychology, 17*, 416–430.

Robertson, I. H., Ward, T., Ridgeway, V., & Nimmo-Smith, I. (1994). *The Test of Everyday Attention*. Bury St. Edmunds, UK: Thames Valley Test Company.

Robertson, I. H., Ward, T., Ridgeway, V., & Nimmo-Smith, I. (1996). The structure of normal human attention: The Test of Everyday Attention. *Journal of the International Neuropsychological Society, 2*, 525–534.

Salthouse, T. A. (1982). *Adult cognition: An experimental psychology of human aging*. New York: Springer-Verlag.

Smith, A., & Nutt, D. (1996). Noradrenaline and attention lapses. *Nature, 380*, 291.

Wilkins, A. J., Shallice, T., & McCarthy, R. (1987). Frontal lesions and sustained attention. *Neuropsychologia, 25*, 359–365.

Wilson, F. C., Manly, T., Coyle, D., & Robertson, I. H. (2000). The effect of contralesional limb activation training and sustained attention training for self-care programmes in unilateral spatial neglect. *Restorative Neurology and Neuroscience, 16*, 1–4.

van Zomeren, A. H., & van den Burg, W. (1985). Residual complaints of patients two years after severe closed head injury. *Journal of Neurology, Neurosurgery and Psychiatry, 48*, 21–28.

van Zomeren, A. H., & Deelman, B. G. (1976). Differential aspects of simple and choice reaction after closed lhead injury. *Clinical Neurology and Neurosurgery, 79*, 81–90.

van Zomeren, A. H., & Deelman, B. G. (1978). Long-term recovery of visual reaction time after closed head injury. *Journal of Neurology, Neurosurgery and Psychiatry, 41*, 452–457.

31

Atypical Attention

Hypnosis and Conflict Reduction

Amir Raz

This chapter attempts to delineate how altered consciousness (e.g., hypnosis) can illuminate our understanding of attention in common wakefulness. The central tenet of this approach is to keep the experimental paradigm relatively pristine but to gain insight into the attentional process by influencing the subjects' "state" instead (Raz & Shapiro, 2002).

Hypnosis has been used clinically for hundreds of years and is primarily a phenomenon involving attentive receptive concentration (Spiegel & Spiegel, 1987). Despite its long use in clinical settings, hypnosis was only certified by the American Medical Association as a legitimate treatment tool in 1958 and as an effective intervention for pain regulation by a National Institutes of Health panel in 1996. Even so, hypnosis has largely remained an elusive concept for science, partly because it is contaminated by folk beliefs and shrouded in layers of misconception, and largely because the way in which it works has never been adequately explained. Fortunately, with the advent of neuroimaging, this state of affairs is gradually changing.

A recent research program has been able to tap attention in novel ways and shed new light on its neural bases by relating hypnosis, suggestion, conflict resolution, and self-regulation (Raz & Shapiro, 2002). An approach particularly conducive to research is the use of posthypnotic suggestion—a condition following termination of the hypnotic experience, wherein a subject is compliant with a suggestion made during the hypnotic episode but does not remember being told to do so. The posthypnotic suggestion is usually summoned on a prearranged signal and can be effective in highly hypnotizable individuals.

It is possible to classify individuals as either highly hypnotizable (HH) or less hypnotizable (LH) based on their susceptibility to hypnotic suggestion as evidenced in performance on standardized scales. Whereas a number of such scales exist (McConkey & Sheehan, 1982), the Stanford Hypnotic Susceptibility Scale Form C (SHSS:C)—partially due to its robust psychometric characteristics—has frequently been the scale of choice in research (Weitzenhoffer & Hilgard, 1962). Hypnotic procedures generate changes in the way at least HH individuals experience themselves and the environment, and these alterations have been shown to affect cognitive processing. Clinicians practicing hypnosis suggest that when one is hypnotized, attentional and perceptual changes may occur that would not have occurred had one been in common awareness. Indeed, hypnotic perceptual alterations in HH are usually accompanied by changes in brain activation (Raz & Shapiro, 2002). Furthermore, HH individuals have been successfully used in assays involving atypical attention (Raz, Fan, Shapiro, & Posner, 2002; Raz, Fossella, McGuinness, Sommer, & Posner, 2003; Raz, Fossella, McGuinness, Sommer, & Posner, 2003; Raz et al., 2003; Raz, Shapiro, Fan, & Posner, 2002a, 2002b, 2002c).

This chapter starts out by reporting on studies showing that HH people can eliminate Stroop interference based on posthypnotic suggestion. When they do so, specific brain changes related to this effect occur. Next, individual differences that might relate to the distinction between high and low hypnotizability are examined. Finally, this chapter discusses hypnotic inductions that might lead to specific deficits and behavioral lesions similar to those found with veridical lesions.

USING POSTHYPNOTIC SUGGESTION
TO REDUCE CONFLICT IN THE BRAIN

Stroop conflict (Stroop, 1935) is an experimental effect elicited when proficient readers name the ink color of a displayed word. Individuals are usually slower and less accurate, indicating the ink color of an incompatible color word (e.g., responding *blue* when the word *RED* is inked in blue) than identifying the ink color of a congruent color name (e.g., responding *red* when the word *RED* is inked in red). This difference in performance constitutes the Stroop conflict and is one of the most robust and well-studied phenomena in attentional research (MacLeod, 1991; MacLeod & MacDonald, 2000).

The dominant view in the literature regards reading as a largely automatic process whereby skilled readers cannot withhold activating a word's underlying meaning despite explicit instructions to attend only to its ink color. Indeed, the standard account maintains that semantic processing of words occurs involuntarily (MacLeod, 1991; Neely, 1991), and that the Stroop task is a model of experimental (cognitive) conflict resolution (Botvinick, Braver, Barch, Carter, & Cohen, 2001).

Some researchers have attempted to explore the Stroop effect under hypnosis (Blum & Graef, 1971; Blum & Wiess, 1986; Dixon, Brunet, & Laurence, 1990a; Dixon & Laurence, 1992; MacLeod & Sheehan, 2003; Nordby, Hugdahl, Jasiukaitis, & Spiegel, 1999; Sheehan, Donovan, & MacLeod, 1988; Spiegel, Cutcomb, Ren, & Pribram, 1985; Sun, 1994; Szechtman, Woody, Bowers, & Nahmias, 1998). However, these assays have largely concentrated on the effect of hypnosis without suggestion and often used nonclassical Stroop paradigms. Historical single-case reports (MacLeod & Sheehan, 2003; Schatzman, 1980), esoteric publications (Sun, 1994), and informal personal communications (T. Wheatley, personal communication, July 5, 2003) proposing hypnotic removal of Stroop conflict have never been rigorously studied.

We examined Stroop interference both in HH and LH subjects with and without a posthypnotic suggestion to see the letters as a meaningless string. As shown in Figure 31.1, we found elimination of Stroop interference in HH but not LH individuals (Raz et al., 2002b). A separate replication of these findings using optical conditions that ensured participants neither looked away nor blurred their vision (i.e., making optical compromise of in-

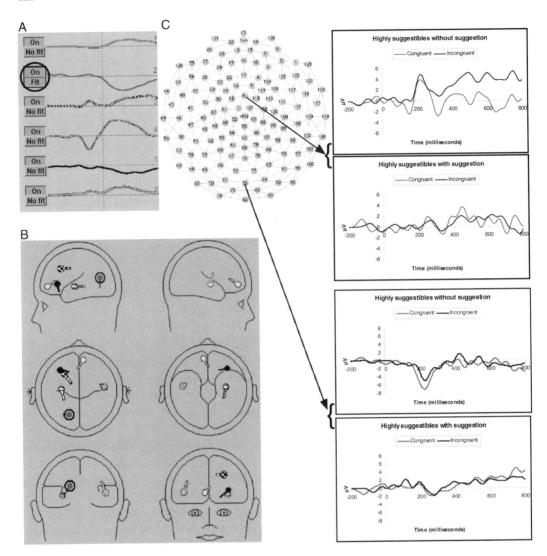

FIGURE 31.1. (A) Regions of significant fMRI activations on Stroop conflict comparing post-hypnotic suggestion with no suggestion in highly suggestible individuals. The Talairach coordinates (x, y, z) for the maximally activated voxel in each of the regions and their Z-value are shown. To relate the fMRI with the ERP data, brain electrical source analyses (BESA) explored the time course of the fMRI generators. (B) The six fixed dipoles placed at locations suggested by the fMRI data. The BESA algorithm provided evidence consistent with independent generators at both the anterior cingulate cortex and cuneus (see Figure 31.1c). (C) Scalp ERPs from a Stroop task showing midfrontal (electrode #6) and midoccipital (electrode #76) activity under both vigilant wakefulness and a specific posthypnotic suggestion rendering words meaningless. These electrodes roughly corresponded with the locations of the anterior and posterior fMRI activations, respectively. All ERPs were relative to a stimulus Stroop word presented at time $t = 0$. Significant differences ($p < .05$) between the suggestion-absent and suggestion-present conditions occurred as early as 200 msec following word presentation.

put stimuli unlikely) proposed the involvement of neural top-down control (Raz, Landzberg, et al., 2003).

Multiple neuroimaging studies using variations of conventional Stroop tasks have activated a network of brain areas including the dorsal anterior cingulate cortex (ACC). Requiring participants to respond to one dimension of a stimulus rather than a strong conflicting dimension (Botvinick et al., 2001; Bush, Luu, & Posner, 2000; MacDonald, Cohen, Stenger, & Carter, 2000), these data have resulted in a popular theory of cognitive control proposing that the ACC is part of a network involved in handling conflict between neural areas (Botvinick et al., 2001; Bush et al., 2000). While some researchers view the ACC through the lens of a conflict-monitoring model (Botvinick et al., 2001; Cohen, Botvinick, & Carter, 2000), others construe it as a regulation model engulfing broader processes of consciousness and self-regulation including executive attention and mentation (Bush et al., 2000).

To unravel the brain mechanism by which the posthypnotic suggestion curtailed Stroop conflict (i.e., how suggestion affected visual processing), we studied HH and LH participants both with and without a suggestion not to see the input as words. We complemented the superior spatial resolution of functional magnetic resonance imaging (fMRI) by scalp electrical event-related potentials (ERPs)—affording high temporal resolution—that were acquired separately while the same participants performed similar Stroop tasks. Data from this combined event-related fMRI and ERPs study recently illuminated the mechanism by which the posthypnotic suggestion to view Stroop words as foreign signs operated in HH subjects. The results show that the elimination of the Stroop conflict resulted in an attenuation of fMRI signal at the ACC and extrastriate areas (Raz et al., 2002a, 2002b, 2002c).

These data are consistent with reports that both attention and suggestion can modulate neural activity for visual stimuli (Kosslyn, Thompson, Costantini-Ferrando, Alpert, & Spiegel, 2000; Mack, 2002; Martinez et al., 1999; Rees, Russell, Frith, & Driver, 1999). For example, by creating a situation in which subjects could look directly at a five-letter word without attending to it (i.e., they had to respond to a superimposed stream of pictures shown in different orientations), an fMRI study reported failure to perceive words even for decidedly familiar and meaningful stimuli placed at the center of gaze (Rees et al., 1999). In addition, positron emission tomography (PET) data showed that HH individuals neither perceived color nor activated extrastriate areas related to color after they had been instructed to see a color pattern in gray scale (Kosslyn et al., 2000). Finally, PET assays of pain showed that specific modulatory hypnotic suggestions could affect activation of different brain structures: whereas suggesting a drop in pain unpleasantness (i.e., pacifying conflict) reduced specific activity in ACC (Rainville, Duncan, Price, Carrier, & Bushnell, 1997), suggesting decreased pain intensity produced activity reduction in somatosensory cortex (Hofbauer, Rainville, Duncan, & Bushnell, 2001). These accounts underline the influence attention and suggestion can impart to conflict situations and top-down cognitive control (Posner & Rothbart, 1998; Rainville, 2002; Rainville, Hofbauer, Bushnell, Duncan, & Price, 2002; Raz & Shapiro, 2002).

The higher temporal resolution afforded by scalp ERPs, whose source was localized more anteriorly, illustrated early reduction of brain waves under the experimental suggestion. Comparing the effects of suggestion (absent vs. present) for the incongruent trials in the HH group, electrophysiological activity differed as early as 100 msec following word presentation. These data revealed that in contrast to no suggestion, the N1—an early ERP component believed to be influenced by attention to a channel of information—was absent under suggestion, and posterior activity was not observed before 250 msec. These findings strongly propose that the absence of conflict was accomplished by changing the way visual input was processed. To relate the fMRI with the ERP data, brain electrical source analyses (BESA) explored the time course of the fMRI generators and provided evidence consistent with independent generators at both the ACC and cuneus.

In addition to data speaking to the reduced conflict-resolution effect, using post-hypnotic suggestion, the experimental design demonstrated how it is practically possible to dissociate attention based on input processing from sensory activity based on the input stream. While this outcome seems to leave as a puzzle how visual input got reduced by the posthypnotic suggestion—one possibility is that all input was reduced; another is that it was word specific—the ERP data tend to support the former.

Furthermore, recent ERP data examining the error-related negativity (ERN), an electrophysiological index closely associated with commission of errors in cognitive tasks involving response conflict (Carter et al., 1998; Falkenstein, Hohnsbein, Hoormann, & Blanke, 1991; Gehring & Fencsik, 2001), showed that while the posthypnotic suggestion reduced conflict, it did not decrease conflict monitoring (Raz, Fan, & Posner, 2004). Compared to the no-posthypnotic-suggestion condition, ACC activation decreased prior to response under suggestion, but then ACC activation increased upon incorrect responses on incongruent trials regardless of suggestion. Thus, it was possible to eliminate conflict resolution (i.e., early ACC diminution) yet maintain conflict monitoring (i.e., ACC activation following incorrect responses).

Finally, recent behavioral data collected from comparing hypnotic and nonhypnotic suggestions using a similar experimental protocol at the University of Connecticut also showed significant reduction, but not elimination, of Stroop conflict under both hypnotic and nonhypnotic suggestions (Pollard, Raz, & Kirsch, 2003). Interpretation of these data proposed that susceptibility to suggestion, not explicit hypnotic procedures, may have been the critical factor underlying Stroop conflict reduction (Braffman & Kirsch, 1999; Kirsch & Braffman, 2001; Pollard et al., 2003).

INDIVIDUAL DIFFERENCES IN ATTENTION AND THE GENETICS OF SUGGESTIBILITY

Using modified Stroop procedures, some researchers have examined HH versus LH subjects outside hypnosis and found reliable differences between the groups (Dixon, Brunet, & Laurence, 1990b; Dixon, Labelle, & Laurence, 1996; Dixon & Laurence, 1992). Stroop interference was significantly larger for the HH subjects compared to the LH subjects. This finding was taken to suggest that outside the hypnotic context, HH subjects processed words more automatically than did LH subjects. However, it may also imply that the baseline efficiency of the executive attention network of HH individuals deviated significantly from the baseline level of LH controls. These findings proposed that HH individuals were perhaps genetically predisposed to elevated levels of executive attention.

Similarly, using non-Stroop executive attention tasks to measure conflict we genotyped participants for a number of genes related to the dopamine system (Fossella et al., 2002) and found that polymorphisms in two genes were significantly related to the efficiency of conflict. These genes were the *dopamine D4 receptor* gene (DRD4) and *monoamine oxidase A* (MAOA) gene. The genetic bases of human suggestibility is currently unclear (Bauman & Bul, 1981; Morgan, 1973; Morgan, Hilgard, & Davert, 1970; Rawlings, 1978). Pioneering recent studies seeking to establish relations between phenotype and genotype found an association between catechol-O-methyltransferase (COMT) high/low enzyme activity polymorphism and hypnotizability (Ebstein, Bachner-Melman, & Lichtenberg, 1999; Lichtenberg, Bachner-Melman, Ebstein, & Crawford, 2004; Lichtenberg, Bachner-Melman, Gritsenko, & Ebstein, 2000; Raz, Fossella, McGuiness, Zephrani, & Posner, in press-a, in press-b).

COMT is a gene that influences performance on prefrontal executive cognition and working-memory tasks (Weinberger et al., 2001). Congruous with both fMRI data identifying signal changes in neuroanatomical loci rich in dopaminergic innervation (e.g., ACC) (Raz et al., 2002a, 2002b, 2002c) and dopaminergic drugs (e.g., propofol) affecting both hypnosis and executive attention (Fiset et al., 1999), valine/methionine heterozygous subjects were more highly suggestible than either valine/valine or methionine/methionine homozygous subjects. The trend of valine/methionine COMT heterozygotes toward higher hypnotizability illuminates data from previous studies examining the role of COMT in executive attention as measured by the Attention Network Test (ANT; Fan, McCandliss, Sommer, Raz, & Posner, 2002) as well as by the Stroop (Sommer, Fossella, Fan, & Posner, in press) and showing enhanced focal attention for carriers of this genotype.

Studies on the ANT found that subjects with the valine/valine genotype showed somewhat more efficient conflict resolution (i.e., less interference) than did subjects with the valine/methionine genotype (Fossella, Posner, Fan, Swanson, & Pfaff, 2002; Fossella et al., 2002). A similar trend was also seen in the Stroop task (Sommer et al., in press). The valine allele of COMT, which confers relatively higher levels of enzyme activity and thus lower relative amounts of extrasynaptic dopamine, has been examined in the context of neuroimaging studies where it correlated with lower activity of the dorsolateral prefrontal cortex (Egan et al., 2001). These data are helpful in the quest to identify persons who are likely to be susceptible to suggestion and classify individual attentional profiles as well as subtypes of suggestibility. Interpretation of these results may imply that the baseline efficiency of the executive attention network of HH individuals differs significantly from the baseline level of their LH counterparts. In this regard, the COMT findings recommend a genetic approach to hypnotizability whereby a genotype may suggest a "biological propensity" that predisposes to an attentional phenotype (e.g., hypnotizability).

MANIPULATING THE SUBJECT: VIRTUAL LESIONS AND BEHAVIORAL LESIONS

In the tradition of neurological science, considerable understanding of the healthy human brain typically relied on insights from pathology and trauma. Studying the deficits seen in lesion models both of nonhuman primates and human patients with well-defined brain injuries has been an influential source of pertinent information. Whereas researchers in social psychology may "push" normal individuals toward the pathological spectrum in their efforts to illuminate behavior (Wegner, 2002), cognitive neuroscientists have largely remained within the traditional approach (i.e., studying patients with specific brain lesions to illuminate the nonpathological brain). The investigation of healthy individuals driven toward the "pathological" domain is evident in both the recent contribution of social psychologists to cognitive science (Wegner, 2003) and the popularity of "virtual lesions" induced by transcranial magnetic stimulation (TMS).

Using both hypnotic and posthypnotic suggestions, we have obtained exploratory "behavioral lesion" data. Our assays examine the behavioral consequences of specific suggestions, agreeable with the behavioral manifestations of patients with lesions (e.g., hemi-inattention neglect), on healthy HH individuals. As a case in point, recent pilot data show that three neglect-naïve HH individuals instructed to "pay more attention to the right side of space" and "feel how drowsy and sleepy" the left side of their bodies have become yielded behavioral responses comparable to those seen in veridical neglect patients on neuropsychological tests (e.g., line bisection, figure drawing, and extinction).

These findings are congruous with other hypnotic accounts. For example, within-vision hypnotic suggestions have been demonstrated to induce scotomas and tunnel vision (e.g., Blum, 1975; Leibowitz, Post, Rodemer, Wadlington, & Lundy, 1980), achromatopsia (e.g., Kosslyn et al., 2000), alexia (Raz et al., 2002b), and agnosia (e.g., Blum & Wiess, 1986). Such phenomena are not limited to vision (e.g., Szechtman et al., 1998).

Thus, behavioral lesions induced by hypnotic or posthypnotic suggestion can similarly be used as a way to supplement data from permanent lesions (e.g., strokes) and temporary lesions (e.g., TMS). Hypnosis is especially suited for targeting the modulatory role of attention and for exploring such effects on sensory and cognitive processes because the risk of harm from hypnosis is low and illuminating attention with hypnosis commonly involves global and systemic effects.

CONCLUSION

Behavioral interventions and their neurobiological impact can be both highly focused and functionally specific (Raz & Michels, 2004). There are converging data showing that at least for HH individuals, posthypnotic suggestion can influence both behavior and focal neural activations via a behavioral intervention. Reducing conflict using posthypnotic suggestion has been shown to affect both the input attributes—proposing a global filtering of visual stimuli—and downstream activity in the ACC, an important part of neural systems related to executive attention and self-regulation.

Atypical assays of attention, whereby normal subjects are transiently transformed into neuropsychological patients, may illuminate neurocognitive issues. Hypnosis presents a behavioral TMS-like variant, and researchers would do well to consider "behavioral lesions" as a promising vehicle to probe attention in novel ways.

REFERENCES

Bauman, D. E., & Bul, P. I. (1981). Human inheritability of hypnotizability. *Genetika, 17*(2), 352–356.

Blum, G. S. (1975). A case study of hypnotically induced tubular vision. *International Journal of Clinical and Experimental Hypnosis, 23*, 111–119.

Blum, G. S., & Graef, J. R. (1971). The detection over time of subjects simulating hypnosis. *International Journal of Clinical and Experimental Hypnosis, 19*(4), 211–224.

Blum, G. S., & Wiess, F. (1986). Attenuation of symbol/word interference by posthypnotic negative hallucination and agnosia. *Experimentelle und Klinische Hypnose, 2*, 58–62.

Botvinick, M. M., Braver, T. S., Barch, D. M., Carter, C. S., & Cohen, J. D. (2001). Conflict monitoring and cognitive control. *Psychological Review, 108*(3), 624–652.

Braffman, W., & Kirsch, I. (1999). Imaginative suggestibility and hypnotizability: an empirical analysis. *Journal of Personality and Social Psychology, 77*(3), 578–587.

Bush, G., Luu, P., & Posner, M. I. (2000). Cognitive and emotional influences in anterior cingulate cortex. *Trends in Cognitive Science, 4*(6), 215–222.

Carter, C. S., Braver, T. S., Barch, D. M., Botvinick, M. M., Noll, D., & Cohen, J. D. (1998). Anterior cingulate cortex, error detection, and the online monitoring of performance. *Science, 280,* 747–749.

Cohen, J. D., Botvinick, M., & Carter, C. S. (2000). Anterior cingulate and prefrontal cortex: who's in control? *Nature Neuroscience, 3*(5), 421–3.

Dixon, M., Brunet, A., & Laurence, J. R. (1990a). Hypnotic susceptibility and verbal automatic and strategic processing differences in the Stroop color-naming task. *Journal of Abnormal Psychology, 99,* 336–343.

Dixon, M., Brunet, A., & Laurence, J. R. (1990b). Hypnotizability and automaticity: Toward a parallel distributed processing model of hypnotic responding. *Journal of Abnormal Psychology, 99*(4), 336–343.

Dixon, M., Labelle, L., & Laurence, J. R. (1996). A multivariate approach to the prediction of hypnotic susceptibility. *International Journal of Clinical and Experimental Hypnosis, 44*(3), 250–264.

Dixon, M., & Laurence, J. R. (1992). Hypnotic susceptibility and verbal automaticity: Automatic and strategic processing differences in the Stroop color-naming task. *Journal of Abnormal Psychology, 101*(2), 344–347.

Ebstein, R. P., Bachner-Melman, R., & Lichtenberg, P. (1999). Genetic and cognitive factors in hypnotizability: Association between the low enzyme activity catechol O- methyl transferase (COMT) MET allele and high hypnotizability. *Molecular Psychiatry, 4*(Suppl.).

Egan, M. F., Goldberg, T. E., Kolachana, B. S., Callicott, J. H., Mazzanti, C. M., Straub, R. E., et al. (2001). Effect of COMT Val108/158 Met genotype on frontal lobe function and risk for schizophrenia. *Proceedings of the National Academy of Sciences USA, 98,* 6917–6922.

Falkenstein, M., Hohnsbein, J., Hoormann, J., & Blanke, L. (1991). Effects of crossmodal divided attention on late ERP components. II. Error processing in choice reaction tasks. *Electroencephalography and Clinical Neurophysiology, 78*(6), 447–455.

Fan, J., McCandliss, B. D., Sommer, T., Raz, A., & Posner, M. I. (2002). Testing the efficiency and independence of attentional networks. *Journal of Cognitive Neuroscience, 14*(3), 340–347.

Fiset, P., Paus, T., Daloze, T., Plourde, G., Meuret, P., Bonhomme, V., et al. (1999). Brain mechanisms of propofol-induced loss of consciousness in humans: A positron emission tomographic study. *Journal of Neuroscience, 19,* 5506–5513.

Fossella, J., Posner, M. I., Fan, J., Swanson, J. M., & Pfaff, D. W. (2002). Attentional phenotypes for the analysis of higher mental function. *The Scientific World, 2,* 217–223.

Fossella, J., Sommer, T., Fan, J., Wu, Y., Swanson, J. M., Pfaff, D. W., et al. (2002). Assessing the molecular genetics of attention networks. *BMC Neuroscience, 3*(1), 14.

Gehring, W. J., & Fencsik, D. E. (2001). Functions of the medial frontal cortex in the processing of conflict and errors. *Journal of Neuroscience, 21,* 9430–9437.

Hofbauer, R. K., Rainville, P., Duncan, G. H., & Bushnell, M. C. (2001). Cortical representation of the sensory dimension of pain. *Journal of Neurophysiology, 86*(1), 402–411.

Kirsch, I., & Braffman, W. (2001). Imaginative suggestibility and hypnotizability. *Current Directions in Psychological Science, 10,* 57–61.

Kosslyn, S. M., Thompson, W. L., Costantini-Ferrando, M. F., Alpert, N. M., & Spiegel, D. (2000). Hypnotic visual illusion alters color processing in the brain. *American Journal of Psychiatry, 157*(8), 1279–1284.

Leibowitz, H. W., Post, R. B., Rodemer, C. S., Wadlington, W. L., & Lundy, R. M. (198). Roll vection analysis of suggestion-induced visual field narrowing. *Perception and Psychophysics, 28,* 173–176.

Lichtenberg, P., Bachner-Melman, R., Ebstein, R. P., & Crawford, H. J. (2004). Hypnotic susceptibility: Multidimensional relationships with Cloninger's Tridimensional Personality Questionnaire, COMT polymorphisms, absorption, and attentional characteristics. *International Journal of Clinical and Experimental Hypnosis, 52*(1), 47–72.

Lichtenberg, P., Bachner-Melman, R., Gritsenko, I., & Ebstein, R. P. (2000). Exploratory association study between catechol-O-methyltransferase (COMT) high/low enzyme activity polymorphism and hypnotizability. *American Journal of Medical Genetics, 96*(6), 771–774.

MacDonald, A. W. III, Cohen, J. D., Stenger, V. A., & Carter, C. S. (2000). Dissociating the role of the dorsolateral prefrontal and anterior cingulate cortex in cognitive control. *Science, 288,* 1835–1838.

Mack, A. (2002). Is the visual world a grand illusion? A response. *Journal of Consciousness Studies, 9*(5–6), 102–110.

MacLeod, C. M. (1991). Half a century of research on the Stroop effect: an integrative review. *Psychological Bulletin, 109*(2), 163–203.

MacLeod, C. M., & MacDonald, P. A. (2000). Interdimensional interference in the Stroop effect: Uncovering the cognitive and neural anatomy of attention. *Trends in Cognitive Sciences, 4*(10), 383–391.

MacLeod, C. M., & Sheehan, P. W. (2003). Hypnotic control of attention in the Stroop task: A historical footnote. *Consciousness and Cognition, 12*(3), 347–353.

Martinez, A., Anllo-Vento, L., Sereno, M. I., Frank, L. R., Buxton, R. B., Dubowitz, D. J., et al. (1999). Involvement of striate and extrastriate visual cortical areas in spatial attention. *Nature Neuroscience, 2*(4), 364–369.

McConkey, K. M., & Sheehan, P. W. (1982). Effort and experience on the Creative Imagination Scale. *International Journal of Clinical and Experimental Hypnosis, 30*(3), 280–288.

Morgan, A. H. (1973). The heritability of hypnotic susceptibility in twins. *Journal of Abnormal Psychology, 82*(1), 55–61.

Morgan, A. H., Hilgard, E. R., & Davert, E. C. (1970). The heritability of hypnotic susceptibility of twins: a preliminary report. *Behavioural Genetics, 1*(3), 213–224.

Neely, J. H. (1991). Semantic priming effects in visual word recognition: A selective review of current findings and theories. In D. Besner & G. W. Humphreys (Ed.), *Basic processes in reading: Visual word recognition* (pp. 264–336.). Hillsdale, NJ: Erlbaum.

Nordby, H., Hugdahl, K., Jasiukaitis, P., & Spiegel, D. (1999). Effects of hypnotizability on performance of a Stroop task and event-related potentials. *Perceptual Motor Skills, 88*(3, Pt. 1), 819–830.

Pollard, J., Raz, A., & Kirsch, I. (2003, July). *The effect of suggestion on Stroop performance.* Paper presented at the Society for Applied Research in Memory and Cognition, Aberdeen University, Scotland.

Posner, M. I., & Rothbart, M. K. (1998). Attention, self-regulation and consciousness. *Philosophical Transactions of the Royal Society London: B (Biological Sciences), 353,* 1915–1927.

Rainville, P. (2002). Brain mechanisms of pain affect and pain modulation. *Current Opinion in Neurobiology, 12*(2), 195–204.

Rainville, P., Duncan, G. H., Price, D. D., Carrier, B., & Bushnell, M. C. (1997). Pain affect encoded in human anterior cingulate but not somatosensory cortex. *Science, 277,* 968–971.

Rainville, P., Hofbauer, R. K., Bushnell, M. C., Duncan, G. H., & Price, D. D. (2002). Hypnosis modulates activity in brain structures involved in the regulation of consciousness. *Journal of Cognitive Neuroscience, 14*(6), 887–901.

Rawlings, R. M. (1978). *The genetics of hypnotisability.* Unpublished doctoral dissertation, University of New South Wales.

Raz, A., Fan, J., & Posner, M. I. (2004). *Posthypnotic suggestion reduces conflict resolution but does not decrease conflict monitoring.* Manuscript in preparation.

Raz, A., Fan, J., Shapiro, T., & Posner, M. I. (2002). *fMRI of posthypnotic suggestion to modulate reading Stroop words.* Paper presented at the annual meeting of the Society for Neuroscience, Orlando, FL.

Raz, A., Fossella, J. A., McGuiness, P., Zephrani, Z. R., & Posner, M. I. (in press-a). Neural correlates and exploratory genetic associations of attentional and hypnotic phenomena. *Hypnose und Kognition, The Official Journal of the Milton Erickson Society for Clinical Hypnosis.*

Raz, A., Fossella, J. A., McGuiness, P., Zephrani, Z. R., & Posner, M. I. (in press-b). Neuroimaging and genetic associations of attentional and hypnotic processes. In U. Halsband (Ed.), *Brain imaging in the neurosciences—An interdisciplinary approach.* Frankfurt am Main, Germany: Peter Lang GmbH-Europäischer Verlag der Wissenschaften.

Raz, A., Fossella, J. A., McGuinness, P., Sommer, T., & Posner, M. I. (2003). *Using genetic association assays to assess the role of dopaminergic neuromodulation in attentional and hypnotic phenomena*. Paper presented at the Cognitive Neuroscience Society, New York.

Raz, A., Landzberg, K. S., Schweizer, H. R., Zephrani, Z. R., Shapiro, T., Fan, J., & Posner, M. I. (2003). Posthypnotic suggestion and the modulation of Stroop interference under cycloplegia. *Consciousness and Cognition, 12*(3), 332–346.

Raz, A., & Michels, R. (2004). *The specious notion of specificity*. Manuscript submitted for publication.

Raz, A., & Shapiro, T. (2002). Hypnosis and neuroscience: A cross talk between clinical and cognitive research. *Archives of General Psychiatry, 59*(1), 85–90.

Raz, A., Shapiro, T., Fan, J., & Posner, M. I. (2002a). Hypnotic modulation of stroop interference: Behavioral and neuroimaging accounts. *Journal of Cognitive Neuroscience, A34*(Suppl.).

Raz, A., Shapiro, T., Fan, J., & Posner, M. I. (2002b). Hypnotic suggestion and the modulation of Stroop interference. *Archives of General Psychiatry, 59*(12), 1155–1161.

Raz, A., Shapiro, T., Fan, J., & Posner, M. I. (2002c, November 9). *Top-down modulation of Stroop interference by posthypnotic suggestion: Behavioral, optical, and neuroimaging accounts*. Paper presented at the 53rd annual meeting of the Society for Clinical and Experimental Hypnosis, Boston.

Rees, G., Russell, C., Frith, C. D., & Driver, J. (1999). Inattentional blindness versus inattentional amnesia for fixated but ignored words. *Science, 286*, 2504–2507.

Schatzman, M. (1980). *The story of Ruth*. New York: G. P. Putnam's Sons.

Sheehan, P. W., Donovan, P., & MacLeod, C. M. (1988). Strategy manipulation and the Stroop effect in hypnosis. *Journal of Abnormal Psychology, 97*(4), 455–460.

Sommer, T., Fossella, J. A., Fan, J., & Posner, M. I. (in press). Inhibitory control: Cognitive subfunctions, individual differences and variation in dopaminergic genes. *Proccedings of the Hanse Institute*.

Spiegel, D., Cutcomb, S., Ren, C., & Pribram, K. (1985). Hypnotic hallucination alters evoked potentials. *Journal of Abnormal Psychology, 94*(3), 249–255.

Spiegel, H., & Spiegel, D. (1987). *Trance and treatment: Clinical uses of hypnosis*. Washington, DC: American Psychiatric Press.

Stroop, J. R. (1935). Studies of interference in serial verbal reactions. *Journal of Experimental Psychology, 18*, 643–661.

Sun, S. (1994). A comparative study of Stroop effect under hypnosis and in the normal waking state. *Psychological Science, 17*(5), 287–290.

Szechtman, H., Woody, E., Bowers, K. S., & Nahmias, C. (1998). Where the imaginal appears real: A positron emission tomography study of auditory hallucinations. *Proceedings of the National Academy of Sciences USA, 95*(4), 1956–1960.

Wegner, D. M. (2002). *The illusion of conscious will*. New York: Bradford Books/MIT Press.

Wegner, D. M. (2003). The mind's best trick: How we experience conscious will. *Trends in Cognitive Science, 7*(2), 65–69.

Weinberger, D. R., Egan, M. F., Bertolino, A., Callicott, J. H., Mattay, V. S., Lipska, B. K., Berman, K. F., & Goldberg, T. E. (2001). Prefrontal neurons and the genetics of schizophrenia. *Biological Psychiatry, 50*(11), 825–844.

Weitzenhoffer, A. M., & Hilgard, E. R. (1962). *Stanford Hypnotic Susceptibility Scale: Form C*. Palo Alto, CA: Consulting Psychologists Press.

32

Clinical and Cognitive Definitions of Attention Deficits in Children with Attention-Deficit/Hyperactivity Disorder

James M. Swanson, B. J. Casey, Joel Nigg, F. Xavier Castellanos,
Nora D. Volkow, and Eric Taylor

The purpose of this chapter is to relate the clinical syndrome of attention-deficit/hyperactivity disorder (ADHD) to cognitive concepts of attention and underlying brain circuits. Doing so requires evaluation of information from multiple levels of analysis, as proposed by Posner and Raichle (1994) and Morton and Frith (1995). Over the past decade or more, several overlapping collaborative groups have used this framework, stimulated by a MacArthur Network on the major mental disorders (see Swanson, Castellanos, Murias, LaHoste, & Kennedy, 1998), a never-funded ADHD center on brain imaging and molecular genetics (see Swanson, Castellanos, et al., 1998), the McDonnell Foundation project on brain development (see Swanson et al., (2001), and an ADHD network on dopamine processes (see Swanson, Volkow, et al., in press). Here, we use this framework again to update and review the characteristics of cognitive deficits manifested by children with clinical diagnoses of ADHD, which we evaluate in light of modern theories, paradigms, and findings from the cognitive neurosciences. Then we use this information to refine the clinical concepts of attention deficits that are associated with ADHD.

CLINICAL DEFINITIONS OF ADHD

Recent evaluations in the United States by the National Institutes of Health (NIH Consensus Committee, 1998) and the American Medical Association (Goldman, Genel, Bezman, & Slanetz, 1998) concluded that more than 5% of the school-age children in the United States meet the criteria for ADHD according to the fourth edition of the *Diagnostic and Statistical Manual of Mental Disorders* (DSM-IV; American Psychiatric Association, 1994), and that an extensive empirical base existed in support of the efficacy of two modalities of treatments that are common in clinical practice: (1) pharmacological, with low oral doses of methylphenidate (e.g., Ritalin, Concerta, Metadate), or amphetamine (Dexedrine, Adderall) and (2) psychosocial, with behavior modification (parent and teacher implemented token systems at home and school).

The generally accepted clinical definition of ADHD is provided by DSM-IV (American Psychiatric Association, 1994). A main component of this clinical definition is a list of 18 symptoms (see Table 32.1), that equally represent a cognitive domain of inattention (nine symptoms) and a hybrid domain of hyperactivity–impulsivity (nine symptoms). The DSM-IV manual provides decision rules to define abnormality based on onset, chronicity, severity, and pervasiveness, as well as an overriding requirement of functional impairment.

In a previous review in honor of the 100th anniversary of Sir George Still's articles in *The Lancet* (Swanson, Castellanos, 1998), we evaluated cross-national differences and concluded that the more stringent decision rules of the tenth edition of the *International Classification of Diseases* (ICD-10, World Health Organization, 1993) could account for a lower prevalence of hyperkinetic disorder (HKD) diagnoses in some countries (about 1–3%) than of ADHD in the United States (over 5%). However, the empirical basis for this conclusion and recommendation was limited (Prendergast et al., 1988). The Multimodality Treatment Study of Children with ADHD (MTA) provided a way to test these suggestions about HKD. The MTA is the largest randomized clinical trial yet conducted of pharmacological and psychosocial treatments for ADHD. Across six sites in North America, 7- to 9-year-old children with ADHD, combined type, by DSM-IV criteria were recruited and entered the study (MTA Cooperative Group, 1999). As part of the McDonnell Foundation program to review the state of the art of human brain development (see Posner, Rothbart, Farah, & Bruer, 2001), an extension of our cross-national collaboration was proposed to rediagnose the MTA sample using ICD-10 criteria (Santosh, 2003). To implement this project, filters were applied to the database of the MTA assessment instruments to evaluate presence of comorbidity, representation of symptom domains, pervasiveness across settings, and degree of impairment. In the MTA sample of 579 confirmed cases with diagnoses of ADHD, combined type, only 145 (about 25% of the sample) met the restrictive ICD-10 criteria for a diagnosis of HKD. Because ADHD, combined type, represents about 60–75% of all referred cases, the rediagnosis of the MTA sample by ICD-10 criteria suggests that only 15–20% of the typical

TABLE 32.1. Domains and Symptoms of ADHD

	9 hyperactivity–impulsivity	
9 inattention symptoms	6 hyperactivity symptoms	3 impulsivity symptoms
• Fails to give close attention to details. • Has difficulty sustaining attention. • Does not seem to listen. • Does not follow through (fails to finish). • Has difficulty organizing tasks. • Avoids tasks requiring sustained effort. • Loses things. • Is distracted by extraneous stimuli. • Is forgetful.	• Fidgets with hands or feet or squirms. • Can't remain seated when required. • Runs about or climbs when inappropriate. • Has difficulty playing quietly. • Is always "on the go" or "driven by a motor." • Talks excessively.	• Blurts out answers. • Has difficulty waiting turn. • Interrupts or intrudes.

cases recognized and treated in the United States may qualify for the refined phenotype defined by the ICD-10 criteria for HKD.

In an analysis of the outcome data from the MTA, Santosh (2003) reported that the HKD subgroup of the MTA sample ($n = 145$) had a larger beneficial response to pharmacological intervention and a smaller response to psychosocial intervention than did the subgroup that did not meet the criteria for HKD ($n = 434$). The analysis of differences in cognitive deficits between these two groups has not yet been conducted or reported.

COGNITIVE DEFICITS

Deficits Identified by Neuropsychological Batteries of Tests

Children with ADHD have normal or near-normal intelligence (e.g., see MTA Cooperative Group, 1999) but still manifest abnormal performance on wide variety of tasks. There are many reviews of this point in the literature, and only a select few are cited here. Pennington and Ozonoff (1996) reviewed the neuropsychological literature and concluded that children with ADHD had performance deficits on the executive function tasks, such as the Tower of Hanoi, Matching Familiar Figures (MFF), Stroop, and Trails B tasks, and a variety of motor inhibition tasks (e.g., go/no-go, stop signal, and continuous performance tasks), but not on nonexecutive function tasks (word span, number span, verbal learning, delayed recall). Sergeant, Geurts, and Oosterlaan (2002) reviewed the literature and concluded that children with ADHD had performance deficits on task that required inhibition, such as the stop-signal task and the Stroop task, but pointed out that these deficits were not specific for the ADHD group as deficits on these tasks were also present in other clinical groups of children without ADHD, such as clinical groups selected on the basis of conduct disorder and reading disorders. Several programs of research have contributed to the large literature on the cognitive deficits associated with ADHD, and some of these are reviewed here, including the program directed by Douglas on "state-regulation deficit" model (Douglas, 1972, 1988; Leth-Steenson, Elbaz, & Douglas, 2000), by Sergeant on the "energetic deficit" model (Sergeant & van der Meere, 1994; van der Meere, 2002), by Barkley on "behavioral inhibition deficit" (Barkley, Grodzinsky, & DuPaul, 1992), by Nigg on "'controlled and automatic processing deficit" (Carte, Nigg, & Hinshaw, 1996; Nigg, Blaskey, Stawicki, & Sachek, in press), and by many others.

In general, this extensive literature indicated that batteries of cognitive tests are not sensitive (clinical ADHD cases are underidentified) or specific (other disorders have similar deficits), so the use of neuropsychological tests to diagnose ADHD is not recommended (Baren & Swanson, 1996; Barkley, 1994; Doyle, Biederman, Seidman, Weber, & Faraone, 2000). However, across many studies in the literature, the consensus of "best" tests for describing cognitive deficits associated with ADHD are the Stroop color–word test, the Logan stop-signal task, and the Posner cued-detection task, which became the components of the Cross-National (X-Nat) battery used in the collaboration generated by the McDonnell Foundation project (Swanson et al., 2000). Some background on why specific tasks were and were not included in the X-Nat battery is provided next.

Deficits Identified by Operational Definitions of Underlying Processes

To go beyond the overall difference between ADHD and control groups on a wide variety of tasks, some investigators have used a different strategy by using a single task that measures a specific cognitive process with objective operations (e.g., in well-controlled conditions of a reaction time paradigm) to test for specific differences between the groups. In one of the first examples of this approach, Sergeant (1988) used an operational definition of sustained attention based on an accelerated vigilance decrement (decline in performance over time). But, instead of providing evidence to support the hypothesis of a sustained attention deficit, this study showed that children with ADHD manifested performance deficits early as well as late in a long block of trials. Because careful investigation did not reveal the defining feature of this cognitive definition (an accelerated vigilance deficit), Sergeant suggested abandoning the reference to a sustained attention deficit as a defining characteristic of the clinical syndrome.

In another early example of this strategy, van der Meere and Sergeant (1988) used a focused attention task of Shiffrin and Schneider (1977) designed to evaluate cognitive inhibitory control and distractibility, characterized by greater than normal interference from irrelevant information, leading to a bias toward premature responses and high error rates (i.e., a speed bias in the speed–accuracy trade-off). Four letters were presented in a square display, with a target letter (L) defined as relevant when appearing on one diagonal ($p = .50$) and requiring a yes response but considered a distractor (foil) when presented on the other diagonal ($p = .11$) and requiring a no response, just as nontarget letters presented on either diagonal ($p = .39$). Compared to the control group, the ADHD group of children tended to make more errors (as expected) but also responded more slowly (about 100 msec slower in the nondistractor [900 vs. 800 msec] and distractor [1,000 vs. 900 msec] conditions) rather than faster as predicted for premature or impulsive responding in a speed–accuracy trade-off model. An analysis of the within-subject correlation of reaction time and errors was performed, but the telltale pattern of a negative correlation of speed and accuracy (i.e., evidence of cognitive impulsivity) was not observed.

Stimulated by collaboration in the MacArthur network, we started a project using the cued-detection paradigm designed to assess covert orienting of attention in children with ADHD (Swanson, Castellanos, et al., 1998). This task measures simple reaction time for the detection of visual stimuli presented on a computer display, with cueing conditions established to vary cue–target interval (100 or 800 msec) and the informative nature of the cue (valid or invalid). Swanson and colleagues (1991) reported an overall deficit due to longer reaction times (by about 100 msec), as well as a specific deficit (an asymmetric abnormal slowing in RT to targets in the right visual field after invalid cues and 800 msec cue–target intervals). This was interpreted as an abnormal selective attention deficit (increased cost). However, Huang-Pollock and Nigg (2003) conducted a meta-analysis of 14 studies that assessed selective attention deficits with variants of the cued-detection task (Posner, Petersen, Fox, & Raichle, 1988). These studies replicated the general finding that ADHD groups had slower reaction times than did the control groups (by about 40–50 msec, with an effect size about 0.25), but the laterality effects (right-sided deficits) and cueing effects (specific deficits after long cues) were inconsistent across studies. This led to the conclusion that children with ADHD do not manifest a specific deficit in the orienting operation of attention as measured by this task. To evaluate a more recent version of this theory of attention based on developments in the cognitive neurosciences, Fan and colleagues (2001) developed the Attentional Network Task (ANT), a single test that can be used in children as well as adults to evaluate the three neuroanatomical networks ("alerting," "orienting," and "executive control") proposed by Posner and Raichle (1994). The initial studies of the ANT evaluated its psychometric properties in normal groups, but recently this task has been used to evaluate subtypes of a clinical group of children with ADHD (Booth, Carlson, & Tucker, 2004). Booth and colleagues (2004) found that subgroups of clinical cases with a diagnosis of

ADHD, combined and inattentive subtypes, differed in terms of "alerting" but not "executive control."

Schachar and Logan (1990) used the Stop task to assess a specific form of motor inhibition in children with ADHD. This task requires the execution of a simple button-press in response to a "go" signal (for children, a letter or a picture of an object such as an airplane), but additional instructions require withholding the response when a "stop" signal occurs (a tone). The presentation of the stop signal is varied from 100 to 500 msec before the expected response to the go signal (the average reaction time [RT]). The percent inhibition is used to locate the RT in the distribution of go trials from which to subtract the stop signal interval to estimate the Stop Signal RT (SSRT). Schachar and Logan found that the average SSRT was greater for a group of children with ADHD than for a control group of children without ADHD. Since its introduction to assess a specific inhibition deficit associated with ADHD, many investigators have used the stop-signal task. Oosterlaan and Sergeant (1998) summarized the literature on the use of this task to assess abnormally long SSRT in children with ADHD and reported an effect size of about 0.6 across 10 studies, and in a collaboration stimulated by the McDonnell Foundation project suggested this task for the X-Nat battery.

New Tasks to Measure Motivational Preference

Although not included in the original X-Nat battery, another test that will likely be in its next revision was developed by Sonuga-Barke, Houlberg, and Hall (1994) to assess a specific motivational style called delay aversion in children with ADHD. This task presented a child with a series of trials to choose between a small reward (1 point) to be delivered after a short delay (1 second) or a large reward (2 points) to be delivered after a long delay (20 seconds). Thus, the child could choose between a small, immediate reward (SIR) and a large, delayed reward (LDR), and the total length of the trial depended on the percentage of choices for the large, delayed reward (%LDR). Sonuga-Barke and colleagues found that the average %LDR was smaller for a group of children with ADHD than for a control group of children without ADHD. This preference was interpreted as a reflection of an "economic choice" to accept the smaller reward over the larger reward in order to avoid an aversive experience of "waiting" for the larger reward and the delay in completion of the task. Since its introduction to assess specific motivational deficit (or difference) associated with ADHD, many investigators have used the delay-aversion task. Sonuga-Barke, Dalen, and Remington (2003) reviewed multiple studies of delay aversion in children with ADHD and showed that the %LDR choices for the smaller-immediate reward produced an effect size of 0.65.

Two "head-to-head" comparisons of ADHD–control differences on the delay-aversion and stop-signal tasks have been reported by Solanto and colleagues (2001) and Kuntsi, Oosterlaan, and Stevenson (2001). They used similar versions of the stop-signal task and the delay-aversion task, with quite different clinical samples. The ADHD sample of the Solanto study was recruited from a subset of the MTA sites in North America and was diagnosed by DSM-IV criteria for ADHD, combined type, while the sample for the Kuntsi and colleagues study was recruited in Europe and was diagnosed by ICD-10 criteria. In both studies, performance measures from two tasks (the stop-signal task and the delay-aversion task) were contrasted for groups of subjects with and without ADHD to evaluate two of the leading theories of ADHD, the core deficit theory based on behavioral inhibition (Barkley, 1994) and the motivational theory based on delay aversion (Sonuga-Barke et al., 1994).

Solanto and colleagues (2001) reported the magnitude of the ADHD versus control differences in performance for a specific measure of inhibition from the stop-signal task (SSRT) and a specific measure of motivation from the delay-aversion task (%LDR). The ADHD group had significantly longer average SSRT (436 vs. 290 msec) and lower average %LDR choice (34% vs. 58%) than the control group, but the magnitude of differences expressed in standard deviation units or effect size (ES) was larger for %LDR (ES = 0.91) than for SSRT (ES = 0.76) and a discriminant analysis revealed that %LDR was better than the SSRT for distinguishing the ADHD from the control group (72% vs. 61% correctly classified). Task performance was also compared to teacher ratings of ADHD symptoms, and the correlations with %LDR were significant for two domains, impulsivity (r = .378) and hyperactivity (r = .278), but the correlations with SSRT were small and nonsignificant for both domains. Thus, the head-to-head, a priori comparison of the theoretically chosen measures of performance favored the motivation delay aversion over the behavioral inhibition hypothesis. In fact, on the stop-signal task, the largest ADHD-control difference was not for the measure of motor inhibition (SSRT) but instead was for an accuracy measure. Even though the groups did not differ significantly on average go RT (764 vs. 769 msec) or probability of omitting a go response (.06 and .05), the overall probability of inhibiting a response was lower for the ADHD than for the control group (.41 vs. .54, ES = .90).

Kuntsi and colleagues (2001), in their head-to-head comparison of the delay-aversion and stop-signal tasks, used subgroups of subjects derived from an epidemiological study of twins in the United Kingdom. Parent and teacher ratings on the Conners scales were used to assess "hyperactivity" related to ICD-10 guidelines, so subgroups were formed based on high ratings from both parent and teacher sources (i.e., pervasive "hyperactivity" or ADHD) and low ratings from both sources (control). The "pervasively hyperactive" group differed from the control group on both SSRT (239 vs. 222 msec) and average %LDR choices (40.3% vs. 53.2%), but the magnitude of the effect was greater for the specific measure of motivation (ES = 0.47) than the specific measure of inhibition (ES = 0.24). However, neither of these predicted measures was the best discriminator of the "pervasively hyperactive" and control groups; instead, measures of speed and accuracy of response to the go stimuli were superior, due to slower (ES = .51, p < .003), more variable (ES = .83, p < .001), and less accurate (ES = .65, p < .002) performance of the ADHD than the control group.

Both of these studies favor the delay-aversion theory over the behavioral inhibition theory of ADHD. The delay aversion theory is based on a difference in motivation, not cognition, and thus may account for discrepancies in clinical and cognitive evaluations of attention deficits in ADHD. However, these studies suggest that both theories may apply to different cases, with the delay-aversion theory applying to more cases (in both of these samples) than the behavioral inhibition theory (see Sonuga-Barke, 2003).

NEURAL ABNORMALITIES

Neural Circuits and ADHD

Despite decades of neuropsychological studies of underlying cognitive processes, specific cognitive deficits have not been identified that are highly correlated with the clinical condition. However, over the last decade, biological studies of brain anatomy have reliably shown abnormalities associated with ADHD. Several research teams have used brain imaging methods to investigate anatomical abnormalities in groups of ADHD children. Using a variety of magnetic resonance imaging (MRI) methods, these studies have documented smaller than normal volumes for several brain regions, including frontal lobes (right frontal white matter), basal ganglia (caudate nucleus and globus pallidus), corpus callosum (rostrum and splenium), and cerebellum (vermis lobules VIII–X). We have summarized the details of these studies elsewhere (see Swanson, Castellanos, et al., 1998), so the specific findings are not presented here. Instead, we have summarized the studies using "effect size" estimates of ADHD versus control differences in brain size for different brain regions. We summarize this large literature in Figure 32.1, where we display the magnitude of the average effect size for ADHD versus control differences in a gray scale, with the darker colors representing large effect sizes (over 10% reduction in size for the ADHD groups compared to the control groups) and the lighter colors representing small effect sizes.

This figure illuminates some major points that can be drawn from this research. First, specific regions (e.g., the caudate nucleus) that contain high density of dopamine receptors are smaller in the ADHD groups than in the control groups (see Figure 32.1a). Second, a difference along a front–back axis may distinguish ADHD and control groups (see Figure 32.1b), with ADHD groups having larger posterior regions (i.e., occipital lobes) and smaller anterior brain regions (i.e., frontal lobes). Third, areas involved in coordinating activities of multiple brain regions (e.g., the corpus callosum and the cerebellum) have specific subregions that are smaller in ADHD than in control groups (see Figure 32.1c). Despite differences in subjects recruited or referred or the specialty of the clinic, as well as differences in technical details of MRI methods, consistency has emerged in the literature of brain anatomy.

Recently, new methods for estimating neuroanatomical differences between groups of children with or without ADHD have been reported by Castellanos and colleagues (2002) and Sowell and colleagues (2003). Castellanos and colleagues used automated techniques and a longitudinal, repeated-measures design to investigate the developmental course of brain anatomy and reported that overall brain size was approximately 3–4% smaller for the group with ADHD than for the group without ADHD. In some brain regions the differences (i.e., smaller caudate regions in the group with ADHD) were present during early childhood but were no longer evident in adolescence, and in other brain regions (i.e., the frontal lobes) the differences previously reported were not detected in this study. Sowell and colleagues used a partially automated method to measure surface anatomy of the cortex and documented that a group with ADHD had smaller prefrontal brain regions than did a group without ADHD, but the differences were localized to more inferior aspects of prefrontal regions and were represented bilaterally instead of predominately in the right hemisphere as in prior reports in the literature.

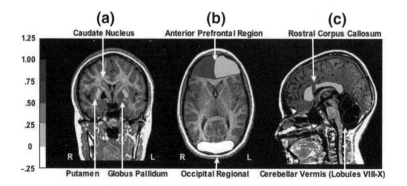

FIGURE 32.1. Effect sizes reported in MRI studies of brains of children with ADHD.

Functional behavioral and brain differences in children with and without ADHD provide additional information about brain structures and their roles in attention deficits in ADHD. Casey and colleagues (1997) provided one of the first studies that related behavioral (performance) measures to anatomical size of brain structures. Using three types of tasks of attention, they showed that performance was correlated with size of the caudate nucleus and volume of white matter in the right frontal lobe and thus linked ADHD–control differences in size to differences in behavior. Vaidya and colleagues (1998) used functional magnetic resonance imaging (fMRI) to assess brain differences in small groups of ADHD and control cases in a within-subject design to assess the behavioral and brain activation effects of stimulant medication versus placebo in subjects performing a go/no-go task. Differences in the diagnostic groups were observed in task activation of the caudate nucleus, as well as different directions of modulation of activity in this brain region by medication (increased in the ADHD group and decreased in the control group). Rubia and colleagues (2001) used fMRI to contrast adolescents with and without ADHD when performing inhibition tasks and in a series of studies revealed differences in function of the caudate nucleus and right frontal areas.

Recently, at the Sackler Institute at Weill Medical College of Cornell University, fMRI has been used to evaluate task activation of brain regions in groups of normal subjects, which is relevant to the understanding of brain regions and neural processes that may underlie attention deficits in children with ADHD. Durston, Tottenham, and colleagues (2003) used functional measures from fMRI to link brain activation during successful response inhibition to performance, using a parametric manipulation of a go/no-go paradigm. An increase in activation of the anterior cingulate, dorsolateral prefrontal, and superior parietal regions was observed on no-go trails as a function of the number of preceding go trials (Durston, Thomas, Worden, et al., 2002). In a second study using similar manipulation within a flanker paradigm, Durston, Davidson, and colleagues (2003) demonstrated that the peak increase in frontal regions occurred before the peak in the parietal region. This finding supported the conflict-monitoring theory that postulates that the anterior cingulate cortex detects or monitors conflict while prefrontal cortex control adjustments may then lead to modulation of superior parietal cortex in top-down biasing of attention. A major advantage of incorporating parametric manipulations in fMRI tasks is that they make it possible to dissociate effects due to differences in performance from effects of interest. In a study comparing young children with ADHD to normally developing children, Durston, Tottenham, and colleagues (2003) used the parametric go/no-go paradigm to show that the children with ADHD activated striatal regions less, regardless of performance. Similarly, Durston, Thomas, Yang, and colleagues (2002) showed that normally developing children (age 7–12) activated regions in frontal cortex more than healthy adults and that activation in key areas correlated with age, suggesting maturational effects. Fan and colleagues (2003) used several versions of tasks that require conflict resolution (e.g., the Stroop color–word and the Eriksen flanker tasks) to compare to regional activation by the ANT task. This study showed that the conflict manipulation of the ANT, Stroop, and Eriksen task all activated the same general brain regions (the anterior cingulate gyrus and lateral prefrontal cortex) found in the Durston study cited previously. Durston and colleagues (2004) showed that intracranial volume was reduced in ADHD subjects, while their siblings displayed an intermediate volume between that of patients and controls, that reductions in right prefrontal gray matter were significant for both patients and their unaffected siblings, and that right cerebellar volume was significantly reduced in patients but not in their unaffected siblings. The finding of reduced intracranial volume in the unaffected siblings of patients with ADHD may suggest an early genetic effect associated with the disorder. Another study by Durston and colleagues (2004) related DRD4 and DAT1 genotype to volumetric measures of prefrontal gray matter and the caudate nucleus in the same group of children. They demonstrate a dissociation where DRD4 preferentially affects prefrontal gray matter and DAT1 preferentially affects caudate volume. Furthermore, these findings were strongest in the unaffected and affected siblings, respectively. These initial studies demonstrate the utility of combining genotyping with structural neuroimaging and begin to define the role allelic variants may play in frontostriatal circuitry underlying cognitive control. The functional implication of reductions in gray matter volume may be interpreted in light of a limited literature on correlations between size of brain structures and performance on neuropsychological tasks (Casey et al., 1997), which showed that measures of cognitive control from performance on response inhibition tasks were related to volume of the prefrontal cortex and basal ganglia in normal groups of children but not in children with ADHD.

In a program of research at Brookhaven National Laboratory, a series of studies have investigated the site of action of methylphenidate (MPH), the most common pharmacological treatment for ADHD. Volkow and colleagues (2001) showed that clinical doses of oral MPH produced a dose-related effect in striatal regions (caudate nucleus) due to dopamine transporter blockade (5 mg ~ 12%, 10 mg ~ 40%, 20 mg ~ 54%, 40 mg ~ 72%, and 60 mg ~ 74% dopamine transporter blockade) that was highly correlated (~.8) with serum concentration of MPH at T_{max}. Volkow and colleagues (1993) showed estimated MPH-induced changes in striatal dopamine with positron emission tomography using [^{11}C]raclopride, a dopamine D_2 receptor radioligand that competes with endogenous dopamine for occupancy of the dopamine D_2 receptors. The study documented that oral doses of MPH increased extracellular dopamine in the brain, due to accumulation of spontaneously released dopamine and MPH-induced dopamine transporter blockade. Recently, Neto, Lou, Cumming, Pryds, and Gjedde (2002) used a similar positron emission tomography technique to replicate this finding and extend it in a sample of adolescents with ADHD, and they also showed increases in striatal dopamine after an oral dose of MPH.

Candidate Genes

We (see Swanson, Wigal, in press, for a review) adopted the dopamine deficit hypothesis of ADHD (Levy, 1994; Levy & Swanson, 2001; Wender, 1971) by choosing as candidate genes the proteins involved in the dopamine synapse. The general understanding of the dopamine synapse suggests that dopamine neurons with cell bodies in the ventral tegmentum area and substantia nigra project to dopamine-receptive neurons, where dopamine is released to traverse the synapse and activates the receptor in the postsynaptic membrane. Once released, a reuptake process involves the dopamine transporter. The regional distribution of dopamine receptors depends on the subtype (D_1, D_2, D_3, D_4, D_5), and colocalization with dopamine transporter is also regionally specific (see de la Garza & Madras, 2000). For example, D_2 receptors are dense in the basal ganglia (caudate nucleus) where the density of dopamine transporter is high, and D_4 receptors are dense in the frontal cortex (e.g., anterior congulate gyrus) where the density of dopamine transporter is low. Based on this, a gene that codes for a dopamine receptor (e.g., the DRD4 gene on chromosome 11) and the dopamine transporter (the dopamine transporter gene on chromosome 5) were chosen as specific candidate genes that may have polymorphisms with variants (alleles) that may be associated with ADHD (e.g., alleles in different proportions in the clinical and control populations). We have reviewed this literature in detail elsewhere (Swanson, Sunohara, et al., 1998; Swanson, et al., 1999, 2000; Swanson, Moyzis, Fossella, Fan, & Posner, 2002; Swanson, Wigal, et al., in press), so we present only a brief review here.

The dopamine transporter gene has a polymorphism created by a 40 base-pair "variable number of tandem repeats" (VNTR) in a noncoding region, and in the human population the primary allelic variants are defined by 9 repeats (in about .25 of alleles) or 10 repeats (in about .75 of allele). Cook and colleagues (1995) reported an increased transmission of the most prevalent allele (10 repeat) in an ADHD sample, and others have replicated this finding (Gill, Daly, Heron, Hawi, & Fitzgerald, 1997; Waldman et al., 1998). The DRD4 gene has a polymorphism created by a 48 base-pair VNTR in a coding region of the gene (exon III), and in the human population the primary allelic variant is defined by four repeats (in about .65 of alleles), with the second most frequent defined by seven repeats (about 10–20% in Caucasian samples) and two repeats (about 5–20% in Asian samples). LaHoste and colleagues (1996) reported that 7-repeat allele was overrepresented in the group with ADHD, and so many others have replicated this finding (Faraone, Doyle, Mick, & Biederman, 2001) that it is now considered to be one of the most reliable genetic findings yet reported about the association of a gene with specific behavior (see Collier, Curran, & Asherson, 2000).

Functional differences between subgroups defined by genotypes of the DRD4 provide additional information about the importance of these candidate genes, as well as some surprising findings. The X-Nat battery was used to test the hypothesis that the 7-repeat allele of the DRD4 gene might be associated with a more pervasive form of ADHD (Swanson et al., 2001). However, in a subset of the MTA sample, all of which had severe behavioral manifestation of symptoms and diagnoses of ADHD, combined type, we observed the opposite pattern. The Stroop color–word, the stop-signal task, and the cued-detection task, all showed that the subgroup defined by the proposed "risk" 7+ genotype (at least one 7-repeat allele present) had normal performance (despite the abnormal behavior that led to diagnosis of a "disorder"). The 7+ subgroup differed in performance from the 7- genotype (no 7-repeat allele present) due to faster (ES ~ 0.6) and less variable (ES ~ 0.8) reaction times on all three tasks.

Recently, Langley and colleagues (2004) used one of the same neuropsychological tasks (the stop-signal task) and the same subgroups based on DRD4 genotype (the 7-present and 7-absent subgroups), and documented a similar pattern for ADHD children in the United Kingdom: the 7-present subgroup had faster response time than did the 7-absent subgroup. In addition, on another test often used to assess cognitive deficits in children with ADHD (the Matching Familiar Figure Test), the 7-present subgroup also respond faster than did a normal control group but tended to make more errors, suggesting "impulsivity" according to the operational definition discussed earlier.

Studies of the dopamine transporter gene have also produced surprising results. First, the most common variant of the 40bp VNTR (the 10-repeat allele, which represents about 70% of all allele in most ethnic groups) has been associated with the clinical diagnosis of ADHD, suggesting that it must combine with another uncommon condition (genetic or nongenetic) to result in the observed prevalence of ADHD (3–5% of the population). This VNTR is in a noncoding promoter region of the dopamine transporter gene, rather than a structural difference (as in the case of the coding-region polymorphism of the DRD4 gene). So it has been suggested that this polymorphism may affect expression and thus density of the dopamine transporter in the brain. Second, the subgroup defined by the 10-repeat/10-repeat homozygotes has been shown to differ from the subgroup defined by the 10-repeat heterozygote genotypes or by the 10-absent genotype. For example,

Cornish and colleagues (2004) selected subgroups with exceptionally high or low ratings of attention and activity, and based on performance on a battery of neuropsychological tests showed that the subgroup with the 10-repeat/10-repeat genotype had deficits in selective attention and response inhibition. In addition to the hypothesis that the 10-repeat genotype is in linkage disequilibrium with a nearby functional variant yet undiscovered, this could suggests that some recessive factor may be operating, in combination with an uncommon genetic or nongenetic factor that produces functional differences associated with dopamine transporter genotype.

CONCLUSIONS

In general, a lack of correspondence has been noted between the clinical concepts of attention deficit from the DSM-IV and ICD-10 manuals and cognitive concepts of attention deficits. Thus, a signature of a specific attention deficit that may underlie ADHD has not been discovered. This should not be surprising, as the clinical criteria for "attention deficit" are based on clinical definitions of Inattention and Impulsivity that differ from the cognitive definitions of these concepts. Within the DMS-IV domain of inattention, the concepts of sustained attention ("difficulty sustaining attention") and distractibility ("distracted by stimuli") are considered important characteristics of the clinical syndrome. However, the expected pattern of performance on cognitive (information processing) tasks due to a sustained attention deficit—an accelerated "vigilance decrement"—is not typical of the performance of groups of ADHD children. Instead, deficits on monitoring tasks are manifested early as well as late in a block of trials. The expected pattern of performance due to distractibility has not been observed, either. On cognitive tasks, irrelevant stimuli do not have greater effects on groups of children with ADHD than on control groups. Thus, the clinical concepts of "sustained attention deficit" and "distractibility" are not confirmed by cognitive assessments of ADHD cases.

The DSM-IV domain of impulsivity suggests premature responding, but in the symptom lists for ADHD the items defining "impulsivity" are related to social interactions ("blurts out answers," "difficulty waiting turn," "interrupts or intrudes"), not to cognitive processes underlying information processing (i.e., a speed–accuracy bias toward speed at the expense of accuracy). However, performance on cognitive tasks has been the focus of many investigations, and in general on standard RT paradigms that evaluate information processing, the expected pattern of performance associated with a speed bias—fast and inaccurate responding—is not manifested by children with ADHD. Instead, the performance of groups of children with ADHD is slow and inaccurate compared to control groups. Thus, in information-processing terms, large groups of children with ADHD do not appear to be "impulsive" at the cognitive level of analysis, while at the behavioral level, the impulsive response style seems to be observed. For example, on the MFF test, children with ADHD tend to respond more quickly and with more errors than do controls, seemingly consistent with a cognitive definition of impulsivity. However, examination of requirements of MFF task and other tasks designed to measure impulsivity reveals that this supposition may not hold at the processing level. On speeded-response tasks (see Posner, 1978), children with ADHD tend to respond slowly and inaccurately. Even when they make fast–inaccurate responses in the MFF paradigm, in which decisions are made whether to "take another look" or not, subjects with ADHD may process the stimulus in a slow, inaccurate manner. The impulsivity symptoms listed in Table 32.1 provide only a partial picture of children whose behavior is typically careless, hasty, and/or reckless when observed in everyday settings such as school classrooms, stores, or homes. This may exemplify the "everyday" lay conception of impulsive behavior, but a multitude of processes have been suggested as contributing to behavioral dyscontrol.

In summary, some basic hypotheses about clinical concepts of attention deficit (i.e., that the clinical symptoms are due to underlying abnormalities in cognitive processes resulting in a deficit in sustained attention, distractibility, and impulsivity) are not supported by careful evaluation of these cognitive concepts based on performance of children with ADHD in standard paradigms from cognitive psychology (i.e., RT studies of mental chronometry). Yet, children with ADHD do have large performance deficits on these cognitive tasks. The characteristics of the manifested deficits are slower speed, lower accuracy, and greater variability in comparison to control groups.

In future collaborative studies, we propose to pursue our finding from recent molecular genetic studies of dopamine genes, which suggested that subgroups defined by genotypes based on the DRD4 and dopamine transporter genes may differ in the pattern of cognitive deficits manifested. For example, the results of studies by Swanson and colleagues (2001) and Langley and colleagues (2003) suggest that the classic pattern of impulsivity (fast and inaccurate responding) might be manifested by the subgroup defined by the 7+ genotype but not the 7- genotype of the DRD4 gene. It is possible that nongenetic etiologies may produce a different pattern of performance on cognitive task (slow and inaccurate responding) that is characteristic of minimal brain damage (see Altman, 1986; Amsel, 1990; Lou, 1996).

Ongoing studies at the Sackler Institute investigate the relationship between variation in dopamine-related genes and brain morphometry. Preliminary studies demonstrate how neuroimaging measures may serve as a biological intermediate phenotype. As illustrated in Figure 32.1 if reductions in brain volume are related to increased genetic risk for ADHD, we expect differences in volume related to genotype for both the subjects with ADHD and their unaffected siblings but not for control subjects. However, if reductions in volume are due to environmental factors, individuals with the disorder are expected to display reductions in volume irrespective of their genotype, whereas individuals at increased genetic risk will either not display reductions in volume or will display reductions in volume as a function of their genotype. In some preliminary studies, this approach has shown some promise.

The finding by Durston and colleagues (2004) of differential reductions in volume between subjects with ADHD and their unaffected siblings who are at increased genetic risk for ADHD may be associated with similar differences in cognitive control between groups. This point could be elucidated in future studies, incorporating carefully designed neuropsychological batteries with structural and functional MRI scans for large numbers of subjects.

In future studies of cognitive deficits associated with ADHD, we propose to include tasks that measure choices to continue to sample information (as in the MFF) as well as tasks that measure speed and accuracy of responding to a discrete stimulus (as in tasks in the X-Nat battery). This will allow us to better define the concepts of "impulsivity" and "inhibition" in our next studies of cognitive deficits associated with ADHD.

Attempts to link the clinical syndrome to "attention deficits" have a long history in the medical literature, dating back to Still's (1902) description of children with impaired "inhibitory volition" and "marked inability to concentrate and sustain attention." This has continued in the modern clinical literature in attempts to identify a core cognitive deficit associated with ADHD. The accumulating evidence from biological studies of brain imaging and molecular genetics point the way for the next steps in the search for attention deficits associated with the clinical syndrome of ADHD.

ACKNOWLEDGMENTS

We would like to acknowledge support by a grant from the MacArthur Foundation (1985–1990), a grant from the McDonnell Foundation (2000–2002), and a Network Grant from the National Institute of Mental Health (2002–2004), which facilitated the work described and summarized in this chapter, as well as support from the Sackler Institute and our institutions that allowed additional but unfunded aspects of the research programs described here.

REFERENCES

Altman, J. (1986). An animal model of minimal brain dysfunction. In M. Lewis (Ed.), *Learning disabilities and prenatal risk* (pp. 241–304). Urbana: University of Illinois Press.

American Psychiatric Association. (1994). *Diagnostic and statistical manual of mental disorders* (4th ed.). Washington, DC: Author.

Amsel, A. (1990). Arousal, suppression, and persistence: Frustration theory, attention, and its disorders. *Cognition and Emotion, 4*(3), 239–268.

Baren, M., & Swanson, J. M. (1996). How not to diagnose ADHD. *Contemporary Pediatrics, 13,* 53–64.

Barkley, R. A. (1994). Can neuropsychological tests help diagnose ADD/ADHD? *The ADHD Report, 2*(1), 1–3.

Barkley, R. A., Grodzinsky, G., & DuPaul, G. J. (1992). Frontal lobe functions in attention deficit disorder with and without hyperactivity: A review and research report. *Journal of Abnormal Child Psychology, 20,* 163–188.

Booth, J. E., Carlson, C. L., & Tucker, D. M. (2004). *The combined and inattentive subtypes of ADHD show different patterns of performance on a neurocognitive measure of alerting.* Unpublished manuscript.

Carte, E. T., Nigg, J. T., & Hinshaw, S. P. (1996). Neuropsychological functioning, motor speed, and language processing in boys with and without ADHD. *Journal of Abnormal Child Psychology, 24,* 481–498.

Casey, B. J., Castellanos, F. X., Giedd, J. N., Marsh, W. L., Hamburger, S. D., Schubert, A. B., et al. (1997). Implication of right frontostriatal circuitry in response inhibition and attention-deficit/hyperactivity disorder. *Journal of the American Academy of Child and Adolescent Psychiatry, 36,* 374–383.

Castellanos, F. X., Lee, P. P., Sharp, W., Jeffries, N. O., Greenstein, D. K., Clasen, L. S., et al. (2002). Developmental trajectories of brain volume abnormalities in children and adolescents with attention-deficit/hyperactivity disorder. *Journal of the American Medical Association, 288,* 1740–1748.

Cook, E. H., Jr., Stein, M. A., Krasowski, M. D., Cox, N. J., Olkon, D. M., Kieffer, J. E., et al. (1995). Association of attention deficit disorder and the dopamine transporter gene. *American Journal of Human Genetics, 56,* 993–998.

Cornish, K. M., Manly, T., Savage, R., Swanson, J., Grant, C., Morisano, D., et al. (2004). Association of the dopamine transporter (DAT1) 10/10-repeat genotype with ADHD-symptoms and response inhibition in a general population sample. *Molecular Psychiatry.*

de la Garza, R., & Madras, B. K. (2000). [(3)H]PNU-101958, a $D_{(4)}$ dopamine receptor probe, accumulates in prefrontal cortex and hippocampus of non-human primate brain. *Synapse, 37,* 232–244.

Douglas, V. I. (1972). Stop, look, and listen: The problem of sustained attention and impulse control in hyperactive and normal children. *Canadian Journal of Behavioral Science, 4,* 258–282.

Douglas, V. I. (1988). Cognitive deficits in children with attention deficit disorder with hyperactivity. In L. M.Bloomingdale & J. A. Sergeant (Eds.), *Attention deficit disorder: Criteria, cognition and intervention* (pp. 65–82). Oxford, UK: Pergamon Press.

Doyle, A. E., Biederman, J., Seidman, L. J., Weber, W., & Faraone, S. V. (2000). Diagnostic efficiency of neuropsychological test scores for discriminating boys with and without attention deficit-hyperactivity disorder. *Journal of Consulting and Clinical Psychology, 68,* 477–488.

Durston, S., Davidson, M. C., Thomas, K. M., Worden, M. S., Tottenham, N. T., Martinez, A., Watts, R., Ulug, A. M., & Casey, B. J. (2003). Parametric manipulation of conflict and response competition using rapid mixed-trial event-related functional MRI. *NeuroImage, 20*(4), 2135–2141.

Durston, S., Hulshoff Pol, H. E., Schnack, H. G., Buitelaar, J. K., Steenhuis, M. P., Minderaa, R. B., Kahn, R. S., & Van Engeland, H. (2004). Magnetic resonance imaging of boys with attention deficit hyperactivity disorder and their unaffected siblings. *Journal of the American Academy of Child and Adolescent Psychiatry, 43*(3), 332–340.

Durston, S., Thomas, K. M., Worden, M. S., Yang, Y., & Casey, B. J. (2002). The effect of preceding context on inhibition: An event-related fMRI study. *NeuroImage, 16*(2), 449–453.

Durston, S., Thomas, K. M., Yang, Y., Ulug, A. M., Zimmerman, R. D., & Casey, B. J. (2002). The development of neural systems involved in overriding behavioral responses: An event-related fMRI study. *Developmental Science, 5*(4), F9-F16.

Durston, S., Tottenham, N. T., Thomas, K. M., Davidson, M. C., Eigsti, I. M., Yang, Y., et al. (2003). Differential patterns of striatal activation in young children with and without ADHD. *Biological Psychiatry, 53,* 871–878.

Fan, J., Flombaum, J. I., McCandliss, B. D., Thomas, K. M., & Posner, M. I. (2003). Cognitive and brain consequences of conflict. *NeuroImage, 18,* 42–57.

Faraone, S. V., Doyle, A. E., Mick, E., & Biederman, J. (2001). Meta-analysis of the association between the 7-repeat allele of the dopamine D_4 receptor gene and attention deficit hyperactivity disorder. *American Journal of Psychiatry, 158,* 1052–1057.

Gill, M., Daly, G., Heron, S., Hawi, Z., & Fitzgerald, M. (1997). Confirmation of association between attention deficit hyperactivity disorder and a dopamine transporter polymorphism. *Molecular Psychiatry, 2,* 311–313.

Goldman, L. S., Genel, M., Bezman, R. J., & Slanetz, P. J. (1998). Diagnosis and treatment of attention-deficit/hyperactivity disorder in children and adolescents. *Journal of the American Medical Association, 279,* 1100–1107.

Huang-Pollock, C. L., & Nigg, J. T. (2003). Searching for the attention deficit in attention deficit hyperactivity disorder: the case of visuospatial orienting. *Clinical Psychology Review, 23,* 801–830.

Kuntsi, J., Oosterlaan, J., & Stevenson, J. (2001). Psychological mechanisms in hyperactivity: I. Response inhibition deficit, working memory impairment, delay aversion, or something else? *Journal of Child Psychology and Psychiatry and Allied Disciplines, 42,* 199–210.

LaHoste, G. J., Swanson, J. M., Wigal, S. B., Glabe, C., King, N., Kennedy, J. L., et al. (1996). Dopamine D4 receptor gene polymorphism is associated with attention deficit hyperactivity disorder. *Molecular Psychiatry, 1,* 121–124.

Langley, K., Marshall, L., van den Bree, M., Thomas, H., Owen, M., O'Donovan, M., et al. (2004). Association of the dopamine D_4 receptor gene 7-repeat allele with neuropsychological test performance of children with ADHD. *American Journal of Psychiatry, 161,* 133–138.

Leth-Steensen, C., Elbaz, Z. K., & Douglas, V. I. (2000). Mean response times, variability, and skew in the responding of the ADHD children: A response time distributional approach. *Acta Psychologica (Amsterdam), 104,* 167–190.

Levy, F. (1994). Attention deficit disorder [Letter]. *Australian and New Zealand Journal of Psychiatry, 28,* 693.

Levy, F., & Swanson, J. M. (2001). Timing, space and ADHD: The dopamine theory revisited. *Australian and New Zealand Journal of Psychiatry, 35,* 504–511.

Lou, H. C. (1996). Etiology and pathogenesis of Attention-deficit Hyperactivity disorder (ADHD): Significance of prematurity and perinatal hypoxic-haemodynamic encephalopathy. *Acta Paediatrica, 85,* 1266–1271.

Morton, J., & Frith, U. (1995). Causal modeling: A structural approach to developmental psychopathology. In D.Cicchetti & D. J. Cohen (Eds.), *Developmental psychopathology* (pp. 357–390). New York: Wiley.

MTA Cooperative Group, Multimodal Treatment Study of Children with ADHD. (1999). A 14-month randomized clinical trial of treatment strategies of attention-deficit/hyperactivity disorder. *Archives of General Psychiatry, 56,* 1073–1086.

Neto, P., Lou H, Cumming, P., Pryds, O., & Gjedde, A. (2002). Methylphenidate-evoked potentiation of extracellular dopamine in the brain of adolescents with premature birth. *Annals of the New York Academy of Science, 965,* 434–439.

National Institutes of Health Consensus Committee. (1998). A diagnosis and treatment of attention deficit hyperactivity disorder (ADHD). *NIH Consensus Statement, 16*(2), 1–37.

Nigg, J., Blaskey, L., Stawicki, J. A., & Sachek, J. (in press). Evaluating the endophenotype model of ADHD neuropsychological deficit: Results for parents and siblings of children with DSM-IV ADHD combined and inattentive subtypes. *Journal of Abnormal Psychology.*

Oosterlaan, J., & Sergeant, J. A. (1998). Response inhibition and response re-engagement in attention-deficit/hyperactivity disorder, disruptive, anxious and normal children. *Behavioral Brain Research, 94,* 33–43.

Posner, M. I. (1978). *Chronometric explorations of mind: The third Paul M. Fitts lectures.* Hillsdale, NJ: Erlbaum.

Posner, M. I., Petersen, S. E., Fox, P. T., & Raichle, M. E. (1988). Localization of cognitive operations in the brain. *Science, 240,* 1627–1631.

Posner, M., & Raichle, M. (1994). *Images of mind.* New York: Scientific American Library.

Posner, M. I., Rothbart, M. K., Farah, M., & Bruer, J. (2001). The developing human brain. *Developmental Science, 4*(3), 253–387.

Prendergast, M., Taylor, E., Rapoport, J. L., Bartko, J., Donnelly, M., Zametkin, A., et al. (1988). The diagnosis of childhood hyperactivity. A U.S.-U.K. cross- national study of DSM-III and ICD-9. *Journal of Child Psychology and Psychiatry and Allied Disciplines, 29,* 289–300.

Rubia, K., Taylor, E., Smith, A. B., Oksannen, H., Overmeyer, S., & Newman, S. (2001). Neuropsychological analyses of impulsiveness in childhood hyperactivity. *British Journal of Psychiatry, 179,* 138–143.

Santosh, J. (2003). *Rediagnosis of the MTA sample by ICD-10 criteria.* Poster presentation at the 156th annual meeting of the American Psychiatric Association, San Francisco.

Schachar, R., & Logan, G. (1990). Are hyperactive children deficient in attentional capacity? *Journal of Abnormal Child Psychology, 18,* 493–513.

Sergeant, J. (1988). From DSM-III attentional deficit disorder to functional defects. In L. M. Bloomingdale & J. Sergeant (Eds.), *Attention deficit disorder: Criteria, cognition, intervention* (pp. 183–198). Oxford, UK: Pergamon Press.

Sergeant, J. A., Geurts, H., & Oosterlaan, J. (2002). How specific is a deficit of executive functioning for attention-deficit/hyperactivity disorder? *Behavioural Brain Research, 130,* 3–28.

Sergeant, J. A., & van der Meere, J. (1994). Towards an empirical child psychopathology. In D. K. Routh (Ed.), *Disruptive behaviour disorders in childhood* (pp. 59–78). New York: Plenum Press.

Shiffrin, R. M., & Schneider, W. (1977). Controlled and automatic human information processing-II. Perceptual and learning, automatic attending and a general theory. *Psychological Review, 84,* 127–190.

Solanto, M. V., Abikoff, H., Sonuga-Barke, E., Schachar, R., Logan, G. D., Wigal, T., et al. (2001). The ecological validity of delay aversion and response inhibition as measures of impulsivity in AD/HD: a supplement to the NIMH multimodal treatment study of AD/HD. *Journal of Abnormal Child Psychology, 29,* 215–228.

Sonuga-Barke, E. J. (2003). The dual pathway model of AD/HD: An elaboration of neuro-developmental characteristics. *Neuroscience and Biobehavioral Reviews, 27,* 593–604.

Sonuga-Barke, E. J., Dalen, L., & Remington, B. (2003). Do executive deficits and delay aversion make independent contributions to preschool attention-deficit/hyperactivity disorder symptoms. *Journal of the American Academy of Child and Adolescent Psychiatry, 42,* 1335–1342.

Sonuga-Barke, E. J., Houlberg, K., & Hall, M. (1994). When is impulsiveness not impulsive? The case of hyperactive children's cognitive style. *Journal of Child Psychology and Psychiatry and Allied Disciplines, 35,* 1247–1253.

Sowell, E., Thompson, P., Welcome, S., Henkenius, A., Toga, A., & Peterson, B. (2003). Cortical abnormalities in children and adolescents with attention-deficit hyperactivity disorder. *Lancet, 362,* 1699–1707.

Still, G. F. (1902). Some abnormal psychical conditions in children. *Lancet, 1,* 1008–1012.

Swanson, J., Castellanos, F. X., Murias, M., LaHoste, G. J., & Kennedy, J. (1998). Cognitive neuroscience of attention deficit hyperactivity disorder and hyperkinetic disorder. *Current Opinion in Neurobiology, 8,* 263–271.

Swanson, J., Gupta, S., Guinta, D., Flynn, D., Agler, D., Lerner, M., et al. (1999). Acute tolerance to methylphenidate in the treatment of attention deficit/hyperactivity disorder in children. *Clinical Pharmacology and Therapeutics, 66,* 295–305.

Swanson, J., Moyzis, R., Fossella, J., Fan, J., & Posner, M. (2002). Adaptationism and molecular biology: An example based on ADHD. *Behavioral and Brain Sciences, 25,* 530–531.

Swanson, J., Oosterlaan, J., Murias, M., Schuck, S., Flodman, P., Spence, M. A., et al. (2000). Attention deficit/hyperactivity disorder children with a 7-repeat allele of the dopamine receptor D_4 gene have extreme behavior but normal performance on critical neuropsychological tests of attention. *Proceedings of the National Academy of Sciences of the United States of America, 97,* 4754–4759.

Swanson, J. M., Castellanos, F. X., Frith, U., Pennington, B. F., Steinfer, D., Spitzer, M., & Spence, M. A. (2001). Psychopathology. *Developmental Science, 4,* 345–357.

Swanson, J. M., Sunohara, G. A., Kennedy, J. L., Regino, R., Fineberg, E., Wigal, T., et al. (1998). Association of the dopamine receptor D_4 (DRD_4) gene with a refined phenotype of attention deficit hyperactivity disorder (ADHD): A family-based approach. *Molecular Psychiatry, 3,* 38–41.

Swanson, J. M., Volkow, N. D., Newcorn, J., Casey, B. J., Moyzis, R., Grandy, D. K., et al. (in press). Dopamine (DA) and attention deficit hyperactivity disorder. In *Dopamine and glutamate in psychiatric disorders.* Totowa, NJ: Humana Press.

Swanson, J. M., Wigal, S. B., Wigal, T., Sonuga-Barke, E., Greenhill, L. L., Biederman, J., et al. (in press). A comparison of once-daily extended-release methylphenidate formulations in children with ADHD in the laboratory school (The COMACS Study). *Pediatrics.*

Vaidya, C. J., Austin, G., Kirkorian, G., Ridlehuber, H. W., Desmond, J. E., Glover, G. H., et al. (1998). Selective effects of methylphenidate in attention deficit hyperactivity disorder: A functional magnetic resonance imaginig study. *Proceedings of the National Academy of Sciences of the United States of America, 95,* 14494–14499.

van der Meere, J. J., & Sergeant, J. (1988). Focused attention in pervasively hyperactive children. *Journal of Abnormal Child Psychology, 16,* 627–639.

Volkow, N. D., Fowler, J. S., Wang, G. J., Dewey, S. L., Schlyer, D., MacGregor, R., et al. (1993). Reproducibility of repeated measures of carbon-11-raclopride binding in the human brain [published erratum appears in J Nucl Med 1993 May; 34(5): 838]. *Journal of Nuclear Medicine, 34,* 609–613.

Volkow, N. D., Wang, G. J., Fowler, J. S., Logan, J., Gerasimov, M., Maynard, L., et al. (2001). Therapeutic doses of oral methylphenidate significantly increase extracellular dopamine in the human brain. *Journal of Neuroscience, 21,* U1–U5.

Waldman, I. D., Rowe, D. C., Abramowitz, A., Kozel, S. T., Mohr, J. H., Sherman, S. L., et al. (1998). Association and linkage of the dopamine transporter gene and attention-deficit hyperactivity disorder in children: Heterogeneity owing to diagnostic subtype and severity. *American Journal of Human Genetics, 63,* 1767–1776.

Wender, P. H. (1971). *Minimal brain dysfunction in children.* New York: Wiley-Interscience.

World Health Organization. (1993). *The ICD-10 classification of mental and behavioural disorders: diagnostic criteria for research.* Geneva, Switzerland: Author.

Author Index

Subject Index

Page numbers followed by an *f* indicate figure, *n* indicate note, and *t* indicate table.

459